INVASIVE FETAL TESTING AND TREATMENT

INVASIVE FETAL TESTING AND TREATMENT

edited by

CHRISTOPHER R. HARMAN, MD

Director, Fetal Assessment Unit
Division of Maternal and Fetal Medicine
Department of Obstetrics, Gynecology & Reproductive Sciences
University of Manitoba
Women's Hospital
Winnipeg, Canada

Boston

Blackwell Scientific Publications

Oxford   London - Edinburgh   Melbourne
Paris   Berlin   Vienna

Blackwell Scientific Publications

Editorial offices:
238 Main Street, Cambridge, Massachusetts 02142, USA
Osney Mead, Oxford OX2 0EL, England
25 John Street, London WC1N 2BL, England
23 Ainslie Place, Edinburgh EH3 6AJ, Scotland
54 University Street, Carlton, Victoria 3053, Australia
Arnette SA, 1 rue de Lille, 75007 Paris, France
Blackwell-Wissenschaft, Dusseldorfer Str. 38, D-10707 Berlin, Germany
Blackwell MZV, Feldgasse 13, A-1238 Vienna, Austria

Distributors:

USA
Blackwell Scientific Publications
238 Main Street
Cambridge, Massachusetts 02142
(Telephone orders: 800-759-6102 or 617-876-7000)

CANADA
Times Mirror Professional Publishing
130 Flaska Drive
Markham, Ontario L6G 1B8
(Telephone orders: 800-268-4178 or 416-470-6739)

AUSTRALIA
Blackwell Scientific Publications (Australia) Pty Ltd
54 University Street
Carlton, Victoria 3053
(Telephone orders: 03-347-5552)

OUTSIDE NORTH AMERICA AND AUSTRALIA
Blackwell Scientific Publications, Ltd.
P.O. Box 87
Oxford OX2 0DT
England
(Telephone orders: 44-865-791155)

Typeset by BookMasters, Ashland, Ohio
Printed and bound by Braun-Brumfield, Inc., Ann Arbor, Michigan

© 1995 by Blackwell Scientific Publications
Printed in the United States of America
95 96 97 98 5 4 3 2 1

Acquisitions: Victoria Reeders
Development: Coleen Traynor
Production: Michelle Choate
Manufacturing: Kathleen Grimes

Library of Congress Cataloging in Publication Data

Invasive fetal testing and treatment / edited by Christopher R.
  Harman.
      p. cm.
    Includes bibliographical references and index.
    ISBN 0–86542–208–7
    1. Prenatal diagnosis. 2. Fetus—Diseases—Treatment. 3. Fetus—
  Abnormalities—Treatment. I. Harman, Christopher R.
  [DNLM: 1. Fetal Diseases—diagnosis. 2. Fetal Diseases—therapy.
  3. Chorionic Villi Sampling—methods. 4. Cordocentesis—methods.
  WQ 211 I62 1955]
  RG626.I58 1995
  618.3′2—dc20
  DNLM/DLC
  for Library of Congress
                                                              94-15786
                                                              CIP

To Pat,

for giving me the confidence to try,

and Frank,

for opening the window.

Contents

Contributors

Hassan Albar, MD
Division of Maternal and Fetal Medicine
Department of Obstetrics, Gynecology and
   Reproductive Services
University of Manitoba
Women's Hospital
Winnipeg, Canada

Nancy Ayres, MD
Department of Pediatrics
Baylor College of Medicine
Houston, Texas

Robert J. Carpenter, Jr., MD
Department of Obstetrics and Gynecology
Baylor College of Medicine
Texas Medical Center
Houston, Texas

Frank A. Chervenak, MD
Department of Obstetrics and Gynecology
Cornell University Medical Center
New York Hospital
New York, New York

Fernand Daffos, MD
Chairman
Institut de Puericulture de Paris
Centre de Diagnostic Prenatal
Paris, France

Steven Edmondson, MD
Department of Obstetrics and Gynecology
The J.S. Abercrombie Section of Pediatric
   Cardiology
Baylor College of Medicine
Houston, Texas

Nicholas Maxwell Fisk, FRACOG,
   MRCOG, DDU
Department of Fetal Medicine
King George V Hospital
Camperdown, Australia

F. Forestier, MD
Service de Medecine et de Biologie Foetales
Institut de Puericulture de Paris
Paris, France

Christopher R. Harman, MD
Director, Fetal Assessment Unit
Division of Maternal and Fetal Medicine
Department of Obstetrics, Gynecology &
   Reproductive Sciences
University of Manitoba
Women's Hospital
Winnipeg, Canada

P. Hohlfeld, MD
Professor, Departement de Gynecologie
   and Obstetrique
University of Lausanne
Lausanne, Switzerland

Jo-Ann Johnson, MD, FRCS(C)
Division of Maternal-Fetal Medicine
Department of Obstetrics and Gynecology
Toronto General Hospital
Toronto, Canada

Phillipa Kyle, MRCOG
Department of Obstetrics and
   Gynecology
University of Cambridge
Rosie Maternity Hospital
Cambridge, England

L. Lynch, MD
Assistant Professor
Department of Obstetrics and Gynecology
Mount Sinai Medical Center
New York, New York

Frank A. Manning, MD
Professor and Head
Department of Obstetrics and Gynecology
Women's Hospital
Winnipeg, Canada

Lawrence B. McCullough, PhD
Baylor College of Medicine
Center for Ethics, Medicine & Public Issues
Houston, Texas

S. Menticoglou, MD
Department of Obstetrics, Gynecology &
    Reproductive Sciences
Women's Hospital
Winnipeg, Canada

Umberto Nicolini, MD
Seconda Clinica
Instituti Clinici di Perfezionamento
Instituto Obstetrico et Ginecologica
Milano, Italy

Mary Pillai, MD
Fellow, Division of Maternal and Fetal
    Medicine
Department of Obstetrics, Gynecology &
    Reproductive Sciences
University of Manitoba

Women's Hospital
Winnipeg, Canada

Charles H. Rodeck, MD
Head, Department of Obstetrics and
    Gynecology
University College and Middlesex School
    of Medicine
University College London
London, England

Janet I. Vaughan, FRCOG, DDU
Locum Consultant in Obstetrics and
    Gynecology
Fetal Medicine Unit
Queen Charlotte's and Chelsea Hospital
London, England

Carl Weiner, MD
Department of Obstetrics and Gynecology
University of Iowa Hospitals and Clinics
Iowa City, Iowa

R. Douglas Wilson, MD
Departments of Medical Genetics and
    Obstetrics and Gynecology
University Hospital, Shaughnessy Site
Vancouver, Canada

Preface

This book is a discussion by practicing physicians about elements of their craft. They are describing problems and solutions that present on a regular basis and which are addressed in an increasingly straightforward fashion. Direct patient testing, in concert with detailed history and physician examination, provide a background for informed decisions about therapy and ongoing follow-up. A reasonable convalescent period usually intervenes before care is transferred to another physician.

This description applies to any well-established branch of medicine, and signifies a mature science which is able to incorporate an individualized approach in a milieu of detailed understanding. It is a measure of the amazing progress over the last decade, that this description applies to *fetal medicine*, in full measure.

We have reached a mature stage of the development of our ability to evaluate (and to *treat*) the fetus as a patient. This point has been attained at startling speed—there is no doubt that fetal medicine is in the log phase of its evolution. Each increment in knowledge has spawned an explosion of related revelations, with an ever-increasing momentum. In the few years since Fernand Daffos demonstrated the utility and ease of ultrasound-guided access to the fetal circulation, we have moved toward a detailed and comprehensive understanding of fetal physiology—an understanding that is changing daily! Ten years ago, a typical volume on fetal physiology was 300 pages long, devoted to epidemiology, theory, intrapartum and neonatal data, and sheep, sheep, and more sheep. In 1993, a number of excellent volumes each contained over 1000 pages of *human* data, an ever-increasing number of journals catalogues the growth of original fetal data, and at least ten international societies devote themselves to the study of fetal physiology in health and disease, and to fetal medicine and surgery.

Against this background of intense interest and rapid growth, the perinatal specialists who have participated in this volume share their state-of-the-art experience. Many of the authors are personally responsible for the progress measured here. They are able to speak from experience with innovative techniques and approaches. They are able to discuss fetal diagnostic and therapeutic measures from a broadening base of fetal data—and not just from the anecdotes and case reports of only a few years ago. As such, this is a second-generation text—we are now able to deal with many *established* modalities on a basis of actual fetal data.

As we move from theory to practice, what appeared obvious has collided with the confusing reality (as in the case of ventriculo-amniotic shunts for hydrocephalus); techniques have come and gone (fetoscopy); and our neonatal colleagues have eliminated the need for daring fetal surgery so recently perfected (open fetal repair of congenital diaphragmatic hernia). Even as this book has been assembled, the lessons learned from antenatal fetal surgery for CDH have been used to *cure* cystic adenomatoid malformation in hydropic fetuses; several groups have detailed their innovations in fixing fetal cardiac abnormalities—or conversely, in removing acardiac twins altogether; not to mention sawing placentas in half with laser beams! It is no wonder that many of our authors reflect this dynamic situation with concerns about the too-rapid acceptance of new techniques or the apparent ease with which old principles have been dropped. The new fetal ethics, so well articulated by Chervenak and McCullough, must continue to grow and evolve to balance us on these shifting sands.

The speed of progress has been breathtaking. I hope the reader can enjoy the opportunity taken here, to catch a breath and survey the steps achieved by this wonderful group of fetal physicians.

Christopher R. Harman

NOTICE

THE ROLE OF INVASIVE FETAL TESTING IN PRENATAL DIAGNOSIS OF HERITABLE DISEASES

1

R. DOUGLAS WILSON

The ability to diagnose heritable genetic diseases in the fetus continues to increase as technology allows the fetus to be examined more closely. With invasive prenatal diagnosis, the fetus can be considered as a patient within a patient.

Invasive prenatal diagnosis includes techniques such as amniocentesis, chorionic villus sampling (CVS), cordocentesis or percutaneous umbilical blood sampling (PUBS), fetal tissue biopsy, fetoscopy, and embryoscopy. *Invasive* implies that specimens are obtained directly from the fetus or indirectly from an associated fetal structure or product by needle or biopsy technique, allowing assessment of specific fetal characteristics.

It is important to emphasize the ethical considerations of prenatal diagnosis. Campbell (1) stated that the primary purpose of prenatal diagnosis is the continuation of normal and wanted pregnancies in which the welfare of mother and fetus is the prime consideration. The emphasis on elimination of handicap should always remain only a modulation of this dominant theme. In addition, it is important to recognize that as invasive prenatal diagnosis techniques are used in the future, not only is prenatal diagnosis possible, but prenatal in utero therapy for diagnosed conditions is probable.

The incidence of genetic disease is common, while individual diseases may be rare. In regard to prenatal diagnosis, genetic disease can be classified into three major categories: congenital anomalies, chromosomal abnormalities, and single gene disorders.

Major congenital anomalies are noted at birth in 2–3% of newborns, while if the period of observation is extended to one year of age, the incidence increases to 5%. The etiology and recurrent risks of congenital anomalies are dependent on whether they are isolated or part of a syndrome sequence or association. The etiology may be sporadic, multifactorial, or due to a specific human teratogen. Evaluation of these factors is important, not only for the prognosis of the fetus or newborn but for predictability in future pregnancies.

Chromosomal abnormalities can be due to nondisjunctional chromosome mechanics, inherited chromosomal rearrangements from carrier parents, or new structural changes with resulting chromosome rearrangement, deletion, or insertion. The most commonly recognized etiology for nondisjunctional chromosomal abnormalities is advanced maternal age. When maternal age at the time of conception is greater than age 34 or 35, as is more commonly stated, at the estimated date of delivery, there are increased risks for a liveborn child with a chromosomal abnormality (Table 1-1) (2,3,4). It is important that the liveborn figures are statistical risks for women who choose *not* to have invasive prenatal diagnosis and take into account those fetuses with chromosomal abnormalities that are lost spontaneously at various gestational ages throughout the pregnancy. The incidence of chromosomal abnormalities at gestational ages when invasive prenatal diagnosis (CVS, amniocentesis) is utilized is shown in Table 1-1.

Single gene abnormalities may be transmitted to the fetus as autosomal dominant, autosomal recessive, or x-linked recessive (rarely dominant) conditions. These can be inherited from carrier parents or as new single gene mutations (usually dominant) from either ovum or sperm. New dominant single gene mutations may occur in advanced paternal age 40 years and are different from risks of advanced maternal age with resulting chromosome nondisjunction. Specific single gene disorders may be present in various ethnic groups. Table 1-2

Table 1-1 Maternal Age at Conception and Fetal Chromosome Risks at Different Gestational Ages

Maternal Age at		Risk of Chromosomal Abnormality		
Conception	Date of Delivery	in Liveborn	at Amniocentesis	at CVS
27	28	1/430	–	–
28	29	420	–	–
29	30	390	–	–
30	31	390	–	–
31	32	320	–	–
32	33	285	–	–
33	34	240	–	–
34	35	180	–	–
35	36	150	1/141	1/89
36	37	125	111	94
37	38	100	88	61
38	39	80	70	58
39	40	80	56	37
40	41	55	44	39
41	42	43	35	23
42	43	34	29	14
43	44	27	22	11
44	45	20	17	7
45	46	–	14	–
46	47	–	11	–
47	48	–	9	–

Adapted from references: (2) Hook EB, Rates of chromosome abnormalities of different maternal ages. Obstet Gynecol 1981;58:282–285; (3) Hook EB, Cross PK, Jackson L, Pergament E, Brambati B. Maternal age-specific rates of 47+21 and other cytogenetic abnormalities diagnosed in the first trimester of pregnancy in chorionic villus biopsy specimens: comparison with rates expected from observations at amniocentesis. AM J Hum Genet 1988;42:797–807; and (4) Hook EB, Cross PK. Maternal age-specific rates of chromosome abnormalities at chorionic villus study: a revision. Am J Hum Genet 1989;45:474–477.

Table 1-2 Genetic Risks: Ethnic Factors

Race	Disease
European	
Northern	cystic fibrosis
Mediterranean	alpha/beta-thalassemia
Ashkenazi Jewish	Tay-Sachs
Black	sickle cell anemia
Asian	alpha/beta-thalassemia

and physiologic health of the fetus are many, in most situations, only one major question is being asked in regard to fetal status. The common indications for genetic invasive prenatal diagnosis are shown in Table 1-3 (5–17).

In most prenatal diagnosis programs, advanced maternal age is the indication for assessment of fetal chromosomes in 80–85% of patients. The indication of a previous pregnancy with a potentially viable or liveborn chromosomal abnormality accounts for 2–5%. Parental chromosomal rearrangements with fetal risks for unbalanced chromosomal abnormalities are present in 0.5–1% of prenatal diagnosis indications.

Fetal structural anomalies identified by ultrasound in the index pregnancy are an increasing indication for prenatal genetic evaluation. For certain fetal anomalies, such as neural tube defects, a past history of a fetus or child by either parent would be an indication for invasive prenatal diagnosis. As ultrasound technology improves, the use of invasive prenatal diagnosis for neural tube indication may decrease, but at present, it is the indication for 3–5% of prenatal diagnoses.

Single gene disorders (molecular, biochemical) are the indication for invasive prenatal diagnosis in approximately 5% of patients. The number of genetic mutations

indicates some of the common ethnic genetic diseases for which patient screening should be considered.

While the number of techniques available to answer questions regarding the genetic

Table 1-3 Indications for Invasive Prenatal Genetic Diagnosis

---

A. Chromosomal Abnormalities

---

1. Advanced Maternal Age
(34 years or greater at conception)

2. Previous History:
    a. stillbirth/liveborn with a chromosomal abnormality (numerical, structural, marker)
    b. parental carrier with significant chromosome rearrangement (translocation, inversion)

B. Single Gene Disorders: Some Common Syndromes (metabolic/biochemical)

Autosomal Recessive:	alpha/beta thalassemia
	cystic fibrosis
	Tay-Sachs disease
Autosomal Dominant:	myotonic dystrophy
	Huntington's chorea
X-linked Conditions:	muscular dystrophy (Duchenne, Becker's)
	hemophilia A/B
	Fragile X mental retardation

C. Congenital Fetal Anomalies Identified in the Index Pregnancy or Previous Pregnancy with NTD

Congenital Anomalies	Increased Fetal Risk for Chromosomal Abnormalities/Incidence
1. CNS: Neural Tube Defects	yes
Hydrocephalus (Isolated)	yes
Encephalocele	rare
Microcephaly	yes
2. Cardiac (Isolated)	4–5%[5]
3. Urinary Tract	
(Obstructive/Parenchymal)	5–9%[6]
4. Cystic Hygroma	60–80%[7]
5. Omphalocele	35–58%[8–12]
Gastroschisis	rare
Diaphragmatic Hernia	4%[13–17]
6. Skeletal: Bone Shortening	yes
Hypomineralization	rare
7. Nonimmune Hydrops	common (5–10%)
8. Multiple Congenital Anomalies	common
9. Intrauterine Growth Retardation (Severe)	common (15%)

that can be identified by molecular DNA or biochemical techniques is rapidly increasing with more than 200 different identifiable disorders (18). Other invasive testing may be required due to maternal disease with teratogenic risks (IDDM, epilepsy).

Other indications for prenatal diagnosis by a noninvasive ultrasound would include a history for either parent of a previous fetus or child with a congenital malformation identifiable by ultrasound (neural tube, cardiac, abdominal wall, or renal anomalies).

Each of the invasive prenatal diagnosis techniques will be discussed with the indications, advantages, disadvantages, and risks. Some diagnostic results may be obtained by a variety of techniques (Fetal karyotype can be obtained from amniocentesis, CVS, or fetal blood sampling), but some prenatal diagnosis techniques will have specific indications for use. The specific use of ultrasound to evaluate congenital malformations will not be discussed in this chapter, but ultrasound technology has allowed the development of these invasive prenatal diagnosis techniques.

Invasive prenatal diagnosis techniques were initially developed in the late 1960s prior to use of ultrasound guidance. Both amniocentesis and transcervical (TC) CVS were initially developed at similar times, but amniocentesis appeared in early trials to be safer and more reliable. Amniocentesis was originally done without ultrasound guidance. As ultrasound became more available, it was used adjunctively, initially to identify a safe site for amniocentesis and subsequently to provide continuous observation of the amniocentesis procedure to decrease the risk of fetal trauma. As ultrasound technology improved and ultrasound guidance of amniocentesis became more commonplace, other techniques of invasive prenatal diagnosis were reintroduced (CVS) or new techniques were

developed (PUBS or fetal tissue biopsy). Fetoscopy was originally developed to allow more direct fetal visualization prior to improved ultrasound visualization. With improved ultrasound technology and greater visualization of the fetus, fetoscopy procedures have declined greatly and, at present, have few indications. Embryoscopy is a new invasive prenatal diagnosis technique designed to allow early visualization of the embryo.

Amniocentesis

Amniocentesis is a second trimester prenatal diagnostic procedure usually performed after 14^{+0} weeks gestation (from the first day of the last menstrual period).

The indications for amniocentesis include advanced maternal age, history of a previous stillborn or liveborn child with a chromosomal abnormality, parental chromosome translocations, history of specific congenital anomalies (neural tube defects), and other biochemical or molecular genetic diseases where results can be obtained from amniocytes or amniotic fluid.

Ultrasound is performed prior to amniocentesis to determine fetal gestational age, location of placenta and amniotic fluid, fetal cardiac activity, and the number of fetuses. In many centers, ultrasound is used concurrently while amniocentesis is performed. The technique is usually performed with a 20–22-gauge spinal needle, and 15–30cc of amniotic fluid is removed. Obtaining the amniotic fluid generally takes less than one minute, and the patient may experience some mild uterine cramping and describe a mild pressure sensation.

The risks of amniocentesis include fetal loss, continued leakage and fetal injury. After amniocentesis, the major risk is fetal loss with or without infection, generally estimated to be one pregnancy loss for every

200 amniocenteses (19,20,21). Other complications following amniocentesis include continued leakage of amniotic fluid, bleeding, and infection. The risk of infection following the procedure is estimated to be very low (1/1000) (22). Fetal injuries at the time of amniocentesis have been reported but, with ultrasound guidance, are very rare.

Increased risks are present when the patient has experienced bleeding prior to the procedure. Amniotic fluid is normally similar in appearance to white wine. If the patient has previously had a history of antepartum bleeding, the amniotic fluid may be brown or dark red due to blood pigments being absorbed across the chorionic membranes. This type of discolored fluid is associated with an increased risk of pregnancy loss due to the previous bleeding episode (23).

The main advantage of amniocentesis is that accurate analysis of the fetal karyotype or other genetic diseases can be obtained from the cultured amniocytes or by measurement of specific substances in the amniotic fluid. Results can generally be obtained prior to 20 weeks gestation.

The major disadvantage of amniocentesis is that the results of the prenatal diagnosis are not available until 17–20 weeks gestational age.

Early Amniocentesis

Early amniocentesis is defined as an amniocentesis performed prior to 14^{+0} weeks gestation. The indication, ultrasound evaluation, and technique are similar to the midtrimester amniocentesis.

Recent concern regarding CVS safety and accuracy has stimulated increased interest in early amniocentesis. Confined placental mosaicism, increased laboratory handling, and risk of congenital malformation are the areas of concern. Confined chorionic mosaicism is discussed in the sec-

tion on CVS. The dissection of maternal decidua from the chorionic villi makes the technique more labor-intensive for laboratory personnel. Fewer cytogenetic specimens can be analyzed for the technologists' time. Recent reports (24–30) have indicated a possible increased risk for fetal craniofacial and limb malformations when CVS is performed at 56–66 days gestation. This finding raises concerns regarding a spectrum of abnormalities, from craniofacial and limb defects on the severe end to more subtle defects that may be more difficult to detect.

Early amniocentesis is feasible, with the majority being performed between 11^{+0} and 14^{+6} weeks gestation (see Table 1-4) (31–51). The technique is usually performed with a 20–22-gauge spinal needle. Variable amounts of amniotic fluid are removed from 1 ml per week of gestation to mean volumes of 25 cc. The timing of the procedure shows that approximately 70% are done between 13^{+0} and 14^{+6} weeks and 90% between 12 and 14^{+6} weeks. Failed or rescheduled procedures range from 1–5%. Laboratory cytogenetic failures range from 0.2–2.9%. The gestational age at early amniocentesis influences the success rate, with one report (37) showing a 32% cytogenetic failure rate at 8^{+0}–11^{+6} weeks gestation and no cytogenetic failures at 12^{+0}–14^{+6} weeks. Total pregnancy loss rates for published studies show spontaneous loss rate ranging from 0.7–6.5% and therapeutic losses ranging from 0.8%–7%. The mean spontaneous loss is 2.7%, and the mean therapeutic loss is 3.1%, for a total pregnancy loss estimate of 5.8%. This value is compatible with the total pregnancy loss rates in the Randomized Canadian Collaborative Trial for Chorionic Villus Sampling and Amniocentesis (52). None of the reported early amniocentesis trials are randomized. Some reports (38,43,51,53) have measured alphafetoprotein (AFP) and acetylholin-

Table 1-4 Published Reports Involving Early Amniocentesis

| Investigator | # Patients | Gestational Age (WKS) | | | | | | Volume (cc) | Trans-placental | AFP/ ACHE | Results (Days) | Needle (Gauge) | Procedure Failure Complications | | | Continuous Ultrasound Guidance |
		<11+0	11+0	12+0	13+0	14+0	15+0						Rescheduled (Number)	Lab Failure (Number)	Total Losses *** (Number)	
Hanson et al (31)	541	—	4	36	149	352	—	25 (15–35)	yes	—	8 (7–10)	20	2.6% (15)	0	SL 4.6% (13) TA 1.0% (3)	no
Müller et al (32)	183	—	—	*30	57	96	—	10–15	—	—	9 (6–12)	22	—	—	SL 1.6%	—
Sandstrum et al (33)	19	—	—	—	—	—	—	10	—	—	10–12	—	—	—	—	yes
Godmilow et al (34)	165	—	—	—	—	—	—	—	—	—	7–19	—	failed 1.8% (3)	1.8% (3)	1.2% (2)	—
Johnson Godmilow (35)	—	—	—	—	—	—	—	—	—	—	—	—	—	—	—	—
†**Williamson**	197	—	4	7	53	133	—	15	yes	—	—	22	resch 3% failed 1.5% (3)	2% (4)	SL 2.5% (5) TA 4.1% (8)	—
†**Weiner Godmilow**	370	—	12	191	117	50	—	10	yes	—	—	22	failed 2.1% (8)	1.0% (4)	SL 6.5%**** TA 1.6%	—
†**Miller**	453	—	0	63	78	256	—	8.8 –25.6	—	—	—	22	resch 0.4%	0	SL 2.7%**** TA 2.6%	—
†**Resta**	495	—	48	273	174	22	—	15	no	—	—	22	20% resch.	0.6% (3)	—	—
Benacerraf et al (36)	108 (3 lost to followup)	—	4	60	25	11	—	10–12	—	—	24–26	22	4.6% (5) unable to do	2.9% (3)	SL 0.9% (1) TA 3.8% (4)	yes
Rooney et al (37)	40	18	7	7	6	2	—	13.9 (1–40)	—	—	6–24	20	—	32% 8–11 wks. 0% 12–14 wks	—	—

Study							Dose					Resched.		SL/TA	
Elejalde et al (38)	615	9	18	77	98	121	292	1 ml/wk	no	yes/yes	19.7	20	resched. 1.12%	0.3%	SL 1.6% (10) TA 0.8% (5)	yes
Evans et al (39)	227	5	10	21	48	143	—	10–15	—	yes/yes	—	22	—	1.3%	SL 0.8% (2) TA 2.6% (6)	yes
Hanson et al (40)	527 (10 lost to followup)	2	9	46	215	255	—	26.3 (5–36)	yes	—	8.8	20	1.5% (8)	0.2% (1)	SL 3.1% (16) TA 1.3% (7)	yes
Lindner et al (41)	135	2	4	16	37	76	—	—	no	AFP	—	20	—	0.7% (10)	SL 0.7% (1) TA 7% (9)	yes
Nevin et al (42)	222	3	2	26	61	130	—	4–17	no	—	10	20	—	0%	SL 1.8% (4) TA 5.0% (11)	yes
Penso et al (43)	407	—	9	179	177	92	—	1ml/wk	yes	yes/yes	14–21	22	3.4%	1.7% (7)	SL 3.9% (15) TA 2.6% (10)	yes
Stripporo et al (44)	505	—	13	42	158	182	110	1 ml/wk	—	—	8–17	22	0	16% (8)	SL 3.2% (16) TA 2.1% (11)	—
Byrne 1991 (45)	324	75	137	69	43	—	—	11	No	—	12 (8–22)	20	—	1.9%	—	yes
Rebello 1991 (46)	114	—	5	23	79	37	—	1 ml/wk	No	—	12.2	20	2.6%	—	—	yes
Hackett et al (47)*	106	—	5	24	42	35	—	1–14	—	—	12.2 (8–30)	20	—	—	SL 1.9% (2)	yes
Liu et al (48)	280	×	×	×	×	×	—	12.3	—	—	11.3	—	—	1.4% (4)	SL 0.7% (2) TA 3.9% (11)	yes
Nevin et al (49)**	500	×	×	×	×	×	—	—	No	—	—	20	—	2%	SL 1.8% (9) TA 4.4% (22)	yes
Shulman et al (50)	150	3	1	4	26	116	—	1 ml/wk	—	—	—	—	—	1.3%	SL 4.7% (7) TA 3.3% (5)	—
Sato et al (51)	604	—	3	25	155	421	—	1 ml/wk	—	Y/Y	—	22	—	0.8%	SL 4.0% (24) TA 4.1% (25)	—

*Same population as Rebello et al. (46)
**Same population as Nevin et al. (42)
***SL spontaneous loss
****TA therapeutic loss
*****Incomplete population followup
†Cited in Johnson and Godmilow (35)

esterase in the amniotic fluid specimens and have published normal values for these earlier gestation weeks.

The early amniocentesis technique attempts to avoid the placenta, but the transplacental approach may be used if no other access is available. Continuous ultrasound guidance for the procedure is used for the early amniocentesis, which may differ from some mid-amniocentesis techniques that use ultrasound only to locate an appropriate location for the procedure.

Randomized trials to compare early amniocentesis with either midtrimester amniocentesis or CVS are necessary prior to the introduction of this invasive technique into clinical prenatal diagnosis programs. Comparison to midtrimester amniocentesis seems more appropriate as gestational age for early amniocentesis appears to be best between 11^{+0}–13^{+6} weeks, which does not correspond with the 9^{+0}–11^{+6} weeks gestational age utilized for the majority of CVS.

Chorionic Villus Sampling

Chorionic villus sampling is considered in detail in the following chapter by Dr. J. Johnson. CVS is usually performed between 9 and 12 weeks gestation using either transcervical or transabdominal techniques. Chorionic villi can be used for chromosomal, metabolic, and DNA analysis. CVS would *not* be appropriate for prenatal diagnosis of congenital malformations, including neural tube defects that have no known chromosomal, metabolic, or molecular basis.

Two large collaborative studies (52) have indicated that TC-CVS, when performed by expert operators, is a relatively safe procedure and may be considered an acceptable alternative to midtrimester genetic amniocentesis. The procedure-related risk of the CVS above the background rate of spontaneous loss is estimated at 1–2% in comparison to 0.5% for amniocentesis. The background rate for spontaneous abortion in the advanced maternal age population is estimated at 4–6% when the pregnancy has been shown to be viable by ultrasound at 10 weeks gestation (54–56).

The major advantage of CVS is the early gestational age at sampling, so if a chromosomal or DNA abnormality is detected and pregnancy termination is requested, both the physical and emotional aspects of pregnancy termination are less than those following amniocentesis. A second advantage is that a large amount of DNA can be extracted directly from villi without cell culturing, allowing an early result for molecular analysis of fetal sex and genetic disorders.

Additional prenatal diagnosis at 16–20 weeks by ultrasound and maternal serum AFP measurement is necessary for CVS patients to give them an overall prenatal evaluation (chromosomal, congenital anomalies) similar to patients undergoing amniocentesis at 15–20 weeks gestational age. Prenatal diagnosis by CVS has been shown to have a high patient acceptance (57) but, in certain areas, has been criticized due to a possibly higher medical cost for the procedure and additional evaluations. Disadvantages of CVS include placental mosaicism and maternal contamination, requiring that two tissue culture procedures be carried out to achieve an acceptable accuracy: a short-term culture (cytotrophoblast cells) and a long-term fibroblast culture (mesenchymal core of villus).

Confined chorionic mosaicism 58 (a complicating factor in 1–2% of CVS samples 52,58–60) is defined as a discrepancy between the chromosomes in the chorionic and fetal tissues, with mosaicism restricted to the cytotrophoblast, the extraembryonic mesoderm, or both of these lineages and a complete absence of mosaicism in the embryo. Chorionic villi at the time of CVS have the structure of tertiary villi, derived from three different cell lineages: polar trophectoderm, extraembryonic mesoderm, and primitive embryonic streak. Although both extraembryonic mesoderm and the embryo proper originate from the inner cell mass (ICM), in mosaicism, the ICM cells that give rise to extraembryonic mesoderm may have a different karyotype from the cells migrating from the primitive streak of the embryo proper. Patients who have confined chorionic mosaicism usually require amniocentesis as an additional prenatal diagnostic technique to define explicitly the genetic complement of the fetus. A second choice would be fetal blood sampling (PUBS) to clarify the discrepancy in some situations. There is some information to indicate that placental mosaicism may have an effect on placental function and may lead to intrauterine growth retardation (IUGR) or even intrauterine death (58). Those fetuses with placental mosaicism should be followed by ultrasound for evidence of growth discrepancies in the second and third trimester. This is an example of how invasive testing for genetic disorders must be integrated and may give rise to the necessity for further invasive testing.

Cordocentesis (Percutaneous Umbilical Blood Sampling)

Cordocentesis (61–63) can be utilized to obtain fetal blood from the umbilical cord from as early as 12 weeks gestation until term.

Fetal karyotyping by PUBS may be indicated when congenital malformations or IUGR are identified by ultrasound. Evaluation of fetal status regarding viral infections, hematological abnormalities, including Rh or immune hemolytic disease, maternal platelet disorders, and inborn errors of metabolism can be performed. In the case of heritable disorders, physiologic assessment can be made by measuring various fetal parameters in fetal blood (Table 1-5) (64–73) and the procedure has both diagnostic and therapeutic implications (Table 1-6).

A wide range of fetal situations and conditions have been studied with PUBS. Within the context of genetic evaluation and other heritable conditions, PUBS can be carried out from 16 weeks gestation to term but has been done as early as 12 weeks. Depending on the indications for the test, 1–3 ml is removed for analysis. For

Table 1-5 Fetal Blood Results at Cordocentesis

Normal Values (Variable Gestational Ages)

albumin (64)
alkaline phosphatase (65)
aspartate amninotransferase (65)
bilirubin (total) (65)
blood gases (pH, pO_2, pCO_2, HCO_3, BE) (66–68)
calcium (65)
cholesterol (65)
coagulation factors (VIIIc, VIII RAg, VII, IX, V, II, XII) (69)
complete blood count (WBC, platelets, RBC, hemoglobin, hematocrit, MCV) (64,65,67,70,71)
differential count (lymphocytes, neutrophils, eosinophils, monocytes, normoblasts) (65,70)
creatinine (65)
gamma-glutamyltransferase (65)
glucose (65,72)
glycine (73)
Hb A/Hb Fac (65)
inhibitors (fibronectin, protein C, alpha-2-macroglobulin, alpha-1-antitrypsin, AT III, alpha-2-antiplasmin) (65)
lactate (66,68)
protein (total) (64)
T cell subset (65)
triglycerides (65)
valine (73)

Table 1-6 Role of Cordocentesis in Prenatal
Heritable Disease

A. Diagnostic Indications	Fetal Blood for:
1. Fetal Anomalies (Single or Multiple)	Chromosomes
2. Fetal Status	CBC, platelets, electrolytes, glucose, lactate, antibodies (immune, nonimmune), blood gases (see Table 1-4)
3. Genetic Risk	Chromosomes (mosaicism), single gene (DNA)
4. Experimental Techniques	PCR (polymerase chain reaction) (DNA hydridization techniques)

B. Therapeutic

1. **Stem Cell Transplantation/Chimeras** (Experimental)

2. **Gene (DNA) Transfer (Future)**

simple karyotyping, 0.5–1.0 ml of pure fetal blood is sufficient. For genetic purposes, a small amount of contamination by amniotic fluid is probably not critical. In diagnosis of some familial disorders by metabolic function, amniocentesis-derived fibroblast cultures remain the principal means of diagnosis because large volumes of blood would be required to make the diagnosis directly. Ongoing advances in microtechniques will continue to add to the list of disorders diagnosable by fetal blood sample.

Currently, the most common indication for PUBS in genetics is to assess fetal chromosomes when single or multiple congenital malformations are identified by ultrasound (74). Fetal chromosomal results are available in 48–72 hours in comparison to amniocentesis results, which may take seven–14 days. Late CVS (75) can also provide rapid chromosomal diagnoses, in some cases in less than 24 hours, when the major differential diagnosis is trisomy 21, 18, or 13. Small chromosomal structural rearrangements may not be as easily detected by direct chorionic villus preparations; therefore, culturing chorionic villus tissue or fetal lymphocytes allows a more accurate cytogenetic diagnosis.

With the increasing number of genetic diseases identified by molecular DNA techniques, the role of PUBS in the identification of single gene disorders in the fetus will increase. At present, molecular DNA diagnoses involve genetic linkage analysis or specific gene mutation analysis and require blood specimens for extraction of DNA from the affected individual (if available) and other unaffected family members. Some genetic disorders (Duchenne muscular dystrophy, cystic fibrosis) have specific gene mutations that can be rapidly screened for in fetal DNA from fetal lymphocytes after family DNA studies have been completed. There are genetic conditions where either the gene has not been isolated or multiple mutations may be present so that linkage analysis of molecular family polymorphisms is still required. The accuracy of the prenatal prediction is based on the specific disease and whether the specific gene mutation or linkage analysis is used. For linkage analysis, genetic recombination or crossing-over must be considered in the interpretation of the results.

The role of PUBS in the evaluation of fetal mosaicism can also be considered.

CVS (59) has been shown to have confined placental mosaicism in 1–2% of cases that require additional invasive testing to assess the clinical significance of the mosaicism. Amniocentesis has a much smaller incidence of mosaicism than CVS (58,59,76). When mosaicism is identified at either CVS or amniocentesis, additional fetal tissue specimens may be required to allow accurate interpretation of the clinical significance for the mosaicism. When mosaicism is identified following CVS, amniocentesis is usually the technique of choice, but PUBS could be considered if a more rapid diagnosis is required. PUBS is more commonly used to assess mosaicism identified at amniocentesis due to later gestational age. By obtaining fetal blood (lymphocytes), a similar cytogenetic evaluation can be obtained as from pediatric or adult chromosome analysis.

The evaluation of mosaicism (two or more karyotypically distinct cell lines) in childhood or adult life requires blood (lymphocytes) and tissue (skin) specimens. It is necessary to establish whether there is a chromosomal abnormality in the constitutional body tissues or the mosaicism is isolated to body areas with no effect on mental, physical, or genetic development. The usual approach in the child or adult is to obtain a blood specimen initially to assess lymphocyte chromosomes. When mosaicism is identified in the lymphocyte cytogenetic preparations, other tissue specimens are assessed, such as by skin fibroblast cultures. On rare occasions, biopsies from other tissues, such as gonads (Turner's syndrome), may be used to assess the extent of mosaicism. In the fetus, the process of mosaicism evaluation is opposite, in that fetal blood is obtained as a secondary evaluation when fibroblast cultures from either amniocentesis or CVS have indicated possible mosaicism.

Embryologically, the mesoderm contributes to hematopoietic stem cells, bone marrow, and epithelial tissues. Epithelial tissues are a combination of ectoderm and mesoderm origin. Therefore, these mesoderm tissues (blood, epithelial tissue) provide primary and secondary specimens to evaluate presence or absence of constitutional chromosomal mosaicism. It is generally felt that skin biopsy fibroblast cultures are more representative of the constitutional chromosomal karyotype for an individual. The technical access to tissue specimens for analysis, blood from newborns or adults and amniotic fluid or chorionic villus tissue from fetuses, is usually the reason for the different approaches to mosaicism in addition to having a second tissue specimen to evaluate.

It is important in this evaluation of mosaicism that there is good communication between the patient, geneticist, perinatologist (obstetrician), and cytogeneticist so that the different factors involved are fully understood prior to the onset of further invasive prenatal procedures.

The role of PUBS in physiological fetal surveillance will become increasingly important as more normative data on the fetus at various gestational ages becomes available (Table 1-5) (64–78). A variety of blood parameters measured routinely in newborn, childhood, and adult abnormalities will allow a wider range of prenatal diagnosis in the high-risk fetal population. At the present time, these procedures are reserved for high-risk pregnancies and would certainly not remove the necessity for newborn screening for inherited metabolic diseases.

A future use for PUBS in the management of heritable diseases will be not only for diagnostic procedures but for therapy as well. The use of PUBS to provide direct access to the fetus may allow hematopoietic stem cell and bone marrow transplantation

(79) and the development of tissue replacement chimeras to allow correction or modification or the morbidity and mortality from certain genetic conditions. The fetus at certain gestational ages is immunologically tolerant and there is no need for immunosuppression. Large amounts of animal research have been undertaken in this area and a small number of human clinical cases have been initiated with no positive outcomes to date (79).

Complications and risks of cordocentesis are uncommon in the context of fetal sampling for genetic evaluation. Premature rupture of membranes (PROM) or premature labor are possible. Fetal trauma or bleeding at the time of the procedure are uncommon and prolonged bleeding of the cord greater than two minutes usually occurs in fewer than 2% of cases (62). The risk of fetal distress or intrauterine death during or following the procedure is 1–5% but depends on the fetal status prior to the procedure.

Additional Fetal Tissue Sampling

Sites for additional fetal tissue sampling include fetal skin, liver, and fluid collections in fetal urinary tract, abdomen, thorax, or cystic hygroma. Techniques to obtain such fetal tissue specimens are similar to freehand ultrasound-guided techniques like amniocentesis and PUBS. Needle insertion into specific fetal areas requires appropriate fetal positioning. Fetal paralysis may be required. Protocols for fetal paralysis for fetal transfusion are published and may vary from center to center. Risks and complications of the procedures are similar to those quoted for PUBS with the risks of fetal death being increased if major congenital malformations and growth retardation are present. The accuracy of the test will be dependent on the tissue being obtained and the specific analysis required. For urinary tract evaluation, fetal urine specimens can be obtained by bladder aspiration for urine osmolality and electrolytes (80). Thoracic and abdominal fluids can be evaluated for cell and protein content (chylothorax). Lymphatic fluid from cystic hygroma can be used for chromosome analysis. Liver (81) and skin (82) have been sampled for evidence of specific genetic syndromes. Liver enzyme assays (81) for glucose-6-phosphatase (glycogen storage disease *type 1*) and ornithine transcarbamoylase (OTC) have been analyzed. Recommendations for these procedures would be similar to those given for the other more commonly invasive prenatal diagnostic procedures.

Radiography

The use of radiography in prenatal diagnosis has decreased significantly with the introduction of real-time ultrasound. In selected situations, there are still appropriate indications for a single plain film of the maternal abdomen, pelvis, and fetus. The most common indication would be when major skeletal abnormalities, such as dwarfism, are suspected by ultrasound. A single X-ray may allow a specific diagnosis to be made prenatally from individual bone involvement and patterning that may be characteristic (83). There appear to be no maternal risks to this procedure, and no studies have shown any increased risk of the fetus developing childhood leukemia.

Amniography uses radiopaque agents injected into the amniotic cavity to outline external and internal fetal structures. X-ray procedures would subsequently be utilized to evaluate the location of the water-soluble iodinated radio contrast materials. There are no significant maternal or fetal risk factors to the contrast material, and maternal or fetal risks of X-ray exposure are similar to the previous discussion.

Fetoscopy and Embryoscopy

Fetoscopy (84) as a prenatal diagnosis technique has few indications now for prenatal diagnosis or treatment. The risk of fetoscopy are greater than the risks of any of the other invasive prenatal diagnosis procedures.

Embryoscopy at the present time is a research technique and may allow early visualization of the embryo. Vaginal ultrasound is able to give similar embryonic and early fetal detail, so it is unlikely that this invasive procedure will have any significant indications.

CONCLUSION

In order to provide comprehensive genetic and heritable disease diagnostics to a general obstetric population, an integrated service is essential. The prenatal team, usually clinical geneticists, cytogeneticists and cytogenetic laboratory, expert ultrasonographers and perinatologists, must collaborate closely with clinical obstetricians, neonatologists, pediatric subspecialists, and so on as well as have the appropriate bioethical support. In most cases, such a team can only be assembled effectively within the confines of a university-based tertiary care prenatal center. The complex nature of prenatal diagnosis suggests facility with a variety of techniques is required (Table 1-7).

The role of invasive fetal testing in prenatal diagnosis allows a more accurate and direct evaluation of the fetal status. Indirect or screening procedures, such as ultrasound and maternal serum AFP, often require diagnostic testing by invasive techniques to confirm suspected diagnoses. It is the hope of workers in the area of prenatal diagnosis that the future will allow not only fetal diagnosis but subsequent in utero fetal therapy to correct or modify the

Table 1-7 Typical Distribution of Prenatal Genetics Tests*

Condition	CVS	Amnio	PUBS	Other
Advanced Maternal Age	20%	70%	10%	—
Specific Disorder	20%	60%	15%	5%
Multiple Anomalies	5%	50%	40%	5%
Intrauterine Growth Retardation	—	20%	80%	—

*Prior to widespread application of early amniocentesis, based on 3000 consecutive cases.

effects of inherited genetic morbidity or mortality.

References

1. Campbell AV. Ethical issues in prenatal diagnosis. Br Med J 1984;288:1633–1634.
2. Hook EB. Rates of chromosome abnormalities at different maternal ages. Obstet Gynecol 1981;58:282–285.
3. Hook EB, Cross PK, Jackson L, Pergament E, Brambati B. Maternal age-specific rates of 47 +21 and other cytogenetic abnormalities diagnosed in the first trimester of pregnancy in chorionic villus biopsy specimens: comparison with rates expected from observations at amniocentesis. Am J Hum Genet 1988;42:797–807.
4. Hook EB, Cross PK. Maternal age-specific rates of chromosome abnormalities at chorionic villus study: a revision. Am J Hum Genet 1989;45:474–477.
5. Romero R, Gianluigi P, Jeanty P, Ghidini A, Hobbins JC. Prenatal diagnosis of congenital anomalies. Connecticut: Appleton & Lange, 1988:p137–138.
6. Wilson RD, Morrison MG, Wittmann BK, Coleman GU. Clinical follow-up of fetal

urinary tract anomalies diagnosed prenatally by ultrasound. Fetal Ther 1988;3:141–151.

7. Edwards MJ, Graham JM. Posterior nuchal cystic hygroma. In: Graham JM, ed. Clinics in perinatology. Philadelphia: WB Saunders, 1990;17(3):611–640.

8. Mayer T, Black R, Matlak ME, et al. Gastroschisis and omphalocele. An eight year review. Ann Surg 1980;192:783–788.

9. Hauge M, Bugge M, Nielsen J. Early prenatal diagnosis of omphalocele constitutes indication for amniocentesis. Lancet 1983;2:507.

10. Nivelon-Chevallier A, Mavel A, Michiels R, et al. Familial Beckwith-Wiedemann syndrome: prenatal echography diagnosis and histologic confirmation. J Genet Hum 1983;5:397–399.

11. Mann L, Ferguson-Smith MA, Desai M, Gibson AM, Raine PAM. Prenatal assessment of anterior abdominal wall defects and their prognosis. Prenat Diagn 1984;4:427–435.

12. Crawford DC, Chapman MG, Allan LD. Echocardiography in the investigation of anterior abdominal wall defects in the fetus. Br J Obstet Gynaecol 1985;92:1034–1036.

13. Greenwood RD, Rosenthal A, Nadas AS. Cardiovascular abnormalities associated with congenital diaphragmatic hernia. Pediatrics 1976;57:92–97.

14. David TJ, Illingworth CA. Diaphragmatic hernia in the southwest of England. J Med Genet 1976;13:253–262.

15. Boles ET, Anderson G. Diaphragmatic hernia in the newborn: mortality, complications, and long-term follow-up observations. In: Kiesewetter WB, ed. Long-term follow-up in congenital anomalies. Proceedings of the Pediatric Surgical Symposium. Pittsburgh: Pediatric Surgical Society, 1989:13–22.

16. Hansen J, James S, Burrington J, Whitfield J. The decreasing incidence of pneumothorax and improving survival of infants with congenital diaphragmatic hernia. J Pediatr Surg 1984;19:385–388.

17. Harrison MR, Golbus MS, Filly RA. The unborn patient. Prenatal diagnosis and treatment. Florida: Grune & Stratton, 1984:257–275.

18. Weaver DD. Catalog of prenatally diagnosed conditions. Baltimore: The Johns Hopkins University Press, 1989.

19. National Institute of Child Health and Human Development, National Registry for Amniocentesis Study Group. Midtrimester amniocentesis for prenatal diagnosis: safety and accuracy. JAMA 1976;236:1471–1476.

20. Simpson N, Dallaire L, Miller J, Siminovitch L, Hamerton J. Prenatal diagnosis of genetic disease in Canada: report of a collaborative study. Can Med Assoc J 1976;115:739–745.

21. Hunter AGW, Thompson D, Speevak M. Midtrimester genetic amniocentesis in Eastern Ontario: a review from 1970 to 1985. J Med Genet 1987;24:335–343.

22. Murken JA, Stengel-Rutkowski S, Schwinger E. In: Enke F, ed. Prenatal diagnosis proceedings, 3rd European conference on prenatal diagnosis of genetic disorders. Stuttgart: Third European Conference on Prenatal Diagnosis of Genetic Disorders 1979;132.

23. Hess LW, Anderson RL, Golbus MS. Significance of opaque discolored amniotic fluid at second-trimester amniocentesis. Obstet Gynecol 1986;67:44–46.

24. Firth HV, Boyd PA, Chamberlain P, MacKenzie IZ, Lindebaum RH, Huson SM. Severe limb abnormalities after chorion villus sampling at 56–66 days' gestation. The Lancet 1991;337:762–763.

25. Mahoney MJ. Limb abnormalities and chorionic villus sampling. The Lancet, 1991;337:1422–1423.

26. Jackson LG, Wapner RJ, Brambati B. Limb abnormalities and chorionic villus sampling. The Lancet, 1991;337:1423.

27. Miny P, Holzgreve W, Horst J, Lenz W. Limb abnormalities and chorionic villus sampling. The Lancet, 1991;337:1423–1424.

28. Firth HV, Boyd PA, Chamberlain P, MacKenzie IZ, Lindenbaum RH, Huson SM. Limb abnormalities and chorion villus sampling. The Lancet, 1991;338:51.

29. MRC Working Party on the Evaluation of Chorion Villus Sampling. Medical Research

Council European trial of chorion villus sampling. The Lancet 1991;337:1491–1499.
30. Anonymous. Chorion villus sampling: valuable addition or dangerous alternative? (Editorial) The Lancet, 1991;337:1513–1515.
31. Hanson F, Zorn E, Tennant F, et al. Amniocentesis before 15 weeks' gestation: outcome, risks, and technical problems. Am J Obstet Gynecol 1987;156(6):1524–1531.
32. Miller W, Davies R, Thayer B, Peakman D, Harding K, et al. Success, safety and accuracy of early amniocentesis (EA). Am J Hum Genet 1987;41:835.
33. Sandstrum M, Stryker JM, Frigoletto FD, Morton CC. Early amniocentesis for chromosome analysis: a preliminary experience. Am J Hum Genet 1987;41(3):847.
34. Godmilow L, Weiner S, and Dunn L. Genetic amniocentesis performed between 12 and 14 weeks gestation. Am J Hum Genet 1987;41:818.
35. Johnson A, Godmilow L. Genetic amniocentesis at 14 weeks or less. Clinical Obstet Gynecol 1988;31(2):345–351.
36. Benacerraf B, Greene M, Saltzman B, Barss V, et al. Early amniocentesis for prenatal cytogenetic evaluation. Radiology 1988;169:709–710.
37. Rooney DE, MacLachlan N, Smith J, et al. Early amniocentesis: a cytogenetic evaluation. Br Med J 1989;299:25–26.
38. Elejalde BR, de Elejalde M, Acuna J, Thelen D, Trujillo C, Karrmann M. Prospective study of amniocentesis performed between weeks 9 and 16 of gestation: its feasibility, risks, complications and use of early genetic prenatal diagnosis. Am J Med Gen 1990;35:188–196.
39. Evans MI, Drugan A, Koppitch C, et al. Genetic diagnosis in the first trimester: the norm for the 1990s. Am J Obstet Gynecol 1989;160:1332–1339.
40. Hanson F, Happ R, Tennant F, et al. Ultrasonography-guided early amniocentesis in singleton pregnancies. Am J Obstet Gynecol 1990;162(6):1376–1383.
41. Lindner C, Huneke B, Masson D, Schlofeldt T, Kerber S, Held KR. Fruhzeitige am-

niozentese zur zytogenetischen diagnostik. Geburtsh u Frauenheilk 1990;50:954–958.
42. Nevin J, Nevin N, Dornan J, Sim D, Armstrong M. Early amniocentesis: experience of 222 consecutive patients, 1987–1988. Prenat Diagn 1990;10:79–83.
43. Penso CA, Sandstrom MM, Garber MF, Ladoulis M, Stryker JM, Benacerraf BB. Early amniocentesis: report of 407 cases with neonatal follow-up. Obstet Gynecol 1990;76:1032–1036.
44. Stripparo L, Buscaglia M, Longatti L, et al. Genetic amniocentesis: 505 cases performed before the sixteenth week of gestation. Prenat Diagn 1990;10:359–364.
45. Byrne D, Marks K, Azar G, Nicolaides K. Randomized study of early amniocentesis versus chorionic villus sampling: a technical and cytogenetic comparison of 650 patients. Ultrasound Obstet Gynecol I 1991;235–240.
46. Rebello MT, Gray CTH, Rooney DE, et al. Cytogenetic studies of amniotic fluid taken before the 15th week of pregnancy for earlier prenatal diagnosis: a report of 114 consecutive cases. Prenat Diagn 1991;11:35–40.
47. Hackett GA, Smith JH, Rebello CTH. Early amniocentesis at 11–14 weeks' gestation for the diagnosis of fetal chromosomal abnormality—a clinical evaluation. Prenat Diagn 1991;11:311–315.
48. Liu CC, Lo FJ, Ho SC, Yang-Feng TL. Early amniocentesis: complemented with in situ amniocyte culture method. Am J Hum Genet (supp) 1991(4);49:1212.
49. Nevin J, Nevin NC, Dornan JC, Fogarty P, Armstrong MJ. Early amniocentesis: clinical and cytogenetic evaluation of 500 cases. Am J Hum Genet (supp) 1991(4);49:1232.
50. Shulman LP, Elias S, Simpson JL. Early amniocentesis: complications in initial 150 cases compared to complications in initial 150 cases of transabdominal chorionic villus sampling. Am J Hum Genet (supp) 1991(4);49:1262.
51. Sato M, Witt D. Early amniocentesis: prospective follow-up of 604 cases. Am J Hum Genet (supp) 1991(4);49:1252.

52. Canadian Collaborative CVS-Amniocentesis Clinical Trial Group. Multicenter randomized clinical trial of chorion villus sampling and amniocentesis. The Lancet 1989;1:1–7.

53. Klapp KH, Nicolaides KH, Hager HD, Voigtlander T, Greiner J, Tariverdian G, Lehmann WD. Untersuchungen zur fruhen Amniozentese. Geburtsh u Frauenheilk 1990;50:443–446.

54. Wilson RD, Kendrick V, Wittmann BK, McGillivray BC. Risk of spontaneous abortion in ultrasonically normal pregnancies. The Lancet 1984;2:920–921.

55. Gilmore DH, McNay MB. Spontaneous fetal loss rate in early pregnancy. The Lancet 1985;1:107.

56. Cashner KA, Christopher CR, Dysert GA. Spontaneous fetal loss after demonstration of a live fetus in the first trimester. Obstet Gynecol 1987;70:827–830.

57. Spencer JW, Cox DN. A comparison of chorionic villi sampling and amniocentesis: acceptability of procedure and maternal attachment to pregnancy. Obstet Gynecol 1988;72:714–718.

58. Kalousek DK, Dill FJ, Pantzar T, McGillivray BC, Yong SL, Wilson RD. Confined chorionic mosaicism in prenatal diagnosis. Hum Genet 1987;77:163–167.

59. Ledbetter DH, Martin AO, Verlinsky Y, et al. Cytogenetic results of chorionic villus sampling: high success rate and diagnostic accuracy in the United States collaborative study. Am J Obstet Gynecol 1990;162:495–501.

60. Wilson RD, Cho K, McGillivray B, Kalousek D, Shaw D, Baldwin V. Chorionic villus sampling: analysis of fetal losses to delivery, placental pathology, and cervical microbiology. Prenat Diagn 1991;11:539–550.

61. Hobbins JC, Grannum PA, Romero R, Reece EA, Mahoney JM. Percutaneous umbilical blood sampling. Am J Obstet Gynecol 1985;152:1–6.

62. Daffos MD, Capella-Pavlovsky MD, Forestier F. Fetal blood sampling during pregnancy with use of a needle guided by ultrasound: a study of 606 consecutive cases. Am J Obstet Gynecol 1985; 153:655–660.

63. Nicolaides KH, Rodeck CH, Soothill PW, Campbell S. Ultrasound-guided sampling of umbilical cord and placental blood to assess fetal well-being. Lancet 1986; 1:1065–1067.

64. Takagi K, Tanaka H, Nishijima S, et al. Fetal blood values by percutaneous umbilical blood sampling. Fetal Therapy 1989;4:152–160.

65. Forestier F. Some aspects of fetal biology. Fetal Therapy 1987;2:181–187.

66. Soothill PW, Nicolaides KH, Rodeck CH, Campbell S. Effect of gestational age on fetal and intervillous blood gas and acid-base values in human pregnancy. Fetal Therapy 1986;1:168–175.

67. Weiner CP, Williamson RA. Evaluation of severe growth retardation using cordocentesis—hematologic and metabolic alterations by etiology. Obstet Gynecol 1989; 73(2):225–229.

68. Nicolaides KH, Economides DL, Soothill MD. Blood gases, pH and lactate in appropriate- and small-for-gestational-age fetuses. Am J Obstet Gynecol 1989;161: 996–1001.

69. Mibashan RS, Rodeck CH, Thumpston JK et al. Prenatal plasma assay of fetal factors VIII and IX. Br J Haematol 1979; 41:611–612.

70. Millar DS, Davis LR, Rodeck CH, Nicolaides KH, Mibashan RS. Normal blood cells values in the early mid-trimester fetus. Prenat Diagn 1985;5:367–373.

71. Fisk NM, Fracog YT, Santolaya J, Nicolini U, Letsky EA, Rodeck CH. Fetal macrocystosis in association with chromosomal abnormalities. Obstet Gynecol 1989;74:611–616.

72. Economides DL, Nicolaides KH, Gahl WA, Bernardini I, Bottoms S, Evans M. Cordocentesis in the diagnosis of intrauterine starvation. Am J Obstet Gynecol 1989; 161:1004–1008.

73. Nicolini U, Hubinont C, Santolaya J, Fisk NM, Coe AM, Rodeck CH. Maternal fetal glucose gradient in normal pregnancies and in pregnancies complicated by alloimmu-

nization and fetal growth retardation. Am J Obstet Gynecol 1989;151:924–927.

74. Nicolaides KH, Rodeck CH, Gosden CM: Rapid karyotyping in nonlethal fetal malformations. Lancet 1986;1:283–286.

75. Basaran S, Miny P, Pawlowitzki IH, Horst J, Holzgreve W. Rapid karyotyping for prenatal diagnosis in the second and third trimester of pregnancy. Prenat Diagn 1988;8:315–320.

76. Wright DJ, Brindley BA, Koppitch FC, Drugan A, Johnson MP, Evans MI. Interpretation of chorionic villus sampling laboratory results is just as reliable as amniocentesis. Obstet Gynecol 1989;74:739–740.

77. Soothill PW, Nicolaides KH, Bilardo K, Hackett GA, Campbell S. Uteroplacental blood velocity resistance index and umbilical venous pO², pCO², pH, lactate and erythroblast count in growth-retarded fetuses. Fetal Ther 1986;1:176–179.

78. Bilardo CM, Nicolaides KH. Cordocentesis in the assessment of the small-for-gestational age fetus. Fetal Ther 1988;3:24–30.

79. Golbus MS, Cowan MJ: In utero stem cell transplantation. In: Proceedings of the fifth annual congress on early fetal diagnosis: recent progress and public health implications. Prague: Fifth Annual Congress on Early Fetal Diagnosis, 1990:81.

80. Golbus MS, Filly RA, Callen PW, Glick PL, Harrison MR, Anderson RL. Fetal urinary tract obstruction: management and selection for treatment. Sem Perinat 1985;9:91–97.

81. Harrison MR, Golbus MS, Filly RA. The unborn patient: prenatal diagnosis and treatment. Orlando: Grune & Stratton, Inc., 1984:139–140.

82. Harrison MR, Golbus MS, Filly RA. The unborn patient: prenatal diagnosis and threatment. Orlando: Grune & Stratton, Inc., 1984:125–126.

83. Wilson RD, Hall JG. Prenatal detection of connective tissue disorders. In: Milunsky A, ed. Genetic disorders and the fetus—diagnosis, prevention, and treatment. 2nd ed. New York: Plenum Press, 1986;710–711.

84. Harrison MR, Golbus MS, Filly RA. The unborn patient: prenatal diagnosis and treatment. Orlando: Grune & Stratton Inc, 1984:125–140.

CHORIONIC VILLUS SAMPLING: INTRODUCTION AND TECHNIQUES

2

J. M. JOHNSON

Prenatal diagnosis of genetic disease in the midtrimester of pregnancy by amniocentesis is a well-established technique that combines the benefits of high diagnostic accuracy with low risks to the mother and fetus (1,2,3). By virtue of its record of safety and accuracy, midtrimester amniocentesis has become the standard against which all other prenatal diagnostic methods are compared. Despite its many positive aspects, however, amniocentesis has several recognized drawbacks. The most significant of these is that the results of genetic analysis are not usually available until the 18–20th week of gestation. This may create a tre- mendous psychological burden for couples in whom selective abortion is indicated. In addition, second-trimester abortion is associated with a higher incidence of maternal medical complications. Accordingly, there has been strong impetus to develop a method of first-trimester prenatal diagnosis.

Chorionic villus sampling (CVS) is a relatively new method of prenatal diagnosis in which tissue for genetic analysis is aspirated from the chorion frondosum under ultrasound guidance. In less than five years of widespread use, CVS has rapidly emerged as a first-trimester alternative to amniocentesis. The principal advantage of CVS compared to amniocentesis is the earlier availability of results, permitting a safer and less psychologically traumatic termination procedure if an abnormality is detected. The advantages and disadvantages of CVS versus amniocentesis are described in Table 2-1. It is important to note that CVS is not a substitute for amniocentesis in the prenatal detection of neural tube defects. Maternal serum alphafetoprotein (AFP) screening is generally advocated at 15–18 weeks of pregnancy following CVS for this purpose. Note also that since anatomy cannot be visualized

Table 2-1 Advantages and Disadvantages of First Trimester Chorionic Villus Sampling vs Second Trimester Amniocentesis

Chorionic Villus Sampling	Amniocentesis
Results available prior to 14 weeks gestation	Results not available until 18–20th week of gestation
Results can be obtained from direct analysis	Most diagnoses require cultured cells
Risks of miscarriage and late fetal loss slightly higher than amniocentesis (1–2%)	Risks well established. Fetal loss rate <0.5%
Cannot diagnose neural tube defects	Amniotic fluid alpha-fetoprotein and acetylcholinesterase possible
Too early to visualize much fetal anatomy	Fetal anatomy sonographically visualized
Chromosomal mosaicism seen more often	Mosaicism is less frequent problem
Laboratory analyses still being established	Laboratory analyses well established
Preferred procedure for diagnosis requiring DNA analysis	Maybe better for cytogenetic abnormalities, such as Fragile-x, breakage syndromes, or structural rearrangements

with certainty in the first trimester, a detailed ultrasound is recommended at 18 weeks gestation to provide reassurance of fetal structural normality in all patients who undergo CVS.

HISTORICAL PERSPECTIVES

The modern era of prenatal diagnosis was introduced in 1952 by Bevus with his report of the technique of amniocentesis (4). In 1961, Liley was the first to demonstrate the utility of amniocentesis in assessing the severity of erythroblastosis indirectly by determining the amount of bilirubin in amniotic fluid in patients sensitized to the Rh factor (5). In 1966, it became clear that fetal cells obtained from amniotic fluid could be cultured and karyotyped (6). This finding stimulated further investigation towards offering second-trimester amniocentesis to women at significant risk for fetal chromosomal abnormalities.

At approximately the same time, Hahnemann et al., reported successful sampling of fetal chorionic villi in the first trimester using a transvaginal hysteroscope (7). His preliminary work was followed by reports from other Scandinavian investigators of techniques for sampling extraembryonic tissue, but the approach was abandoned in favor of amniocentesis because of a high frequency of short-term complications (8).

In the early 1970s, Chinese investigators began performing blind aspirations of chorionic villus material in the first trimester for the purpose of fetal sex prediction. Their report in the *Chinese Medical Journal* in 1975 was the first to describe CVS in a large group of women (n=100) with continuing pregnancies (9). They achieved a relatively high success rate (94%) with a remarkably low spontaneous abortion rate (6%). Because the procedure was done for sex selection and this practice was discontinued, CVS did not receive significant attention until 1982, when a report by Kazy et al. described its benefits for genetic diagnosis and emphasized the role of ultrasound guidance in successful sampling (10).

A series of articles from other investigators quickly followed, establishing the feasibility of CVS for cytogenetic, biochemical, and molecular prenatal diagnosis (11,12,13). In 1985, Brambati and coworkers in Milan, Italy reported a technique for rapid laboratory analysis of uncultured villi, by which a case of Trisomy 21 was diagnosed at 11 weeks gestation five hours after CVS (14). This report spurred intensive efforts by investigators around the world towards further evaluation of the method. The Milan group were also the first to recognize the problem of maternal cell contamination in villus cultures and were able to minimize the problem using careful initial tissue dissection. Since then, CVS has developed rapidly, and enough experience has now been gained to delineate its safety, accuracy, and reliability.

FIRST TRIMESTER DEVELOPMENT

A complete understanding of CVS is not possible without an appreciation of normal intrauterine anatomy and first-trimester development. In the preimplantation stage, the blastocyst consists of an inner cell mass and an outer layer of enveloping cells. The embryo proper is believed to be derived from a small number of cells of the inner cell mass, while the remaining cells form the amnion, allantois, and yolk sac (15). The cells from blastocyst wall develop into the trophoblast, which then differentiates into the chorion and placenta.

With implantation, chorionic villus projections invade the maternal decidua, extending outward from the gestational sac and completely enveloping it as a delicate fringe. By the sixth menstrual week of gestation, the villi opposite the side of implantation have begun to degenerate.

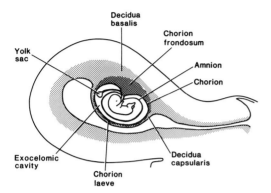

Figure 2-1A Intrauterine anatomy at approximately 10 weeks gestation.

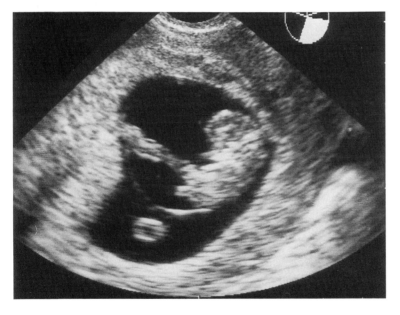

Figure 2-1B Transvaginal ultrasound picture of an embryo at 9.6 weeks gestation. The umbilical cord can be seen inserting into the echogenic chorion.

As the gestational sac enlarges, these villi are removed from the maternal blood supply leaving the underlying chorionic membrane denuded, which is called the smooth chorion or chorion laeve (Figure 2-1A). The chorion laeve's covering layer of decidua (decidua capsularis) eventually abuts the decidua on the opposite uterine wall. In contrast, villi along the site of implantation rapidly proliferate into the maternal decidua and uterine wall. A soft thickened area of villi, 1.0–1.5 cm in thickness, is present by the ninth week of gestation. This is the *chorion frondosum*, which eventually develops into the placenta and can be visualized as an area of increased echogenicity on ultrasound (Figure 2-1B). The chorion frondosum is the opti-

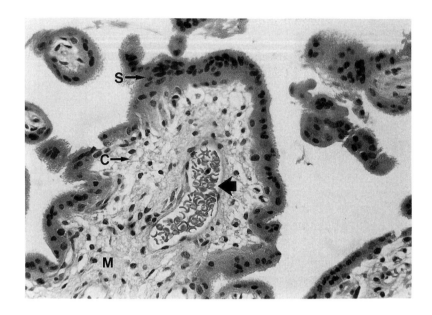

Figure 2-2 Histologic cross-section of first trimester chorionic villi. The arrow shows a villous capillary with a nucleated red blood cell. (S=syncytiotrophoblast, C=cytotrophoblast, M=mesenchymal core) Courtesy of Dr. Susan Ritchie. Department of Pathology University of Toronto.

mal site for obtaining a chorionic villus sample for prenatal diagnosis. Because the chorionic villi have the same genetic constitution as the fetus, samples of this tissue should reflect the chromosomal, biochemical, and DNA status of the fetus. Only a small amount of villi are required for most diagnoses (10–20 mg), which represents less than 1% of the villi destined to become the functioning placenta.

Microscopically, chorionic villi consist of a central mesenchymal core covered by a trophoblastic epithelium. The epithelium has two layers, an inner cytotrophoblast that is single-celled and a peripheral syncytiotrophoblast that is multinucleated (Figure 2-2). Whereas cytotrophoblast cells undergo mitosis, the nuclei of the syncytiotrophoblast do not(16). The mesenchymal core is composed of loose stromal tissue in a connective tissue matrix. Villus capillaries containing fetal blood course through the center (Figure 2-2). Direct chromosomal analysis using chorionic villi is possible because of the spontaneously dividing cells present in the cytotrophoblast layer. Cultured preparations, which yield improved chromosome morphology, can be obtained by culturing the mesenchymal core.

INDICATIONS FOR CVS

The most common indication for offering CVS is late maternal age (≥80%), which is defined as ≥35 years of age at the time of delivery. The remaining indications are described in Table 2-2. CVS is also useful for rapid karyotyping in cases of ultrasound-identified fetal abnormalities diagnosed af-

Table 2-2 Indications for Chorionic Villus Sampling

1. **Late Maternal Age (≥ 35 Years)**
2. **Previous Trisomic Offspring**
3. **Parental Chromosome Rearrangement**
4. **X-linked Recessive Disorders**
5. **Mendelian Disorders**

ter 18 weeks gestation when fetal blood sampling is either not possible or unavailable. In these cases, the procedure would be performed by the transabdominal route.

Since chorionic villi are an excellent source of fetal DNA, CVS has become the main technique for prenatal diagnosis by DNA analysis (17). Increasing numbers of genes are being cloned and probes developed to diagnose diseases by this technology. DNA analysis is now available for hemoglobinopathies (sickle cell disease, alpha-thalassemia, most beta-thalassemias) and for most families with hemophilias (A and B), Duchenne muscular dystrophy, and cystic fibrosis (17). Minute amounts of DNA, theoretically even from a single cell, can be analyzed by replicating the genetic material using the polymerase chain reaction, and it can be expected that this methodology will be increasingly used in the future (18). It is even now possible to diagnose rubella infection in the first trimester by detecting rubella antigen or ribonucleic acid sequences in chorionic villi using monoclonal antibodies or a cloned complementary DNA probe (19).

Many inborn errors of metabolism can be identified by CVS if the deficient enzyme is expressed in the villi; it is usually in much the same range as in cultured amniocytes. The villi can be assayed directly to give the result within a day, except in a few conditions in which culture is required. However, certain difficulties have been encountered and specific precautions are necessary to ensure reliable results. For example, there may be discrepancies in enzyme expression between direct assays of chorionic villi, cultured chorionic villi, and cultured amniotic fluid cells. The activity of alpha-L-iduronidase is quite low in direct assays, but greatly increased in cultured villi (20). The opposite finding is seen in glycogen storage disease *type II*, in which alpha-glucosidase activity is much higher in fresh tissue. For other disorders, the presence of naturally occurring isoenzymes may make the diagnosis difficult. An example is the high level of arylsulfatase C in trophoblasts, which makes the diagnosis of meta-chromatic leukodystrophy (deficiency of arylsulfatase A) difficult (20). Thus, the reliability of CVS in the diagnosis of metabolic disorders depends on obtaining sufficient tissue free of maternal cell contamination, understanding the expression of the enzyme in question, and using amniocentesis for confirmation of all enzymatic diagnosis in which experience with CVS is limited.

TECHNIQUES OF CHORIONIC VILLUS SAMPLING

Several techniques have been described for performing CVS, but only two methods are currently in widespread use. These include the transcervical catheter aspiration technique (transcervical CVS, or TC-CVS) and the transabdominal needle aspiration technique (transabdominal CVS, or TA-CVS). At present, more than 80% of CVS worldwide is performed via the transcervical route; however, transabdominal CVS is gaining increased popularity.

Transcervical Chorionic Villus Sampling

Transcervical CVS is usually performed between nine and 12 weeks of gestation.

Figure 2-3 Prototype chorionic villus sampling catheter manufactured by Portex Ltd. (Hythe, Kent, England CT216JL)

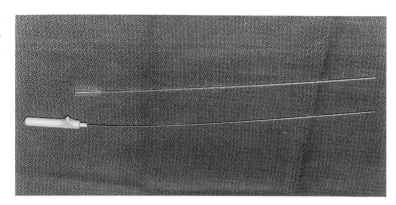

Prior to the procedure, a real-time ultrasound examination determines the viability and gestational age of the fetus and the location of the chorion frondosum. The patient is then placed in the lithotomy position, a speculum is inserted, and the cervix and vagina are cleansed with an antiseptic solution. A number of different transcervical catheters are available, all of which contain a malleable metal obturator that may be preformed to negotiate the cervicouterine angle and the pathway of intended biopsy site. The Portex catheter, which may be considered a prototype for CVS catheters, consists of a 1.45-mm (16-gauge) polyethylene catheter with a 1-mm malleable stainless steel stylet (Figure 2-3).

Under ultrasound guidance, the catheter is passed through the cervix and placed within the villi of the chorion frondosum (Figure 2-4A,B). The metal obturator is removed and a 20-cc syringe containing medium is attached to the catheter. Negative suction is applied to the syringe with simultaneous "to and fro" movements of the catheter. The catheter is then withdrawn under continuous negative suction and the sample examined immediately under a dissection microscope. Villi have a distinctive frond-like appearance with bud-like projections, and blood vessels can usually be seen coursing along their surface

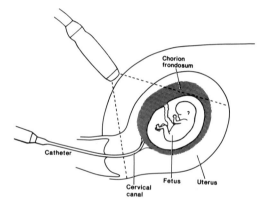

Figure 2-4A Schematic diagram of transcervical chorionic villus sampling.

(Figure 2-5). If the amount of chorionic villi is determined to be inadequate for diagnostic purposes, the procedure is repeated. A fresh sterile catheter is used for each additional pass in order to minimize the risk of intrauterine infection. In general, no more than three passes are attempted, and the fetal heart rate (FHR), sac configuration, and appearance of the chorion frondosum are visualized carefully after each pass. The only discomfort reported by most patients is the pressure of the ultrasound transducer on the full bladder and the placement of the tenaculum on the cervix, if one is used. Vaginal spotting is common following transcervical procedures but usually

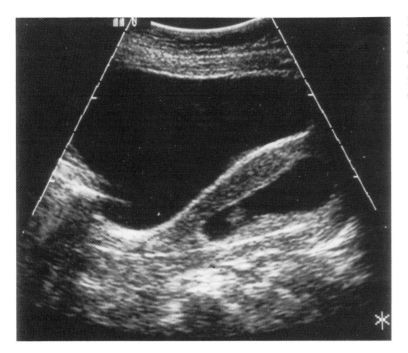

Figure 2-4B Ultrasound picture of transcervical chorionic villus sampling. The echogenic catheter is visualized within the chorion frondosum.

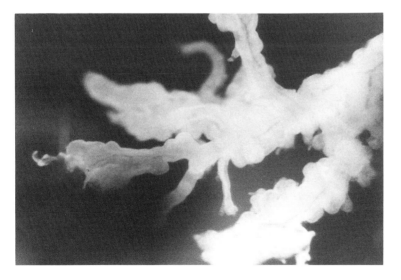

Figure 2-5 Chorionic villi as they appear under the dissection microscope (10 ×). Note the blood vessels coursing along the surface of the villi and the distinctive bud-like projections.

subsides within three days. Patients are advised to avoid strenuous activity and intercourse until all vaginal spotting has ceased. Should a flu-like syndrome develop within the first week after the procedure, patients are asked to report immediately because it may indicate an intrauterine infection.

Transabdominal Chorionic Villus Sampling

In this technique, as with transcervical CVS, an ultrasound examination is first performed to determine fetal viability, gestational age, and location of the chorion frondosum. The abdomen is then draped and prepped in a fashion similar to that for an amniocentesis. An 18- or 20-gauge needle is inserted through the maternal abdomen and uterine wall, and guided into the chorion frondosum using ultrasound (Figure 2-6A). A 20-cc syringe is attached to the needle and negative suction is applied to the syringe while simultaneously moving the needle tip back and forth within the chorion to sample several sites. The ultrasound transducer is manipulated so as to maintain the tip of the needle under visualization at all times (Figure 2-6B). If an insufficient sample is obtained (<10 mg tissue), then a new needle is reinserted. We favor

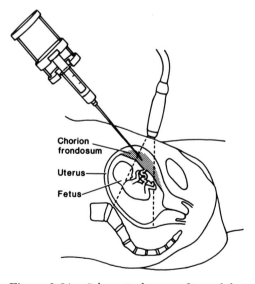

Figure 2-6A Schematic diagram of transabdominal chorionic villus sampling. An aspirating device attached to the syringe facilitates negative suction. (Cameco syringe holder, Precision Dynamics, San Fernando, CA)

this "freehand" technique because of its flexibility and the ability to adjust the needle pathway. An aspirating device attached to the syringe (Figure 2-6A) facilitates negative suction and permits better control of the needle tip. An alternative approach is to employ a needle-guiding device attached to the transducer with a double needle system, as described by Smidt-Jensen et al. (21). In this system, an 18-gauge guide needle with a 21-gauge aspiration needle is used. This offers the advantage that multiple aspirations can be performed through the guide needle. Most real time machines are equipped with an on-screen template of the needle track that can be used to target the sampling site if this approach is utilized.

At our institution, the selection of the route of CVS (transcervical or transabdominal) is at the discretion of the operator and depends on a number of factors. These include the location of the chorion, the position of the uterus and bladder, and the presence of uterine or cervical abnormalities. For example, in patients with posterior, low-lying placentas, we favor the transcervical route, whereas for patients with anterior or high-posterior fundal placentas, we favor the transabdominal approach. The maternal bladder plays a critical role in facilitating both procedures. A full bladder, for example, will help to straighten the cervicouterine angle in a patient with an anteverted uterus, facilitating passage of a transcervical catheter. On the other hand, emptying the bladder to varying degrees may increase the anteversion of the uterus, thereby allowing access to a posterior or fundal placenta by the transabdominal route. It should be noted that in some patients, emptying the bladder may allow loops of bowel to become superimposed between the uterus and anterior abdominal wall. This compromises the ultrasound

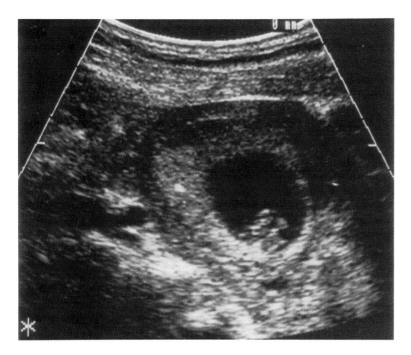

Figure 2-6B Ultrasound picture of transabdominal CVS. The needle tip is visible with the chorion frondosum.

visualization, and may preclude access to the placenta by the transabdominal route. In this circumstance, we would allow the bladder to fill again and attempt the procedure transcervically.

The presence of uterine or cervical abnormalities may also influence the route of CVS. Cervical stenosis, low-lying myomata, or cervical polyps may preclude transcervical sampling, but not necessarily transabdominal sampling. Conversely, if myomata of the anterior uterine wall were present, transcervical CVS may be preferable. Overall, we feel the two procedures are complementary and that having both available enhances a woman's overall chance of successful sampling. This is supported by our own data, where we achieved an overall rate of successful sampling of 97% using both procedures compared to 93% (p<0.05) when only the transcervical route was offered (22).

A third approach, the *transforniceal approach*, has also been described and may have a role in select cases. In this technique, a 20-gauge needle is inserted through the posterior fornix and uterine wall and into the chorion frondosum under transabdominal ultrasound guidance. We have performed this approach successfully in patients with extremely retroverted uteri and posterior placentas in whom access by conventional routes was not possible.

RELATIVE AND ABSOLUTE CONTRAINDICATIONS TO CVS

A complete obstetric and gynecologic history should always be obtained on patients prior to undergoing chorionic villus sampling. Any history of operative procedures, particularly involving the cervix, or of uterine fibroids, pelvic infection, or any problems, such as bleeding,

Table 2-3 Contraindications to Chorionic Villus Sampling

Absolute Contraindications	Relative Contraindications
Presence of intrauter-ine device	Abnormal sono-graphic evaluation
Active bleeding	Uterine myomata (de-pending on posi-tion)*
Cervical stenosis*	Previous operation on the cervix*
Untreated endocer-vicitis or pelvic inflammatory dis-ease*	Maternal coagu-lopathy
Active genital herpes simplex*	? Presence of blighted ovum (vanishing twin)

*Transabdominal technique may be utilized.

during the present pregnancy should be elicited. Any cervical or vaginal infections should be investigated and treated prior to sampling. The absolute and relative contraindications to CVS are described in Table 2-3.

An abnormal ultrasound appearance of either the embryo or gestational sac may indicate an impending spontaneous abortion warranting postponement or cancellation of the CVS procedure, with re-evaluation of the pregnancy in 7–10 days, depending on the findings.

Uterine contractions are frequently visualized sonographically in early gestation and have a similar appearance to fibroids. As they may pose a mechanical barrier to transcervical or transabdominal CVS, it is advisable to postpone the procedure for a short period until the uterine wall has relaxed.

Bleeding in the first trimester of pregnancy is a relative contraindication to CVS. As these patients are at increased risk of spontaneous abortion, they should be counselled as such. Signs of placental abruption or retroplacental hematoma should be looked for sonographically. Such findings may warrant postponement or cancellation of the procedure. If there is active bleeding at the time of the scheduled procedure, a similar decision should be made, particularly if the cervix is open. In cases where the cervix is closed, the bleeding has been slight, and there is no bleeding or ultrasound abnormalities noted at the time of the procedure, CVS may be performed.

The presence of an intrauterine device should be considered an absolute contraindication to CVS because of the increased risk of developing intrauterine infection with a foreign body in the uterus.

If there is cervical stenosis for any reason, transcervical procedures may be traumatic to the endocervical canal, which may increase the risk for endocervicitis and miscarriage. In these cases, transabdominal CVS should be considered.

In cases where the mother is Rh-sensitized, and the fetus must be Rh-positive because the father is homozygous, CVS may be contraindicated. There is an increased risk of accelerating the maternal antibody response through transfer of fetal erythrocytes with CVS. The chorion frondosum is very well vascularized from both the fetal and maternal standpoint. Capillary vessels containing fetal blood cells run through each healthy villus. These villus projections are surrounded by the maternal lacunae, which are miniature reservoirs of maternal blood. Theoretically, disruption of the villus branches may cause spillage of fetal red blood cells from the capillaries into the maternal lacunae. With an Rh-negative woman and an Rh-positive fetus, sensitization may occur. This concern is supported by studies that show a rise in the concentration of maternal serum alphafetoprotein (MSAFP) in patients following chorionic villus sampling (24). If this rise represents fetal blood traversing the intervillus space, then sensitization is possible. In a study by Warren et al., 49% of 161 patients showed a significant rise in MSAFP after transcervical aspiration (25). The magnitude of the rise correlated with the number of attempts at biopsy. These and other authors advocate that all Rh-negative women should be given Rh immunoglobulin following CVS (23–25).

A history of cervical incompetence or DES-exposure does not appear to be a contraindication to CVS. In fact, CVS may be a desirable option in these patients as it allows the chromosomal status of the fetus to be determined prior to placement of cervical cerclage.

CHORIONIC VILLUS SAMPLING AND TWIN GESTATION

The discovery of twins at the time of any prenatal diagnostic procedure calls for specific counselling prior to performing the procedure. As the risks of finding an affected fetus as well as the risks associated with the procedure are altered as the number of gestations increases, the couple may require additional time to consider their options in the light of this new information. The option of selective termination should the fetuses be discordant for a genetic disorder should be discussed. Selective termination appears to be reasonably safe at gestations applicable to reporting of CVS results (i.e. <16 weeks), with retention of the pregnancy and no maternal problems in the majority. Of special consideration

with regard to CVS is that patients need to understand the risk of diagnostic error from a mixed or unrepresentative sample and that monozygotic twins cannot necessarily be distinguished from having sampled only one chorion frondosum. Many centers continue to offer midtrimester fetal blood sampling to confirm or clarify abnormal results from twin CVS.

Chorionic villus sampling in multiple pregnancy requires that separate samples of villi from each gestational sac be obtained. If a well-defined, separate chorion frondosum can be identified for each fetus, the approach is relatively straightforward. The tissue can be obtained by either two transcervical passes of the catheter or a combined transcervical and transabdominal approach. If the placentas are fused, there is an increased risk of obtaining a mixed sample. Brambati and colleagues have suggested that such patients should not undergo CVS unless separate umbilical cord insertions can be identified sonographically (26). TA-CVS may be necessary to ensure precise villus sampling near the cord insertion of one or both fetuses. In addition, the couple should be counselled regarding these risks prior to performing the procedure.

If the cytogenetic results indicate the fetal sex is discordant, then it is likely that each gestational sac has been sampled. When the results are concordant for fetal sex, there are three possibilities: 1) that the twins are dizygotic and of the same sex, 2) that they are monozygotic, or 3) that the villi sampled represent only one gestational sac. Cytogenetic or DNA polymorphism may be helpful to distinguish those that are dizygotic, but distinguishing monozygotic twins from a sampling deficiency cannot always be be done.

A final consideration is that of the "vanishing twin" phenomenon, thought to occur in approximately 2.8% of all pregnancies (27). If a blighted ovum is suspected or diagnosed sonographically along with a viable twin, special care must be taken to avoid the chorion frondosum surrounding the nonviable sac. Since chorionic villi belonging to the blighted sac may remain viable for sometime after the demise of the embryo, the patient should be counselled that one cannot rule out the possibility of cross-contamination from the dead twin. Because of this potential complication, consideration should be given to offering the patient amniocentesis.

The *fetal loss rate* associated with CVS in twin gestation has been evaluated by Wapner et al. in a group of 158 pregnancies involving 316 fetuses (28). The total fetal loss rate, based on the number of fetuses, was 6.8%, which is significantly grater than that reported with singletons. In this group, there was ony one case in which fetal sex was erroneously assigned, with no other apparent diagnostic errors.

RISKS OF CHORIONIC VILLUS SAMPLING

Procedure-related risks of CVS include fetal loss, threatened abortion, intrauterine infection, perforation of the amniotic sac, and unexplained mid-trimester oligohydramnios. The potential impact of CVS on subsequent fetal growth and development is also of concern since the procedure is performed during a time frame that includes embryogenesis.

Fetal Loss with Transcervical CVS

The *fetal loss rate* associated with transcervical CVS has been evaluated in several large series, and a figure of 3.3% (range 1.9%–5.2%) is quoted based on the outcome of over 12,000 cases from five centers (30). This figure, however, should be weighed in relation to the background loss rate at the gestation at which the procedure is performed and the age distribution of the patients. The only randomized comparison between CVS and amniocentesis that is available at present is the Canadian Collaborative CVS and Amniocentesis Trial (31). In this study, patients eligible for prenatal diagnosis because of late maternal age were randomized to either CVS (9–12 weeks gestation) or amniocentesis (15–17 weeks). There were 89/1169 (7.6%) total losses (spontaneous, induced abortions and late losses) in the CVS group and 82/1174 (7%) in the amniocentesis group for an excess of 0.6% for those women undergoing CVS (NS) (30). This data is consistent with that reported in the National Institute of Health Collaborative Trial in the United States, which evaluated the safety and accuracy of CVS in 2,278 women compared with 671 who underwent amniocentesis (31). Both groups were recruited in the first trimester, however were not randomized. The rate of fetal loss was 7.2% in the CVS patients and 5.7% in the amniocentesis patients. After adjustments for differences in gestational and maternal age, the total loss rate for women in the CVS group exceeded that of the amniocentesis group by 0.8% (31). Thus, although we cannot be certain by how much CVS increases fetal loss rates above some natural background rate, we can be confident that the difference in loss rates between CVS and amniocentesis is not statistically significant. The *timing of fetal losses* was similar in both the amniocentesis and CVS patients, with most occurring before 20 weeks (30,31). In the Canadian study, however, a shift towards later losses was noted in the CVS group, where a perinatal mortality rate of 1.3% was reported, compared with 0.6% in the amniocentesis patients

(NS) (31). The greatest imbalance in the frequency of stillbirths was after 28 weeks, when there were six in the CVS group and only one in the amniocentesis group. No factors have been identified to explain these late losses, which may have been an incidental finding since similar trends have not been observed in other studies (29,31). No differences in perinatal morbidity were noted, with mean birthweights, incidence of small for gestational age infants, and proportion of preterm births being similar in both groups.

A potential drawback of these collaborative studies is that CVS was a new technique at the time they were conducted, and significant variability existed in operator experience as well as in procedure and laboratory techniques. Since that time, considerable expertise has been gained in the method, reducing the impact of these variables. At our institution, CVS has been offered as a clinical service since the completion of the Canadian Collaborative Trial, with consistent, experienced operators and laboratory personnel. Review of our experience over a recent 16-month period revealed a total fetal loss rate of 9.2% (51 of 554) (22). This is slightly higher than the fetal loss rate in the Canadian trial (7.6%, NS), which can be explained by the fact that our data included indications other than late maternal age in 24% of cases. This placed the group at higher risk of having an abnormal result, accounting for the higher induced abortion rate (6.4% vs 2.2% in the Canadian trial) (22,30). Excluding these induced abortions, the fetal loss rate (including spontaneous abortions, stillbirths, and neonatal deaths) was 2.7% compared to 5.4% in the Canadian trial (22,30). This spontaneous loss rate is lower than the expected background loss rate because terminations following the diagnosis of an abnormality has likely removed some of the cases from the CVS group that were destined to abort spontaneously. The data indicate, however, that CVS is associated with acceptably low fetal loss rates. The mean procedure to fetal loss interval was 28 days (range seven–57) in the patients who had spontaneous abortions prior to 20 weeks (n=7), and 72 days for the three patients (0.5%) who had a fetal loss beyond 20 weeks (22).

Fetal Loss with Transabdominal CVS

Although experience with transabdominal CVS is less, preliminary data suggest fetal loss rates are not in excess of those with transcervical CVS, and may, in fact, be lower. Data from the International CVS Registry shows an observed fetal loss rate with transabdominal CVS in over 4,000 cases of 2.3% compared with 3.5% in women who underwent transcervical CVS (29). This data is confirmed by the largest randomized study comparing transabdominal and transcervical CVS published to date, by Brambati et al. (32), who report a total fetal loss rate of 3.3% and 3.9% with transabdominal and transcervical CVS respectively. The preliminary results of the U.S. National Institute of Health Collaborative Trial comparing transabdominal and transcervical CVS also show no significant difference in fetal loss rates between the two procedures (33). The experience with transabdominal CVS at our institution is consistent with these studies (34). There were fewer large samples obtained with transabdominal CVS; however, there were no significant differences in the incidence of samples less than 10 mg, which is considered sufficient for diagnostic purposes in the vast majority of cases. In our own series, the mean sample size was significantly smaller with transabdominal CVS (15.3 mg versus 21.2 mg for transcervical CVS); however, there was no difference in the rate of successful culture or in the obtaining of a result. Transabdominal CVS was consistently associated with a lower rate of immediate complications, with less than 5% experiencing bleeding and/or spotting compared to as high as 25% with transcervical CVS.

These data indicate that transabdominal CVS is a safe and useful alternative to transcervical CVS. The main *advantages* of the procedure include a slightly lower fetal loss rate and a much reduced incidence of immediate complications such as bleeding. This is likely because the fine-gauge needle used with transabdominal CVS causes less placental trauma than the relatively large-bore transcervical catheter. For this reason, transabdominal CVS can be performed safely from approximately nine weeks gestation to term, unlike transcervical CVS, which has a fairly narrow window of optimal safety (between nine and 13 weeks). Transabdominal CVS also appears to be associated with a shorter operator/learning period, particularly for those individuals previously trained in ultrasound-guided needle insertion techniques, e.g., amniocentesis. There also appears to be a lower incidence of maternal cell contamination with transabdominal CVS, possibly reflecting the "cleaner" samples obtained TA-CVS (34).

The disadvantage of transabdominal CVS is that inserting a needle into the uterus in early gestation appears to be associated with significantly greater maternal discomfort than passing a catheter through the cervix (36). A study evaluating patient acceptance of CVS has shown, however, that this factor does not appear to adversely influence patient acceptance of the method, which was found to be equal among patients undergoing transabdominal and TC-CVS (35).

The only randomized study comparing TA-CVS, TC-CVS, and amniocentesis was recently published by a group of Danish investigators (36). In this study, a total of 3,347 women were randomized to either TA-CVS, TC-CVS, or amniocentesis. Excluding induced abortions and preprocedure losses, the total fetal loss rate was 2.4% for TA-CVS, 6.8% for TC-CVS, and 1.8% for amniocentesis patients (36), suggesting that the fetal loss rate with TA-CVS was not significantly different from amniocentesis. However, in their hands, there was a major difference between TA- and TC-CVS (36). In addition, the incidence of failed transcervical samplings was 3.2% versus 1.9% for the transabdominal patients in their series, and significantly more transcervical patients (5.4%) were changed to transabdominal sampling because of an a priori evaluation of sampling obstacles than vice versa (1%). The group concluded that when choosing a prenatal diagnostic procedure, the choice must be between TA-CVS and amniocentesis if risk is considered the criterion. These particular data, however, likely reflect the experience and bias of the operators, as similar conclusions have not been reached by others (32,34).

Other Risks with CVS

The risk of *intrauterine infection* following CVS potentially poses a serious threat to both the mother and the fetus. In the largest series reported of CVS, the incidence of infection ranged from 0.2–0.5%, and all occurred following transcervical procedures (29). The clinical presentation most commonly consisted of a flu-syndrome occurring within hours to several days following the procedure. The clinical course tended to be insidious, with days to weeks elapsing before patients suddenly developed high fevers with the signs of septic abortion. Appropriate therapy consists of antibiotic coverage for both aerobes and anaerobes followed by uterine evacuation. There have been two case reports of septic shock following CVS; in one case, recovery did not occur until a complete abdominal hysterectomy and bilateral salpingo-oophorectomy was performed (37,38). One case of maternal peritonitis has been reported by Brambati et al. following transabdominal CVS, presumably related to needle perforation of the bowel (22). Otherwise, intrauterine or other infections have not been reported with transabdominal CVS.

Preventive measures against intrauterine infection include adherence to strict aseptic technique and use of a fresh sterile catheter whenever more than one pass is required for transcervical aspiration. Patients with documented vaginitis or cervicitis should be treated prior to the procedure and consideration should be given to the transabdominal approach. Patients and their physicians must be alerted to the symptoms associated with intrauterine infection and ensure extremely close follow-up should a flu-like syndrome develop.

Spontaneous rupture of the membranes during the procedure or thereafter is also a rare event, occurring less than 0.5% of the time (29). The vast majority of cases will result in a spontaneous abortion. There have also been several reports of midtrimester *oligohydramnios* (16–20 weeks) in patients who have had CVS (20,26,29,39). Almost all had a history of persistent vaginal spotting or wetness after the procedure (20). While the etiology of this is uncertain, it is possible that damage of the membranes may occur if the catheter is advanced too close to the gestational sac, traumatizing the membrane and leading to later loss of fluid. Introduction of vaginal organisms may also play a role in damage to the membranes. There have been no reports of an increased incidence of *congenital abnormalities* associated with CVS in any of the large collaborative trials (26,29–34,36). Special mention is needed regarding recent reports of limb abnormalities.

CVS and Limb Abnormalities

In 1991, Firth et al. (40) reported a cluster of babies with severe limb abnormalities born to women who had undergone transabdominal CVS between 56–66 days of gestation. These included four cases of oromandibular limb hypogenesis syndrome and one case of a terminal transverse limb reduction defect in a series of 289 patients (1.7%). The spectrum of anomalies present in these five cases was less consistent with abnormal morphogenesis than with *incomplete* morphogenesis, in which an insult, e.g., vascular insult, disrupts the development of a normal embryo. Furthermore, they all occurred within a fairly narrow gestational range (days 56–66). All were performed by the transabdominal route, sample sizes varied from three to 50 mg, and the karyotype was normal in all cases (40).

As a result of this publication, many institutions (including our own) made a policy to avoid transabdominal CVS prior to 66 days of gestation (8.6 weeks).

Subsequent to this publication, a flurry of letters and articles appeared in the literature both supporting and refuting this association.

In terms of the large collaborative trial data, subsequent analysis (from the European Collaborative Trial, the Canadian Collaborative Trial, and the NIH Trial in the United States) did not support this association. However, 100% ascertainment of cases could not be guaranteed. In addition, several other reports have also not supported this association. Dolk et al. published an article in *The Lancet* in 1992 concerning this possible association (41). They conducted an investigation in seven European

Registration of Congenital Abnormalities and Twins (EUROCAT) Registries, which included more than 600,000 births. They compared cases of limb reduction abnormalities to cases of other anomalies reported, with regard to respective exposure rates for CVS. There were 336 cases of limb reduction of which four (1.2%) had CVS exposure. There were 11,883 cases of other congenital anomalies identified, 78 (0.66%) of which had CVS exposure, giving an odds ratio of 1.8 (95% confidence intervals 0.66–4.99). This increase was not statistically significant, the confidence intervals being wide. Their conclusion was that the EUROCAT data do not give any evidence of a risk associated with early or late CVS, although the wide confidence intervals around the odds ratio suggest a limited power of the study. They suggest that if there is a risk as high as that cited in Firth et al., it must be associated with either a specific procedure or exposure timings, which are infrequent in these EUROCAT Registry areas (41).

Jackson et al. reported in the *CVS Newsletter* in 1991 the results of over 78,000 CVS procedures, both transabdominal and transcervical (42). There were 28 distal limb defects, which was not above the expected incidence (approximately one in 2,000). Again, they report they could not be assured of 100% ascertainment.

Mahoney reviewed 9,588 pregnancies, both transabdominal and transcervical, 10% of which were performed prior to 66 days of gestation (44). They had no cases of oromandibular limb hypogenesis syndrome. There were seven limb reduction defects, again not above the expected incidence (44).

A more recent publication by Burton et al. reported 436 CVS procedures performed between January 1989 and November 1990 (45). Of 391 liveborn infants, there were four transverse limb reduction defects, which is similar to the incidence reported by Firth et al. In their cluster, three of the procedures were performed transcervically and one transabdominally. As a consequence of their experience, they have discontinued offering CVS.

Recently, an NIH consensus panel with representation from Europe, the United States, and Canada met to discuss the issue. Although the official report is not yet available, the statement will recommend that prenatal diagnosis programs offering CVS should advise women about this possible association. They state that while the expected incidence of transverse limb reduction defects is in the range of one in 2,000 in the general population, the incidence in women undergoing CVS may be one in 1000.

Due to incomplete ascertainment and the fact this is likely a spectrum of anomalies ranging from perhaps stippled nails to frank transverse limb reduction, prospective studies are needed to confirm or refute this association. The experience by Firth et al. of the oromandibular limb hypogenesis syndrome has not been repeated by other centers. It appears that the most common abnormality is a transverse limb reduction. The possible mechanism with CVS might be that of an ischemic insult with interruption of embryonic blood supply resulting in peripheral limb reduction defects.

We recommend that each center define its own policy concerning this problem. Patients should be given the information so they can make an informed decision about whether to proceed with CVS. In addition, centers should be aware of the possible association of these anomalies with the gestational age at which the test is performed, the experience of the operator, and the method, e.g., transabdominal or transcervical. Consideration should be given to withholding

CVS prior to 10 weeks gestation for the transabdominal route and 9.6 weeks gestation for transcervical CVS.

ACCURACY OF CVS

While CVS is considered an accurate and reliable method of prenatal diagnosis, incorrect diagnoses have been reported (46–49). The most common sources of diagnostic error include maternal cell contamination and confined placental mosaicism. A review of villus morphology and CVS laboratory techniques is required to understand these problems. As described previously, chorionic villi consist of three major components: 1) an outer layer of hormonally active, invasive syncytiotrophoblast, 2) a middle layer of cytotrophoblast from which the syncytiotrophoblast is derived, and 3) an inner mesodermal core containing blood capillaries for oxygen and nutrient exchange (Figure 2-2). After collection, the chorionic villi are exposed to trypsin to digest and separate the cytotrophoblast and underlying mesodermal core. The cytotrophoblast has a high mitotic index, with many spontaneous mitoses available for immediate chromosome analysis. The liquid suspension is dropped onto slides and used for the direct chromosome preparation. The remaining villus core is placed in culture and is typically ready for harvest and chromosome analysis within six to 12 days.

Maternal Cell Contamination

Chorionic villus samples typically consist of a mixture of placental villi and maternal decidual cells and blood. Although specimens are thoroughly washed and dissected under the microscope following collection, some maternal cells may remain and grow in culture, resulting in maternal cell contamination. This type of error is likely to go unnoticed if the fetus is female. If the fetus is male or a female with an abnormal karyotype, however, a mosaic karyotype will result from the admixture of normal fetal cells. Early investigators estimated the rate of maternal contamination in CVS to be as high as 27% based on discrepant results in which the fetus was known to be a male (48). At present, careful dissection and the use of enzymatic digestion of the chorionic villi cells prior to tissue culture has reduced the incidence to 1–2% (49). Maternal cell contamination is seen almost exclusively in villus cultures. The problem is not seen in direct chromosome preparations because in contrast to cytotrophoblasts, maternal decidua has a low mitotic index. Spontaneous maternal mitoses are, therefore, a rare occurrence. The phenomenon is also rare in amniocentesis (0.3%) (46). This is because amniocentesis is associated with very little trauma to maternal tissues, and sampling is performed within the amniotic sac.

The diagnosis of maternal cell contamination is based on the finding of discordant results between the direct and cultured preparations, with the culture showing a female karyotype. In these cases, amniocentesis and ultrasound should be offered to the patient to clarify the results. The use of chromosome polymorphisms may also be of use in distinguishing maternal cell contamination from the rare instances of true XX/XY mosaicism or chimerism.

Confined Placental Mosaicism

The second major source of diagnostic error associated with CVS is confined placental mosaicism (CPM), the result of nondisjunction occurring during embryogenesis, leading to the presence of aneuploid cells in the extraembryonic tissues that are not present in the fetus itself (50). The most common type of CPM in CVS specimens involves abnormalities in the direct preparation with normal results in the long-term culture and in the fetus. This type of abnormality results from a postzygotic non-disjunctional event occurring in the trophoblast cell line. Because the vast majority of cells in the developing blastula are trophoblasts, it is not surprising that this type of event is the most frequently seen. Usually in this situation, the long-term culture and fetus will be normal so that analysis based on a direct preparation alone will give a *false-positive* (falsely abnormal) result. If the postzygotic nondisjunctional event were to occur in the cells of the inner cell mass that will migrate into the villi and contribute to the extraembryonic structures, then the long-term culture would contain abnormal cells, whereas the direct preparation and fetus would be normal. This is a very rare occurrence (48). The finding of mosaicism in both the direct and long-term culture with a normal fetal karyotype is also a rare event. This type of discrepancy would be explained by a nondisjunctional event occurring early in fetal development, giving rise to a mixture of abnormal cells in both the extraembryonic and trophoblastic cell lines, but sparing the embryonic cell line. Another possible explanation is that of selection against the abnormal aneuploid cell line in the fetus leading to their eventual loss with weaker selective pressures in the extraembryonic tissue allowing for persistence of the abnormal cell line (49). Finally, there have been a few (one per 1,000) *false-negative results* in which none of the abnormal cells present in the fetus were observed at CVS (50–52). Most of these reports, however, occurred when only a direct preparation was done.

The overall incidence of chromosomal mosaicism reported in CVS samples ranges from 0% to 4.4%, with the average being 1.1% (one per 100 samples) (49). This is four times the frequency of mosaicism recorded for amniocentesis, and ten times greater than the level of mosaicism observed in newborn surveys (53,54), indicating that most mosaicism in CVS is unrelated to the fetal karyotype (49). Indeed, mosaicism detected at CVS is rarely confirmed in the fetus (2.3 per 1,000 CVS), so other explanations, particularly pseudomosaicism and CPM, are more likely (49). Since the highest levels of mosaicism are reported with the direct preparation, this eliminates the possibility of pseudomosaicism. Confirmation of mosaicism in the placenta, however, occurs at a fairly high rate (71%) (49). Thus, it would appear that CPM is responsible for the majority of mosaic results in CVS. The phenomenon of confined placental mosaicism emphasizes the advantages of analyzing chromosomes in both direct preparations and cultured cells in CVS and the potential hazards of limiting analysis of one cell lineage.

The frequent occurrence of equivocal cytogenetic results from CVS, because of mosaicism, can present difficulties in genetic counselling. The following *guidelines* are, therefore, recommended. When mosaic results are reported in the direct preparation, the patient should be advised to wait for the long term culture results. If the culture results are normal, CPM should be suspected and the couple can be advised to continue the pregnancy. If the culture reveals mosaicism, further testing, such as amniocentesis or fetal blood sampling, is warranted, particularly when the abnormality involves chromosomes associated with a potentially viable, but abnormal fetus, e.g., 18,13,21 or sex chromosomes). Detailed ultrasound examinations may also provide information on the status of these fetuses. If the pregnancies continue to term, it is helpful to examine the placenta both anatomically and cytogenetically for evidence of a resorbed twin or confined placental mosaicism.

The relationship of confined placental mosaicism and fetal outcome remains to be determined. Initially, investigators reported an association between CPM and adverse perinatal outcome, including a higher incidence of intrauterine growth retardation, fetal demise and perinatal morbidity (55). It was hypothesized that this association was due to altered placental function in fetal development caused by the presence of abnormal cells in the placenta. However, more recent reviews have different conclusions. Vejerslev and Mikkelsen have reviewed over 11,000 cases of CVS and found mosaicism confined to the placenta in 99 cases (56). The spontaneous abortion rate in patients with CPM was not statistically different from that reported by the central CVS Registry (29,56). In another study, follow-up of 124 cases of confined placental mosaicism in which the pregnancies were allowed to continue failed to demonstrate any association with small for gestational age infants (57). Schreck et al. also report no increased incidence of perinatal morbidity or mortality in a group of 18 patients with CPM compared to 91 control patients (49).

Because of the frequency of chromosomal mosaicism in CVS and its attendant need for further testing, e.g., amniocentesis, fetal blood sampling, a discussion of mosaicism should be included in counselling prior to CVS. The higher frequency of discrepant results in direct CVS preparations also emphasizes the prudence of delaying decision-making until results of CVS culture have been obtained. Although the observation of mosaicism clearly complicates genetic counselling, it does not appear to be associated with adverse fetal outcome (50).

PATIENT ACCEPTANCE OF CVS

Since patient attitudes and acceptance of diagnostic procedures play an important role in determining the extent of their use, the importance of evaluating these factors is evident. A recent study conducted through the prenatal diagnosis clinic at the University of Toronto evaluated 253 consecutive women (101 CVS, 152 amniocentesis) to determine their attitudes towards and their acceptance of their prenatal diagnostic experience (35). The results showed that the women seeking prenatal diagnosis tended to be highly educated (65% with one or more year of post-secondary education) with planned pregnancies (78%) living as married couples (88% married) (35). For the women who chose CVS, the most important factors influencing their decision was the shorter waiting period for results and the method of termination. Their doctors' recommendation of CVS and the increased privacy associated with early testing were also important factors. For the women who chose amniocentesis, no single factor was identified as the most important, but physician advice and lack of knowledge concerning the availability of CVS were the most important of the factors identified. Both amniocentesis and CVS patients found the procedure to be less uncomfortable than they had anticipated. This was determined on the basis of a pain scale that the patients filled out immediately before and after the procedure, where 0 was the least painful and 10 was the most painful. The principal causes of procedure discomfort were the insertion of the needle and the removal of the sample for amniocentesis and the pressure of the ultrasound transducer on the bladder for CVS. Factors such as position on the table, exposure of the genitals, and abdominal preparation were not significant causes of procedural discomfort. Of the three procedures, TA-CVS was the most uncomfortable, followed by amniocentesis, and transcervical CVS was associated with the least discomfort. Overall, patient acceptance and satisfaction was highest when they felt they were adequately counselled prior to the procedure, well-informed during the procedure and provided with follow-up advice afterwards (these included patients with abnormal results). It was also determined that in patients undergoing prenatal diagnosis, maternal fetal bonding increases significantly once the rest results are known and that this increase occurs at least five weeks earlier for CVS patients than for amniocentesis patients (59).

FUTURE DIRECTIONS

The introduction of CVS has had a major impact in the field of prenatal diagnosis. It has been shown to be a reasonably safe and reliable technique with widespread applications and a high degree of acceptance among women undergoing the procedure. Despite these advantages, CVS has several limitations. These include a slightly higher fetal loss rate than with amniocentesis and a higher incidence of equivocal results, e.g., mosaicism, requiring clarification through further testing. Because of the need for both direct and long-term cultures to achieve optimal diagnostic accuracy, CVS is a very labor-intensive and costly procedure. This has resulted in limited availability of CVS, which tends to be confined to tertiary level centers. For these reasons, there has been increased impetus to develop a new alternative to both CVS and amniocentesis, namely early amniocentesis.

Early amniocentesis (EA) is defined as an amniocentesis performed prior to 15 weeks gestation. EA may be considered an alterna-tive to midtrimester amniocentesis for patients who want earlier testing but who present too late for CVS, who do not wish to have the additional risks with CVS or to whom CVS is not available. It is also a useful alternative to midtrimester amniocentesis for earlier clarification of equivocal CVS results. Although there are fewer cells in the amniotic fluid in early gestation, there appears to be a higher percentage of viable cells, and cytogenetic analysis does not appear to be a problem (58).

Early studies found that amniocentesis prior to 16 weeks was associated with a higher incidence of failure to obtain fluid, repeat taps or bloody taps, and a higher incidence of culture failures (1,59). Since that time, major advances in ultrasound technology and improved laboratory methodologies have made early amniocentesis a feasible alternative. Preliminary current data are encouraging, with total fetal loss rate of approximately 2% (range 0–4.6%) (58,60–62), slightly higher than midtrimester amniocentesis, but less than that of CVS.

SUMMARY

In summary, CVS has become a well-established tool in the armamentarium of the obstetrician involved in prenatal diagnosis. Although research in prenatal diagnosis continues to focus on ways to provide earlier testing with faster results, it is unlikely that safe techniques for obtaining tissue earlier than nine weeks with CVS will be developed. This is especially true in light of the recent data suggesting an increased incidence of congenital anomalies with invasive testing prior to this time (40). While CVS has proved useful for cytogenetic, biochemical, and DNA diagnosis, unfortunately, it has not achieved its initial promise of providing rapid and reliable cytogenetic diagnosis. Because of the lower incidence of mosaicism in amniocentesis culture, the trend of the future may be towards offering early amniocentesis for cytogenetic diagnosis, reserving CVS for those disorders requiring biochemical or DNA analysis. With continued advances in DNA technology, however, in particular polymerase chain reaction (PCR), and in situ hybridization techniques, it may be possible to obtain accurate, same day results from prenatal diagnosis specimens, either amniotic fluid or CVS without the need for culture. These exciting new possibilities will provide even more alternatives in the area of prenatal diagnosis in the future.

References

1. Canadian Medical Research Council 1977. Diagnosis of genetic disease by amniocentesis. No. 5. Supply Services, Ottawa, Canada, 1977.
2. National Institute of Health and Development Amniocentesis Registry. The safety and accuracy of mid-trimester amniocentesis. U.S. Department of Health, Education and Welfare, 1978; No. 78-190.
3. Medical Research Council 1978. An assessment of the hazards of amniocentesis. Br J Obstet Gynaecol 1978 (Suppl. 2); 85:.
4. Bevus DCA. The antenatal prediction of hemolytic disease of the newborn. The Lancet 1952;i:395–398.
5. Liley AW. Liquor amnii analysis in the management of the pregnancy complicated by Rhesus sensitization. Am J Obstet Gynecol, 1961;82:1359–1370.
6. Steel NW, Bragg WR. Chromosome analysis of human amniotic fluid cells. The Lancet 1966;i:383.
7. Hahnemann N, Mohr J. Antenatal fetal diagnosis in the embryo by means of biopsy from extraembryonic membranes. Bull Eur Soc Hum Genet 1968;2:23–29.
8. Kullander S, Sandahl B. Fetal chromosome analysis after transcervical placental biopsies during early pregnancy. Acta Obstet Gynecol Scand 1973;52:355–359.
9. Tiatung Hospital of Anshan Steel Works Department of Obstetrics and Gynecology. Fetal sex prediction by sex chromatin of chorionic villi cells during early pregnancy. Chin Med J 1975;1:117–126.
10. Kazy Z, Rozovsky IS, Bakharev VA. Chorion biopsy in early pregnancy: a method of early prenatal diagnosis for inherited disorders. Prenat Diagn 1982;2:39–45.
11. Niazi M, Coleman DV, Loeffler FE. Trophoblast sampling in early pregnancy: culture of rapidly dividing cells from immature placental villi. Br J Obstet Gynaecol 1981;88:1081–1085.
12. Williamson R, Esdall J, Coleman DV, et al. Direct gene analysis of chorionic villi; a possible technique for first trimester antenatal diagnosis of hemoglobinopathies. The Lancet 1981;2:1125–1127.
13. Old JN, Ward RHT, Karagozlu F, et al. First trimester fetal diagnosis for hemoglobinopothies: three cases. The Lancet 1982; 2:1413–1419.
14. Brambati B, Simoni G. Fetal diagnosis of trisomy 21 in the first trimester of pregnancy. The Lancet 1983;1:586.
15. Markert CL, Petters RM. Manufactured hexaparental mice show that adults are derived from three embryonic cells. Science 1978;202:56–58.
16. Watanabe M, Ito Y, Yamamoto M, et al. Origin of mitotic cells of the chorionic villi in direct chromosome analysis. Hum Genet 1978;44:191–193.
17. Williamson R, Eskdale J, Coleman DV, et al. Direct gene analysis of chorionic villi: a possible technique for the first trimester diagnosis of hemoglobinopathies. The Lancet 1981;ii:1125–1127.
18. Shehab FF, Doherty M, Cai S, et al. Detection of sickle cell anemias and thalassemias. Nature 1987;329:293–294.
19. Ho-Terry L, Londesborough P, Rees KR, et al. Diagnosis of fetal rubella infection by

nucleic acid hybridization. J Med Virol 1988; 24:175–178.

20. Hogge WA. Chorionic villus sampling. In: Harrison MR, Golbus MS, Filly RA, eds. The unborn patient: prenatal diagnosis and treatment. 2nd Ed. Philadelphia WB Saunders, 1991;53–57.

21. Smidt-Jensen S, Hahnemann N. Transabdominal fine-needle biopsy from chorionic villi in the first trimester. Prenat Diagn 1984;4:163–169.

22. Scheufler PW, Johnson JM, Beatty RB, et al. Chorionic villus sampling since the Canadian Collaborative Trial: what have we learned? Soc Obstet Gynaecol Can 47th Annual Meeting. Toronto, Canada 1991.

23. Blakemore KJ, Baumgarten A, Shoenfeld-Dimaio N, et al. Rise in maternal serum alpha-fetoprotein concentration following chorionic villus sampling and the possibility of isoimmunization. Am J Obstet Gynecol 1986;155:988–993.

24. Warren RC, Butler J, Morsman JM, McKenzie C, Rodeck CH. Does chorionic villus sampling cause fetomaternal hemorrhage? The Lancet 1985;4:691.

25. Brambati B, Oldrini A. Methods of chorionic villus sampling. In: Brambati B, Simoni G, Fabro S, eds. Chorionic villus sampling; fetal diagnosis of genetic diseases in the first trimester: clinical and biochemical analysis. Vol. 21. New York: Marshall Dekert, 1986:94.

26. Brambati B, Oldrini A, Ferrazzi E, et al. Chorionic villus sampling: an analysis of the obstetric experience of 1,000 cases. Prenat Diagn 1987;7:157–169.

27. Landy HG, Weiner S, Corson SL, et al. The "vanishing twin": ultrasonographic assessment of fetal disappearance in the first trimester. Am J Obstet Gynecol 1986;155:14–19.

28. Wapner RJ, Johnson A, Davis G, Jackson LG. Prenatal diagnosis in multiple pregnancy: a comparison between CVS and amniocentesis. Soc Perinat Obstet 9th Annual Meeting, New Orleans, Louisiana. Am J Obstet Gynecol 1989;146:159.

29. Jackson L. CVS Newsletter. Philadelphia, Jefferson Medical College, 1988 (Feb 1–8).

30. Canadian Collaborative CVS-Amniocentesis Clinical Trial Group. Multi-centered randomized clinical trial of chorionic villus sampling and amniocentesis. First report. The Lancet 1989;i:2–6.

31. National Institute of Child Health and Human Development. Safety and efficacy of chorionic villus sampling for early prenatal diagnosis of cytogenetic abnormalities. N Engl J Med 1989;320:609–617.

32. Brambati B, Manzani A, Tului L. Transabdominal and transcervical chorionic villus sampling: efficacy and risk evaluation of 2,411 cases. Am J Med Genet 1990;35–164.

33. US National Institute of Child Health and Human Development Chorionic Villus Sampling and Amniocentesis Study Group. A randomized comparison of transcervical and transabdominal chorionic villus sampling. N Engl J Med 1992;327:594–598.

34. Scheufler P, Johnson JM, Beatty RB, et al. Transabdominal chorionic villus sampling: successful integration into an existing CVS program. Soc Obstet Gynecol 47th Annual Meeting, Toronto, Canada 1991.

35. Caccia N, Johnson JM, Robinson GE, Barna T. The impact of prenatal testing on maternal-fetal bonding: Chorionic villus sampling vs. amniocentesis. Am J Obstet Gynecol 1991;165:1122–1126.

36. Smidt-Jensen S, Permin M, Philip J. Sampling success and risk by transabdominal chorionic villus sampling, transcervical chorionic villus sampling and amniocentesis: a randomized study. Ultrasound in Obstet Gynecol 1991;1:86–90.

37. Barela AI, Kleinman GE, Golditch IM, et al. Septic shock with renal failure after chorionic villus sampling. Am J Obstet Gynecol 1986;154:1100–1102.

38. Blakemore KJ, Mahoney MJ, Hobbins JC. Infection and chorionic villus sampling. The Lancet 1985;2:339.

39. Turnpenny PD, Hakin MM, Chwites RJ, et al. Oligohydramnios sequence in a liveborn infant following chorionic villus sampling. Prenatal Diagnosis 1990;10:675–676.

40. Firth HV, Boyd PA, Chamberlain P, et al. Severe limb abnormalities after chorionic villus sampling at 56 to 66 days gestation. The Lancet 1991;337:762–763.
41. Dolk H, Bertrand F, Lechat MF. Chorionic villus sampling and limb abnormalities. The Lancet 1992;339:876–877.
42. Jackson L, et al. CVS Newsletter, 1991.
43. Mahoney MJ. Limb abnormalities and chorionic villus sampling. Lancet 1991;337: 1422–1423.
44. Froster UG, Baird PA. Limb-reduction defects and chorionic villus sampling. The Lancet 1992;339:66.
45. Burton BK, Schulz CJ, Burd LI. Limb anomalies associated with chorionic villus sampling. Obstet Gynecol 1992;79:726–730.
46. Martin AO, Simpson JL, Rosinsky BJ, Allias, S. Chorionic villus sampling and continuing pregnancies II: cytogenetic reliability. Am J Obstet Gynecol 1986;154: 1353–1362.
47. Hsu LYF. Prenatal diagnosis of chromosome abnormalities. In: Milunsky A, ed. Genetic disorders and the fetus. New York: Plenum Press, 1986:169–170.
48. Cheung SW, Crane JP, Beaver AJ, et al. Chromosome mosaicism and maternal cell contamination in chorionic villi. Prenat Diagn 1987;7:535–542.
49. Schreck RR, Falik-Borenstein Z, Hirata G. Chromosomal mosaicism in chorionic villus sampling. Clinics in Perinatology 1990; 17:867–888.
50. Eichenbaum SZ, Krumins EJ, Fortune DW, et al. False-negative findings on chorionic villus sampling. The Lancet 1986;2: 391–392.
51. Linton G, Lilford RJ. False-negative findings on chorionic villus sampling. The Lancet 1986;2:630.
52. Martin AO, Alias S, Rosinsky B, et al. False-negative finding on chorionic villus sampling. The Lancet 1986;2:391.
53. Hamerton JL, Canning N, Ray N, et al. The cytogenetic survey of 14,069 newborn infants. Clin Genet 1975;8:223–243.
54. Jacobs PA, Melville N, Ratcliffe S. A cytogenetic survey of 11,680 newborn infants. Amn Hum Genet 1974;37:359–376.
55. Kalousek DK. The role of confined chromosomal mosaicism in placental function and human development. Growth 1988;54:1–8.
56. Vejerslev LO, Mikkelsen M. The European collaborative study on mosaicism in chorionic villus sampling: data from 1986 to 1987. Prenat Diagn 1989;9:575–588.
57. Schwinger E, Seidl E, Klink F, et al. Chromosomal mosaicism of the placenta—a cause of developmental failure of the fetus? Prenat Diagn 1989;9:639–647.
58. Hanson FW, Florn EM, Tennant FR, et al. Amniocentesis before 15 weeks gestation: outcome, risks and technical problems. Am J Obstet Gynecol 1987; 156:1524.
59. National Institute of Health and Development Amniocentesis Registry. The safety and accuracy of mid-trimester amniocentesis. U.S. Department of Health, Education and Welfare, 1978; No. 78-190.
60. Elejalde B, de Elejalde M, Acuna J, et al. Prospective study of amniocentesis performed between weeks 9 and 16 of gestation: its feasibility, risks, complications and use in early genetic prenatal diagnosis. Am J Med Genet 1990;35:188–196.
61. Golbus MS, Loughman WD, Epstein CJ. Prenatal genetic diagnosis in 3,000 amniocenteses. N Engl J Med 1979;300:157–163.
62. Benacerraf B, Greene M, Satzman B, et al. Early amniocentesis for prenatal cytogenetic evaluation. Radiology 1988;169:709–710.

CORDOCENTESIS: CLINICAL CONSIDERATIONS

3

FRANK A. MANNING

The advances in assessment and care of the human fetus have been dramatic in recent years. The introduction of chronic invasive monitoring in the experimental animal fetus opened the way to an understanding of the complexities and marvel of human fetal development. The advent of ultrasound imaging methods made it possible to extend the animal data to the human. The remarkable and constant improvements in imaging methods, moving from initial crude composite bistable images to the now sophisticated contemporary methods of dynamic imaging in grey scale, Doppler shift analysis, color flow mapping, and in the immediate future, three-dimensional imaging, have made it possible to collect structural and functional information with great precision and detail. The practicing perinatologist can now "see" the fetal patient as clearly, indeed, often more clearly, than is possible in the neonate. Until recently, what was lacking in perinatal medicine was the ability to augment this rich source of physical data on the fetus with details regarding its intrinsic chemistry. In many ways, this limitation defined the dividing line between fetal and neonatal medicine. In the past decade, this limitation has gradually disappeared since it has become possible to obtain fetal blood for analysis.

The first attempts at obtaining fetal blood in the human were based on direct visualization of fetal vessels using a modified pediatric cystoscope (1). This fetoscopy approach was modified and refined by others (2,3). However, the technique was severely limited since it was of considerable technical difficulty and was associated with a fetal loss rate of as high as 5% (2). As a result, the application of fetoscopic fetal blood sampling never became widespread nor generally accepted as a useful clinical method. The overt limitations common to fetoscopy

were circumvented abruptly and dramatically with the introduction of ultrasound-guided percutaneous fetal blood sampling (referred to interchangeably as PUBS or cordocentesis). It was the innovative approach of Daffos et al. by which fetal blood was sampled from the placental insertion of the umbilical vein via a needle guided by dynamic ultrasound from the maternal abdomen that marked the true potential of this means of fetal assessment (4). Unlike the previous fetoscopic approach, the technique reported by Daffos was shown to be relatively safe and could be done with relative technical ease. As a result, the method of PUBS has now become a standard in the armamentarium of fetal evaluation and risk assessment. The clinical application of PUBS is now widespread, having moved out from the select academic centers to become used in day to day clinical practice. Concurrently, the scope of applications for the method has also broadened and continues to increase. In the present day, the applications of PUBS now mirror the use of blood sampling in the extrauterine patient, being a means of both establishing the diagnosis and monitoring of the severity and progression of existing fetal disease. Paradoxically, access to immediate and reliable information regarding fetal hematological, biochemical, and blood gas and acid-base status has confirmed the validity of some aspects of morphological, morphometric, and functional fetal assessment, precluding the need for invasive testing in many instances. Thus, for example, the precision by which the assessment of fetal functional activities predict the presence and severity of fetal hypoxemia and acidemia has been confirmed by direct analysis of cord blood values, and as a result, the role of direct measurement of fetal blood gases and pH has been obviated (5,6,7).

CORDOCENTESIS:
TECHNICAL CONSIDERATIONS

Cordocentesis is a technique by which a needle is guided by ultrasound through the maternal abdomen such that the tip is observed to strike and enter the lumen of a vessel within the umbilical cord thereby permitting access to the fetal circulation and sampling of pure fetal blood. The technique may be applied from as early as 12 weeks gestation but commonly is used at or beyond 18 weeks gestation. The technical aspects of the procedure are best considered by components.

Preprocedural Preparation (Table 3-1)

Cordocentesis is an invasive fetal procedure known to be associated with measurable fetal risk and the remote, but real, risk of maternal morbidity. Accordingly, it is essential to provide the parents with a complete description of the indications for the procedure, the benefits that may accrue to mother and/or fetus from the information obtained, and the potential complications that may occur. It is useful to determine prospectively the management to be taken in the event of a complication. This latter point is of some considerable importance in the use of this procedure for rapid karyotyping of the third-trimester fetus with structural anomaly(ies) and for assessment of the very immature, but potentially viable, growth-retarded fetus. In either instance, it should be determined prospectively whether intervention will occur if a life-threatening fetal complication should arise.

The procedure may be done either in an outpatient setting or in proximity to a delivery suite, the choice depending on fetal age and the planned management should a fetal

Table 3-1 Prerequisites for Cordocentesis

I Logistics

  A) Equipment
   1) Ultrasound Machine

   - high resolution dynamic imaging system
   - transducer selection optional (section, linear, curvilinear)
   - gated pulsed Doppler highly desirable, but not essential
   - color Doppler not essential and not often of clinical value
   - transducer-fixed needle guide optional

   2) Sampling Needles/Syringes

   - a range of variable length 20–22-gauge spiral needles
   - Teflon-coated echo reflective needles optional
   - transponder needle optional
   - 5–10 heparin flushed 1–3 cc plastic syringes
   - 3–5 heparin flushed saline-filled 1 cc plastic syringes

   3) Sample Site Confirmation Method

   - bed-side Singh test available (0.1 M NaOH solution)
   - cell sorter (Coulter counter) optional (not essential)
   - specific red cell antigen anti-sera (for fetuses previously transfused with adult blood)

  B) Personnel

   - at least two operators, one of whom (preferably both) with experience in dynamic ultrasound and needle manipulation
   - some methods rely on a single operator to manipulate both the U/S and the needle, using an assistant to draw the sample. Other methods rely on one operator for ultrasound needle guidance and the other for needle manipulation and sampling
   - a laboratory technician for immediate (bedside) confirmation of sample source

Table 3-1 *Continued*

C) Resources

- suitable outpatient facility for the immature fetus (<26 weeks)
- immediate access to operative/delivery suite for the mature fetus (>26 weeks)
- access to postprocedural fetal heart rate monitoring

II Preoperative Preparation

- informed written consent
- preoperative maternal anxiolytic therapy, e.g., diazepam optional
- preoperative prophylactic antibiotics, e.g., ampicillin/Cloxacillin optional, but highly recommended
- pancuronium should be immediately available (use is optional)
- fresh O negative adult packed RBC should be available

complication occur. The procedure is best done by a team of two working in tandem. There are two common ways of splitting the duties. In one model, both the ultrasound imaging and the needle manipulation are done by one operator and the other's role is to remove the stylet and take the samples once the needle is appropriately placed. In the other model, one member operates the ultrasound to guide the needle while the other manipulates the needle and takes the samples. Neither method has a clear advantage over the other; the method chosen depends on operator experience and preference. The administration of a mild sedative to the mother, e.g., diazepam, is occasionally warranted, but for most patients, preprocedural anxiety is eased by providing a description of the procedure. In particular, it is useful to give the patient some estimate of the expected duration and the probability of success. In the majority of cases, the entire procedure can be accomplished within 10

minutes and the average interval between placement and removal of the needle is less than two minutes. Most patients agree that the discomfort/pain is similar to that of amniocentesis, as a point of comparison in the preprocedure explanation. In experienced hands, a second needle insertion is unusual, occurring less than 3% of the time (8).

The value of antibiotic prophylaxis is uncertain and use is not uniform. In a recent series of 750 procedures by Weiner et al. (9), prophylactic antibiotics were not used. In three cases, postprocedural culture-proven amnionitis occurred (*Staphylococcus epidermidis* in all cases) and was suspected on clinical grounds in two cases. In the Manitoba experience of more than 1000 procedures (10) in which prophylactic antibiotics were used routinely, there have been no cases of either proven or suspected amnionitis. The true value, if any, of antibiotic prophylaxis can only be determined by a prospective randomized trial. When used, the usual choices are either ampicillin alone (500 mg PO about one hour before the procedure, then q8h for two doses) or in combination with cloxacillin in similar dosages.

Immediate transient and complete fetal paralysis can be induced by intravascular injection of pancuronium, the usual dose being 0.2–0.3 mg per Kg estimated fetal weight. Fetal paralysis is frequently required for the longer intravascular transfusion procedures but is almost never necessary for the much shorter diagnostic procedures. Although some groups advocate routine use of fetal paralysis (9) most do not. Given the relatively short time required to take the sample once the needle is in the fetal vessel (usually a matter of 15–30 seconds) the risk of dislodgement by fetal movement is extremely unlikely. In a personal experience in excess of 1000 procedures this complication has only been encountered on two occasions, in both in-

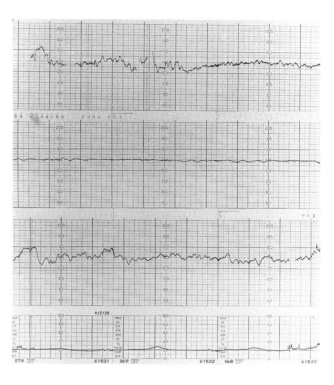

Figure 3-1 Pancuronium effect on fetal heart rate. The upper panel shows normal accelerations and variability in the fetal heart rate of a 34-week fetus. The middle tracing shows a sharply reduced variability, absence of accelerations, modest elevation in baseline heart rate, and the presence of a vaguely sinusoidal pattern. This change in fetal heart rate characteristics, completely reversed within 3 1/2 hours as shown in the bottom panel, is a typical result of paralysis using pancuronium intravenously at doses of 0.1–0.3 mg/kg of estimated fetal weight.

stances with a transamniotic approach to a posterior cord insertion site. If pancuronium is used it is important to advise the patient that fetal movements will not occur until several hours later. Induced fetal paralysis results in a mild tachycardia and a near total loss of heart rate variability or even a sinusoidal-like heart rate pattern (Figure 3-1); these observations should not be interpreted as indicative of fetal compromise.

Procedure Performance (Table 3-2)

Site Selection

The initial step in performing the procedure is target identification. As a general clinical rule, the majority of the time involved in PUBS procedure is spent in identifying the target (the typical time ratio between site selection and the actual needling procedure is about 10/1). The ideal target is a segment of the umbilical vein at a site where it is relatively fixed and, therefore, not liable to move away or turn at contact with the needle. There are three sites where these conditions are met: at or near the insertion of the umbilical vein into the placental substance (Figure 3-2), at the opposite end of the cord, that is at the umbilicus (Figure 3-3), or at the intrahepatic portion of the umbilical vein (Figure 3-4). In practice, the placental insertion is always the preferential target, and attempts at sampling from the intrahepatic portion of the umbilical vein are rare, generally reserved for those cases in which the placental insertion site is either obscured or inaccessible. It is also possible to puncture fetal vessels in a free portion of the cord, although this approach is usually reserved for fetuses in whom access at a fixed site is not judged to be clinically feasible or when visualization

Table 3-2 Cordocentesis: Procedural and
Monitoring Considerations

1) Site Selection
- key step to the procedure
- umbilical vein at the placental insertion site is
  the preferential target
- free loop, intrahepatic umbilical vein and cardiac
  chambers are secondary targets
- confirm depth from maternal abdomen to target
2) Needle Entry/Guidance
- always maintain a perpendicular needle entry to
  maternal abdomen
- U/S guidance may be either by adjacent
  perpendicular or remote tangential method
- the needle tip should be guided to just above the
  target (1-2 mm) then advanced briskly at a
  controlled distance
3) Confirmation/Sample Procedure
- remove stylet and observe needle hub for back
  flow
- apply gentle suction by syringe (excessive
  suction does not help and may compound the
  sampling procedure)
- take the planned sample volume before
  confirmation of position
- give 0.1–0.3 cc saline flush to confirm needle
  position (by ultrasound)
4) Postprocedure Monitoring
  a) Immediate
  - confirm presence or absence of bleeding from
    puncture site
  - record duration of postpuncture bleeding
  - observe fetal heart rate
  - maternal blood sample for Kleihauer-Betke
    test
  b) Longer Term
  - continuously monitor fetal heart rate for 2–4
    hours postprocedure
  - repeat U/S assessment 24–48 hours
    postprocedure

of the fixed sites are rendered difficult due
to oligohydramnios.

The prime 'target' for access to the fetal
circulation varies by series. Most clinical
studies have sited the placental insertion of
the cord as the preferred site(8,10). However, in Weiner's report (9) the placental insertion site was used in only 60% of cases
(450 procedures), and a free loop of cord
was selected in 38% (283 procedures). The
fetal abdominal cord insertion site and the
intrahepatic portion of the umbilical vein is
rarely used since visualization and access
are often difficult and since fetal movement
in response to the painful stimulus compounds the procedure. In the Weiner series,
these sites were used in only 2% of cases.

Placental Cord Insertion Site. The placental insertion site is the most easily accessible and
commonly used site for PUBS. The insertion and origins of the cord vessels in the
placenta are initially approximated by systematic survey of the fetal placental surface.
This placental cord insertion site is almost
always eccentric in location and may occasionally appear to be at the periphery of the
placenta. A central location of the cord insertion is unusual. There is usually a large
vascular lake, invariably maternal in origin,
that creates an echolucency just above the
cord insertion site (Figure 3-5). In the course
of sampling, it is important to ensure that
the needle is guided past this vascular structure so as to avoid contamination of the
sample with maternal blood. The fetal vessels are fanned out across the fetal surface of
the placenta and can be traced back to the
site where they enter and exit the placenta at
the cord root (see also Figure 3-17). The cord
root can usually be identified with certainty,
being characterized by the visible branching
of the umbilical vein at the placental surface
and the approximation of the arteries and
vein in the cord substance (Figure 3-6).

Occasionally, a portion of free cord,
which can be confused with the cord root,
will lie in proximity to the fetal surface of
the placenta. This error is avoided by confirming the branching of the vein into the
placental substance, a feature unique to the
cord root and by observing the effect of

Figure 3-2A Ideally-visualized cord insertions on the placental surface. Anterior insertion, showing the classic "Windsor knot" cord insertion, with the umbilical vein in the centre, flanked by two entwining umbilical arteries (small arrows).

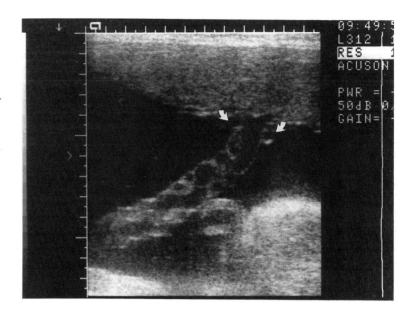

spontaneous fetal movement on the cord position. Free loops of cord will usually be displaced by fetal movement, whereas while the cord root may become stretched and distorted, its actual position relative to the placental surface does not change. In practice, it is often of value to use fetal movement effects on the cord to aid in selecting the placental insertion site. Range-gated Doppler ultrasound in either a

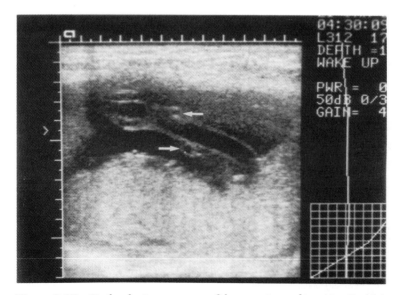

Figure 3-2B Similar classic appearance of the posterior cord insertion. In this instance, note the relatively wide separation of the two coils of arteries (small arrows).

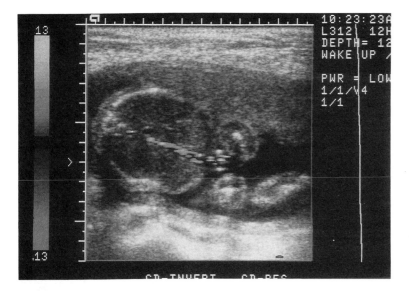

Figure 3-3 Color Doppler showing the umbilical cord insertion into the fetal skin, with a linear illustration of the intrahepatic portion of the umbilical vein. Smaller echoes at the 10:00 position directly adjacent to the spine illustrate both aorta and inferior vena cava as they approach the heart. In order to achieve this linear representation, the transducer must be angled upward and posteriorly, mimicking the course of the umbilical vein.

two-dimensional or color imaging display can be used as an adjunct to identifying the placental cord insertion site, but neither technique offers much, if any, practical clinical advantage. The ideal target is a portion of the umbilical vein lying free within the amniotic fluid, so as to ensure a pure fetal blood sample but close enough to the fixed placental insertion site so as to remain relatively tethered. The umbilical vein is selected because it is the largest of the fetal vessels and, therefore, the easiest to hit with the needle and because it is relatively thin-walled and, therefore, the easiest to penetrate. In practice, this ideal site to enter the umbilical vein is no more than 2 cm from the

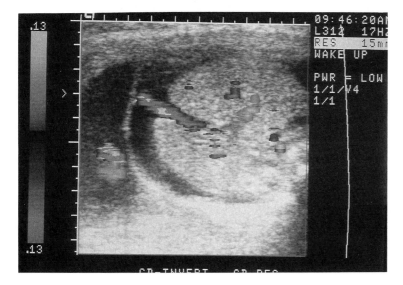

Figure 3-4 Proximal course of the umbilical vein as it crosses from the skin surface, through a moderately large pocket of fetal ascites (blue), and then into the substance of the liver (red, as it changes direction). While the anatomic landmarks are similar to those in Figure 3-3, access is easier, considering the anterior angulation of the target, larger diameter vessels, and higher degree of visualization due to contrast provided by excess amniotic fluid and ascites.

Figure 3-5 Large venous lake (arrow) directly adjacent to the cord insertion (shown by the color Doppler). Care must be taken to traverse the chorion and enter the substance of the cord and to confirm the obtaining of a pure fetal sample by infusion of saline down the vessel.

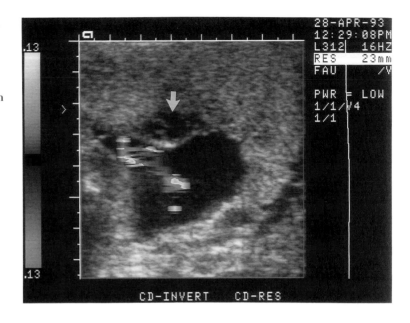

cord insertion site (and usually less). It is technically possible to obtain fetal blood from branches of umbilical vein, either within the placental substance at the cord insertion site or along the surface of the pla-centa, but such an approach greatly increases the likelihood of contamination of the sample by maternal blood. In practice, sampling from these sites should be avoided except as a last resort. In theory,

Figure 3-6 Umbilical cord in cross-section floating freely in the amniotic fluid (upper right) and once the vessels have divided along the surface of a posterior placenta (center).

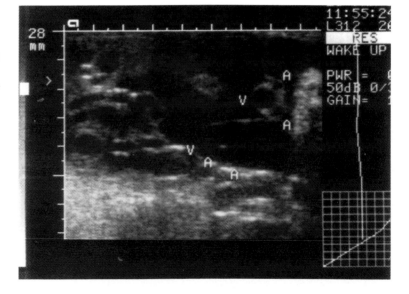

sampling from a fetal artery might be safer since there are two arteries and inadvertent occlusion of one is unlikely to cause fetal demise. The fetal arteries are, however, small and thick-walled and, therefore, more difficult to access. In day-to-day practice, arterial samples are usually only obtained by accident, that is, after missing the vein and penetrating the artery.

Cordocentesis tends to be easiest when the placenta is anterior but can be done with any placental position. When the placenta is implanted on the posterior uterine wall, the cord insertion site may be obscured by the fetus, although in practice, this occurrence is quite unusual. Placing the mother on her side will often cause the fetus to drift towards the dependent side and aid in visualization of the target. When the placenta is posterior, it may often be necessary to guide the needle past the fetal limbs. If a limb obstructs the path to the cord insertion, the needle may be advanced so as to touch the limb. This stimulus usually evokes a withdrawal response, allowing the needle to pass onward.

Ultrasound Needle Guidance

The entry site on the maternal abdomen should be nearly directly above the cord insertion. This site is identified and marked on the skin surface, usually by indenting the skin with a needle hub. The site is then cleaned with an antiseptic solution, then draped with sterile towels and infiltrated with local anesthesia. A 20- or 22-gauge spinal needle is used for the fetal sampling. The length of the needle selected will vary by the maternal habitus and the estimated distance of the fetal target from the maternal skin surface. The length of the standard spinal needle is 8.9 cm, and in more than 85% of cases, this is of sufficient length to reach the target. A longer needle may be re-quired if the mother is grossly obese, if there is hydramnios, or if the placenta is posterior and the cord insertion site more than about 8 cm from the maternal skin surface. In general, the longer the needle, the more difficult it is to guide it along the projected path. Accordingly, it is clinically useful to use the shortest needle possible (avoiding the obvious problem of failing to reach the target). Special needles modified to enhance echo-reflectance of the distal portion and tip are commercially available, but in practice, these needles offer little, if any, practical advantage, and they are more expensive.

The needle is advanced under continuous ultrasound guidance, either freehand or by use of a rigid needle guide fixed to the ultrasound transducer. Most operators use the freehand approach since it is less cumbersome and permits minor adjustments in the course of the procedure. The disadvantage of the freehand approach is that the needle may be deflected from the planned trajectory, usually occurring as a result of a uterine contraction, and that lateral motion of the tip increases the risk of laceration of the vessel wall. Weiner et al. (9) have suggested that the complication rate with PUBS might be significantly higher with this approach than when using a rigid guide. By either method, the needle is guided under continuous dynamic ultrasound imaging. The needle can be guided using either a sector, linear, or curvilinear transducer, the selection depending primarily on the personal preference and experience of the operator. Needle imaging and guidance can be done in one of two ways:

Adjacent Perpendicular Ultrasound Guidance Approach

By this technique, the ultrasound transducer is placed in a sterile plastic bag containing contact gel (nonsterile) and then positioned such that the transducer is nearly directly over the selected target site. Sterile mineral oil on the maternal skin surface provides ultrasonic continuity between skin and sterile plastic bag. The needle is passed through the maternal skin in the perpendicular alongside the transducer and advanced until the needle tip is felt to enter the uterine wall. At this juncture, the transducer is angled through a short arc until the needle tip is identified by its bright echo (Figure 3-7). The tip is then continuously imaged as it passes downwards towards the cord insertion site. Care must be taken to avoid confusing a portion of the needle shaft with the tip of the needle. This error is easily avoided

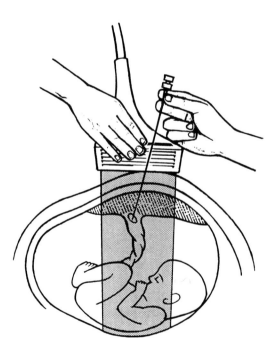

Figure 3-7 Schematic drawing of the "perpendicular" intersection of the needle tip with the ultrasound beam. In this case, the bright tip of the needle is visualized and guided to the target while the remainder of the needle shaft is not visualized.

by angling the ultrasound beam down the shaft until the much brighter terminal needle tip echo is seen; the shaft has a linear, indistinct profile, while the tip is brighter and definitely oval when imaged properly. If there is difficulty visualizing the needle tip, rotation of the needle 90 degrees will bring the open lumen of the tip across the beam, enabling localization. The tip is advanced towards the target until it is placed within about 2–3 mm above the intended entry site (Figure 3-8). At this point, the features of the target are again briefly assessed to ensure there has not been any major change and to confirm the distance to the target and the route the needle tip will follow. The needle tip is then advanced slowly and deliberately until it is seen to reach the cord substance visible by a slight indentation in the cord and slight motion away from the needle pressure. A brief final check of the needle position relative to the vein is made (accounting for any angulation introduced with the foregoing maneuvers), and then, the needle tip is advanced more briskly a distance of about 1–3 mm. The needle tip can usually be seen to indent the vein, often appearing to cause a transient occlusion of the lumen as the vessel walls collapse under pressure. As the needle enters the vessel, the lumen suddenly reappears, and there is usually a very brief echo resulting from turbulent blood flow created by the needle tip. In the mature fetus (>32 weeks), it is occasionally possible to feel the resistance on the vessel wall as the needle penetrates it, but more commonly, there is no recognizable sensation. In the immature fetus, there is no sensation of needle entry at all, and it is possible to transfix the cord without any tactile awareness.

Remote Tangential Needle Guidance Approach

By this method, the ultrasound transducer is placed some distance away from

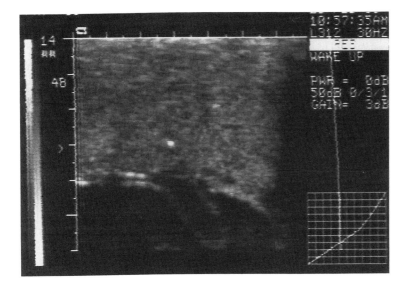

Figure 3-8 Serial photographs taken a few seconds apart (note the time in the upper righthand corner), as the needle is advanced into the umbilical vein at its origin on the surface of this anterior placenta. In this case, the ultrasound beam is at right angles to the shaft of the needle, and only the tip, the bright white dot, is visualized. Frequent referencing of the needle tip by small increments of rotation of the transducer confirm that this is not an unusually bright echo derived somewhat in mid-shaft. In general, however, only the needle tip gives such a bright echo, allowing certainty as to needle placement.

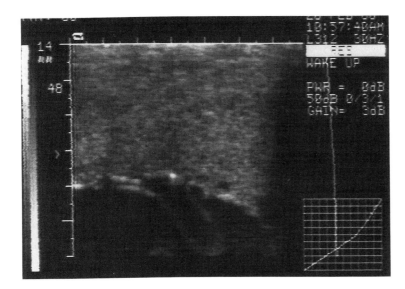

the proposed needle entry site and angled such that the needle is seen longitudinally (Figure 3-9). The needle enters the maternal skin in the perpendicular plane and is advanced towards the target site. The ultrasound transducer is angled such that the shaft and tip of the needle are in constant view (Figure 3-10). The technique of needle entry is similar to the adjacent perpendicular method. This method has

Figure 3-8 (continued)

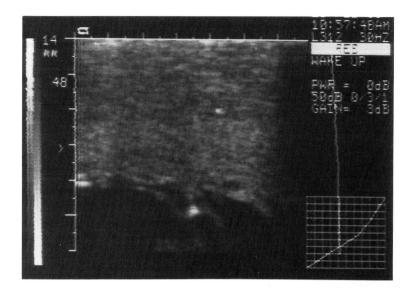

the advantage of providing a better overall view of the needle course but has the disadvantage of a less well-defined view of the entry site.

Confirmation of Correct Vascular Insertion and Blood Sampling

Once the needle tip is assumed to be placed in the fetal vessel, the stylet should be removed and a heparin-flushed 1-cc tuberculin syringe attached. This is a critical time in the procedure since it is essential to rigidly maintain the position of the needle tip, and, in particular, lateral motion of the needle should be avoided. The needle tip should be carefully observed during the removal of the stylet and attachment of the syringe. If inadvertent movement of the needle tip occurs it is usually an advancement and not a withdrawal. Occasionally when the stylet is removed, a bead of blood will be observed to well up into the needle hub, seen first as a backflow of the saline column in the stylet and followed by a color change, then a free flow of blood. The presence of this finding does not confirm that

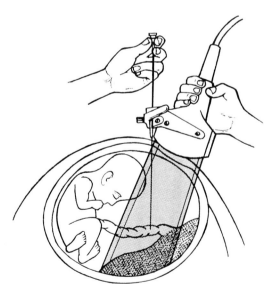

Figure 3-9 Longitudinal intersection of the ultrasound beam with the needle. In this method, the ultra-sound beam (usually curvilinear) intersects the entire shaft of the needle.

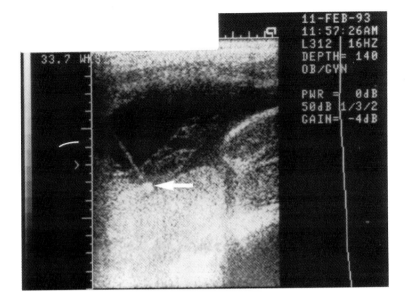

Figure 3-10 Longitudinal placement of this linear transducer shows most of the shaft of the needle being inserted into the umbilical cord immediately adjacent to its origin on the surface of a posterior placenta. The needle shaft is seen clearly, and the tip of the needle (arrow) remains brighter with this view. Due to the broad distribution of echoes from the needle tip, the view shown is not sufficient to prove that the needle is actually in the vessel, as this image can be obtained with the needle either in front of or behind the cord. This absence of depth of field is the one drawback of this method of needle visualization. (Courtesy of Dr. G. Ryan, Mount Sinai Hospital, Toronto)

the tip is within a fetal vessel since the same effect will occur if the tip is within a maternal vessel. Further, the appearance of blood in the hub is of no value in determining if the tip lies within a fetal vein or artery since either may produce this effect. In contrast, the failure to observe blood in the hub does not indicate that the tip is not freely placed in the lumen of a fetal vessel. Frequently, blood will not flow back despite the tip being free within the lumen of the vessel.

Once the 1-cc syringe is firmly attached to the needle hub, gentle suction should be applied. If the needle tip is free in the vessel, blood can be easily aspirated. If blood does not return freely with gentle suction, the needle tip is not correctly placed. A common error in the inexperienced is to assume that increasing the suction pressure is of some advantage if there is no initial return; such is never the case and this technique

should be avoided. If free flow is not achieved, the needle should be slowly rotated while maintaining gentle suction. If blood is still not aspirated, the needle position should be reassessed. In practice, the most common reason for failure to obtain a sample is the result of the needle tip either passing through the vessel into the cord substance beyond or lodging against the vessel wall. Either problem is overcome by slight withdrawal of the needle while maintaining suction. The increments of needle withdrawal can only be learned by experience, but as a general rule, they ought to be extremely small and deliberate. When the needle tip is through the vessel wall, it will drag the wall with it as the needle is withdrawn, and as a result, the luminal space becomes very narrowed, leaving a very small margin of error. If no return is obtained by this technique, it may be assumed that either the needle passed tangential to the vessel and lodged in the cord substance or the vessel moved away as the needle advanced. In either instance, if blood is not aspirated with rotation and graduated withdrawal, the tip should be withdrawn to the original position a few millimeters above the target and the situation reassessed. The needle should never be advanced blindly.

Once free flow of blood in the needle is established, the planned sample volume should be taken even before the appropriate needle site position is confirmed. This approach is strongly recommended since it limits the time of the procedure and, therefore, the risk of needle dislodgement. Samples should be collected in syringes that have been flushed with a 1/1000 heparin solution. This method will ensure there is sufficient residual heparin in the syringe to prevent coagulation of the sample and is used for all samples except where the assay specifically prohibits it. The sample volume will vary according to the indications for the procedure and fetal age and is usually in the range of 3–5 cc. Once the sample is collected

and passed off, the source is confirmed. There are several methods used to confirm that sample is fetal in origin.

The first and most direct step is to inject a small bolus of normal saline (0.1–0.3 cc) down the needle. If the needle tip is freely placed in the umbilical vein, the saline flush is seen as a transient bright echo that appears first at the needle tip and then disappears quickly down the vein (Figure 3-11). This ultrasound effect is absolutely characteristic and, when observed, is certain evidence that the sample is fetal in origin. The failure to see this effect does not always indicate inappropriate placement since visualization will depend on imaging the vessel near the injection site. If the umbilical vein is imaged some distance downstream from the injection site, the saline flush may be diluted and may no longer be visible or may take a few seconds to reach the imaged segment. If the needle tip is in an artery, the saline flush is considerably more difficult to identify (Figure 3-12). When observed, the flush is seen to flow towards the placenta and to disappear very rapidly across the

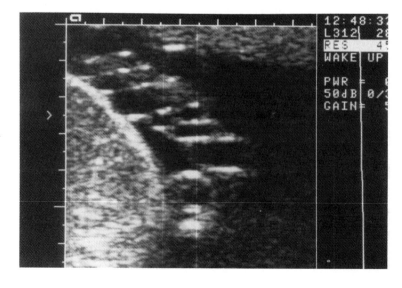

Figure 3-11A Saline flush, remote from the needle insertion into the umbilical vein at its origin on the surface of this anterior placenta. After the saline was injected, the flush became visible as a marked increase in turbulence within the vein (arrow, see Figure 3-11B).

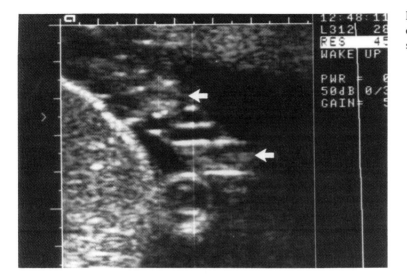

Figure 3-11B Clearly outlining the arteries, which show no such turbulence.

placental surface. If the needle tip is in a maternal placental lake, the saline flush will appear to be contained into a relatively small area within the placental substance and swirl around without egress. Color Doppler is of no value in confirming appropriate needle placement, and the saline flush cannot be seen by this method.

The origin of the sample can also be rapidly determined at the bedside by the Singer, or alkaline precipitation, test (APT). A drop of sample blood is added to a test tube containing a 0.1 molar sodium hydroxide solution and mixed. Fetal blood will not denature rapidly in this solution and at one minute, the solution will remain pink in

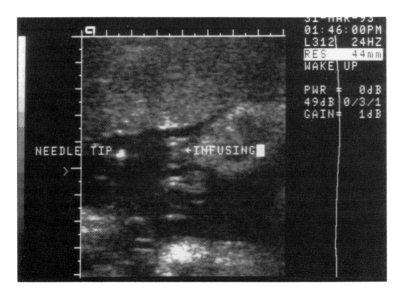

Figure 3-12 Intra-arterial infusion of saline may be somewhat more difficult to see. In this case, the needle tip is placed in an umbilical artery, which loops out of the picture, and then emerges in cross-section a few centimeters to the right, as labelled. The circular opacity indicates turbulence within one of the umbilical arteries.

color. Maternal (adult) blood will rapidly denature and the solution will turn a brownish green color. These color changes are best compared against a control tube containing adult blood. This test is simple and reliable in most instances and can be used in lieu of the more elaborate and expensive cell sorting systems (Coulter counter method). The APT is not sufficiently sensitive to accurately detect or quantitate admixtures of maternal and fetal blood. This test cannot be used in fetuses previously transfused with maternal blood, as for example in alloimmune disorders.

The Kleihauer-Betke acid elution method can be used to confirm the sample source, and in the case of admixture, to determine with great accuracy the proportion of blood from the mother and fetus. This technique is time-consuming and cannot be used at the bedside. The accuracy of the Kleihauer-Betke test is greatest before the mid-third trimester since after this time, there is increase in the population of fetal cells containing adult hemoglobin (11). It is similarly of little use in sample verification when the fetus has had multiple transfusions of adult blood.

Alternately, the presence of maternal blood and serum in the sample can be confirmed by assaying the beta HCG concentration. In pure fetal blood, this peptide occurs in almost negligible concentrations, whereas in maternal blood, the concentration is high. The usual ratio of HCG concentration between fetal and maternal blood is about 1:400 (11). Detection of contamination of the sample by amniotic fluid cannot be determined easily at the bedside and may be difficult under any circumstances. The presence of amniotic fluid in the sample can confound the determination of fetal coagulopathies and may invalidate biochemical measurements. The possibility of amniotic fluid contamination should be suspected

whenever the initial sample appears to be diluted, when some streaming of the saline flush is seen into the amniotic cavity, or whenever there is wide variation in the hemoglobin concentration of serial samples. The presence of amniotic fluid contamination can be confirmed by combined analysis of the AFP or beta-HCG concentration of the sample. AFP appears in high concentrations in fetal blood and much lower concentrations in amniotic fluid, whereas the opposite occurs for HCG. Alternately, a smear may be made of the sample and then scanned for the presence of desquamated epithelial cells. The serum bilirubin concentration is also a useful indicator of serodilution. In practice, the occurrence of amniotic fluid contamination is unusual, and when it occurs, it is usually very obvious.

Postprocedural Monitoring

Once the sample has been obtained and confirmed to be fetal in origin, the needle is removed. In practice, it is usual to observe the cord entry site at the time of the needle removal. As the tip leaves the cord substance, there is usually a plume of fetal blood observed to project into the amniotic fluid (Figure 3-13). Sustained bleeding may be seen in up to 43% of cases. This bleeding at the venous puncture site may initially appear vigorous and under pressure. The blood may project into the amniotic fluid and be seen to reflect off fetal parts or the surface of the placenta. Usually after about a minute, there is a subtle but progressive diminution in the shape and height of the ultrasound plume followed rapidly by a rapid disappearance of the plume effect, replaced by intermittent echo-reflective droplets seen to fall towards the dependent aspect of the amniotic cavity. There may be intermittent fluctuations in the visible amount of bleeding, but the general pattern is towards subsidence. Bleeding from an arterial puncture site initially ap-

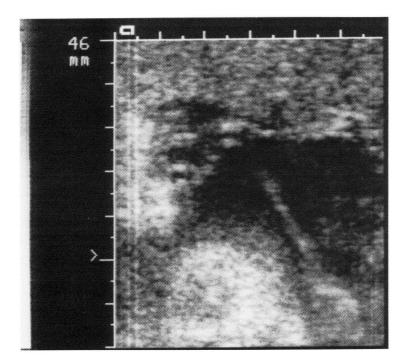

Figure 3-13A Backbleeding after the needle has been removed from its transamniotic insertion into the umbilical vein. The plume of fetal blood is first a thin straight line ricocheting off an adjacent fetal limb some distance away.

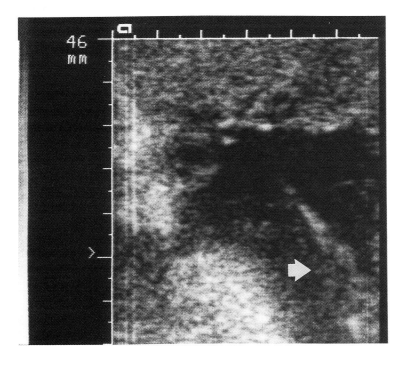

Figure 3-13B The plume becomes more ragged and feathery (arrow) as the speed of bleeding diminishes, and it is followed until its complete cessation.

Figure 3-13C Total duration of backbleeding in this instance was 103 seconds, from a 22-gauge needle puncture.

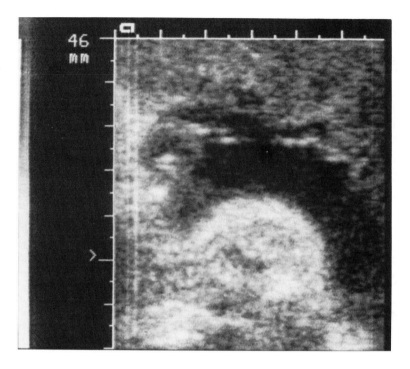

pears similar to venous bleeding. Bleeding from an arterial puncture site does not usually subside slowly but rather quite suddenly ceases. The ultrasound characteristics of bleeding from puncture sites in the cord have recently been described (12). Extremely small rates of flow from a needle in a water bath can be visualized without difficulty by a properly-placed ultrasound transducer (Figure 3-14): with proper care, intra-amniotic bleeding will not be missed. The average duration of observed bleeding after cordocentesis was 137 seconds, being longer after umbilical vein puncture (mean 144 seconds) and shorter in duration with arterial puncture (mean 95 seconds). The duration of bleeding is not different between puncture by a 20- or 22-gauge needle. A bleeding duration of greater that 300 seconds is very abnormal and is usually an indication for fetal volume replacement by immediate intrauterine (intravascular or intracardiac) transfusion. Prolonged post-procedural bleeding should alert the clinician to the possibility of fetal thrombocytopenia.

The fetal heart rate should be assessed immediately after the needle is withdrawn and for a few minutes thereafter. The heart rate can usually be determined by observing the umbilical artery pulsations. Typically, there is no visible change in heart rate after the procedure. A slowing of the fetal heart rate is of considerable concern, and the mother should be placed immediately on her side and 100% oxygen administered by a rebreathe mask (see section on complications). A fetal tachycardia is less worrisome unless there is evidence of active bleeding from the cord puncture site.

A maternal blood sample for Kleihauer-Betke testing should be drawn immediately

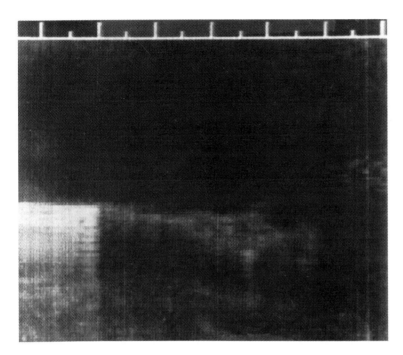

Figure 3-14 In vitro water bath experiment showing needle tip (bright multiple linear echoes at left), and the turbulence produced by injection of 0.001 ml of red cells, illustrating the easy visualization of minute amounts of backbleeding.

before and after the procedure. Provided the fetal condition remains stable after the procedure, this test can be run at the routine pace. In the event of fetal tachycardia, the test result should be expedited so as to detect significant fetomaternal hemorrhage.

The need for intermediate monitoring of fetal condition after PUBS is variable depending on the fetal age, and the indications for the procedure and the results of assessment immediately after the procedure is concluded. In general, if postprocedural bleeding abates rapidly and the fetal heart rate remains within normal limits, there is no need for prolonged monitoring and the patient may usually be discharged directly. If there are any concerns regarding the amount of fetal bleeding or fetal heart rate stability, more prolonged continuous FHR monitoring and intermittent dynamic ultrasound assessment is indicated.

COMPLICATIONS OF CORDOCENTESIS

A number of complications, both minor and life-threatening, have been reported for cordocentesis (Table 3-3).

Procedure-related Perinatal Mortality

The overall mortality for the procedure will depend on the clinical population. Perinatal death is more common among fetuses with structural and/or karyotypic anomalies. Daffos, who has among the largest experiences with the method, observed 21 fetal deaths in 1320 procedures giving a gross loss rate of 1.6% (13). Nine of these deaths occurred in either malformed or infected fetuses. The fetal death rate among fetuses in whom perinatal survival was possible was 0.9% (12 deaths). Boulot el al., in a

Table 3-3   Cordocentesis: Complications

Fetal Death	
Overall	2–3%
Procedure-related	0.5–10%
Bradycardia	
Life-threatening Hemorrhage (Intra-amniotic, Intraplacental, Cord Hematoma)	0.5%
Infection	< 0.5%
Premature Labor	
Overall	3–4%
Procedure-related	?0%

series of 322 cases, reported a procedural mortality of 3.1% (10), and Weiner et al.(9), in a series of 594 cases done solely for diagnosis, reported a procedural death rate of 0.8%. Therefore, it may be assumed that the death rate associated with cordocentesis is in the range of about 1%.

Fetal Bradycardia

Fetal bradycardia, defined as a heart rate at or below 100 bpm., is observed in up to 6.1% of procedures and is the most commonly recognized procedural complication (9). Postprocedural bradycardia occurs more commonly after arterial puncture (incidence 19%), in the growth-retarded fetus (incidence 17.2%), and after intravascular transfusion (incidence 7.7%). The pathophysiological basis for this complication is not always clear but is most likely the result of either acute segmental spasm of the vessel wall at and around the puncture site or extrinsic compression of the vessels in the cord occurring secondary to extravasation of blood from the puncture site into the cord substance. In most instances, the bradycardia is transient, lasting only from a few sec-

onds to a few minutes. From the clinical perspective, the bradycardia may be considered innocuous; despite a slow baseline rate, there is evidence of a gradual increase in heart rate. The bradycardia is sinister if the rate remains fixed or falls and the duration of the episode exceeds 15 minutes. Postprocedural bradycardia is more common following arterial puncture and may be associated with reduced or absent umbilical artery diastolic velocity waveforms, and is more common, and possibly more dangerous, when there is a single umbilical artery.

The treatment of bradycardia is initially expectant, placing the mother in a lateral position and administering oxygen by face mask. The FHR should be monitored continuously, usually using a standard FHR monitor. In the fetus sufficiently mature to effect a successful transition to neonatal life, preparations for emergency delivery should be made. If the heart rate is not demonstrating some recovery by about five minutes after onset of the complication, the patient should be transferred to an operating theatre. If by 10 minutes there are no signs of recovery, then delivery should be instituted. In the immature fetus, there is little that can be done other than to continue maternal oxygen therapy.

Fetal Hemorrhage

While the observation of some bleeding from the puncture site is common, the observation of sustained and life-threatening bleeding is relatively rare. The in vitro discrimination between blood and amniotic fluid is very high; volumes of as little as 0.001 ml/min can be recognized by this method (Figure 3-14). However, measurement of total volume of blood loss by subjective ultrasound methods is not entirely reliable. In vivo cord perfusion studies have demonstrated that the bleeding rate from a

22-gauge puncture site is highly variable and loss per minute may range from as little as 0.3 ml to as great as 18.4 ml/per minute. In vitro, the rate of blood loss is related directly to the cord perfusion rate (12). In vivo, the cord perfusion rate is usually not known, but the duration of bleeding may be determined with some precision. The percentage loss of fetal blood volume based on combined in vitro and in vivo data may be calculated to range from less than 5% to greater than 60%.

Clinical observations support these estimates. According to repeated or serial sample data, in most instances, provided the duration of postprocedural bleeding falls within the normal range, the hematocrit will either remain stable or decrease marginally. Sustained bleeding may be associated with hypovolemic collapse and death. In the Manitoba experience (12) there have been nine fetuses that exhibited sustained postprocedural bleeding (=>300 seconds) (12). In each instance, FHR was grossly abnormal and other acute fetal biophysical variables were absent. Two of these fetuses were greater than 32 weeks gestation and were delivered by prompt cesarian section. Both were grossly anemic at birth (hematocrit <15%) and were hypotensive but responded to blood volume replacement and survived. In three of the seven immature fetuses, immediate access to the fetal circulation was established (two by umbilical venipuncture, one by intracardiac puncture), and the fetuses were transfused with emergency 0-negative blood. All three fetuses survived. In four fetuses (all of whom were profoundly anemic in the first place), vascular access could not be reestablished and death occurred within 30 minutes. Fetal exsanguination culminating in death has been reported by others (8,14). The risk of serious fetal bleeding (Figure 3-15) is generally considered to be increased in the presence of fetal thrombocytopenia (15) although not all investigators have found this association (9). Concern regarding fetal

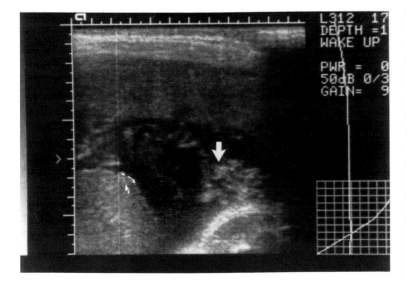

Figure 3-15 Transamniotic puncture of the umbilical vein was performed for fetal platelet count at 24 weeks gestation in a patient being treated for neonatal alloimmune thrombocytopenia. Experience suggests that fetuses severely affected with this disorder have abnormal vessel wall characteristics, making the vessel possibly more prone to tearing at the point of needle insertion. In this instance, torrential bleeding followed removal of the needle and resulted in the formation of a large frothy clot hanging from the needle insertion site (arrow).

exsanguination is generally indicated when the duration of bleeding persists beyond five minutes or there are other fetal signs, such as a persistent tachycardia and an impression of incomplete filling of the ventricles.

The treatment of sustained fetal hemorrhage is relatively straight-forward. Supportive measures, such as maternal positioning and administration of oxygen by face mask, should be instituted in all cases. In the mature fetus, immediate delivery is the treatment of choice. The neonatal support team should be forewarned that the perinate will be hypotensive and anemic. If the fetus is immature or it is not possible to effect delivery of a mature fetus, the only treatment option is immediate fetal transfusion. The intravascular route selected will vary. In practice, if the umbilical vein is not easily accessible, it is prudent to move directly to intracardiac puncture and transfusion. It is important to make this decision early in the course of clinical management because with delay, the umbilical vessels will collapse and become inaccessible and cardiac puncture will become more difficult. Ideally, the transfusion should be matched against maternal sera. In practice, however, this complication is usually so severe that transfusion with O negative blood is the most practical option.

Fetomaternal hemorrhage occurs commonly after PUBS, and in some studies, the incidence reaches nearly 60% (16). The volume of fetal blood lost into the maternal circulation is usually less than 2.5 ml, but occasionally, massive hemorrhage can occur. It follows that Rh immunoglobulin should be administered to every Rh-negative nonsensitized patient after every procedure. In practice, there is usually a delay of up to a day or more between the procedure and the recognition of fetal bleeding by Kleihauer-Betke testing. If the test result is positive, demonstrating a bleed of significance (usually =>10 ml of fetal blood), the fetus should be reassessed immediately by ultrasound and a maternal blood sample for repeat Kleihauer-Betke testing done. If on repeat ultrasound assessment the fetus appears grossly normal with a normal biophysical profile score, management is conservative. If the fetal biophysical profile score is abnormal (=<6/10) or there is evidence of fetal ascites, preparations should be made for either immediate intravascular transfusion or delivery.

Fetal bleeding may also occur into the cord substance and the subchorionic placental plate (Figure 3-16). Bleeding into the cord substance can result in either extrinsic compression of the vessels or segmental vascular spasm. The incidence of cord hematoma formation is reported as approximately 10%, but in most of these cases the hematoma is small and without serious or persistent fetal effects (17). Sustained vascular spasm and intimal damage can result in cord thrombosis. If this occurs in the vein, the effects are dramatic and lethal. Arterial thrombosis is compatible with continued fetal survival.

Infection and Premature Labor

Amnionitis is a rare but recognized complication of cordocentesis (9), and may result in either fetal death or premature labor or neonatal sepsis. Life-threatening maternal sepsis and adult respiratory distress syndrome has been reported as a complication of cordocentesis (18).

Uterine contractions commonly occur with passage of the needle through the myometrium, visible by ultrasound as a slight change in uterine echo reflectance and a minor distortion of the placental surface anatomy. Occasionally, the contraction

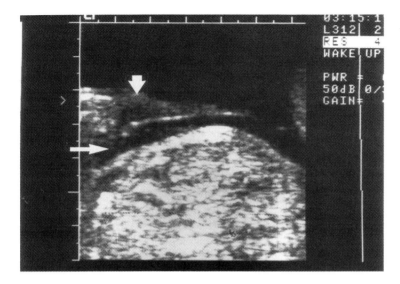

Figure 3-16 Subchorionic bleeding following cordocentesis. The fetus (20 weeks gestation) was both severely anemic and thrombocytopenic, with severe alloimmune erythroblastosis. On removal of the needle, there was prompt elevation of the chorion by rapid blood loss (horizontal arrow). Some of this blood leaked out the puncture hole into the amniotic fluid and coalesced into a filmy clot (vertical arrow). Cardiovascular collapse followed, requiring intracardiac resuscitation, which was successful.

may be more intense and prolonged, a phenomenon that is more likely to occur after the needle is manipulated within the myometrium or there have been several attempts at needle placement. The effect of these strong uterine contractions on the cord insertion site can be quite dramatic, resulting in buckling of the placenta and movement of the target by as much as 5 cm. Further, the occurrence of a contraction can lift the needle back out of the vessel. This technical complication is most common during intravascular transfusion and is rarely a problem with the shorter diagnostic procedures. Persistence of uterine contractions following a PUBS is not uncommon, occurring in about 7% of cases (19). Persistence of postprocedural contractions culminating in either rupture of membranes and/or premature delivery is uncommon. In the Daffos series of 1320 procedures, the incidence of premature delivery was 3.8%, a rate that was not different from that observed in the general population (13).

CORDOCENTESIS: CLINICAL INDICATIONS

Cordocentesis is a relatively new clinical method, and as a result, its range of applications is still being developed and investigated. The procedure is invasive with measurable fetal (and maternal) risks and, therefore, its application must always be carefully considered. In particular, it is important to avoid the use of this method when other diagnostic options are available. The indications for the procedure will vary by the referral population. The contemporary indications for cordocentesis are as follows (Table 3-4):

Table 3-4 Cordocentesis: Clinical Indications

Assessment of alloimmune pregnancy
Cytogenetic studies
Diagnosis of fetal infection
Assessment of inherited or acquired fetal disorders
Fetal blood gas and acid base studies

Assessment of the Alloimmune Pregnancy

In most series, assessment of the fetus at risk for alloimmune anemia is among the most common indications for PUBS. The procedure offers several obvious clinical advantages in the assessment of the fetus at risk for alloimmune disease. Firstly, analysis of fetal blood permits determination of fetal blood type and, therefore, absolute determination of fetal risk for alloimmune anemia; the confirmation that the fetus does not have the offending red cell antigen obviates the need for serial monitoring and repeated amniocentesis. Secondly, in the affected fetus, the degree of fetal anemia can be determined directly and accurately and the presence and efficacy of the fetal erythroblastic compensation determined. From these data, the need for and timing of intravascular transfusion can be determined. Thirdly, serial analysis of fetal hemoglobin concentration in transfused fetuses permits a rational approach to the frequency of repeat transfusions. The disadvantages of PUBS in the management of the fetus at risk for alloimmune anemia are considerable. In addition to the generic risks of the procedure, there are unique added risks in the sensitized pregnancy. Transplacental hemorrhage is a common, and in many cases, unavoidable complication of cordocentesis. While the volume of the bleed is usually small and insignificant to the fetus, the stimulatory effects on the maternal immune system are usually dramatic. Titer rises more than 100-fold can occur, which may prove lethal to the affected fetus.

The use of PUBS in the management of the alloimmune fetus should be highly selective. Maternal antibody titers and serial measurement of amniotic fluid bilirubin concentration, while not as precise as direct measurement of hemoglobin, are nonetheless a highly effective means of management of the fetus at risk. To date, there is no evidence that any clinical advantage is gained by substituting the more risky procedure of PUBS in place of these time-honored and proven methods. However, there are exceptions to this general statement. PUBS is valuable in the assessment of the fetus whose father is heterozygous for the offending red cell antigen. PUBS is indicated in those rare cases in which there is ultrasound evidence of fetal anemia despite a stable maternal titer or a reassuring amniotic fluid bilirubin concentration. Serial PUBS may also be of value in avoiding unnecessary transfusion in the fetus capable of mounting effective compensation to persistent alloimmune hemolysis.

Cytogenetic Studies

Fetal lymphocyte culture is a rapid means for determination of the fetal karyotype, usually yielding a reliable result within two to four days. In contrast, amniocyte culture is slower and less reliable, yielding a result usually within seven to 14 days, or even as long as 28 days. In most clinical circumstances, there is no urgency for a result, and the longer time period required for amniocyte culture is acceptable. Therefore, PUBS should not be considered as a substitute for the less risky procedure of amniocentesis. CVS is another alternative, with intermediate turnaround time.

In some clinical circumstances, PUBS is the method of choice for cytogenetic studies. PUBS is indicated when cytogenetic results of amniocentesis or chorionic villus biopsy have yielded either no result or an equivocal result (mosaicism) and may be the method of choice in investigation of a fetus at risk for fragile X syndrome. The use of PUBS in the assessment of the fetus with a structural anomaly should be individualized. In the immature anomalous fetus, there is no advantage in PUBS for cytogenetic studies and amniocentesis is the method of choice. In the abnormal fetus in whom intervention (either delivery or an in utero corrective procedure) is considered, feasible PUBS is usually the method of choice for cytogenetic studies.

Assessment of Intrauterine Infection

Fetal blood analysis is useful in the investigation and diagnosis of fetal infection, discussed in detail by Fernand Daffos in Chapter 4 (20–25). Some caution is required in interpretation of fetal immunological responses to infectious agents as the presence and nature of these responses may vary with fetal age. The humeral immune system does not become responsive until about 20 weeks gestation, and the typical antibody response seen in extrauterine life may not be as evident in fetal life. The presence of specific IgM is definitive evidence of fetal antigen exposure but does not indicate active ongoing infection. Fetal IgG antibody is not of value since it is not possible to differentiate maternal from fetal sources. The identification of the infectious agent by direct visualization, culture or DNA technology is definitive evidence of fetal infection. Fetal cellular responses to infection are nonspecific and cannot be used for diagnosis. The mean total fetal white cell count ranges from 4200–4500/cc and tends to remain relatively unchanged throughout fetal life (11). The differential count demonstrates a relatively high proportion of lymphocytes (approximately 80%) and the neutrophil count is relatively low (approximately 7%). The alterations in white cell count produced by infection will vary by the nature of the infection but, in general, are inconsistent and not of diagnostic nor prognostic value. Low fetal platelet count, elevated bilirubin, or elevated fetal liver enzymes are supportive, but not conclusive, of fetal infection.

Assessment of Congenital Fetal Disorders

PUBS may be used to identify numerous fetal genetic diseases. Fetal coagulopathies, including hemophilia A and B, von Willebrand's disease, and congenital thrombocytopenias can now be diagnosed by fetal blood analysis (8,26–28). Fetal hemoglobinopathies including alpha- and beta-thalassemia and sickle cell diseases may be diagnosed by analysis of fetal blood (29,30). Fetal immune disorders, including chronic granulomatous disease and variants of severe combined immune deficiency syndrome, can be diagnosed by analysis of fetal blood (31). Fetal blood analysis may also be used in the diagnosis of a wide range of inherited metabolic disorders, e.g., hypophosphatasia, amino acid disorders, mucopolysaccharidoses, glycogen storage diseases.

Other Applications

Cordocentesis has proven a useful tool in assessing fetal blood gas and acid-base status in normal and pathological circumstances. The normal distribution of fetal pO_2, pCO_2, pH and bicarbonate has been described in detail (33,34). The relationship between fetal blood gas status and abnormalities of fetal biophysical activities and blood flow velocity waveforms has been described (5,7,35). However, the routine use of PUBS in the assessment of the fetus at risk for asphyxia is not a common practice.

PUBS may be of value in assessing the etiology and severity of intrauterine growth retardation (IUGR) (Chapter 5). Karyotypic malformations occur more frequently in growth-retarded fetuses particularly those exhibiting early onset symmetrical growth restriction. A cytogenetic diagnosis can usually be obtained with less risk by amniocentesis in these cases; PUBS should be reserved for those cases when an immediate answer is required. Numerous biochemical, hematological, and blood gas abnormalities are reported in growth-retarded fetuses (36,37). In our practice, PUBS is of limited value in the management of IUGR since most of the critical decisions can be made by noninvasive fetal assessment methods. In individual cases, PUBS is instrumental in diagnosis and subsequent evaluation of therapy, in a long list of congenital and intrauterine-acquired metabolic, endocrinologic, and family-specific disorders.

The role of cordocentesis in the evaluation and management of twin gestation is not clear at present. The technique may be useful in early identification and quantification of twin-to-twin transfusion.

Integrated Application of Cordocentesis

While there are many opportunities to expand the data available in a given clinical situation by access to the fetal circulation,

the foregoing delineation of risk reminds us that there may be a price to obtaining this information. It is important to remember at the outset that the frequency of karyotypic abnormalities is usually quite low and that fetal mortality from technical problems of PUBS for purely genetic sampling is most regrettable. Thus, in many instances, the extra time necessary to obtain karyotype results by amniocentesis culture may be preferable to persisting at a difficult cordocentesis.

Several anatomic variants may also present technical challenge (Figures 3-17–3-20). In some instances, the difficult cord must be approached in any case, based on the likelihood of a treatable, but life-threatening fetal disorder. In many other instances, however, the technical difficulty should call for re-evaluation of the risks of the procedure, which may be markedly elevated on an individual basis.

Only through the careful application of medical and ethical principles can the oper-

Figure 3-17 (See earlier text.) Asterisk denotes a straight portion of umbilical vein mimicking a classic cord insertion into the center of this anterior placenta. In fact, the spherical object illustrated is just a free loop of cord, and the actual cord insertion (at least 5 cm distant from this image) is not shown in this picture. An attempt at puncturing the cord at the point indicated by the asterisk would likely be unsuccessful as this loop of cord will be highly mobile and not readily pinned against a posterior object.

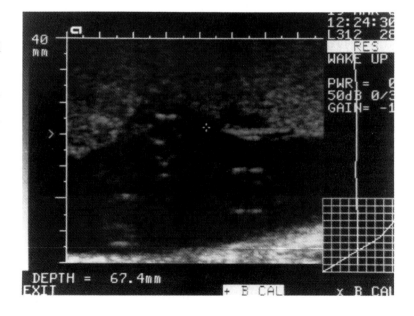

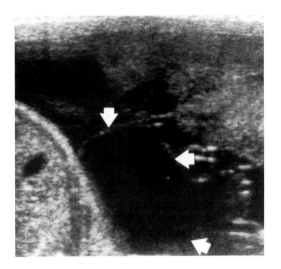

Figure 3-18 Cord insertion on the surface of an anterior placenta, with relationships distorted by the presence of a large allantoic cyst (arrows).

ator avoid taking unnecessary risks just to get a sample.

SUMMARY

The advent of the ability to sample fetal blood with minimal risk has opened broad new vistas for understanding fetal responses in health and disease, in prenatal diagnosis of intrinsic and acquired disease, and in development of effective methods for fetal treatment. In less than a decade, this method of fetal assessment has become a standard technique and its application is widespread. The addition of fetal blood analysis to the already well-developed ultrasound-based abilities to assess fetal structural and functional integrity now make it possible to identify and evaluate fetal disease with far greater certainty than was imaginable a few years ago. In many ways, it may now be argued that this combination of methods will vault fetal medicine into the same category of diagnostic and

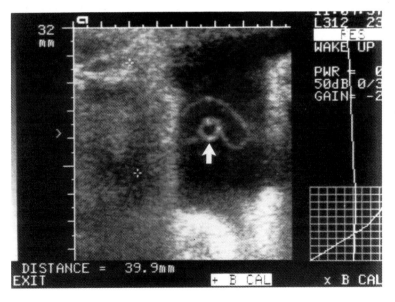

Figure 3-19 Single umbilical artery (arrow). Special care should be made to obtain venous vascular entry in the case of, for example, the anomalous fetus with a single umbilical artery. Whether or not these vessels are more likely to go into spasm is not known, but since there is only one artery, the consequences of severe spasm are likely more deleterious.

Figure 3-20 Color Doppler flow mapping of vasa
previa, with a completely
membranous cord insertion.
AP = anterior portion of the
placenta. PP = posterior
portion of the placenta.
AB = amniotic band. B =
tip of maternal bladder. af =
amniotic fluid pocket. Note
the course of the umbilical
vein (blue) and the tightly-
paired umbilical arteries
(red) through the mem-
branes between the two
portions of the placenta.
Despite the most obvious
indications for cordocentesis in such a case, only if
life-saving treatment was
absolutely mandatory,
should such a vessel be approached with a needle!

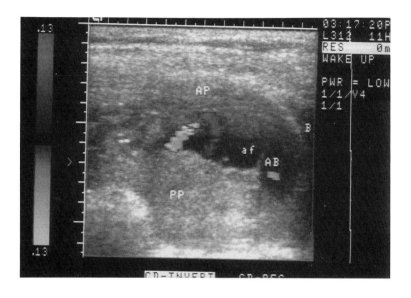

therapeutic precision as is usual and expected in extrauterine medicine.

References

1. Valenti C. Endoamnioscopy and fetal bi-
    opsy: a new technique. Am J Obstet Gynecol
    1972;114:561–564.
2. Hobbins JC, Mahoney M, Goldstein, LA. A
    new method for intrauterine visualization
    by the combined use of fetoscopy and ultra-
    sound. Am J Obstet Gynecol 1974;188:
    1069–1072.
3. Rodeck CH, Campbell S. Umbilical cord
    insertion as a source of pure fetal blood
    for prenatal diagnosis. The Lancet 1979;
    i:1244–1245.
4. Daffos F, Capell-Pavlovsky M, Forestier F.
    A new procedure for fetal blood sampling
    in utero: preliminary report of 53 cases. Am
    J Obstet Gynecol 1983;146:985–987.
5. Vintzileos AM, Campbell WA, Rodis JF,
    et al. The relationship between fetal bio-
    physical assessment, umbilical velocimetry

    and fetal acidosis. Obstet Gynecol 1991;
    77:622–626.
6. Manning FA, Snijders R, Harman C, et al.
    Fetal biophysical profile score VI: correla-
    tion with antepartum umbilical venous fe-
    tal pH. Am J Obstet Gynecol 1993;169:
    755–763.
7. Ribbert LSM, Snijders RJM, Nicolaides KH.
    Relationship of fetal biophysical profile and
    blood gas values at cordocentesis in se-
    verely growth-retarded fetuses. Am J Ob-
    stet Gynecol 1990;163:569–571.
8. Daffos F, Capella-Pavlovsky M, Forestier F.
    Fetal blood sampling during pregnancy
    with use of a needle guided by ultrasound:
    a study of 606 consecutive cases. Am J Ob-
    stet Gynecol 1985;153:655–660.
9. Weiner CP, Wenstrom KD, Sipes SL, et al.
    Risk factors for cordocentesis and fetal in-
    travascular transfusion. Am J Obstet Gy-
    necol 1991;165:1020–1025.
10. Boulot P, Deschamps F, Lefort G, et al. Pure
    fetal blood samples obtained by cordocen-
    tesis: technical aspects of 322 cases. Prenat
    Diag 1990;10:93–100.

11. Forestier F, Cox WL, Daffos F, et al. The assessment of fetal blood samples. Am J Obstet Gynecol 1988;158:1184–1188.

12. Segal M, Manning FA, Harman CR, et al. Bleeding after intravascular transfusion: experimental and clinical observations. Am J Obstet Gynecol 1991;165:1414–1418.

13. Daffos F. Fetal blood sampling. In: Harrison MR, Golbus MS, Filly RA, eds. The Unborn Patient: Prenatal Diagnosis and Treatment. Philadelphia: WB Saunders 1990: 75–81.

14. Rightmire D, Ertmoed EE: Fetal exsanguination following cord blood sampling. Am J Obstet Gynecol 1991;164:339.

15. Bowman J, Harman C, Menticoglou S, Pollock J. Intravenous fetal transfusion of immunoglobulin for alloimmune thrombocytopenia. [Letter] The Lancet 1992;340: 1034–1035.

16. Nicolini U, Kochenour N, Greco P, et al. Consequences of fetomaternal hemorrhage after intrauterine transfusion. Br Med J 1988;297:1379–1381.

17. Pielet BW, Socol ML, MacGregor SN, et al. Cordocentesis: an appraisal of risks. Am J Obstet Gynecol 1988;159:1497–1500.

18. Wilkins I, Mezrow G, Lynch L, et al. Amnionitis and life-threatening respiratory distress after percutaneous umbilical blood sampling. Am J Obstet Gynecol 1989; 160:427–428.

19. Ludomirski A, Weiner S. Percutaneous fetal umbilical blood sampling. Clin Obstet Gynecol 1988;31:19–26.

20. Daffos F, Forestier F, Capella-Pavlovsky M, et al. Prenatal management of 746 pregnancies at risk for congenital toxoplasmosis. N Engl J Med 1988;318:271–275.

21. Morgan-Capner P, Rodeck CH, Nicolaides KH, et al. Prenatal detection of rubella-specific IgM in fetal sera. Prenat Diag 1979; 5:21–26.

22. Lange IR, Rodeck CH, Morgan-Capner P, et al. Prenatal diagnosis of intrauterine cytomegalovirus infection. Br Med J 1982; 284:1673–1674.

23. Cuthbertson G, Weiner CP, Giller RH et al. Prenatal diagnosis of second trimester cogenital varicella syndrome by virus-specific immunoglobulin. J Pediatr 1987; 111:592–595.

24. Naides SJ, Weiner CP. Antenatal diagnosis and palliative treatment of nonimmune hydrops fetalis secondary to fetal parvovirus B19 infection. Prenat Diag 1989;9: 105–114.

25. Knisely AS, O'Shea PA, McMillan P, et al. Electron microscopic identification of parvovirus virions in euthyroid-line cells in fatal hydrops fetalis. Pediatr Path 1988; 8:163–170.

26. Daffos F, Forestier F, Kaplan C, et al. Prenatal diagnosis and management of bleeding disorders with fetal blood sampling. Am J Obstet Gynecol 1988;158: 939–946.

27. Hoyer LW, Lindsten J, Blomback RM, et al. Prenatal evaluation of a fetus at risk for von Willebrand's disease. The Lancet 1979; ii:191–192.

28. Bussel JB, Berkowitz RL, McFarlane JG, et al. Antenatal treatment of alloimmune thrombocytopenia. N Engl J Med 1988; 319:1374–1378.

29. Cao A, Furbetta M, Angius A, et al. Prenatal diagnosis of betathalassemia: experience with 133 cases and the effect of fetal blood sampling on child development. Ann NY Acad Sci 1980;344:165.

30. Weatherall DJ, Old JM, Thein SL, et al. Prenatal diagnosis of the common hemoglobin disorders. J Med Genet 1985;22: 422–430.

31. Newburger PE, Cohen HJ, Rothchild SB, et al. Prenatal diagnosis of chronic granulomatous disease. N Engl J Med 1979; 300:178–183.

32. Harman CR, Manning FA, Bowman JM, Pollack J, Menticoglous S. Fetal umbilical venous blood gases and pH in anemic fetuses: changes with maternal hyperoxygenation. Am J Obstet Gynecol 1994 (in press).

33. Soothill PW, Nicolaides KH, Rodeck CH, et al. Blood gases and acid-base status of the human second trimester fetus. Obstet Gynecol 1986;68:173–176.

34. Soothill PW, Nicolaides KH, Rodeck CH. Fetal blood gas and acid-base parameters. Rodeck CH, ed. Fetal Medicine. Oxford: Blackwell Scientific, 1989: 57ff.

35. Bonnin P, Guyot B, Bailliart O, et al. Relationship between umbilical and fetal cerebral blood flow velocity waveforms and umbilical venous gases. Ultras Obstet Gynecol 1991;2:18–22.

36. Soothill PW, Nicolaides KH, Bilardo C, et al. Uteroplacental blood velocity resistance index and umbilical venous pO_2, pCO_2, pH, lactate, and erythroblast count in growth-retarded fetuses. Fetal Therapy 1986; 4:174–179.

37. Soothill PW, Nicolaides KH, Campbell S. Prenatal asphyxia, hyperlactemia, hypoglycaemia, and erythroblastosis in growth-retarded fetuses. Br Med J 1987;1: 1051–1053.

FETAL INFECTIOUS DISEASES: INVESTIGATION AND THERAPIES

4

F. DAFFOS
F. FORESTIER
L. LYNCH
P. HOHLFELD

Congenital infections can be the cause of diseases in the neonate and are sometimes responsible for severe handicaps. Under specific circumstances, they can be prevented and treated. We do not intend to describe all these infections. We have selected five, rubella, cytomegalovirus, varicella, toxoplasmosis, and parvovirus, for their importance from a practical point of view.

RUBELLA

The syndrome of congenital rubella was first described in 1941 by an Australian ophthalmologist (1). The virus of rubella is among the most pathogenic agents that can affect an embryo or a fetus. The most frequently encountered injury is neurosensory deafness. Before vaccination became the rule, rubella was responsible for 16% of the cases of deafness of central origin (2). Many other injuries, including cardiac malformations (persistent ductus arteriosus, ventricular septal defect) as well as eye lesions (cataract, microphthalmia, glaucoma, retinopathy) can be associated with it. The lesions of the central nervous system, including microcephaly, encephalitis, or mental retardation, can be extremely serious. These malformations are generally associated with intrauterine growth retardation (IUGR) and a dysfunction of the hematopoietic system (3). Lastly, 10 to 15% of the rubella infections contracted during the first trimester result in spontaneous abortion (4).

Risks to the Fetus

The risk of fetal infections and malformations varies with the different stages of pregnancy (5). The risk of infection is about 66% up to 12 weeks and 45% between 13 and 18 weeks of amenorrhea.

It is more difficult to assess the risk of fetal malformation, but serious and multiple damage is the rule when the infection occurs before 11 weeks of gestation (6). During the early second trimester, the global percentage of malformations is about 35%. After the 17th week of pregnancy, no further severe damage is observed and the children only present subclinical forms of congenital rubella (7). It is not possible, however, to evaluate the possible long-term effects on neuropsychiatric development.

Prenatal Diagnosis and Subsequent Approach

Diagnosis is made by fetal blood sampling at or after the 22nd week of pregnancy by detection of specific anti-rubella IgM. IgM can be synthetized by the fetus by the 12th week of amenorrhea, but the presence of these antibodies can be found constantly only after the 22nd week. The diagnosis is also based on the presence of other biological signs, such as erythroblastosis, variable anemia, thrombocytopenia, and increased gamma-GT, LDH, and interferon (8). Direct detection of the virus can also be done by culture.

Maternal reinfections may occur, especially in patients with very low levels of antibodies after vaccination. Reinfections can be serologically defined as a significant increase of the IgG with or without the appearance of IgM. In such cases, the risk of fetal infection is low but exists (9), and cases of severe lesions have been described after reinfection (10). Therefore is it highly recommended to obtain a rubella serology for all patients, including women who had positive IgG during a previous pregnancy, at the beginning of the pregnancy. It is also essential to perform further serological tests in cases of exposure, even for positive patients.

We performed 119 prenatal diagnoses of congenital rubella. Fifty-four were done for maternal seroconversion before 12 weeks, 31 were positive (57%), 30 pregnancies were terminated, one was continued. (At birth, congenital rubella infection was confirmed, but the baby had no clinical damage.) Twenty-three prenatal diagnoses ruled out fetal infection (43%). One case was a misdiagnosis. This mistake occurred at the beginning of our experience, when our knowledge of fetal immune response was limited. Fetal blood sampling was performed too early (before 22 weeks).

Sixty-five diagnoses were performed for maternal infection between 13 and 18 weeks of amenorrhea. Thirty-six of them were negative (56%), and all the babies were healthy at birth. Twenty-nine were positive (44%). In 15 cases, the mothers requested termination of the pregnancy. Fourteen pregnancies were continued, and one of the babies had severe deafness at birth.

Prevention

Active immunization by vaccination is the only efficient way of preventing congenital rubella. Two strategies have been suggested: vaccination for all children or selective vaccination of all females of childbearing age. Generalized vaccination stops virus transmission, reduces the risks of an epidemic, and in an indirect way, protects non-vaccinated females. Selective vaccination protects the subjects at risk, limits the use of the vaccine, and allows the virus to circulate among the population. At the present time, the first solution seems to yield better results (11). One should never forget, however, that over 50% of congenital rubella syndrome appear in multiparae (3), which underscores the importance of vaccinating sero-negative women in the postpartum period. Postpartum vaccination alone would reduce the cases currently on record by more than half.

Vaccination is contraindicated during pregnancy, but it does not mean that the pregnancy should be terminated after such a vaccination. The risk of fetal infection varies from 3–20%, according to the vaccine utilized (3), but no case of congenital rubella has ever been described following a vaccination. Theoretically vaccination is 95% effective, and, in practice, 85%.

Passive immunization by injection of specific immunoglobulins can be performed in cases of exposure during pregnancy. It is obviously useless if it is administered once the rash has appeared. Patients treated in this way may sustain a subclinical infection, and their serological condition should, therefore, be checked regularly. However, there is no evidence that passive immunization prevents fetal infection or damage.

CYTOMEGALOVIRUS (CMV)

Cytomegalovirus is the most frequently observed congenital infection, with an incidence varying from 0.2–2.2% of live births, depending on the populations studied(12). The contagiousness of CMV is relatively low and its transmission requires prolonged and close contact (sexual intercourse, oropharyngeal secretions, or transfusion of blood products). The infection is most often asymptomatic during pregnancy, and in Europe, 45% of pregnant women are positive at the beginning of pregnancy. In the United States, 55% of pregnant women in higher income groups and 85% of those in lower income groups are seropositive (13).

Risks to the Fetus

The risk of primary infection during pregnancy for seronegative women ranges from one to four percent. In 40% of the cases, the virus will be transmitted to the fetus. Eighty-five to 90% of the infected infants are asymptomatic at birth, and only 10% of these are likely to develop sequelae, most commonly hearing loss. The other 10 to 15% of the infected infants have symptoms at birth (14), including petechiae, thrombocytopenia, increased conjugated bilirubin, hepatosplenomegaly, chorioretinitis, microcephaly, and intracerebral calcifications. Pass (15) published the long term follow-up of 34 children suffering from cytomegalic inclusions disease: 10 of them were dead before the age of two years (most had died at the age of three months), 16 had microcephaly, and cerebral palsy was extremely frequent. Twelve of them had impaired hearing or vision and the IQ of 10 of the 24 survivors was under 80.

The transplacental transmission of CMV does not depend on the time when the mother was infected. Fetal infection has been described after primary infection during the first, second, and third trimesters of pregnancy (4), but the risk of symptoms and sequelae seems to be notably higher when the infection occurs during the first 27 weeks (16). There may be recurrences and reinfections, and the risk of fetal infection, then, is the same as with primary infections. In such cases, however, the risk of fetal damage is very low, if one considers that in areas where all pregnant women are seropositive, no handicaps caused by CMV are observed (17). However, cases of fetal damage have been reported (18). We have performed 16 prenatal diagnoses of CMV in our departments. Indications were maternal seroconversion in eight cases, severe unexplained IUGR in three, and ultrasound abnormalities suggestive of congenital CMV in five. Prenatal diagnosis confirmed the fetal infection in seven cases, three of which were terminated. Of the remainder, one

baby was healthy at birth and three died of massive CMV infection.

Prenatal Diagnosis

Prenatal diagnosis is based on fetal blood sampling and amniocentesis at 20 to 23 weeks. The virus itself can be isolated in amniotic fluid or fetal blood with the former being more reliable. Other nonspecific signs of infections, such as thrombocytopenia, elevated gamma-GTP and total IgM may also be seen. It can be assumed that infected fetuses with untrasonographic signs of brain injury or evidence of hematopoietic or hepatic disease have an extremely high probability of severe disease and sequelae.

Prevention

Vaccination is not widely available and consists of a live attenuated virus, which should not be administered during pregnancy. Passive immunization is not possible since exposure to the infection cannot be identified in most cases. Given the particularities of CMV infection and the lack of prophalaxis or treatment, routine screening of pregnant women during pregnancy does not seem to be justified. One might consider testing early in pregnancy for it would permit diagnosis of a primary infection if clinically suspected. A further serological assay could also be considered at 20 weeks in selected cases since the most severe infections occur during the first half of pregnancy. This could be applied to sero-negative women whose profession entails close contact with children, e.g., hospitals, day-care centers. The only mode of transmission of the CMV that can be prevented by the obstetrician is infection resulting from transfusions. Any pregnant woman receiving blood transfusions during pregnancy should receive CMV-negative blood, whatever her serological status may be.

For all these reasons, CMV congenital infections will probably remain a major cause of handicap in years to come. Nowadays, the number of seriously affected children is about equal to the number of congenital rubellas observed in nonepidemic years before vaccination was performed.

VARICELLA

Primary varicella is rarely an adult's disease. Approximately 95% of pregnant women are immune. Its incidence can be estimated at one to five cases in 10,000 pregnancies. However, maternal morbidity and mortality is relatively high. Out of 118 cases described in the medical literature, 20% had pneumonia, 10% of which resulted in the mother's death (19). But, it should be pointed out that only the most serious cases are described in the literature.

Risks to the Fetus

The virus is seldom transmitted to the fetus (1–2% of the cases). The syndrome of congenital varicella consists of typical malformations, such as cutaneous scars, hypoplasia of the hands and feet, cerebral cortical atrophy, mental retardation with convulsions, eye lesions, such as chorioretinitis or cataract, and IUGR. The risk of congenital varicella syndrome seems to be limited to first and early second trimester infections. All the cases of congenital varicella syndrome described have followed infections occurring between the seventh and the 21st week of pregnancy.

The pathogenesis of the lesions observed in cases of congenital varicella is not clear. Higa (20) hypothesized that these injuries

are not caused by the direct action of the virus but could result from the occurrence of genuine intrauterine fetal shingles.

The immunity conferred by varicella is stable, and further infections are practically non-existent. The risk of maternal varicella zoster is probably negligible because viremia is less frequent and the fetus is protected by the presence of maternal antibodies. Nevertheless, some cases of congenital varicella syndrome have occurred following a zoster infection (17).

Prenatal Diagnosis and Subsequent Approach

In view of the small risk observed, termination of pregnancy is not indicated in cases of maternal varicella. Prenatal diagnosis by fetal blood sampling may be justified considering the severe central nervous system lesions observed in cases of fetal infection. Maternal varicella near the time of delivery carries a risk of neonatal varicella. In such cases, the risk of fetal infection ranges from 25–30%. The severity of neonatal varicella depends on the time of maternal infection with respect to delivery and on the development of maternal IgG. Maternal varicella occurring from five to 21 days before delivery and developing in the infant during the first four days of its life will have a variable outcome with a good prognosis. When it occurs four days before to two days after delivery, which means that the child will develop the disease five to 10 days after birth, the infection can be very severe, with a very high risk of morbidity or mortality. The difference between benign neonatal disease during the first four days of life and the more severe manifestations of neonatal varicella at five to 10 days of life can easily be accounted for. In the first case, the maternal antibodies are present with a very high concentration in fetal blood and protect the infant, whereas in the second case, the concentration of maternal antibodies in fetal blood is too low to ensure adequate protection.

Prevention

Passive immunization is currently available and should be administered within 24–72 hours to sero-negative pregnant patients who have been exposed to varicella.

Once the rash is present, immunoglobulins should only be used at term if delivery is anticipated within four to five days.

Acyclovir crosses placental barrier (21) and has been proposed by some authors for varicella occurring near delivery (22). However, the fetal effects are unknown, thus it cannot be recommended early in pregnancy.

TOXOPLASMOSIS

Toxoplasmosis is a parasitic disease caused by a protozoan, *Toxoplasma gondii*. The cat is the only natural host. However, the toxoplasma can infect many animals, (including humans). Humans can be either directly infected from cat feces or indirectly by ingestion of undercooked meat from parasitized animals. Infection is frequent but most often asymptomatic, except in cases of immunodeficiency. For pregnant women, the consequences of infection may be serious if the parasite is transmitted to the fetus. In Europe, about 50% of the women of childbearing age are immune to the disease.

Risks to the Fetus

The risk of fetal infection is 7% (23), but it varies with the time of seroconversion and regularly increases from the beginning to the end of pregnancy (Table 4-1). Transmission to the fetus results from placental infection and secondary passage into the fetal

Table 4-1 Incidence of Fetal Infection in Cases of Acquired Toxoplasmosis According to Gestational Age

Periconceptional Maternal Infection	1.2%
• Maternal infection between 6 and 16 weeks	4.5%
• Maternal infection between 21 and 35 weeks	17.3%
• Maternal infection between 21 and 35 weeks	28.9%

circulation. On the other hand, the earlier the fetus is infected, the more serious are the sequelae. Severe congenital toxoplasmosis is a rare but most dangerous form of the disease, especially when the fetus has been infected during the first trimester of pregnancy. It is characterized by multisystemic damage and causes, in particular, destruction of cerebral tissue often associated with cerebral ventricle dilatation.

Prenatal Diagnosis and Treatment

Prenatal diagnosis is based on ultrasound examination, amniocentesis, and fetal blood sampling (24). It can be performed as of 18 to 20 weeks of amenorrhea. The analysis of fetal blood allows the detection of indirect biological signs of infection, i.e., leukocytosis, eosinophilia, thrombocytopenia, elevated levels of total IgM, and gamma-glutamyltransferase, and specific fetal IgM. Parasitological tests include inoculation of fetal blood and amniotic fluid into mice and fibroblast cultures.

According to the prenatal diagnosis, three different approaches may be proposed. If the fetus is not infected, the treatment with spiramycin should be continued in order to avoid later contamination from an infected placenta, and ultrasound examinations will suffice until delivery.

Spiramycin is an antibiotic whose activity in toxoplasmosis has been experimentally and clinically documented (25). Its tissue concentration in the placenta is excellent, and it passes through the fetoplacental barrier having been found in fetal blood sampled for prenatal diagnosis (26). When toxoplasmosis occurs during pregnancy, spiramycin reduces the risk of fetal infection by 60% (27). Its purpose is not to treat an already infected fetus but to prevent the parasite from passing into the fetal circulation. The lapse of time between maternal seroconversion and the onset of spiramycin therapy seems to be of importance, as a prolonged interval is more often associated with the presence of severe fetal lesions on prenatal diagnosis (23). A dose of 3g/day is necessary to obtain adequate placental concentrations. This treatment involves no particular risk, with excellent tolerance even when it is administered over long periods of time. No hepatotoxicity has ever been reported, nor any interference with other drugs.

If the fetus is infected following toxoplasmosis acquired during the first trimester or if the ultrasound reveals cerebral damage, termination of the pregnancy should be considered. A study of 1200 cases of seroconversion during pregnancy (23) showed that termination was only necessary in a very low percentage (2.7%) of cases. All the other cases of confirmed fetal infection should be treated with specific and anti-*T.gondii* drugs. This treatment is reserved for the cases where fetal infection has been demonstrated by prenatal diagnosis [Table 4-2 (outlines the therapeutic protocol)]. Pyrimethamine 50mg/day is the most active agent against toxoplasmosis (28). This drug behaves as a folic acid antagonist, which explains its toxicity in tissues with high metabolic activity, particularly hematopoietic cells. Administration of folinic acid 15 mg/day can correct or prevent hematological disorders without affecting treatment efficacy since this substance does not seem to be absorbed by the parasite. It is advisable to check platelet and leucocyte counts as well as hemoglobin concentration.

Sulfadiazine is commonly prescribed. Its antitoxoplasmic action can be achieved in nontoxic doses. Its use would be ill-advised in cases of G_6P_D deficiency, allergy to sulfa drugs and leukopenia (28). The combination of pyrimethamine and sulfadiazine is the treatment presently preferred. This regimen is used in three-week courses alternating with spiramycin. The synergistic action of these two drugs is excellent (29). The pyrimethamine-sulfadiazine combina-

Table 4-2 Treatment in Cases of Toxoplasmosis Acquired During Pregnancy

Therapy	Dosage	When	Indications
Spiramycin	3g/day	Start as soon as seroconversion is documented and continue throughout pregnancy regardless of the prenatal diagnosis results	In all cases of seroconversion during pregnancy
Pyrimethamine	50mg/day	Not before prenatal diagnosis	Only for infected
Sulfadiazine	3g/day	3 week courses	fetuses

tion has also been used and is effective against *Toxoplasma gondii,* but it is seldom prescribed because of possible side effects (Lyell syndrome).

In the above-mentioned study, the intrauterine treatment of infected fetuses allowed the delivery of 53 healthy children, 44 had subclinical toxoplasmosis and nine had benign signs. These children underwent follow-up for periods from six months to four years. None of them developed a severe toxoplasmosis, and they all had normal psychomotor development.

Such an approach to diagnosis and treatment is beneficial in many ways. First of all it avoids a large number of unecessary terminations of pregnancy. The treatment, which may prove dangerous and is in any case considered ill-advised before 16 weeks of pregnancy, is reserved for infected fetuses. It also allows a more accurate follow-up during the first year of the child's life. If the mothers receive a "blind" treatment, it becomes impossible at the time of birth to tell the noninfected children from those who have been cured. Then, it becomes mandatory to treat all the children during at least eight months, knowing that this treatment is totally useless for some 93% of them. Lastly, children who receive intrauterine treatment have favorable outcomes without significant sequelae.

Prevention
___

It is most important to warn sero-negative pregnant women about the precautions they should take (Table 4-3).

Finally, serological screening during pregnancy should allow detection of seroconversions, prenatal diagnosis, and adequate treatment.

Table 4-3 Prevention of Toxoplasmosis: Advice to Pregnant Women Whose Serological Tests Are Negative

- Cook meat at 60° C + (Industrial deep-freezing also seems to destroy parasites efficiently)
- When handling raw meat, do not touch eyes or mouth
- Carefully wash hands after handling raw meat, dirt, or vegetables soiled by dirt
- Wash fruit and vegetables before eating
- Wear gloves when gardening
- Avoid all contacts with things that may have been contaminated by cat feces
- If the cat's litter has to be changed, put on gloves and disinfect often with boiling water

PARVOVIRUS

The pathogenic effect of parvovirus, particularly B19, on the fetus has been recognized for less than 10 years. The classical maternal symptoms are the typical facial rash and arthralgias, which are not very specific and usually do not lead to prenatal diagnosis.

Most often, prenatal diagnosis is considered once fetal hydrops is diagnosed on ultrasound. This is a consequence of acute fetal anemia due to the direct effect of the virus on the red blood cell precursors. B19 develops only in erythroid precursors (BFU-E) and results in acute anemia and fetal death in 10–30% of cases (30).

Prenatal Diagnosis
___

Prenatal diagnosis is easily performed on fetal blood, which demonstrates an aplastic anemia and the presence of the virus (electron microscopy or DNA analysis).

Evolution of Pregnancy

Most hydropic fetuses will die of cardiac failure if in utero treatment is not instituted. However, spontaneous in utero recoveries have been reported without any sequelae at birth. Correction of the anemia by fetal blood transfusions is the only available treatment (31).

References

1. Gregg NM. Congenital cataract following German measles in the mother. Trans Ophtalmol Soc Aust. 1941;334–345.
2. Peckham CS, Martin JAM, Marshal WC, et al. Congenital rubella deafness: a preventable disease. The Lancet 1979; 1:258–261.
3. Preblud SR, Alfort CA. Rubella. In: Remington JS, Klein JO, eds. Infectious disease of the fetus and newborn infant, (3rd ed). Philadelphia: WB Saunders Company, 1990:196–240.
4. Enders G. Infektionen und impfungen in der Schwangerschaft. Erhan and Schwarzenberg. München 1988.
5. Enders G, Nickerl-Pacher U, Miller E, et al. Outcome of confirmed periconceptional maternal rubella. The Lancet 1988;i: 1445–1447.
6. Miller E, Cradock-Watson JE, Pollock TM. Consequences of confirmed maternal rubella at successive stages of pregnancy. The Lancet 1982;2:781.
7. Grillner L, Forsgren M, Barr B, et al. Outcome of rubella during pregnancy with special reference to the 17–24th week of gestation. Scand J Infect Dis 1983;15:321–325.
8. Daffos F, Forestier F, Grangeot-Kéros L, et al. Prenatal diagnosis of congenital rubella. The Lancet 1984;11:1–3.
9. Hornstein L, Levy U, Fogel A. Clinical rubella with virus transmission to the fetus in a pregnant woman considered to be immune. N Engl J Med 1988;21:1415–1416.
10. Enders G, Jonatha W. Prenatal diagnosis of intrauterine rubella. Infection 1987;3: 162–164.
11. Rudd P, Peckham C. Infection of the fetus and the newborn: prevention, treatment, and related handicap. Clin Obstet and Gynecol 1988;2:56–71.
12. Stagno S, Pass RF, Dworsky ME et al. Congenital and perinatal cytomegalovirus infections. Sem Perinatol 1983;7:31–42.
13. Stagno S, Whitley RH. Herpes virus infections of pregnancy: Part I. Cytomegalovirus and Epstein Barr Virus Infections. N Engl J Med 1985, 313:1270–1274.
14. Stagno S. Cytomegalovirus. In: Remington JS, Klein JO, eds. Infectious disease of the fetus and newborn infant (3rd ed). Philadelphia: WB Saunders.
15. Pass RF, Stagno S, Myers GJ, et al. Outcome of symptomatic congenital cytomegalovirus infection: results of long-term longitudinal follow-up. Pediatrics 1980; 66:758–762.
16. Stagno S, Pass RF, Cloud G, et al. Primary cytomegalovirus infection in pregnancy. JAMA 1986;256:1904–1908.
17. Schopfer K, Lauber E, Krech U. Congenital cytomegalovirus infection in newborn infants of mothers infected before pregnancy. Arch Dis Childhood 1978;53:536–539.
18. Harris S, Ivarison S, Svonberg L. Secondary maternal cytomegalovirus infection causing symptomatic congenital infection. N Eng J Med 1981;305:284.
19. Gershon A. Chickenpox, measles and mumps. In: Remington JS, Klein JO, eds. Infectious disease of the fetus and newborn infant, (3rd ed). Philadelphia: WB Saunders, 1990:395–345.
20. Higa K, Dan K, Manabe H: Varicella zoster infections during pregnancy: hypothesis concerning the mechanisms of congenital malformations. Obstet Gynecol 1987;69:214–222.
21. Greffe BS, Krasny HC, Dooley SL, et al. Transplacental passage of acyclovir. J Pediatr 1986;108:1020–1021.
22. Haddad J, Messer J, Willard et al. Acyclovir et grossesse: aspects actuels. J Gynecol Obstet Biol Reprod 1989;18:679–683.
23. Hohlfeld P, Daffos F, Thulliez P, et al. Fetal toxoplasmosis: outcome of pregnancy and infant follow-up after in utero treatment. J Pediatr 1989;115:765–769.

24. Daffos F, Forestier F, Capella-Pavlovsky M, et al. Prenatal management of 746 pregnancies at risk for congenital toxoplasmosis. N Engl J Med 1988;318:271–275.
25. Kernbaum S. La spiramycine. Utilisation en thérapeutique humaine. Sem Hôp Paris 1982;58:289–297.
26. Forestier F, Daffos F, Rainaut M, et al. Suivi thérapeutique foetomaternel de la spiramycine en cours de grossesse. Arch Fr Pédiatr 1987;44:539–544.
27. Desmont G, Couvreur J. Congenital toxoplasmosis: a prospective study of 78 pregnancies. N Engl J Med 1974;290:1110–1116.
28. Marcon P, Thulliez P. Traitement de la toxoplasmose congénitale. J Pediatr Puéricult 1988;4:210–214.
29. Couvreur J. Traitement de la toxoplasmose congénitale. Le Pédiatre 1987;102: 5–16.
30. Peters MT, Nicolaides KH. Cordocentesis for the diagnosis and treatment of human fetal parvovirus infection. Obstet Gynecol 1990, 75: 501–504.
31. Soothill P. Intrauterine blood transfusion for nonimmune hydrops fetalis due to parvovirus B19 infection. The Lancet 1990; 336:121–122.

THE BIOCHEMICAL ASSESSMENT OF THE HUMAN FETUS: NORMS AND APPLICATIONS

5

CARL P. WEINER

Safe access to the fetal circulation has opened many new possibilities for both the direct evaluation and treatment of fetal disease. One such possibility is laboratory assessment. There has been sufficient study to safely state that the fetus responds to both normal and abnormal alterations in its environment in a manner that enhances the chance of survival. Knowledge of that response permits the fetologist to more accurately diagnose the cause and determine the impact of the disorder. Armed with an accurate biochemical assessment of the fetus prior to therapy, the fetal response can then be monitored in a more sophisticated fashion than previously possible.

This chapter focuses on several areas where the biochemical assessment of the fetus is presently or potentially of value: growth dysfunction, fetal heart rate abnormalities (exclusive of arrhythmias), nonimmune hydrops fetalis and fetal hyper/hypothyroidism. Other applicable disorders, such as fetal hemolytic disease and cardiac arrhythmias, are discussed in separate chapters of this book.

NORMAL

The interpretation of fetal biochemistry requires knowledge of the norm. Though an obvious premise, such knowledge has been difficult to acquire since truly normal fetuses are not often subject to blood sampling. Even a busy fetal diagnosis and treatment unit will test many abnormal fetuses before obtaining data on one normal fetus. The difficulty acquiring an adequate sample size is compounded by the fact that many laboratory parameters change with gestation. Further, the concentrations of several biochemical parameters differ in the umbilical vein and artery, requiring that the vessel sampled be identi-

fied definitively. Few of the pioneering studies of the human fetus took the vessel sampled into account. When considered, erroneous identification of the vessel was possible since the vessel pressure was not measured.

While nomograms exist for a variety of laboratory parameters, many have been based on populations that included either a poorly defined population, samples obtained at delivery, or fetuses with a variety of problems assumed by the authors not to impact upon the study variable (1–12). The latter requires an assumption that cannot be substantiated until the true normal is known, and results based on samples obtained at either hysterotomy or cesarean section may have been influenced by such factors as the maternal fasting condition or transient maternal hypotension. The latter alters placental perfusion.

The most accurate nomograms will be based on normal fetuses evaluated either because of maternal alloimmunization and found to be antigen-negative or because of maternal primary infection and found to be uninfected (13–16). Unfortunately, some of these studies either did not consider gestation at all, or did not span a wide enough range, (13,14). Figures 5-1–5-18 are nomograms developed at the University of Iowa for a variety of potentially useful fetal parameters available in most hospitals based solely on documented healthy fetuses.

Indications for Fetal Biochemical Assessment

Intrauterine Growth Deficiency

Depending upon the definition employed, one out of 10 fetuses will be small for gestation; about two-thirds of these will actually have reduced body mass and the remainder appropriately grown but short. Growth deficiency is the largest diagnostic

Effect of Gestation on Total RBC Count

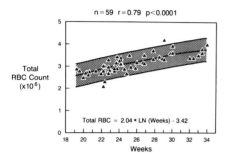

Figure 5-1   95% prediction interval for the normal fetal RBC count across gestation (17).

Effect of Gestation on Hematocrit

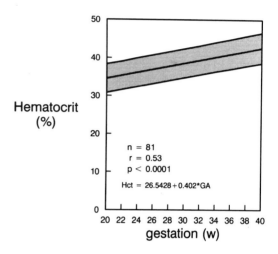

Figure 5-3   95% prediction interval for the normal fetal hematocrit count (g/dL) across gestation (16).

Effect of Gestation on Hemoglobin

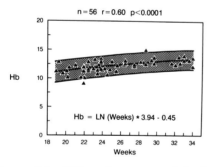

Figure 5-2   95% prediction interval for the normal fetal hemoglobin concentration (g/dL) across gestation (17).

Effect of Gestation on the WBC Count

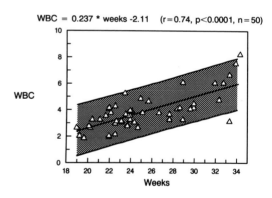

Figure 5-4   95% prediction interval for the normal fetal WBC count ($\times 10^3$) across gestation (17).

Effect of Gestation on
Platelet Number

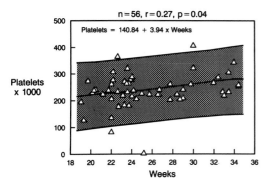

Figure 5-5 95% prediction interval for the normal fetal platelet count ($\times 10^6$) across gestation (17).

Effect of Gestation on the
Mean Platelet Volume (fL)

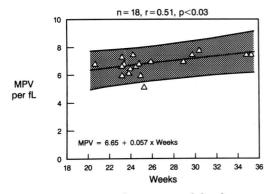

Figure 5-6 95% prediction interval for the normal fetal mean platelet volume count (fL) across gestation (17).

Effect of Gestation on
Total Protein

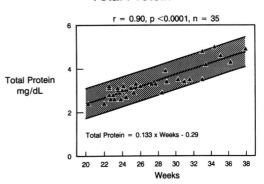

Figure 5-7 95% prediction interval for the normal fetal total protein concentration (mg/dL) across gestation (17).

Effect of Gestation
on Albumen

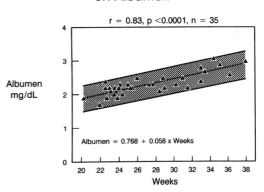

Figure 5-8 95% prediction interval for the normal fetal albumen concentration (mg/dL) across gestation (17).

Effect of Gestation on LDH

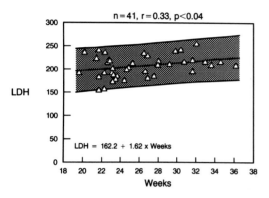

Figure 5-9 95% prediction interval for the normal fetal total LD concentration (IU/ml) across gestation (17).

Effect of Gestation on AST

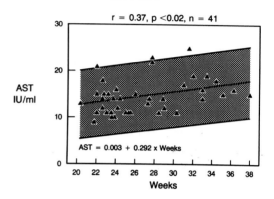

Figure 5-11 95% prediction interval for the normal fetal total AST concentration (IU/ml) across gestation (17).

Relationship Between LDH and UVpH

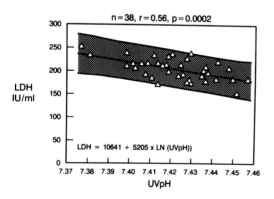

Figure 5-10 95% prediction interval of the relationship between normal fetal LDpH gestation (17).

Effect of Gestation on ALT

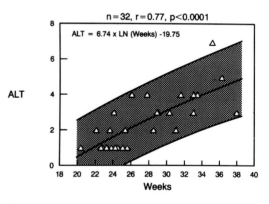

Figure 5-12 95% prediction interval for the normal fetal ALT concentration (IU/ml) across gestation (17).

Effect of Gestation on Normal Fetal GGT

(n = 26)

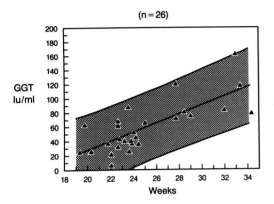

Figure 5-13   95% prediction interval for the normal fetal GGT concentration (IU/ml) across gestation (17).

Effect of Gestation on UVpH

n = 59, r = -0.23, p = 0.08

UVpH = 7.449 + 0.001 x Weeks

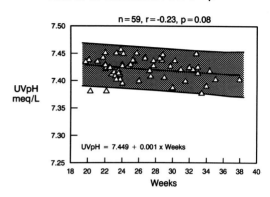

Figure 5-15   95% prediction interval for the normal fetal UVpH (meq/L) across gestation (17).

Effect of Gestation on the Total Bilirubin

Total Bilirubin = Weeks * 0.059 + 0.194

— REGRESS

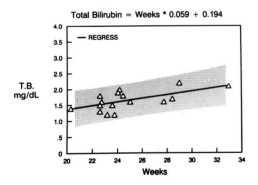

Figure 5-14   95% prediction interval for the normal fetal total bilirubin (mg/dL) across gestation (15).

Effect of Gestation on the UVpCO₂

n = 58, r = 0.34, p = 0.009

$UVpCO_2$ = 29.36 + 0.21 x Weeks

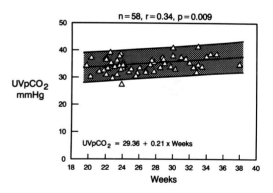

Figure 5-16   95% prediction interval for the normal fetal UVpCO₂ (mmHg) across gestation (17).

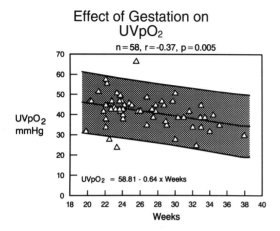

Figure 5-17 95% prediction interval for the normal fetal UVpO$_2$ (mmHg) across gestation (17).

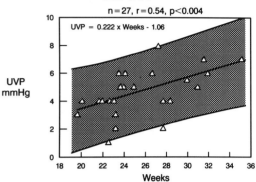

Figure 5-19 95% prediction interval for the normal fetal UVP (mmHg) across gestation (17).

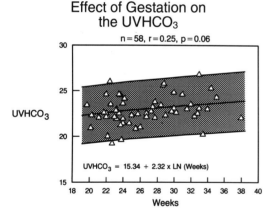

Figure 5-18 95% prediction interval for the normal fetal UVHCO$_3$ (meq/L) across gestation (17).

group of patients for the fetologist and potentially the largest group amenable to antenatal therapy. Assuming that the antenatal diagnosis of fetal growth deficiency can be made accurately (presently a tenuous assumption discussed in a companion chapter), it should be asked which fetuses are potential candidates for blood sampling? All? The answer is a certain "No!" There is little, if any, clinically important informa-

tion gained by the phlebotomy of a structurally normal fetus with late-onset growth deficiency. They are almost always asymmetric in character and the result of placental dysfunction (18). Delivery, even if one to two weeks preterm, subjects the fetus to less risk than cordocentesis (PUBS). Unfortunately, the postnatal workup is usually inadequate to determine whether they are in fact malnourished and not infected. Since they appear "normal," the diagnosis of growth deficiency is usually based on weight.

PUBS is clearly indicated for the evaluation of the fetus with either severe, early onset, i.e., detectable prior to 32 weeks, or symmetric growth deficiency (whenever detected). The differential diagnosis includes a karyotypic abnormality (about 20%), congenital infection (about 10%), maternal or fetal systemic disease (less than 1%), and by exclusion, uteroplacental dysfunction (about 70%) (personal experience). Though a karyotype may be obtained from a variety of fetal tissues, only a fetal blood sample allows a comprehensive approach to all possibilities. At the University of

Iowa, this diagnosis requires both a fetal abdominal circumference centile < 2.5 and an estimated fetal weight centile < 10. Such stringency is necessary to minimize the likelihood of subjecting a normally grown fetus to the risk of PUBS.

Though the karyotype is essential, the central diagnostic problem is differentiating growth deficiency secondary to congenital infection from that secondary to uteroplacental dysfunction. The accurate diagnosis of fetal infection requires the use of both direct (culture, electron microscopy, and serology) and indirect laboratory markers (quantitative IgM, liver enzymes, complete blood count, etc.). Fetal serology is woefully insensitive as the sole element for the identification of congenital infection in a symptomatic fetus. Unfortunately, we remain without a laboratory marker highly predictive of either viral or parasitic infection. Polymerase chain reaction technology may ultimately supply the solution.

i. Respiratory Blood Gases

Hypoxia (with or without metabolic/ metabolic-respiratory acidosis) often accompanies severe growth deficiency. This is true whether the etiology is a chromosome abnormality, congenital infection, or uteroplacental dysfunction (19,20). Clearly, "birth asphyxia" does not necessarily occur at birth. Approximately one-half of growth-restricted fetuses without a chromosome abnormality have evidence of increased placental resistance (based on Doppler velocimetry). A lower, but not insignificant, percentage of fetuses small because of congenital infection also have evidence of increased placental resistance. Preliminary study suggests this results from viral placentitis. Different from the course observed with uteroplacen-

tal dysfunction, the placental resistance may decline as the placental inflammatory response to the virus decreases. We have yet to observe hypoxia in a growth-deficient fetus with normal umbilical artery Doppler velocimetry. We have, however, seen a metabolic acidosis characterized by a large anion gap in association with a normal umbilical artery resistance index and a chronic viral infection.

Which vessel should be sampled in the process of evaluating severe, early-onset growth deficiency? Theoretically, the umbilical artery would supply the most information about the fetus and the umbilical vein the most information about the placenta. However, primary fetal acidosis is very rare. If the umbilical venous respiratory blood gases are abnormal, one can safely assume that the umbilical artery will also be abnormal. Since the risk of a procedure-related bradycardia is increased manifoldly by the combination of umbilical artery puncture and severe growth deficiency, our practice is to always target the umbilical vein.

In uteroplacental dysfunction, the lower the fetal pO_2, the higher the fetal pCO_2 and the lower the fetal pH (20, 21). Fetuses with markedly abnormal umbilical blood gases usually have abnormal, noninvasive fetal surveillance tests, e.g., nonstress test, contraction stress test, and biophysical profile, (personal observation, 22–24). The clinical dilemma is whether or when to act on a modestly abnormal fetal blood gas documented during the evaluation of a severely growth deficient fetus whose noninvasive surveillance tests are acceptable.

Before any decision is made, the possibility of a technical error must be considered. How was the sampled vessel identified? Was the pressure measured? Would the values obtained be acceptable if instead of the umbilical vein, the umbilical artery had been punctured? Was the cordocentesis performed with the woman positioned with her uterus displaced off the great vessels? Was there a fetal bradycardia at the time of the blood sampling? Knowing that the amniotic fluid phospholipid profile was predictive of neonatal lung maturity would help. At the University of Iowa, we have not delivered the very preterm fetus whose lung studies were immature if the antenatal surveillance tests were otherwise acceptable. Others have reached the same conclusion (25). These fetuses are intensively monitored in the hospital since overt fetal distress can develop in a short period of time. It could be argued that it is wrong to give greater weight to an indirect test when a direct measurement is available. However, current perinatal morbidity and mortality estimates are based on the results of noninvasive tests. Stated differently, we know what an abnormal contractor stress test or biophysical profile means. We do not know what a mild metabolic acidosis means. Additional study is necessary to determine whether a chronic but "mild" metabolic acidosis is a greater danger to the fetus than prematurity.

It has been proposed that the fetus hypoxic secondary to presumed uteroplacental dysfunction be given a "trial" of maternal hyperoxygenation (26). If fetal oxygenation improves, then the pregnancy can continue. Maternal hyperoxygenation is enticing, but still unproven, therapy. Some, but not all, investigators have observed an increase in cerebral artery resistance and a decrease in umbilical artery resistance, suggesting improved oxygenation. In our experi-

ence, maternal hyperoxygenation has not prolonged the duration of pregnancy complicated by placental dysfunction. Treated fetuses, except one, have each developed overt fetal distress as diagnosed by conventional noninvasive parameters within a short interval of time (usually less than a week). Further, hyperoxygenation alters the distribution of fetal blood flow and may have untoward metabolic side effects (27). One explanation for the lack of success could be the selection of candidates. Some investigators did not adequately document that the etiology of growth deficiency was uteroplacental dysfunction. At Iowa, we have reserved oxygen therapy for the very preterm fetus with hypoxia (usually associated with absent umbilical artery diastolic blood flow). In this instance, it may be the extent of placental damage is already too great for the oxygen to increase a clinically significant amount. One report lacking fetal blood gases reached a similar conclusion based on Doppler studies (28).

Another scenario where PUBS has been suggested for the measurement of respiratory blood gases is to aid the interpretation of an unusual or confusing FHR tracing (29). For example, a woman at 30 weeks gestation appears to have late decelerations on the fetal heart rate monitor. Bearing in mind that a blood sample provides information at only one point in a continuum of events and that fetuses with significant metabolic acidosis usually have abnormal noninvasive surveillance tests, PUBS can only rarely be justified for this indication. If the pH is only modestly low, you are left in the same quandary discussed in the above paragraph. And, though a normal pH would be reassuring, the fact that it is normal does not rule out the possibility of fetal hypoxia during contractions and the development of acidosis as the contractions continue.

There are two practical alternatives to PUBS in this situation. First, supplemental maternal oxygenation by mask. If the fetal heart rate decelerations resolve with oxygen and then recur when the oxygen is discontinued, there is little question that the decelerations reflect hypoxia. The second alternative is to perform a contraction stress test until the interpretation of the tracing is no longer ambiguous.

ii. Hematologic Parameters

Hematologic parameters are affected by each of the three major causes of severe, early onset fetal growth deficiency. In fetuses undergrown because of uteroplacental dysfunction, the hematocrit increases as the pO_2 decreases; erythropoietin is modestly elevated. Therefore, it would appear that the polycythemia is a compensatory response to hypoxemia.

In addition to increased red cell number, the size of the red cell (mean corpuscular volume, MCV) in growth-restricted fetuses is inversely proportional to oxygen content independent of gestational age. In the healthy fetus, the MCV is unrelated to oxygen content. Gestational age is the major determinant of MCV (30,31). The MCV of fetuses with either trisomy or triploidy is elevated *independent* of both gestation and oxygen content. Thus, the control of erythropoiesis (and ultimately the MCV) is dysfunctional in trisomic/triploid fetuses. Though fetal disorders other than trisomy/triploidy are also associated with an elevated MCV, the positive predictive value of a high MCV for trisomy/ triploidy ranges between four and 18% (the latter in growth-retarded fetuses) (31). This exceeds the positive

predictive value of a low maternal serum alpha-fetoprotein level for trisomy. Perhaps most important, a normal MCV almost eliminates the possibility of trisomy or triploidy (but not for other karyotypic abnormalities).

The effect of congenital infection, even the same virus, upon hematologic parameters is highly variable. For example, human B-19 parvovirus can cause pancytopenia, isolated anemia, anemia secondary to disseminated intravascular coagulopathy, and anemia secondary to heart failure from myocardiopathy (unpublished, 32–34). The fetal immunologic response depends upon the infectious agent, the stage in gestation the infection occurs, and, likely, the fetal genetic makeup.

Significant thrombocytopenia is common in fetuses with either congenital infection or trisomy/triploidy, whereas the platelet count is only modestly reduced in fetuses growth-deficient secondary to uteroplacental dysfunction. The decreased platelet number associated with uteroplacental dysfunction may reflect decreased synthesis since the platelet size is reduced for gestation. With time, thrombocytopenia secondary to infection tends to resolve.

Both leukopenia and, less commonly, leukocytosis occur in fetuses with congenital infection. In our experience, leukocytosis with a left shift is uncommon in preterm fetuses; rather, it seems to evolve with chronicity.

One recent report documented by serial fetal blood samples the evolution of the fetal response to cytomegalic virus (35). It should be pointed out that the fetal serology became negative prior to delivery. The loss of an identifiable IgM response has been observed in fetuses with other viral infections (including varicella and parvovirus B19) when the time between infection and delivery is long enough.The normal level of fetal IgM is undetectable (< 7 mg/dL).

iii. **Lactate and Other Metabolites**

During normal human pregnancy, lactate concentration remains constant with advancing gestation (20). The severity of fetal hypoxia and the resistance to blood flow in uterine arcuate arteries correlates directly with the concentration of lactate (20,21,36). Further, the concentration of glucose is inversely related to the severity of hypoxia (21). This suggests that the low glycogen stores at birth typical of malnourished neonates is the cause rather than the result of hypoglycemia. While the measurement of lactate does not presently have a clinical role in the biochemical evaluation of the undergrown fetus, it may in the future. Several instances have been reported where lactate appeared to rise before the fetal heart rate tests became abnormal (37). If the concentration of lactate proves to be a sensitive marker for mild hypoxia, it might be useful in the identification of fetuses who are candidates for oxygen therapy.

Fetuses undergrown on the basis of placental dysfunction have other metabolic abnormalities. The triglycerides are elevated while insulin and glucose concentrations are reduced (5). Nonesterified free fatty acid concentration is unaltered. For reasons not germane to the present discussion, the elevated triglyceride concentration likely results from decreased utilization secondary to either impaired fat oxidation or reduced uptake into adipose tissue. The effect of maternal oxygenation upon the concentrations of fetal lactate, glucose and triglyceride have not as yet been re-

ported in the growth restricted fetus. pH of the growth restricted fetus has been observed to decline with glucose administration. This information will likely have bearing on any future attempts at *in utero* hyperalimentation.

iv. **Other Tests**

Modest elevations in lactic dehydrogenase (LD) and the transaminases (AST, GGT, and ALT) are common in growth-deficient fetuses (38). Dramatic elevations are less common. Enzyme abnormalities occur via one of two mechanisms. First, though frequently referred to as "liver function tests," LD and AST are produced by many tissues and are generally regarded as nonspecific indicators of cell injury. GGT is produced throughout the biliary tree and in other organs; it is often elevated in patients with hepatic or renal abnormalities. In appropriately-grown fetuses, the rise in LD with gestation is more strongly related to the declining pH than gestational age (Figure 5-10). However, in growth-deficient fetuses, there is a direct correlation between each of these enzymes (as opposed to LD alone) and umbilical venous pH. It is possible that cell turnover is increased in the growth-deficient fetus because of uteroplacental dysfunction. As a result, these enzymes are diffusely increased.

Second, hepatitis is rather common in the congenitally infected fetus whether the agent be viral or parasitic (33, 39). Serial testing of affected fetuses may demonstrate improvement or resolution of the inflammatory process over time. With the development of effective antiviral agents, it is likely that the efficacy of antenatal therapy will be monitored by serial measurements of these enzymes as in the postnatal patient.

The "stress" of substrate deprivation results in increased catecholamines.

Umbilical artery and vein concentrations of norepinephrine and epinephrine are increased in direct proportion to the degree the blood gases are abnormal (40). Though the standard deviation around the norm is quite wide, the measurement of norepinephrine and epinephrine may yet prove to be clinically useful. Coupled with lactate, a normal catecholamine concentration would argue against the existence of significant fetal stress and suggest that the diagnosis of growth deficiency is erroneous. Further, antenatal therapy, whether it be fetal hyperalimentation or maternal hyperoxygenation should lead to a reduction in catecholamine concentration if efficacious.

Nonimmune Hydrops

Nonimmune hydrops is but a symptom which may result from a myriad of causes. I define hydrops as anasarca and specifically exclude from the diagnosis a fetus with a single, localized fluid collection. The challenge to the fetologist is to determine what the etiology is, whether it is potentially amenable to antenatal therapy, and whether the fetus is responding to therapy prior to resolution of the hydrops. An in-depth laboratory assessment can greatly aid this process.

Following a detailed ultrasound examination in search of structural and functional abnormalities, the first invasive step is to determine the umbilical venous pressure. An elevated pressure suggests a high afterload and would be consistent with pump failure (secondary to either structural abnormalities or myocarditis) or obstructed cardiac return. A normal umbilical venous pressure suggests that the cause of hydrops is not cardiothoracic in origin. For example, if the etiology of the hydrops is thought to be a hydrothorax, measure the umbilical venous pressure before and after draining the fetal chest. If the pressure was increased because of obstructed cardiac return, it should return to normal with drainage of the chest as the mediastinum shifts back toward the midline. Fetal myocarditis is also associated with an elevated atrial natriuretic peptide (ANP) (33). If therapy improves ionotropy, ANP will decline. After the measurement of the fetal pressure, the laboratory parameters are then used to reduce the scope of the differential diagnosis.

Fetal Hyper/Hypothyroidism

Graves' disease is an autoimmune disorder where a thyroid-stimulating immmunoglobulin G (TSlgG) directed against the thyrocellular receptor for TSH produces primary hyperthyroidism. As many as 25% of neonates whose mothers have Graves' disease exhibit symptoms of thyrotoxicosis (41). With a perinatal mortality rate between 15–25%, affected fetuses can have high output cardiac failure, growth deficiency, postnatal craniosynostosis, and persistent neurologic and developmental abnormalities (42). The fetus is presumably at low risk for perinatal Graves' disease if the maternal TSIg is absent.

Definitive treatment for maternal disease is ablation of the thyroid [either surgical or medical (iodine-131)]. Unfortunately for the fetus, ablation does not eliminate TSIg. Palliative maternal therapy includes medication, such as propylthiouracil, to inhibit the synthesis of thyroxine and reduce the peripheral conversion of T_4 to T_3. These medications cross the placenta and likewise inhibit fetal thyroid synthesis.

It is difficult to determine whether and to what degree a fetus is affected by either TSIg or medication. Growth dysfunction, tachycardia, and other signs of fetal stress are nonspecific. Further, stillbirth secondary to fetal hyperthyroidism may occur in the absence of either fetal tachycardia or IUGR. Though it has been suggested that the fetal endocrine status can be assessed by measuring the amniotic fluid concentration of thyroid hormone, this has proven unreliable (43). Only by examining the fetal thyroid profile can therapy be optimized. Normal values for T_4, T_3, and TSH have recently been published (9). There are now several reports where maternal therapy for Graves' disease was altered to treat the fetus (44,45).

The inability to accurately assess the fetal effect of maternally administered antithyroid drugs leads to the practice of prescribing the lowest dose possible for maternal control so that the risk of fetal hypothyroidism is kept low. As a result, the fetologist is more likely to be referred a hyper- rather than hypothyroid fetus. Acquired fetal hypothyroidism does occur either from misuse of antithyroid medication, the presence of TSH-receptor blocking antibodies, or marked fetal sensitivity to the medication. On occasion, a fetal goiter severe enough to obstruct the trachea may occur. More often than not, fetal hypothyroidism (either acquired or congenital) is sonographically asymptomatic. Direct fetal evaluation is necessary to make the diagnosis. When indicated, exogenous thyroxine can be administered either by injection into the amniotic fluid for absorption after swallowing or by fetal intramuscular of thyroxine in an oil base for slow absorption (46,47).

CONCLUSION

Primary care fetal medicine requires both a diagnosis of the disease and an understanding of the fetal response to it. Biochemical assessment is a necessity. Much has been learned, much remains unknown. It is clear that the fetus is not an inert passenger. Rather, the developing human responds to a variety of environmental changes in a manner to enhance its survival. Understanding those responses has already improved perinatal morbidity and mortality.

References

1. Nicolaides KH, Rodeck CH, Millar DS, Mibashan RS. Fetal haematology in rhesus isoimmunisation. Br Med J 1985;290: 661–663.
2. Nicolaides KW, Rodeck CH, Mibashan RS, Kemp JR. Have Liley charts outlived their usefulness? Am J Obstet Gynecol 1986;155:90–94.
3. Soothill PW, Nicolaides KH, Rodeck CH, Campbell S. Effect of gestational age on fetal and intervillous blood gas and acid-base values in human pregnancy. Fetal Ther 1986;1:168–175.
4. Bozzetti P, Buscaglia M, Cetin I, et al. Respiratory gases, acid-base balance and lactate concentrations of the midterm human fetus. Biol Neonate 1987;51:188–197.
5. Economides DL, Crook D, Nicolaides KH. Investigation of hypertriglyceridemia in small-for-gestational age fetuses. Fetal Ther 1988;3:165–172.
6. Weiner CP, Heilskov J, Pelzer GD, Grant SS, Wenstrom KD, Williamson RA. Normal values for human umbilical venous and amniotic fluid pressures and their alteration by fetal disease. Am J Obstet Gynecol 1989;161:714–717.
7. Nicolini U, Tannirandorn Y, Gonzalez P, et al. Continuing controversy in alloimmune thrombocytopenia: fetal hyperimmunoglobulinemia failed to prevent thrombocytopenia. Am J Obstet Gynecol 1990;163:1144–1146.
8. Greenough A, Nicolaides KH, Lagercrantz H. Human fetal sympathoadrenal responsiveness. Early Hum Dev 1990;23:9–13.
9. Thorpe-Beeston JG, Nicolaides KH, Felton CV, Butler J, McGregor AM. Maturation

of the secretion of thyroid hormone and thyroid-stimulating hormone in the fetus. N Engl J Med 1991;324:532–536.

10. Moniz C, Nicolaides KH, Keys D, Rodeck CH. γ-glutamyl transferase activity in fetal serum, maternal serum, and amniotic fluid during gestation. J Clin Pathol 1984; 37:700–703.

11. Moniz CF, Nicolaides KH, Bamforth FJ, Rodeck CH. Normal reference ranges for biochemical substances relating to renal, hepatic, and bone function in fetal and maternal plasma throughout pregnancy. J Clin Pathol 1985;38:468–472.

12. Moniz CF, Nicolaides KH, Tzannatos C, Rodeck CH. Calcium homeostasis in second trimester fetuses. J Clin Pathol 1986; 39:838–841.

13. Forestier F, Daffos F, Galactéros F, Bardakjian J, Rainaut M, Beuzard Y. Hematological values of 163 normal fetuses between 18 and 30 weeks of gestation. Pediatr Res 1986;20:342–346.

14. Forestier F, Daffos F, Rainaut M, Bruneau M, Trivin F. Blood chemistry of normal human fetuses at midtrimester of pregnancy. Pediatr Res 1987;21:579–583.

15. Weiner CP. Human fetal bilirubin and fetal hemolytic disease. Obstet Gynecol 1992;166: 1449–1452.

16. Weiner CP, Williamson RA, Wenstrom KD, Sipes SL, Grant SS, Widness J. Management of fetal hemolytic disease by cordocentesis: i. Prediction of fetal anemia. Am J Obstet Gynecol 1991;165:546–553.

17. Weiner CP, Sipes SL, Wenstrom KD. The effect of gestation upon normal fetal laboratory parameters and venous pressure. Pediatr Res (submitted).

18. Weiner CP. Pragmatic application of sonography to the evaluation of abnormal fetal growth. Ultrasound Quarterly (in press).

19. Weiner CP, Williamson RA. Evaluation of severe growth retardation employing cordocentesis - hematologic and metabolic alterations by etiology. Obstet Gynecol 1989;73:225–229.

20. Nicolaides KH, Economides DL, Soothill PW, Blood gases, pH, and lactate in appropriate- and small-for-gestational-age fetuses. Am J Obstet Gynecol 1989;161: 996–1001.

21. Soothill PW, Nicolaides KH, Campbell S. Prenatal asphyxia, hyperlacticaemia, hypoglycaemia, and erythroblastosis in growth-retarded fetuses. Br Med J 1987;294: 1051–1053.

22. Nicolaides KH, Sadovsky G, Visser GHA. Heart rate patterns in normoxemic, hypoxemic, and anemic second-trimester fetuses. Am J Obstet Gynecol 1989;160:1034–1037.

23. Visser GHA, Sadovsky G, Nicolaides KH. Antepartum heart rate patterns in small-for-gestational-age third-trimester fetuses: correlations with blood gas values obtained at cordocentesis. Am J Obstet Gynecol 1990; 162:698–703.

24. Ribbert LSM, Snijders RJM, Nicolaides KH, Visser GHA. Relationship of fetal biophysical profile and blood gas values at cordocentesis in severely growth-retarded fetuses. Am J Obstet Gynecol 1990;163:569–571.

25. Nicolini U, Nicolaides P, Fisk NM, et al. Limited role of fetal blood sampling in prediction of outcome in intrauterine growth retardation. The Lancet 1990;336:768–772.

26. Nicolaides KH, Campbell S, Bradley RP, Bilardo CM, Soothill PW, Gibb D. Maternal oxygen therapy for intrauterine growth retardation. The Lancet 1987;i:942–945.

27. Gull I, Charlton V. The effect of maternal hyperoxygenation on fetal metabolism. Proceedings, Society for Gynecologic Investigation 1991;abstract #575.

28. Arduini D, Rizzo G, Romanini C, Mancuso S. Hemodynamic changes in growth-retarded fetuses during maternal oxygen administration as predictors of fetal outcome. J Ultrasound Med 1989;8:193–196.

29. Hobbins JC, Grannum PA, Romero F, Reece EA, Mahoney MJ. Percutaneous umbilical blood sampling. Am J Obstet Gynecol 1985;152:1–6.

30. Nicolaides KH, Snijder RJM, Thorpe-Beeston JG, Van den Hof MC, Gosden CM,

Bellingham AJ. Mean red cell volume in normal, anemic, small, trisomic, and triploid fetuses. Fetal Ther 1989;4:1–13.

31. Sipes SL, Weiner CP, Wenstrom KD, Williamson RA, Grant SS. The association between fetal karyotype and mean corpuscular volume. Am J Obstet Gynecol 1991; 165:1371–1376.

32. Anand A, Gray ES, Brown T, Clewley JP, Cohen BJ. Human parvovirus infection in pregnancy and hydrops fetalis. N Engl J Med 1987;316:183–186.

33. Weiner CP, Naides SJ. Antenatal diagnosis and palliative treatment of nonimmune hydrops fetalis secondary to fetal parvovirus B19 infection. Prenat Diagn 1989; 9:105–114.

34. Sahakian V, Weiner CP, Naides SJ, Williamson RA, Scharosch LL. Intrauterine transfusion of nonimmune hydrops fetalis secondary to human parvovirus B19 infection. Am J Obstet Gynecol 1991;164: 1090–1091.

35. Watt-Morse M, Laifer S, Hill L. Serial cordocentesis in the evaluation of intrauterine cytomegalovirus infection. Am J Obstet Gynecol 1991;164:296 (abstract #180).

36. Soothill PW, Nicolaides KH, Bilardo C, Hacket G, Campbell S. Uteroplacental blood velocity resistance index and umbilical venous pO_2, pCO_2, pH, lactate and erythroblast count in growth-retarded fetuses. Fetal Ther 1986;1:176–179.

37. Pardi G, Buscaglia M, Ferrazzi E, et al. Cord sampling for the evaluation of oxygenation and acid-base balance in growth-retarded human fetuses. Am J Obstet Gynecol 1987;157:1221–1228.

38. Wenstrom KD, Weiner CP, Williamson RA. Effect of gestational age and disease on fetal liver function. Proceedings, Society of Perinatal Obstetricians, 1990. Abstr. 199, p212.

39. Daffos F, Forestier F, Capella-Pavlovsky M, et al. Prenatal management of 746 pregnancies at risk for congenital toxoplasmosis. N Engl J Med 1988;318:271–275.

40. Weiner CP, Robillard JE. Atrial natriuretic factor, digoxin-like immunoreactive substance, norepinephrine, epinephrine, and plasma renin activity in human fetuses and their alteration by fetal disease. Am J Obstet Gynecol 1988;159:1353–1360.

41. Zakarya M, McKenzie JM, Hoffman WH. Prediction and therapy of intrauterine and late-onset neonatal hyperthyroidism. J Clin Endocrinol Metab 1986;62:368–371.

42. Hollingsworth DR. Grave's disease. Clin Obstet Gynecol 1983;26:615–634.

43. Landau H, Sack J, Frucht H, Palti Z, Hochner-Celnikier D, Rosenmann A. Amniotic fluid 3-, 3′-, 5′-triiodothyronine in the detection of congenital hypothyroidism. J Clin Endocrinol Metab 1980;50:799–801.

44. Wenstrom KD, Weiner CP, Williamson RA, Grant SS. Prenatal diagnosis of fetal hyperthyroidism using funipuncture. Obstet Gynecol 1990;76:513–517.

45. Porreco RP, Bloch CA. Fetal blood sampling in the management of intrauterine thyrotoxicosis. Obstet Gynecol 1990;76:509–512.

46. Davidson KM, Richards DS, Schatz DA, Fisher DA. Successful in utero treatment of fetal goiter and hypothyroidism. N Engl J Med 1991;324:543–546.

47. Perelman AH, Johnson RL, Clemons RD, Finberg HJ, Clewell WH, Trujillo L. Intrauterine diagnosis and treatment of fetal goitrous hypothyroidism. J Clin Endocrinol Metab 1990;71:618–621.

INVASIVE TECHNIQUES IN THE MANAGEMENT OF ALLOIMMUNE ANEMIA

6

C. R. HARMAN

Management of alloimmune fetal erythroblastosis, "Rh Disease," is the epitome of fetal medicine. Scientific and clinical breakthroughs have been incorporated to produce sustained improvements in results over several decades (Figure 6-1) (1). Sequencing of the D-antigen protein (2) marks the culmination of red blood cell (RBC) research that began with demonstration of the Rhesus factor 50 years ago (3). Postpartum Rh immunoglobulin prophylaxis (4), expanding to routine antenatal and event-specific prophylaxis, has reduced sensitization of Rh-negative women to less than 2/1000 (5). In pregnancies where sensitization has not been prevented, fetal monitoring by amniocetesis (6) or cordocentesis (PUBS) (7) means that therapy is initiated selectively and early in the course of disease. Ultrasound-guided intraperitoneal fetal

transfusion (IPT) (8), added a further drop to Rh disease mortality. With the advent of intravascular fetal transfusion in 1984 (9,10), effective access was gained to the sickest of these—the moribund hydrops (11).

In essence, this chapter is a "progress report" on this multidisciplinary effort, an effort that has led to remarkable success in *fetal* approaches to *fetal* disease based on explicit understanding of *fetal* pathophysiology. While some facets remain under discussion, e.g., the role of fetal erythropoietin, much has been learned in the course of intrauterine treatment to modify our concepts of disease process based on the modest fetal blood samples available before, during, and after IVT. A broad range of studies has detailed data on hematologic hemodynamic, cardiovascular, circulatory, biochemical, respiratory, and behavioral aspects of fetuses under treatment. Key aspects of physical (ultrasound) examination have been correlated with disease severity. A small amount of follow-up data is also now available about IVT survivors (12).

Clearly, comprehensive review of this wealth of material would require a volume of its own. While reference to fetal disease processes is integral in practical application, physiology discussions will be kept at a minimum. The role of this chapter is to detail the clinical context and current technical essentials of investigation of the alloimmunized pregnancy and of intrauterine treatment of the anemic fetus.

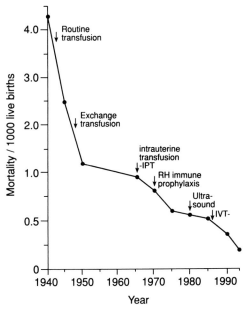

Figure 6-1 Progress in management of alloimmune fetal anemia. Note the change in the ordinate scale below 1.0/1000. The progress continues, but the *major* impacts are decades old.

THE MANITOBA RH PROGRAM

As one of the longest-standing dedicated Rh programs, the publicly-funded province-wide program in Manitoba has experienced this progress first-hand. Clinically based, the program has focused on maximizing the impact of Rh-immune globulin prophylaxis (5,13–15) including the development of *pure* anti-D IgG for both intravenous and intramuscular use (16). This Rh-immune globulin in preparation (WinRho), the standard for use in our program, contains no IgM, IgA, or trace proteins.

Application of the principles described in the classic paper on Rh-prophylaxis by Professor Bowman (5) includes many unusual situations (17) (Table 6-1). Even when optimal application occurs, however, prevention may not be complete, prophylaxis may fail for a variety of reasons (Table 6-2) (18–22). Noting that the largest proportion (31% in total, under "Inappropriate Management") of Rh-sensitization remains due to unexplained omission of Rh-IgG, several *new* factors now result in the presentation of highly sensitized women at early stages of their first or second pregnancy. The relative

Table 6-1 Indications For Rh-Immune Globulin

(D-Negative Woman, Unsensitized, with All *Pregnancy Events When the Fetus/Baby Is Not Proven Rh-Negative.)*

Any Instance of:
Spontaneous abortion (with or without D&C)
Therapeutic abortion (any method)
Chorion villus sampling
Genetic amniocentesis
Amniocentesis for lung profile

Treat, Additional RhIG Depending on Kleihauer Test:
Antepartum hemorrhage
Molar pregnancy
Large transplacental hemorrhage
Stillbirth
Obstetric manipulation
Manual removal of placenta

Routine Prophylaxis (None of the Above Has Occurred):
28 weeks gestation, and
40 weeks, if undelivered, or
Delivery of Rh-positive baby

Table 6-2 Causes of Sensitization Leading to IVFT (130 Fetuses Requiring Intrauterine Treatment)

Total Unavoidable	*71 Patients*	*54.6%*
Atypical Antibodies		10%
No Program Available		
Prior to Routine Delivery Prophylaxis		5%
Prior to Routine Antenatal Prophylaxis		10%
Immigrants		6%
Pregnancy Hemorrhage*		12%
Sensitization <28 weeks		5%
Grandmother Theory**		3%
Prior D+ Transfusion		4%
Failed Prophylaxis	*12 Patients*	*9.2%*
(Received appropriate dose/timing RhIg) Most likely sensitized by failure of:		
Antenatal prophylaxis		5%
Postpartum prophylaxis		4%
Total Avoidable	*47 Patients*	*36.2%*
Inappropriate Management		
Spontaneous abortion untreated		6%
Therapeutic abortion untreated		12%
Failed to receive prophylaxis (Antenatal)		12%
Failed to receive prophylaxis (Delivery)		1%
IV Drug Abuser — "Boosting"†		5%
Patient Refused Prophylaxis Previous Pregnancy		2%

*Clinically-diagnosed hemorrhage, in 50% prophylaxis was attempted, but unsuccessful.
**Sensitization of the mother when *she* was a fetus, by maternal-fetal hemorrhage. Antibody detected in early first pregnancy, no prior exposure except D+ "grandmother" of the fetus requiring IVT.
†Intravenous injection of partner's (antigen-positive) blood to obtain "better" drug effect.

importance of "atypical" blood group antigens (notably Kell, but including c, Duffy, Cellano, C^w) has also increased in our referred population, with both decreased Rh sensitization and improved referral for Kell alloimmunization (23–26). Thus, a meticulous Rh-program, careful attention to other red cell alloimmunization, and centralized referral form the clinical setting for the "investigation and treatment" arm of the Winnipeg program—the University of Manitoba Intrauterine Transfusion (IUT) Team.

The IUT team began with the first intrauterine fetal transfusion in North America January 2, 1964 (27) by the intraperitoneal route that had recently been described by Liley (28). A total of 870 intraperitoneal transfusions on 364 fetal subjects have been done since by this multidisciplinary team. The advent of ultrasound-directed procedures in 1980 and refinement in pre- and post-transfusion monitoring in 1980–85 saw further improvements in IPT survival rates (Figure 6-2), culminating with a series in which no non-hydropic fetus died (8).

On May 29, 1986, our team performed the first IVT in Canada on a fetus who

was deteriorating rapidly despite serial IPT (11). Our experience with the intravascular approach is summarized in a case-controlled evaluation of the two principal techniques—IPT and IVT (29). Since our first IVT, we have converted almost entirely to the intravascular approach and have now treated 131 fetuses with over 620 procedures for alloimmune anemia. Of these, 129 (611 total procedures) have been delivered and form the basis of this review (Table 6-3) (30). Not included in these statistics, but benefitting directly, are fetuses undergoing transfusion for nonimmune anemia and alloimmune fetal thrombocytopenia.

Only a few months prior to our first IVT, we had begun PUBS for restricted diagnostic groups in which detection was *only* possible by fetal blood sampling. In our view (at that time), this did *not* include Rh or other alloimmune problems; it was only after significant positive experience with IVT that fetal blood sampling became a routine monitoring tool in our approach. Since late 1986, we have performed over 250 cordocenteses for evaluation of fetal alloimmunization, also shown in Table 6-3. We continue to use amniocentesis for ΔOD 450 (31) in our monitoring protocol, although we do not rely on Liley's original predictive data (32) as newer values have become available (6,33,34); literally thousands of "Rh amnios" contribute to our current approach.

This, then, is the clinical context of a data base, spanning more than 30 years. A consistent approach has been in place for a decade in ultrasound assessment of fetal disease status, which always has included Biophysical Profile Scoring. Therapeutic success has improved as techniques have been modified. Our team is a referral resource for many tertiary groups, both in performing IUT (Figure 6-3) and latterly in consultation regarding technical problems.

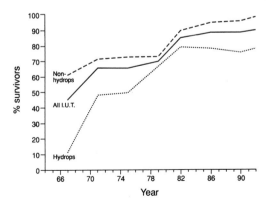

Figure 6-2 Survival rates for fetuses treated with intrauterine transfusion. In 1986, conversion from IPT to IVT took place.

Table 6-3 Invasive Procedures—Alloimmunization University of Manitoba Intrauterine Transfusion Team 1964–93

Fetal Blood Sampling—Cordocentesis	Procedures	Fetuses
Total sampled	263	162
Antigen negative—not affected	36	36
Antigen positive—not anemic	111	46
Antigen positive—anemic*	116	80
(Treated:Serial IVT-74;		
Neonatal-6**)		
Intravascular Fetal Transfusion (IVT)	589	129
Intracardiac Fetal Transfusion (ICT)	11	10
Intraperitoneal Fetal Transfusion (IPT)		
Pre-Ultrasound era		
(Jan. 2, 1964–1980)	657	278
Ultrasound era (1980–1986)	202	75
IVT era (May 29, 1986—Present)	11	11

* <5th Percentile for gestation. Not hydropic.
** ≥ 36 Weeks gestation, delivered and treated as neonates.

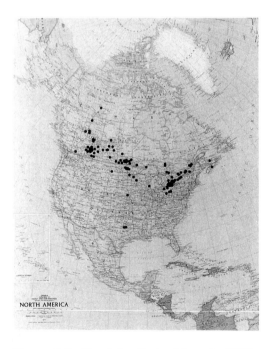

NORTH AMERICA

Figure 6-3 Hospitals referring fetuses for IVT by the Manitoba Team.

These factors suggest the usefulness of a one-center review, based on our current experience and practice. Where possible, techniques and observations from other groups are included, but the reader must be aware of differences from center to center. Finally, the three segments—fetal blood typing, pretreatment testing, and intrauterine transfusion—are presented in a chronological framework, but the discussion will clearly demonstrate that these are often very separate and seldom follow a rigid progression.

FETAL BLOOD TYPING IN SENSITIZED PREGNANCIES

Rationale

There are dangers to all invasive procedures; with alloimmune disease, these are compounded by the potential for early, severe disease that makes such efforts technically more difficult. But, delaying until the procedure is "easy" may mean accelerated hydrops and irreversible fetal compromise. There are many fetuses in our series who had procedures deferred because an ultrasound showed a "perfectly normal" fetus that was followed by profound hydrops in as little as one week.

Early procedures are dangerous; delay is ill-advised. Knowing the fetal blood type in this situation is invaluable. The logic is obvious. An antigen-positive fetus is at a level of danger indicated by the mother's history, antibody type, and strength, justifying early, albeit dangerous, attention. The negative fetus would be in no danger whatsoever from his mother's sensitization. Except for a single procedure to determine blood type, he would be spared the inherent risks of testing and therapy.

Prior to the PUBS era, serial amniocentesis and even *serial intraperitoneal fetal transfusions* (when the amniocentesis failed to exclude severe hemolysis) were done in some pregnancies ultimately delivered of Rh-negative babies (1). Such inadvertent "treatment" was an unavoidable consequence of having to apply statistics instead of direct knowledge to serious alloimmunization. If the father is heterozygous, the "odds" are 50:50 that the fetus is affected; the likelihood is 90:10 that high ΔOD 450 readings are the product of serious fetal hemolysis; and the risks from intraperitoneal fetal transfusion were of 5–8% fetal mortality *per procedure*. Knowing the fetal blood type eliminates the chance of applying such dangerous therapy unnecessarily.

On the other hand, fetal blood typing is currently not without risk. It is unlikely that a fetus will exsanguinate or have other lethal consequences at PUBS, but there is a defined risk of infection, rupture of membranes, and so on, regardless of the reason for the procedure. In such cases, the antigen-negative fetus incurs needless morbidity. More critically, any procedure that obtains fetal blood has the potential for producing transplacental hemorrhage and serious aggravation of antibody titer, with dire consequences for the antigen-positive fetus. Of course, those consequences will be carried over to *all* subsequent positive fetuses in the form of a permanently elevated maternal antibody level. Thus, although the information is useful, the potential cost means that fetal blood typing is *not* applied in every case at risk for alloimmune disease. We do not, for example, have a routine of fetal blood typing at 20 weeks in all Rh-negative sensitized women.

The choice for fetal blood typing involves factors that are not all strictly medical (Table 6-4). In some cases, financial or emotional hardships, or even apparent futility in the most severely affected, e.g., previous hydrops at 14–15 weeks, might indicate pregnancy termination of a positive fetus. For continuing pregnancy with a positive fetus, necessary family arrangements should be made; the management plan should be established; the ancillary needs are different in every situation, and information is pivotal.

If the father is heterozygous (*known* in the case of atypical blood group alloimmunization or *predicted* in Rh disease), if there are significant family considerations, or if previous fetuses were not severely affected, and/or the placenta is anterior, we tend to type the fetus. If the placenta is posterior with a difficult cord insertion, if travel to the hospital is not a problem, and especially, if preliminary amniocentesis were suggestive of an unaffected fetus, we tend to follow with detailed ultrasound surveillance and serial amniocentesis, without ever doing a fetal blood type.

In many cases, other testing, e.g., genetics, is indicated, and fetal blood typing can be done; this information *is* valuable and

Table 6-4   Fetal Blood Typing

Advantages

Negative Fetus
   Allow pregnancy continuation
   Avoid multiple amniocenteses
   Avoid inappropriate I.U. treatment
   "Normal" pregnancy care and delivery
   Reduced anxiety, expense, travel

Positive Fetus
   Allow pregnancy termination*
   Early definition of at-risk fetus:
   Family—Financial and logistic planning
   I.U.T. Team—Investigation and treatment
                     planning
               —Initiate adjunctive therapies*

Disadvantages

All Fetuses	Non-immune procedural
	complications
	Cost

Positive Fetus Aggravation of sensitization

I.U. = Intrauterine.
*In certain circumstances—see text.

should be obtained where possible in the heterozygous situation. A separate blood-typing procedure is not recommended when the fetus is certain to be positive, e.g., *certain* homozygous father, when previous disease was early and/or hydropic, i.e., when a rise in titer might cause acceleration of antibody production to an extreme level, when there is suggestive evidence of a positive fetus, e.g., a titer rise early in the current pregnancy, or when the monitoring center and the IUT team are geographically far apart.

Procedures for Fetal Blood Typing

Fetal blood may be obtained for typing in a variety of ways. Properly accredited laboratories should be able to do complete blood typing on fractions of milliliters; forensic methods allow for D-typing of only a few hundred red cells on a single thread (35). Several methodological variations have been used to sort, verify as fetal, and, ultimately, determine blood group type, of minute numbers of fetal red cells. Microagglutination using fluorescent markers (36), antigen-specific binding using an immunogold-silver developing process (37), microscopic evaluation of antibody-mediated rosette formation (38–39), or cellular assays using monocyte monolayer techniques (40) (see Figure 6-4) all can identify Rh-positive or Kell-positive fetuses in immunized mothers. Precise steps to eliminate maternal or trophoblast contamination depend on the sampling, and while several of these techniques were developed in the context of CVS, they can be applied to samples obtained by any route. These methods pale in comparison to the sensitivity of DNA amplification by (polymerase chain reaction [PCR]) as described with very recently-developed processes. With PCR, it is the Rh+D gene, determined from the nuclear DNA of the nucleated fetal or trophoblast cells, that indicates Rh-positivity (as opposed to the D-antigen determined from the cell membrane of fetal red blood cells, in the former methods). If fetal DNA/PCR proves completely reliable and can always be done using fetal cells from the maternal circulation, none of the invasive procedures and none of the associated cautions will be relevant.

Fetoscopy

The earliest consistently successful, highly-detailed fetal blood typing was done in the late 1970s and early 1980s by fetoscopic needle puncture, with blood grouping routinely possible on the small fetal blood samples obtained (41). Some of the variations in expression now understood about fetal versus adult red cell antigens were also described. It may be notable that this group found that fetoscopy was no more likely than amniocentesis (about 30%) to cause significant provocation of antibody production, compared with their own experience (75% aggravation) in ultrasound-guided PUBS (42).

Cordocentesis

Routine cordocentesis is used, with one difference: sample purity is not critical. Antigenicity can be determined in samples contaminated with up to 50–60% maternal blood or large amounts of amniotic fluid. For example, if the PUBS procedure fails or is halted due to bradycardia, maternal discomfort, etc., if there is even a small pinkish tinge, 10 ml of centrifuged amniotic fluid will yield a perfectly-adequate pellet of fetal or mixed RBC for typing. A Kleihauer is done to demonstrate a reasonable proportion of fetal cells in ensuring reliability of an antigen-negative result.

Amniocentesis

Amniocyte cultures cannot reliably express Rh or other RBC antigens. If blood-tinged fluid is obtained at genetic amniocentesis (or during Rh surveillance using serial amniocentesis), it is tested as above for the D-antigen. We do not recommend it through an anterior placenta but do routinely perform genetic amniocentesis when the placenta is not traversed in sensitized women, with the appropriate indications. Early genetic amniocentesis at 10–14 weeks may offer enhanced opportunity for blood typing, considering the higher concentration of multipotential cells of yolk sac origin.

Searching for minute quantities of fetal blood in amniotic fluid may not be necessary, however, if recent reports are substantiated. Of 15 samples of amniotic fluid analyzed by PCR (using the newly-developed Rh gene primers for the CE and D loci respectively (2), there was 100% concordance with fetal blood obtained by cordocentesis (43). Cells from only 2 ml of centrifuged amniotic fluid suffice, apparently requiring minimal technical refining to be processed with the DNA primers. This new development using amniocentesis appears to be ideal for fetal blood typing— minimal invasiveness and high accuracy.

Chorionic Villus Sampling

Direct fetal blood typing using red cells from stem villi has been reported by a number of groups (36–39). In one typical report, fetal blood typing was 100% accurate, although there were a few technical problems and pregnancy termination was elected in 3/5 positive cases, based on this testing (38). Reasonably large series have been evaluated, demonstrating the reliability of this approach in determining blood type. PCR-based technology may be useful here; not all CVS samples have enough actual fetal blood cells for typing. Detection of the Rh-positive gene in trophoblast is preliminary at this point (43). Expression of the Rh protein, the D-antigen on the surface of trophoblast, has been argued for many years, but this is not clinically applicable. There is, however, a significant risk of aggravating sensitization by CVS (44–45), and consideration should be given to waiting for amniocentesis, e.g., until 13–14 weeks.

Most studies have dealt with the ability to detect and type fetal blood obtained incidental to CVS done for karyotype. More controversial might be CVS used specifically to determine blood type so the parents could decide whether or not to continue the pregnancy (38,39). Meticulous counselling would be key in such a process to ensure truly informed consent and would have to include knowledge that continuation of an antigen-positive pregnancy after CVS, e.g., Rh-positive but continued because 46,XX was identified, may be at even higher risk. The PCR-facilitated methodology above (43) was also applied with 100% concordance to CVS samples. Although this enhances accuracy and eliminates the need to obtain actual fetal RBC with the CVS, it is no less invasive.

Fetal Blood Typing From Maternal Blood Samples

Occasionally, spontaneous or accidental transplacental hemorrhage (TPH) may provide the information necessary. If serial Kleihauer examinations show persistence/slow decline of fetal cells after TPH, the fetus is almost certainly antigen-negative. Fetal Rh-positive cells in the circulation of a highly-sensitized woman disappear within a matter of minutes, whereas fetal red cells from an Rh-negative fetus would persist for many days. Of course, this is purely an incidental test; deliberately provoking fetomaternal bleeding in the sensitized woman would be pure negligence!

Recently published work showing fetal blood typing on maternal blood samples, i.e., not using invasive techniques, is an exciting advance (46). In this report, 21 Rh-negative women were studied utilizing Rh-gene primers. With PCR amplification, determinations were made based on discrete migration of the Rh (D) DNA compared to known positive and negative controls. The test is binary: D-positive DNA is either present or absent; the Rh-negative condition is absolute absence of the gene. The data are presented in detail (Table 6-5) due to their critical importance. Unfortunately, the preliminary work is not 100% concordant. In fact, only 16 of 21 were correctly typed (8/10 positive fetuses, and 8/11 negative fetuses were correctly identified). Although details are limited, it seems cor-

Table 6-5   Fetal Rh Typing from Maternal Blood Samples*

Gestation**	Baby	PCR	Antibody†
16	+	+	None, ABO
17	+	−	None
22	+	+	348, ABO
31	+	+	P, ABO
31	+	+	P
32	+	+	P
32	+	+	5.8
33	+	+	53
37	+	−	P
38	+	+	None
16	−	−	None
16	−	−	None
16	−	−	None
18	−	−	None
18	−	+	None
32	−	−	P, ABO
32	−	−	P
34	−	+	None
36	−	+	None
37	−	−	None
41	−	−	P

*Data from Lo et al (46).
PCR = polymerase chain reaction.
†All mothers Rh-negative. Numbers indicate sensitized women with absolute anti-D level (IU/ml) as shown.
P = passive antibody from antenatal prophylaxis present at time of testing.
ABO = ABO incompatibility between mother and fetus.
**Weeks gestation when maternal sample drawn.

rect typing *was* achieved in all five cases of alloimmunization. The incorrect results follow no particular pattern. Errors occurred at early and late gestations, with and without maternal–fetal ABO incompatibility, and apparently not influenced by the presence of passive antibody in maternal circulation after antenatal prophylaxis. In a larger series, one would require paternal blood type and volume/number of fetal cells per 10 ml maternal sample, to evaluate practicality as well as basic accuracy.

This technology might be very significantly enhanced by flow cytometry to enrich the yield of (47,48) presumably fetal nucleated red blood cells. The DNA of any circulating fetal cells might be expected to be detected by this powerful technology, leaving open the possibility of trophoblast cells from the current pregnancy or even fetal lymphocytes from previous pregnancies, being reflected in the results (49,50). The authors do not offer explanation for the three false-positives; if this test were used to determine termination of pregnancy, perfect concordance would be needed. Larger numbers are required before the benefits and pitfalls of this methodology can be assessed accurately. In many cases, i.e., all Rh-negative fathers and all homozygous Rh-positive fathers, totalling over 50% of the population, the history will tell us the fetal Rh, and accurate population-based statistics can be used to predict paternal status (51). Hopefully, these reservations will be addressed by technical improvements, making this interesting research an accurate tool and, therefore, of immense value.

Finally, it is emphasized that fetal blood typing by any means is not critical to the unsensitized woman, who can be adequately protected by winRho 99+% of the time, and is of no relevance at all to the weakly-sensitized woman, who cannot be protected, but who is at minimal risk of severe fetal disease.

INVASIVE FETAL MONITORING— INDIVIDUALIZED PATIENT CARE

A number of avenues of information are available to the team managing seriously-sensitized pregnancies, both indirect, maternal, historical, statistical, and direct, fetal examination and fetal testing. These data are of gradually increasing sensitivity and specificity as the fetal blood stream is approached (Table 6-6), and ultimately the data from cordocentesis will define the extent to which this particular fetus is anemic. It is facile to suggest that the information available from indirect sources

Table 6-6 Indications for Invasive Fetal Testing

Test to Determine IF *Treatment is Necessary*

Antibody Specificity
D, c, Kell, C, e, Fy^a, K(cellano)C^w

Antibody Strength
For D: Albumin titer ≥1:16
      Absolute anti-D level ≥ 2 μg/ml
      (10 IU/ml)
Kell: Indirect Coombs' titer 1:4
All others: Indirect Coombs' 1:16

Antibody Pattern (Serial Testing)
Late-appearing IgM-IgG conversion
Recent 2-dilution rise from any level

Test to Determine WHEN *Treatment Should Begin*

History
Previous affected infant, heterozygous father
Homozygous father, previous infant no/mild effect
Homozygous father, albumin titer ≥1:64
Homozygous father, previous infant ≥ moderate disease

Fetal Blood Type Positive
Previous affected infant, new antibody rise
Fetal blood typing done, albumin titer ≥1:64

Evidence of Significant Fetal Hemolysis
Ultrasound examination
Amniotic fluid spectrophotometry
Cordocentesis results

NON HYDROPS

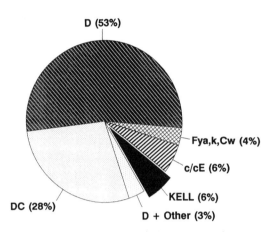

D (53%)

Fya,k,Cw (4%)

c/cE (6%)

KELL (6%)

DC (28%)

D + Other (3%)

HYDROPS

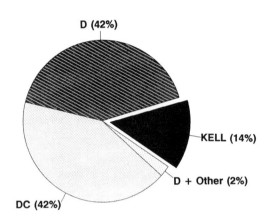

D (42%)

KELL (14%)

D + Other (2%)

DC (42%)

Figure 6-4 Distribution of alloimmune antibodies in pregnancies requiring intrauterine transfusion. Note the relatively large proportion of fetuses hydropic because of Kell alloimmunization. Kell alloimmunization comprises 11% of our overall IVT population, 14% of those hydropic, and 33% of Class 4 hydrops.

is not valuable. It would be foolish to insist, for example, PUBS as the first step in monitoring the fetus when there is an anti-E indirect Coombs' titer of 1:8. This antibody seldom causes severe fetal disease. No data should be discarded just because it is not absolute; the most comprehensive assessment includes information from all sources.

Antibody Assessment

Although not invasive, antibody assessment information is integral to the timing and methods of fetal testing. Collaboration of an experienced serology lab is critical as is a detailed understanding of local factors. In our population of fetuses referred with hydropic alloimmunization (Figure 6-4), for example, Kell sensitization plays a prominent role, whereas serious anti-Kell disease in Oxford was only four in 350,000 deliveries (52). Experience with Kell alloimmu-

nization suggests antibodies are not reliable in determining risk; we have seen fetal hydrops with anti-Kell indirect Coombs' titers as low as 1:4 (23). This variability, however, is not a feature of the Rh system or other atypical antibodies. Thus, the investigation must place Kell in a special category before generalizing about antibody-disease relationships.

It seems obvious that maternal antibody strength is related to severity of fetal disease, but proof of that relationship remains elusive. Titration (21) or absolute quantitation (21,52–54) produce general impressions of risk and a retrospective relationship between disease severity and antibody strength. Various "cutoff" values have been suggested [4 IU/ml,(53) 10 IU/ml (1,21), 10–20 IU/ml (53) or 15 IU/ml (54)], below which severe disease is rare, but at higher levels, the relationship between strength and impact is unreliable. There is inherent difference between one antibody's kinetics

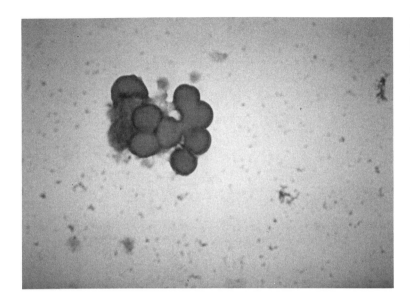

Figure 6-5 Photomicrograph from monocyte monolayer, showing Rh-positive fetal RBC engulfed by a maternal monocyte. (Photomicrograph courtesy of Dr. Ken Moise, Baylor University).

and the next, and then there are many variables: many fathers are heterozygous; maternal titers remain high or even rise slightly with an antigen-negative fetus; low titers produce significant disease in at least some women; there are dramatic differences between one pregnancy and the next with only minor changes in titer; there may be sudden rises in titre late in pregnancy, producing unexpectedly severe disease; and there are striking differences depending on the blood group under study.

IgG subclasses have immunopathologic significance, and may show clinical gradation: IgG_3 was not seen with hydrops and IgG_1 was associated with infrequent/later hydrops (6% hydropic at 28 weeks), while combined IgG_1IgG_3 (21% hydropic, as early as 20 weeks) was most severe (55). IgG_1 and IgG_1IgG_3 had similar rates of serious hemolysis requiring antenatal therapy (59% and 62%, respectively), so clinical discrimination is not reliable.

Cell-mediated responses against D-positive cells are facilitated by anti-D, so an in vitro system (monocyte monolayer assay) has been used to evaluate the antibody (Figure 6-5). Prediction of disease severity has been accurate (40), variable (56), or inconclusive (57); the technique is time-consuming and difficult, and not easily duplicated (58).

Our experience includes undisputed cases of D-alloimmune hydropic stillbirth in women who subsequently had titers only 1:8 in albumin (although the level may have been higher at the moment of stillbirth). Clearly, such data are not discarded in evaluation. Historical factors are always critical in initiating surveillance and in deciding between cordocentesis and amniocentesis. On the other hand, history would be irrelevant in the absence of a persistent titer against a clinically-important antigen, when a new father/partner is antigen-negative, or when the putative titer, e.g., anti-C 1:8, is not in a range to produce the reputed effect, e.g., hydropic stillbirth at 24 weeks. The critical point of difference between first-sensitized pregnancy and subsequent sensitized pregnancy is underscored in the arguments in current literature (7,54,59–65). This acrimonious echange illustrates several points:

1. Different methodologies, different experience, and different expertise give rise to different approaches by different teams;
2. Any attempt to be dogmatic about a *single* best approach is likely to fail the test of time;
3. A balanced approach with utmost concern to avoid aggravation of mild/ moderate disease, while detecting severe disease early, likely requires a broad range of data. Antibody, type, strength, chronological pattern and historical factors are integrated with paternal zygosity to assign relative risk. In all cases, recent change in status, e.g., early pregnancy titer rise, supersedes previous reassuring information and favors earlier testing.

With these principles in mind, any suspicious factor should prompt early fetal testing to determine the need for transfusion, or where the need is already established, e.g., homozygous father and previously affected infant, to determine when transfusion should begin (refer again to Table 6-6). In general, we use either amniocentesis or PUBS in the former case, and PUBS exclusively in the latter case.

Amniocentesis For ΔOD 450

Background

Bilirubin enters amniotic fluid in proportion to fetal hemolysis, quantifiable by its deflection of absorbance of light at 450nm–ΔOD 450. Liley's classic application to data on severe erythroblastosis (32) has endured three decades of clinical evaluation, with success when it has been applied appropriately. Liley defined his zones by relating known outcomes to observed ΔOD 450. Zone lines were chosen to demarcate two zones of certainty: below the Zone 1–2 boundary, i.e, Zone 1 fluids, no babies severely affected; above the Zone 2–3 boundary, i.e., Zone 3 fluids, no babies unaffected; and one zone, between the two lines, where outcome was not certain. In its simplest form, it is very difficult to dispute this relationship.

Zone 2 is a stumbling point–most fetuses in the upper portion (above 80% Zone 2) are affected, but some are not, hence, Whitfield's action line, an acknowledgement of the curvilinear nature of amniotic fluid bilirubin over the course of normal pregnancy, with extrapolation back to 23 weeks gestation (66) (vs Liley's original 28-week minimum). It is interesting that this report of amniocentesis in severe Rh disease allowed procedures as early as 20 weeks.

The inherent dangers of IPT, especially without ultrasound, justified this approach. If potentially lethal procedures were to be undertaken, the threshold, i.e., Zone 3 boundary, had to be high enough to be certain that poor outcome was otherwise destined. If some fetuses became severely affected before action was taken because the ΔOD was below Zone 3, i.e., falsely reassuring values, about 5% of cases, this was an inevitable consequence of not wanting to treat unnecessarily. Conversely, even with these high thresholds, about 10% of intrauterine procedures were done according to high ΔOD 450, falsely alarming values, when ultimately the fetus was only mildly affected. Other groups have suggested these proportions are about 11% (52) in each direction or even as high as 10% false-reassuring, 54% falsely alarming values (67).

High-resolution ultrasound and ultrasound criteria for description of severe fetal disease (68) have meant that hydrops fetalis is no longer overlooked when ΔOD 450 is low. Secondly, greater success with IPT meant progressively earlier application and, as a result, demands for earlier standards. These demands, (a) greater precision (b) among fetuses who were anemic without physical disease (c) earlier in pregnancy are NOT requirements that can be met by Liley's data. It is not necessary to misappropriate the Liley curve or subject it to detailed statistics. *It was not designed to measure hemoglobin, but to suggest the likely outcome of untreated alloimmune disease.*

Interpretation of ΔOD 450

In response to these concerns, modifications were made to the original Liley diagram (Figure 6-6) (23,33,66,67,69–71). These attempts at reconciliation of the Liley principle with expanding knowledge of fetal hemolysis, are not at all in agreement. It seems safe to say that the application of amniotic fluid spectrophotometry at gestations before 24–26 weeks is subject to considerable variation.

Why do amniotic fluid bilirubin levels fluctuate during the mid-trimester? There are many reasons for this, not all completely understood. It is not proven, for example, by which routes bilirubin actually enters amniotic fluid. Many more surfaces (fetal integument, mucous membranes, cord and placental vessels, and perhaps even early membranes) are permeable at the beginning of pregnancy than allow bilirubin transmission later. The animal model includes excretion of bilirubin via the tracheal bronchial tree (72), proven in icteric human fetuses. Fetal urine does not contain significant bilirubin and remains crystal clear, even in the moribund hydrops, even at very early gestation. Early pregnancy bleeding and contributions via the yolk sac and membranes during the extrafetal development of the gastrointestinal tract are also probable

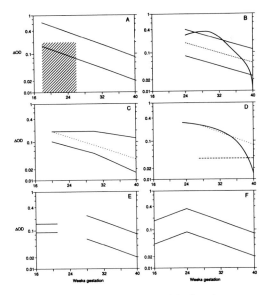

Figure 6-6   Some of the "modified" Liley curves that have been published. **6-6A**   Nicolaides (67) and Joshi (69) both used simple extrapolation of the Liley zones back from the data-based limit of 28 weeks of the Liley zones. There are no observational data to substantiate this extrapolation. **6-6B**   Steyn et al. (70) modified the Whitfield (66) action line, and extended the Liley (32) zones back to 24 weeks. **6-6C**   Reiss et al. (71) used their data (not published) to construct a new set of lines. **6-6D**   The Whitfield (66) action line, which reflects the curvilinear nature of amniotic fluid bilirubin levels throughout pregnancy. **6-6E**   Ananth (33) and Queenan have shown early second-trimester data that has effective correlation with ultimate fetal disease. This is shown on the same graph as the original Liley (32) zones. **6-6F**   The original modification proposed by Bowman (23) expressing an arc-shaped contour of amniotic fluid bilirubin levels. This theoretical postulate led to the research and development of the curve we now use, shown in Figure 6-7.

sources for amniotic fluid bilirubin in early pregnancy.

It is not surprising that a wide variety of results have been obtained in constructing a normal curve at this gestation. In Figure 6-6, the recommendations look more like opinions than the result of detailed data analysis, for example, the completely linear "extrapolated" Liley curve displayed by Nicolaides (Figure 6-6A) despite the clearly curvilinear normal human data he provides. The points in Nicolaides' study (67) and large studies by Ananth et al. (73) and Albar et al. (6), demonstrate a slightly rising slope of ΔOD 450 values for normal pregnancy between 14–16 and 20–22 weeks; after levelling off between 20–22 and 24–26 weeks, values decline, as depicted by Liley. A curvilinear equation would clearly provide the best statistical regression.

The curve now in use at our institution is based on 610 amniocentesis results, with percentile curves shown in Figure 6-7 (34). We use the dashed line, which joins the 80% Zone 2 limit of Liley zones, the 87.5th percentile of our own normative data. The Liley Zone 1 line connects with the 32.5th percentile curve again at 28 weeks gestation. To date, we have evaluated this curve prospectively in 32 alloimmunized patients. Affected pregnancies show an angulation from the level of the first amniocentesis. Isolated single readings, even at markedly elevated levels (0.25 or greater), when obtained at <20 weeks, are not reliable indicators of anemia on an immediate basis. Two representative cases are shown. It is clear, even in these cases using a "new" curve, that trend analysis is critical in discerning which individuals require invasive fetal treatment.

As in many centers, the data are derived from local patients and probably have limitations in application elsewhere. Further, the reservations regarding amniotic fluid and the various sources of bilirubin and

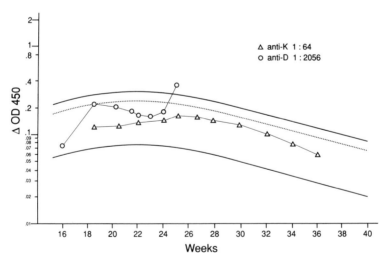

Figure 6-7 The "Bowman curve" (34) with representative amniotic fluid ΔOD 450 profiles. The upper curve (open circles) shows the sudden ΔOD 450 rise at 24 weeks, associated with the appearance of accelerating hydrops ultimately reversed with a series of IVT. In the second case (triangles), severely immunized against Kell, serial ΔOD 450 did not cross the 80% Zone 2 line, IVT was not necessary, and a healthy baby was delivered at 37 weeks, requiring two exchanges for elevated bilirubin. Action on an isolated level in several instances in either curve would have resulted in inappropriate action; trend analysis is critical.

other contaminants that may influence absorbance at 450nm, are not removed simply by having a larger number of data points! That a relatively smooth curve is found, appealing from a biologic point of view, suggests that this may be a reasonable pattern to expect. Clearly, in the patient at 20 weeks with a suspicious single fluid, e.g., ΔOD 450 = 0.280, a high antibody titer, and a significant past history, one would move to PUBS and/or fetal transfusion, provided a suitable target was present. On the other hand, in the same patient, ΔOD 450 = 0.100 would be relatively reassuring, and we do weekly ultrasound examinations and repeat amniocentesis in 10–14 days. As noted above, the population examined prospectively using this curve is relatively small, but no glaring errors have yet appeared. The key, of course, is to integrate all available information about the fetus, and using the discriminants between amniocentesis and cordocentesis as described below, avoid fetal deterioration.

Finally, antigen-negative fetuses, i.e., father heterozygous, with previously-affected infants, displayed an early trend suggestive of unaffected status. Regardless of first ΔOD 450 level, if the absolute value at repeat amniocentesis was significantly lower, it was highly predictive of a negative fetus. The data are not yet numerous enough at 16–20 weeks to allow rigid application of this apparent principle.

Technical Factors

Amniocentesis for ΔOD 450 is done under ultrasound direction. If the placenta is completely anterior and must be traversed, cord vessels are not accessible (generally before 18 weeks), *and* there are travel or family imperatives prohibiting serial ultrasound, we consider passage of a 27-gauge needle at the extreme limits of the placenta, far from the cord insertion. With all these

conditions, transplacental amniocentesis in a sensitized patient is seldom advocated. This practice explains why our incidence of transplacental hemorrhage following amniocentesis for the monitoring of Rh-alloimmunization is very low (1.8% of >2000 amniocenteses) (74). With a posterior placenta and accessible amniotic fluid, we have no compunction about serial amniocentesis. Some, e.g., C. P. Weiner, have argued that an amniocentesis is just as likely to cause infection, ruptured membranes, aggravation of sensitization, and other complications as in PUBS (63). That is certainly not our experience, although we agree with his low estimate of cordocentesis complications. Amniocentesis is an extremely safe procedure with no mortality in >2000 amniocenteses in second and third trimester.

The needle tip is clearly visualized in the amniotic space and 5–8 ml aspirated. Any traces of bleeding after needle removal are monitored until cessation, although in most cases this is maternal. If blood is obtained, e.g., as a result of sudden fetal activity pushing the cord against the needle, or if an initially-clear sample becomes blood-stained, a sample is aspirated and the needle tip is carefully visualized to determine the origin of the blood. Any blood-tinged fluid is retained for Kleihauer test and fetal blood group. Standard centrifugation will remove the red cells, allowing both blood typing on the red cells and reliable ΔOD 450 measurement on the fluid.

Amniocentesis is begun in most situations at 18 weeks gestation. With history of serious fetal anemia or hydrops before 18 weeks, the situation becomes quite experimental and we do not attempt fetal monitoring. In those rare situations, we will move directly to early IPT until PUBS becomes technically feasible. (Although Nicolaides has never seen a case before 17 weeks, we are aware of four hydropic deaths in three women at 16 5/7, 17 1/7, and 15 4/7 and 16 4/7 weeks, respectively (75), so such exigencies *are* needed.)

The interval for repeat amniocentesis depends on history, antibody titer, ΔOD 450, and any effect the procedure or passage of time has on antibody level. It is essential to continue serial ultrasound examination, and to repeat maternal antibody titration in the interval.

Problems

Trend analysis is the essential ingredient of ΔOD 450 interpretation, and failure to adhere to this principle is the most common error of ΔOD 450 evaluation. In addition to difficulties in interpretation at early gestation, a number of errors may be introduced. Fetal urine is perfectly clear, ascitic fluid is bright amber with a high protein content and very low absorption above 575nm, while a number of contaminants may interfere (Table 6-7).

Other Amniotic Fluid Parameters of Interest

The presence of pure *heme pigment* should not be disregarded as residual from previous amniocenteses. Until proven otherwise by cordocentesis, a pure heme pigment peak (at

405 μ, Figure 6-8) denotes sudden accelerated hemolysis, so rapid that conversion to bilirubin is overwhelmed (21). *Arginine vasopressin* may be present in amniotic fluid of decompensating anemic fetuses (76). Amniotic fluid *erythropoietin* (EPO) bears a linear relationship to fetal anemia and serum EPO, but initial studies have shown only moderate predictive accuracy (77–79). In the appropriate clinical circumstances, karyotype or viral studies may be indicated when the fluid values (severe) are out of proportion to the maternal sensitization (mild), suggesting alternate diagnosis.

Complications

In current experience, we have not had a single serious immediate complication. This includes >2000 amniocentesis procedures, with up to 10 procedures (from 18 to 40 weeks) in some individuals. Although fetal hemorrhage from cord laceration, chorioamnionitis, direct fetal injury, or uterine injury appear in the world literature, selection considering the factors in Table 6-8 must mean these are all exceedingly rare. Referral to a secondary center may be required, but fluid can be shipped (in light-proof container to avoid bilirubin degradation) without difficulty. Procedure and tests are low-cost.

Table 6-7   Interference With ΔOD 450 Readings

Contaminant	Absorption	Consequence
Fetal Serum (Traumatic Amniocentesis)	450nm	False elevation
Bilirubin (Fetal GI Obstruction)	450nm	False elevation
Heme Pigments (Intra-amniotic Bleeding with Hemolysis)	580, 540, 415 (oxyhemoglobin) 405 (methemalbumin)	No readable peak Falsely low
Meconium Pigments	420 peak, panspectral increase	No readable peak

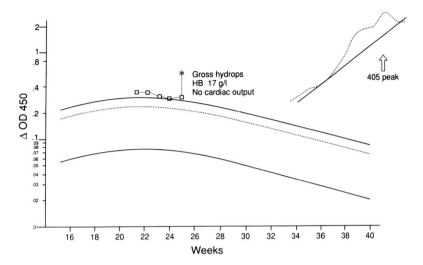

Figure 6-8 ΔOD 450 trend. Fetus found to be severely hydropic at last visit, referred immediately for IVT. (▲ = ΔOD 450, * = ΔOD 450 on amniotic fluid obtained at time of attempted IVT.) Class 4 hydrops with no cardiac output, fatal outcome. Insert shows: Amniotic fluid spectrophotometry showing a heme pigment peak. In this case, the peak at 405nm distorted the 450 peak. This 405 peak was due to hemolysis proceeding so rapidly that complete metabolism to bilirubin was not possible. In automated systems, such variants may be omitted, leading to erroneous (optimistic) interpretation. This fetus was in the midst of a hemolytic crisis.

Maternal immune consequences of amniocentesis in our institution do not substantiate claims by proponents of routine cordocentesis. Bowell et al. (42) suggest that amniocentesis is likely to cause elevation of maternal antibody titers in as many as 44%, while this has only occurred in 3.1% of our cases (Table 6-8) (31). Note the difference between this percentage, which reflects the number of pregnancies monitored by amniocentesis in which the maternal titer rose, and the rate of proven TPH, 1.8% of procedures, by maternal Kleihauer test *five* minutes postamniocentesis. This is another area where the experience of individual teams may cause adoption of rigid guidelines. We remain flexible, using the procedure with lowest risk of fetal injury and/or maternal antibody provocation. We do not share the enthusiasm of Weiner et al. (80) that cordocentesis can be accomplished without *any* maternal antibody provocation, but at the same time, will switch immediately from serial amniocentesis to PUBS when there is the slightest doubt about the ΔOD 450 trend, the antibody strength, or fetal ultrasound appearance. Guidelines for when to switch procedures are summarized in Figure 6-9.

Cordocentesis

Background

With the demonstration of safe access to the fetal circulation, a wealth of data has become available on investigation and management of the anemic fetus. The contributions of Nicolaides, Daffos, Rodeck, Berkewitz, and Weiner, and many others cannot be chronicled completely here. Clearly, cordocentesis provided a "quantum leap" in understanding

Table 6-8 Factors Favoring Initial Choice of Monitoring Method (Note All the Reasons to Switch to Cordocentesis in Figure 6-9)

Serial Amniocentesis
 Posterior lateral or fundal placenta
 No previous hydropic disease
 Normal amniotic fluid volume
 Gestation <20 weeks
 Geographic isolation
 Maternal anxiety

Cordocentesis (PUBS)
 Anterior placenta
 Previous hydropic disease
 Fetal blood typing needed
 Gestation >20 weeks
 Changes in antibody level

Consider Maternal Immune Provocation

	TPH	AB RISE
Amniocentesis	1.8%	3.1%
Cordocentesis	33%	26.5%

TPH = Transplacental hemorrhage. AB = antibody.

fetal disease and our ability to treat it. Although many parameters measurable in PUBS samples may be of pathophysiologic interest, prognostic value, or of great *individual* sensitivity, the primary values we utilize are hemoglobin/hematocrit, serum bilirubin level, nucleated red cell count, and the red cell smear.

First Samples

On the first occasion, of course, fetal blood typing and direct Coombs' test are performed. Even a contaminated specimen may be used for typing because the antigen-positive fetus will be detectable against the background of antigen-negative adult cells. The direct Coombs' test is an indicator of antibody strength, but a variable predictor of progression of anemia. When the Coombs' test is complete in <1 minute, but the fetal hemoglobin is within the normal range (de-

fined by gestational age, Figure 6-10), we rely on serial ultrasound with intermittent PUBS but on serial amniocentesis if correlation between the ΔOD 450 and fetal hemoglobin level is satisfactory. Thus, the Coombs' test influences us but has not been predictive enough to mandate a fixed schedule of PUBS or exclude the possibility of subsequent anemia, i.e., excluding further cordocentesis. Our primary differences from the recommendations by Weiner et al. (7) probably are based on the fact that we sample few patients with modest maternal antibody titration (1:8–1:32 by indirect Coombs).

First and Subsequent Cordocenteses

Cordocentesis without intravascular fetal transfusion is not considered for hydropic fetuses. In nonhydropic fetuses, we usually perform PUBS as a separate procedure, with the patient and team available for IVT on short notice. On some occasions, when (a) there are suspicious ultrasound findings, (b) ΔOD 450 values have been alarming, (c) previous PUBS was highly suggestive of accelerating disease, or (d) previous pregnancies have shown potential for severe anemia, the patient is prepared as for intravascular fetal transfusion, but infusion is withheld until the hemoglobin value is known at the bedside ("cordo-IVT"). In either the isolated cordocentesis or "cordo-IVT," the cutoff value for proceeding to transfuse a fetus is based on the gestational age guidelines and is agreed upon *prior* to the procedure.

 Hematologic values. Since hemoglobin is the actual oxygen-carrying entity, we prefer its measurement. To be precise, this is the measurement of total hemoglobin present in fetal red cells and not measurement of fetal hemoglobin exclusively. (This may explain

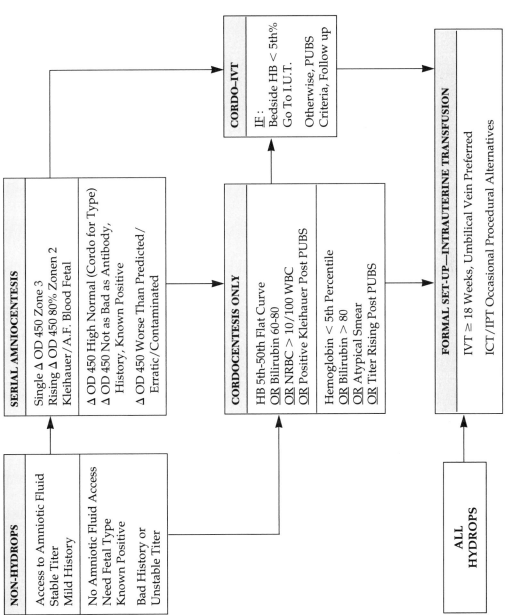

NON-HYDROPS

Access to Amniotic Fluid
Stable Titer
Mild History

No Amniotic Fluid Access
Need Fetal Type
Known Positive

Bad History or
Unstable Titer

SERIAL AMNIOCENTESIS

Single Δ OD 450 Zone 3
Rising Δ OD 450 80% Zonen 2
Kleihauer/A.F. Blood Fetal

Δ OD 450 High Normal (Cordo for Type)
Δ OD 450 Not as Bad as Antibody,
History, Known Positive

Δ OD 450 Worse Than Predicted/
Erratic/Contaminated

CORDOCENTESIS ONLY

HB 5th-50th Flat Curve
OR Bilirubin 60-80
OR NRBC > 10/100 WBC
OR Positive Kleihauer Post PUBS

Hemoglobin < 5th Percentile
OR Bilirubin > 80
OR Atypical Smear
OR Titer Rising Post PUBS

CORDO–IVT

IF :
Bedside HB < 5th%
Go To I.U.T.

Otherwise, PUBS
Criteria, Follow up

FORMAL SET-UP—INTRAUTERINE TRANSFUSION

IVT ≥ 18 Weeks, Umbilical Vein Preferred

ICT/IPT Occasional Procedural Alternatives

**ALL
HYDROPS**

Figure 6-9   Thresholds determine the need and timing of switching from one invasive modality to another.

Figure 6-10 Normal hemoglobin range defined by 250 nonanemic fetuses with normal outcome who underwent cordocentesis for various reasons throughout gestation. Plots show fetal hemoglobin levels of fetus in Case Summary #1 (stars) and another fetus with posterior placenta, serial cordocentesis (open squares). There was no change in maternal antibody level. She ultimately required induction of labor, three exchanges at 36+ weeks for anemic baby - HB 66g/l.

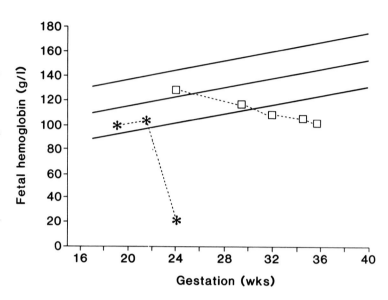

why the linear regression of fetal hemoglobin concentration has a slightly lower slope than the regression of fetal hematocrit; as an increasing amount of adult hemoglobin is present, the cells are at the same time becoming smaller, as term approaches.)

Fetal hemoglobin concentration rises throughout gestation. Based on >250 nonanemic fetuses, our equation was used to generate the normative distribution shown (Figure 6-10). This is very similar to distributions published by others, which is interesting in view of the widely disparate geographic, cultural, and socioeconomic factors (7,81). We utilize the fifth percentile as our indicator to proceed directly with transfusion during "cordo-IVTs." After isolated cordocentesis, hemoglobin level <fifth percentile or abnormalities in other indices as noted below mandate return within 24 hours for the first IVT.

The use of fetal hemoglobin or hematocrit to define the severity of fe-

tal disease is a point not yet proven. It might appear obvious that anemia can only be defined by hemoglobin concentration or hematocrit, but it is not certain that the extent of *measured anemia* is absolutely concordant with the *severity of disease*. This concept is important when one assesses methods of monitoring and management of the anemic fetus.

Our cutoff level was chosen in order to avoid transfusing fetuses who do not require it and is not based on evidence that that level is critical for fetal well-being. It is notable that Weiner uses the same statistical basis for election of transfusion and that the cutoffs used by Nicolaides and many other groups reflect the distribution of sick fetuses rather than the critical nature of fetal anemia of a given extreme. Although paradoxical, it may well be that fetal anemia is not the gold standard of fetal alloimmune hemolytic disease.

Fetal serum bilirubin. Fetal serum bilirubin is easily measured in uncontaminated samples of fluid, and we use it as a test of amniotic fluid or maternal serum contamination of the sample. After a difficult procedure where visualization was less than perfect, or after IVT which required needle repositioning, serum bilirubin can provide reassurance that testing and/or transfusion was done in the same vessel consistently throughout. Our experience is that only very large, very rapid IVT produce any pre-/post-procedure changes. Equivalent (high) pre-/post-levels suggest proper needle placement throughout. Serum bilirubin is evaluated in standard laboratory fashion, and although there may be a slight gestational trend (82), we apply the same simple guidelines throughout pregnancy.

If total bilirubin is >80 mmol/L, preparation is made for immediate fetal transfusion regardless of the current hemoglobin level. This is one instance in which the hemoglobin has been found to be an inaccurate estimation of fetal condition, specifically of the rate of hemolysis. On three occasions (2.4%) of fetuses requiring serial IVT, *hemolytic crisis* has been rapid, evidenced by very high fetal serum bilirubin associated with overt damage on the RBC smear. In such a situation, we regard the hemoglobin level as suspect until another explanation for the elevated serum bilirubin is found. This frequency (<3% false-reassuring fetal hemoglobin levels) is an overstatement of any unreliability that may exist as it deals only with the minority of patients who have required transfusion. In general, concordance between hemoglobin and serum bilirubin is good.

Fetal bilirubin between 60 and 80 nmol/L indicates accelerated hemolysis and the need for successive PUBS, usually weekly. Values between 40 and 60 are indeterminant, requiring integration of all available information and selection of a repeat sampling interval, usually between two and four weeks. If the value does not exceed 40 mmol/L, hemolysis is likely present at a low level, if any, and the bilirubin value is not used to adjust the necessity or frequency of subsequent testing. Intervals depend on patient accessibility (for weekly ultrasound examinations) and obtaining maternal antibody titers in the interval (at least one titer seven days following each cordocentesis), evaluated on the background of the patient's antibody characteristics and history.

Nucleated red blood cell count (83). In normal gestation, the nucleated red blood cell count (conventionally expressed as NRBC/100 WBC) decreases progressively. This parameter is less reliable than others and may be highly variable from one fetus to the next, given the unique character in each individual of the anemia–tissue oxygen-erythropoietin-NRBC loop. Further, if fetal bleeding at PUBS is excessive or repetitive sampling attempts result in uterine hypertonicity, an elevated NRBC count may be procedure-related, as the NRBC count obtained the next day (at the time of IVT) is substantially lower (unpublished observations). The literature suggests variable success in using either the reticulocyte count (83) or the NRBC count (7) in the *prediction* of fetal anemia. Generation of NRBC of all lineages is an immediate response of the severely anemic fetus and *correlates* well with the extent of fetal disease, but the *predictive* element is not reliable enough to initiate therapeutic action in itself.

Red cell characteristics. Using mean corpuscular volume (MCV) may be a way of overcoming variation between reticulocyte count, NRBC counts, and so on. As earlier/younger red cells (and ultimately, RBC precursors) become more prominent, MCV will rise. In the early stages of fetal anemia, this parameter may reflect subtle decreases in circulating lifetime of fetal red cells; as older (smaller) cells are hemolyzed, average cell size will rise. On occasion, we have noted unusual numbers of aberrant forms (anisocytosis, schistocytosis, and other deformed cells), as is seen in typical mechanical hemolysis in nonfetal patients. These are indicative of extremely rapid hemolysis associated with unusually high-serum bilirubin, but not always with low hemoglobin concentration. Only if the red cell smear is overtly aberrant do we disregard the reassurance of a normal hemoglobin value and proceed with serial PUBS at short interval.

Technical Factors

Isolated cordocentesis is a routine procedure, without premedication or prophylaxis. Diligent antisepsis is practiced (We have never had a case of chorioamnionitis.) and to minimize the chance of TPH, we almost always use two operators. One directs the procedure using continuous ultrasound (one hand on the keyboard the other in a sterile sleeve), while the other manipulates the 22-gauge spinal needle and withdraws the specimens. We do not use a needle guide but choose the most vertical approach available and change direction as little as possible. We approach the vessel directly in the

path of the needle (We have had no episodes of artery spasm.) but will choose the umbilical vein 1–2 cm from the surface of the placenta if possible.

Other Fetal Blood Parameters of Interest

Blood gases and pH are done routinely during IVT and may be valuable in assessing the procedure-related compromise when the procedure is complicated and/or recovery is delayed. Prediction of acceleration of anemia has not been demonstrated. In all fetuses above threshold for transfusion (and in many fetuses *below* the threshold we choose for transfusion), biochemical, cellular, hormonal, blood gas, enzymatic, and many other parameters are unperturbed by fetal anemia. In early experimental anemia, the first changes are at the level of erythrocyte and endothelial metabolism. Serum *carboxyhemoglobin* elevation may be an early sign, although one not likely to achieve universal application due to its technical strictures. In general, the variable expression of such factors when related to specific fetal hemoglobin levels suggests that: (1) not all fetuses have the same effect from the same degree of anemia, and (2) most fetuses have very few effects at all of mild to moderate anemia, and some of those may, in fact, be positive, e.g., the enhanced cardiac output which often attends significant but still moderate anemia (70–100 g/l) (84,85).

Complications

The major concern is of aggravation of maternal sensitization. We have had no serious fetal complications, although the literature includes hemorrhage, chorioamnionitis, bradycardia, lethal hematoma, and an estimated mortality of one to three per 1000. Isolated PUBS is not used in hydrops, and the risk of lethal hemorrhage in nonhydrops must be exceedingly small. PUBS is a fairly expensive procedure, with expensive tests which must be done on site; both procedure and tests require referral to a tertiary center, with those additional attendant costs (monetary and otherwise).

AMNIOCENTESIS VERSUS CORDOCENTESIS— WHY ALL THE FUSS?

We favor amniocentesis in many situations but utilize cordocentesis freely. We see no reason to become rigid in this and reject the position that only PUBS can provide reliable data. It is true that cordocentesis provides digital laboratory data much more in harmony with our medical/scientific background than the relatively loose interpretive nature of ΔOD 450. Many advances have been made based on data from PUBS and on occasion, PUBS may produce surprisingly low results in the face of normal amniocentesis values. This is not a reason to abandon amniocentesis and subject every woman with sensitization to cordocentesis. The cautions against PUBS are clear in many references, with a much higher rate of transplacental hemorrhage and subsequent aggravation of maternal sensitization, including the development of antibodies against *new* red blood cell antigens, in many centers. Case histories are illustrative here.

Case History #1 (See Figure 6-10)

This Rh-negative woman had high levels of anti-DC and was managed in collaboration with our institution in her third pregnancy. In the first pregnancy, she did not receive antenatal Rh prophylaxis, delivered a term infant who was Rh-positive and unaffected, had no antibodies present at the time of delivery, and received postpartum Rh prophylaxis. At the beginning of the second pregnancy, she had anti-D IgG, 1:64 (albumin), and was induced at 36 weeks for an infant who was well after two exchange transfusions and phototherapy. In the third pregnancy, anti-D was 1:128, an anterior placenta prevented safe amniocentesis, and she underwent cordocentesis at 19+ weeks. This showed fetal hemoglobin 100 g/L, in the normal range for gestation, associated with serum bilirubin 47 mmol/L, and three NRBC/100 WBC. The second cordocentesis 2 1/2 weeks later showed hemoglobin 102 g/L, serum bilirubin 48 mmol/L, and similar RBC findings. On the first occasion, postprocedure Kleihauer was negative. On the second occasion, the maternal antibody titer had risen to 256, and Kleihauer evaluation showed a small number of fetal cells in the maternal circulation five minutes after cordocentesis. Thinking that the first procedure possibly further aggravated by the transplacental hemorrhage identified at the second procedure, had caused increased maternal sensitization, we requested (but did not receive) repeat maternal blood sample after one week. The patient returned after two weeks for her scheduled repeat cordocentesis. The fetus was moribund and hydropic, with a terminal heart rate tracing. Attempts at intrauterine resuscitation were futile; hemoglobin measurement from the fetal right ventricle was 22 g/L. The profound ability of serial cordocentesis to cause exacerbation of maternal antibody production to very rapidly lethal disease was proven in this case, with post-stillbirth measurement of maternal antibody titer >2056. The patient subsequently underwent a further pregnancy with an Rh-positive, severely-affected infant. IVT began at 23 weeks, resulting in healthy delivery of an intact survivor. On that occasion, the placenta was posterior, antibody production was not aggravated over the course of therapy, and antibody level remained at 64.

Case Study #2

This patient was strongly Rh-sensitized by emergency Rh-positive transfusion in childhood. The first pregnancy was delivered at 34 weeks gestation with escalating hemolysis demonstrated by serial amniocentesis. That infant required multiple exchange transfusions and phototherapy but ultimately did well. In the second pregnancy, initial antibody titer was 1028, and because the husband was heterozygous for D, cordocentesis was done at 22 weeks for fetal blood typing and assessment of anemia. Kleihauer test 10 minutes after the procedure was negative. Normal values were obtained for 22 weeks: hemoglobin 122 g/L, bilirubin 36 mmol/L, NRBC count 7/100 WBC. The cordocentesis was described as a "difficult" procedure, and one of the samples had a low pH, suggesting contamination by amniotic fluid. Our team was consulted with regard to subsequent surveillance. Maternal antibody titration after seven days showed a rise to 4096. The patient was immediately referred to our unit. On arrival, she had a dead, hydropic fetus. Antibody titration at that time showed a further rise to >16000. Our impression was that the Kleihauer had simply been too long after the procedure to note fetal cells entering the maternal circulation, causing this profound rise in antibody titer and leading to fetal demise.

Case Study #3

This 38-year old woman had therapeutic abortion not protected with Winrho, resulting in serious anti-CD sensitization, with a titer of 1:64 (albumin). After further miscarriages, she was referred to our team at 18 weeks gestation with a normal-looking fetus. Initial amniocentesis was 0.105, the titer was still 1:64, the husband was most likely homozygous. Serial amnio-

centesis was elected as the monitoring method as the placenta was posterior and geographic isolation was a significant factor, and she was returned to the referring center. By 25 weeks, ΔOD 450 was 0.100, the placenta was bulky, there was possible scalp edema (there were definitely no ascites); the fetus was very active. Cordocentesis was undertaken at the referring center, ultimately with death of the fetus, who was proven to be significantly anemic—Hb 58 g/L. Although this was a devastating experience, even worse was the effect on maternal sensitization—her titer rose to 1:65,536 (absolute level 342 µg/ml, 1710 IU/ml). Two further pregnancies resulted in documented hydropic death *before 17 weeks gestation* despite plasmapheresis, maternal immune globulin infusion (86) and our intention to do intraperitoneal and/or intravascular transfusion at 16+ weeks.

These cases are not presented to discourage the gathering of detailed and definitive data on affected fetuses. They are presented to illustrate that even the most conscientious approach may cause some harm. None of these cases was sufficiently unique that in retrospect one realizes that the interval should have been less, the cordocentesis should not have been done in the first place, or transfusion should have been commenced regardless of the normal, reassuring findings. In the first two cases, two weeks elapsed between procedures (and, in fact, between ultrasound examinations—a potentially serious error). It has been our policy since that time to recommend weekly ultrasound examinations in *all* fetuses whose direct Coombs' reaction is complete in <1 minute.

It has been our experience, including nine years using cordocentesis in evaluation of alloimmune disease, that both procedures have their uses, their liabilities, and complementary value. Although many situations do favor PUBS (Table 6-8), the initial phase of monitoring in many patients is still by amniocentesis. Accessibility and costs, as well as the rare direct complications, probably favor amniocentesis, but these are relatively minor issues in the large majority of cases, and decisions are made primarily on the basis of the management issues cited. The formulation of a randomized controlled trial to study the advantages and disadvantages of the two techniques, as if they were artificially separate and exclusive, is neither possible nor necessary.

Monitoring Summary

The threshold for invasive monitoring is based on antibody type and character, heavily influenced by history of previously-affected infants and of the profile of the antibody itself during the index pregnancy. Albumin titer of 1:16, corresponding roughly to an indirect Coombs' titer of 1:32 or greater, and corresponding to an absolute anti-D level of 2 µg/ml (10 IU/ml), is our threshold for antibody strength. If it is normal, the fetal physical examination allows invasive monitoring by whichever route is desirable; however, if the physical examination is abnormal, there is no indication for temporizing by testing, and immediate fetal treatment is indicated. In the nonhydropic fetus, isolated PUBS would be elected when there is a significant chance (based on paternal zygosity) that the fetus is antigen-negative or mildly affected, versus "cordo-IVT," when the fetus is known antigen-positive, but the severity of anemia is not yet determined. These decisions will be greatly influenced by the availability of fetal blood grouping. Thresholds to proceed with transfusion according to PUBS results or at the bedside, when a low hemoglobin is reported during cordo-IVT, are shown for

our institution. The diagram shown in Figure 6-9 summarizes this approach, which uses thresholds to prompt moving to the next step.

EXAMINATION OF THE FETUS
IN ALLOIMMUNE DISEASE

Many elements of fetal ultrasound surveillance in alloimmune disease have been credited with unique properties in predicting anemia. Individual, *isolated* measurements of umbilical vein diameter, the pericardial space, umbilical arterial or venous velocimetry, QRS complex width, mean heart rate variation, total fetal activity, or any other parameter does not have the reliability to *predict* the onset of anemia requiring treatment (87–89). To be sure, all the above have at least one reference demonstrating *correlation* with hemoglobin level. In many cases, however, it is apparent that the correlation is secondary to gestational age. As an alloimmune pregnancy progresses, the fetus generally becomes more anemic; as gestation progresses, most of the above parameters increase; it is likely inevitable that there will be statistical correlation.

This does not mean that some of these observations are without merit; it means that none of them should be used in isolation. We have, indeed, seen cases, for example, where the umbilical vein is dilated >1.5 cm (90). This is associated with gross cardiac dilatation, venous pulsation, and fetal hypertension as evidenced by direct measurement and by indirect observation of the bouncing cord as it lies in the amniotic fluid. The abdominal circumference is >80th percentile for gestation, and 6/8 fetuses with this finding were hydropic. To extract the large umbilical vein diameter from this total picture is to give it undue credit.

Key elements of the comprehensive fetal physical examination are discussed below. Note, however, that while one gains an impression of approaching disease, which helps in deciding between amniocentesis, cordocentesis, or cordo-IVT, the impressions are *subjective* and based on a total assessment of the fetus and his situation. In a seriously immunized pregnancy, it is never our policy to use a "normal" fetal physical examination to justify deferral of invasive monitoring. This is important: 15% of fetuses referred with hydrops fetalis to our team have had amniocentesis procedures deferred because "the fetus looked completely well," only to have gross hydrops on the return scan two weeks later. The intention of the scan is to find early signs of hydrops and accelerate action, not to delay necessary plans because the exam is normal—the normal-appearing fetus may have a hemoglobin as low as 45 g/L!

Similar experiences have led some to conclude there is no value in ultrasound examination of the fetus (7,52,83). This is difficult to test. We use suspicious ultrasound findings as reason to accelerate intervention and evaluate the physical findings of severe fetal disease by an ultrasound classification system based on the progression of findings in hydropic disease, diagrammed in Figure 6-11 (31).

Class 0 fetuses are controls, undergoing PUBS for suspected alloimmune disease, shown to be antigen-negative or antigen-positive with no hemolysis, a weak direct Coombs' test, and normal outcome not requiring exchange transfusion. None of these fetuses had any evidence, in either placental or fetal physical findings, suggestive of "accelerated alloimmune disease."

Class 1 fetuses had amniocentesis for monitoring because none were overtly hydropic, all with elevated ΔOD 450. They all progressed to PUBS and were antigen-positive, Coombs' complete <1 minutes, exceeding the threshold for initiation and serial treatment by IVT. Abdominal circumference measurements were accelerating in nature. Umbilical arterial Doppler velocimetry was above the gestational age-corrected 90th percentile in 27%, but the group mean was at the 50th percentile. Markers suggestive of early hemodynamic stress included visible pericardial effusion in 35% (but not >3 mm in any case) (Figure 6-12A), biventricular outer diameter greater than expected in one-third; bounding umbilical cord, increased ventricular excursion, "hyperdynamic heart action," inferior vena cava pulsations, and increased maximum blood flow velocity in the ascending aorta. All parameters were noted with increased frequency, but for none of these was

	ULTRASOUND APPEARANCE				ABNORMAL BPS <6/10
Class	Placenta	Ascites	Effusions	Anasarca	
0	−	−	−	−	−
1	+	−	−	−	−
2	+	+	−	−	−
3	+	+	+	+	−
4	+	+	+	+	+

Figure 6-11 Ultrasound classification of severe fetal alloimmune disease. (+ = Abnormal sign present.)

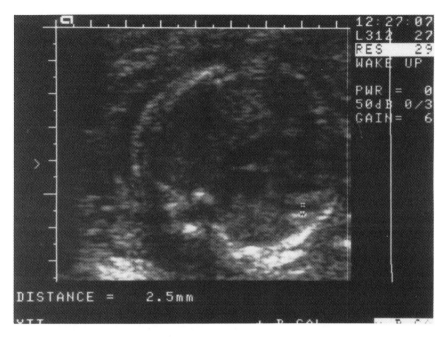

Figure 6-12A Subjective ultrasound observations in Class 1 disease. Small pericardial effusion, in association with subjectively hyperdynamic cardiac action, and increased S:D ratio.

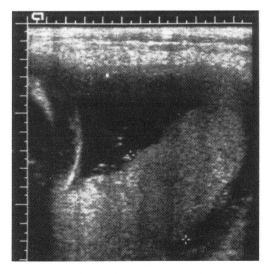

Figure 6-12B Hydramnios and early placental distension in Class 1 disease.

the frequency >50%. Serum bilirubin ranged from 41 mmol/L (the only fetus below 60 mmol/L) to 185 mmol/L. NRBC count was >10/100 WBC in only 6%. In 80%, amniotic fluid measured >8 cm in maximum vertical pocket depth, increased placental thickness, and loss of detailed placental architecture (Figure 6-12B). Hemoglobin levels ranged from 120 g/L (the threshhold for IVT at 33+ weeks) to one case at 45 g/L and a second at 52 g/L, both 31+ weeks.

Class 2 fetuses have early signs of hydrops fetalis. Hydramnios, loss of placental architecture, increased overall uterine volume, and increased uterine tone were universal. Ascites was unequivocal >5 mm in all cases, but of varying extent (Figures 6-13A, 6-13B). Particular care was taken not to confuse the appearance with so-called pseudoascites (91). In 50% there was exaggerated occipital scalp thickness, not exceeding 7 mm (Figure 6-13C), and none had peripheral edema. Doppler indices were more likely to be elevated (Figure 6-13D), biventricular outer diameter (BVOD) was greater than expected in >50% (Figure 6-14), but there were no cases of pericardial effusion >3 mm. The remainder of the fetal cardiac examination was similar to Class 1, although higher frequencies of all subjective findings were noted. Hematologic

Figure 6-13A Class 2 ultrasound features. Progression in the amount of ascites. By the time severe ascites has developed, there are usually other generalized signs, constituting progression to Class 3.

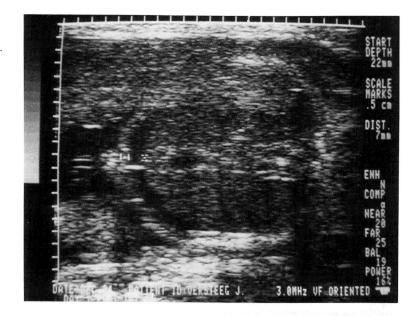

Figure 6-13B

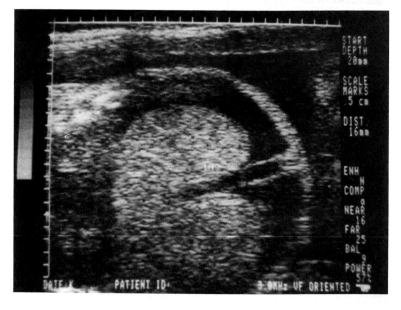

and biochemical parameters overlap significantly with Class 1 disease. The ascites disappeared relatively quickly after treatment.

Class 3 fetuses have severe physical disease with all the gross manifestations of accelerated hydrops fetalis. All had massive ascites, scalp edema, and body edema, especially notable in hands and face and upper body, illustrated in Figure 6-15A-D. The placenta was usually grossly enlarged (Figure 6-15D). Doppler velocimetry usually,

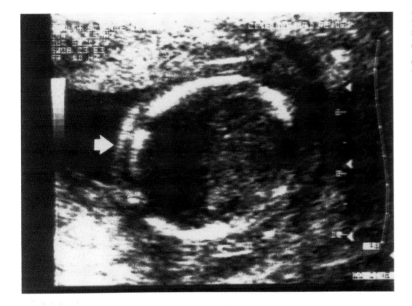

Figure 6-13C Shows early scalp edema, seen in 50% of Class 2 fetuses, but not associated with general anasarca, by definition.

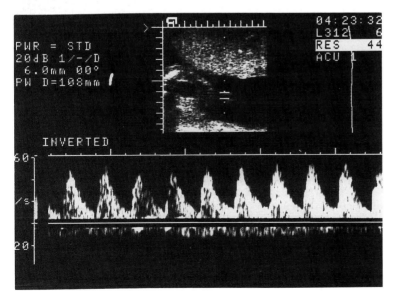

Figure 6-13D Increased S:D ratio reflecting serious anemia (fetal hemoglobin level 46 g/L at 28 weeks gestation).

Figure 6-14 Distended fetal heart with biventricular outer diameter (BVOD) enlarged for the gestational age of 24 weeks.

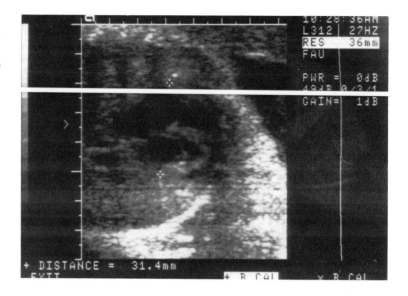

but not always, showed markedly elevated S:D ratio, with unusually high peak systolic velocity measurable in the ascending aorta in 80%. A number of fetuses had reduced heart rate variation on computerized analysis prior to transfusion, and the other subjective echocardiographic findings were also increased. The one redeeming feature of these fetuses prior to transfusion was that they were active, with a normal Biophysical Profile Score despite the presence of obviously life-threatening disease. Despite this severity of disease and fetal hemoglobins, which ranged as low as 13 g/L (22 weeks) to

Figure 6-15 Class 3/4 physical findings. **6-15A** Gross scalp and face edema, virtually obscuring the normal facial features. O = orbit, F = forehead, C = cheek. This "Buddha face" returned to normal after a series of 8 IVT, with a healthy survivor at term.

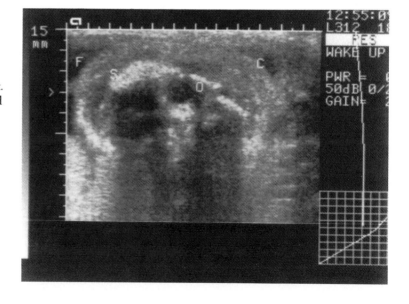

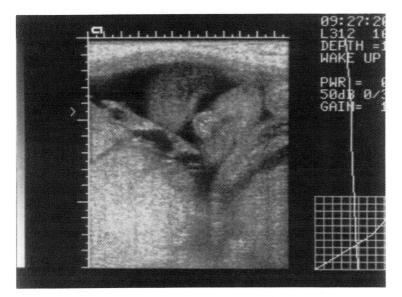

Figure 6-15B This fetus also has gross facial edema, using her distended placenta (lower left) as a pillow. Note also the large pleural effusion (arrow).

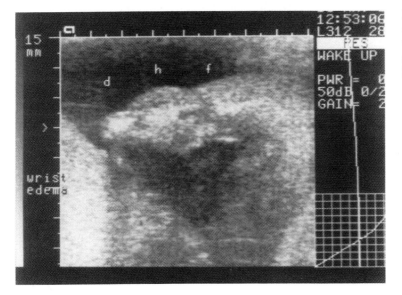

Figure 6-15C Peripheral edema showing almost-unrecognizable features of the left arm. d = digits, h = hand, f = forearm.

55 g/L (28 weeks), they had normal umbilical venous gases, normal pH, and normal cardiac output in response to their first transfusion.

In Class 4 fetuses, findings were occasionally more severe, especially at later gestation (Figure 6-16), but the primary difference added to these severe physical findings was the abnormally reduced fetal behavior. In Class 4 fetuses, there were exceptionally few movements with reduced tone and no fetal breathing movements; by definition, all had abnormal Biophysical Profile Scores. Hemoglobin values ranged

Figure 6-15D Class 3 fetuses have enormously-swollen placentas, frequently associated with uterine hyperdisten-sion, and maternal signs and symptoms of extrinsic renovascular compression ("mirror syndrome").

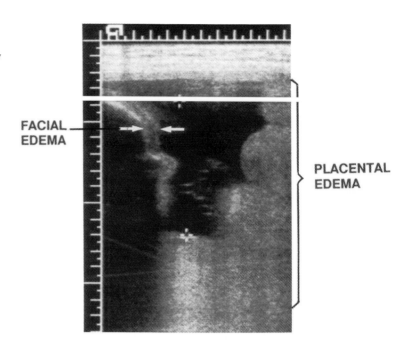

from 8 g/L (0.8 g/dL) at 21 weeks to 52 g/L at 25 weeks.

Correlation between the severity of disease and findings in the initial pretransfusion blood samples obtained is illustrated in Figures 6-17–6-19. There was a wide range of hemoglobin concentrations in Class 1 (non-hydropic) fetuses and significant overlap among the other classes. Biochemical markers and other fetal hematologic mark-

Figure 6-16 Exaggerated findings in a Class 4 placenta show extreme placental buckling due to edema and invagination of the cord insertion some 3 cm below the surface of the placenta.

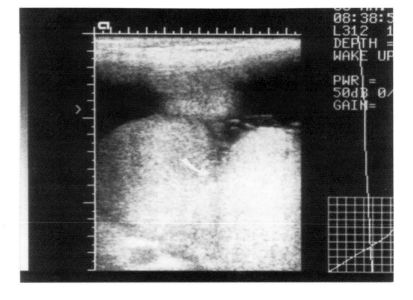

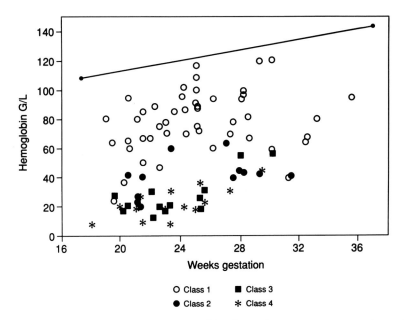

Figure 6-17 Fetal hemoglobin at pre-IVT blood sampling versus gestational age. The mean normal fetal hemoglobin concentration is shown at the top. Note the broad range of fetal hemoglobin found in Class 1 disease and the significant overlap of hemoglobin measurements in fetuses with markedly different severity of physical disease.

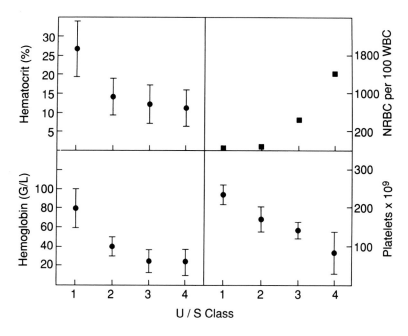

Figure 6-18 Ultrasound class plotted against fetal hematocrit, NRBC count, platelet count, and mean hemoglobin for each class. Ultrasound evidence of progressive physical disease correlates with progressive hematologic derangement.

Figure 6-19 Ultrasound class versus biochemical markers. Bilirubin actually declines as hemolysis peaks; the fetus is so anemic that even total hemolysis generates little in the way of bilirubin. As liver function is impaired, serum albumin falls. Only in the extremes of fetal disease does systemic homeostasis falter, exemplified by umbilical venous pH. Finally, there is a progressive linear relationship between the Log serum erythropoietin concentration and the physical manifestations of fetal disease.

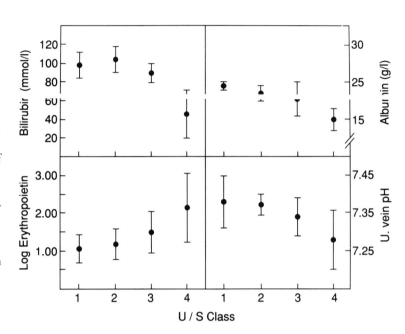

ers showed significant progression with accelerating disease, also reflected in a progressive rise in serum erythropoietin concentration (92,93). This relationship allows the possibility that an underlying factor in severity of fetal disease is erythropoietin overdose.

As emphasized about other parameters, the *correlations* between ultrasound class and direct hematological and biochemical parameters are evidence of a natural relationship, as opposed to comprising a system for prediction. No one knows whether the gold standard for the measurement of fetal disease ought to be the hemoglobin level or the extent to which the fetus is physically compromised. Hemoglobin concentration and physical disease are clearly linked (Figure 6-17), but this linkage is *not* complete. Two interpretations are possible: (1) the hemoglobin value indicating severe disease is correct, and the fetus who does not appear profoundly ill does not reflect the pathophysiology of disease; or (2) factors other

than the hemoglobin concentration, per se, are critical in determining the level at which the fetus is able to continue to function normally. The most important utility of the classification system, however, relates directly to fetal function and prognosis. The Class 4 (moribund hydrops) distinction, based on an abnormal Biophysical Profile Score in a severely-affected fetus, indicates the need for *immediate* intrauterine resuscitation, supportive maternal measures, and continuous monitoring. This is a situation that is highly unstable, prone to disruption by even mild uterine contractions, which, of course, are more frequent in accelerated disease. Emphatically, these are not cases that will wait overnight. We transfuse such fetuses immediately on arrival to our fetal surgical theater and repeat IVT frequently.

Doppler Ultrasound

Doppler ultrasound has many useful applications in evaluation and treatment of severe alloimmunization, but there are finite limitations of Doppler flow velocimetry. There is correlation between hemoglobin concentration and an increase in maximum systolic flow velocity with a corresponding increase in the ratio between systolic and diastolic velocities in early phases of serious anemia. But, changes in resistance patterns are variable as disease progresses. In some cases of overt cardiac failure, ratios remain the same while maximal velocities diminish substantially. This phenomenon is seen only in Class 3/4 structural disease, associated with profound anemia. Other cases suggest markedly increased placental resistance (on the basis of gross placental edema) with absent end-diastolic velocity. When therapy is successful in such extreme cases, normal diastolic velocities and other normal parameters of umbilical blood flow have also returned, pointing out resolution of placental as well as fetal changes.

Our knowledge of changes in hemodynamics as anemia progresses, but before hydrops supervenes, is somewhat speculative. It would appear that the expert observer can discern increased cardiac work, evidenced functionally by increased maximal systolic velocity and increased Doppler velocimetry ratios, supported by structural evidence of minor pericardial effusions, exacerbated cardiac contractility, and possibly increased outflow tract velocities (84,85,89,94–96). Whether these vary from one fetus to the next or reliably predict when to intervene is quite unclear. Whether these findings are a response to perceived deficits, i.e., the fetus somehow "senses" early anemia, or the result of increased cardiac efficiency with thinner blood is unknown. Papers dealing with this topic suggest that Doppler velocimetry provides specific relation with fetal anemia. In practice, with prospective application, these correlations have *not*

proven reliable predictors. This information is not ignored and may form the basis for accelerating repeat PUBS cordo-IVT when taken in the context of the individual case.

Doppler ultrasound occupies an essential role during intravascular fetal transfusion. Color flow mapping makes definition of fetal vessels for cordocentesis and IVT a relatively efficient process. While color Doppler is basically useless during the transfusion (the lack of resolution of the vessels being prohibitive in terms of continuous observation of turbulence, for example), semi-quantitative color Doppler is useful in post-IVT monitoring to ensure circulatory stability.

Intratransfusion observations are of significance in reducing the chance of volume overload. Post-IVT monitoring with Doppler velocimetry is not rewarding, however (Figure 6-20). There is apparently no correlation between Doppler velocimetry and post-IVT hemoglobin concentration, either short-term or long-term. This may be because Doppler changes in alloimmune hemolytic disease are more due to cardiac responses to anemia than related to blood viscosity; both factors function at the same power order in the Doppler equation. This is a significant feature of Doppler velocimetry in the progressively anemic fetus: factors usually understood to be constant and, therefore, not considered in evaluating Doppler flow velocity waveforms, i.e., in the IUGR fetus, are all extremely variable in alloimmune disease. Vessel diameter is probably increasing with progressive anemia; this is the first response in nonfetal patients as hemoglobin drops. Vessel compliance may also be significantly increased. Blood viscosity is progressively lower. Cardiac function is significantly altered by falling viscosity, decreased oxygen delivery, altered resistance (first falling because

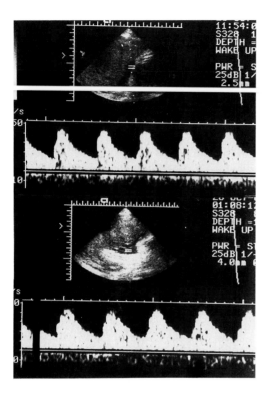

Figure 6-20 Umbilical artery Doppler velocimetry before and after a 100 ml fetal transfusion that raised the fetal hemoglobin from 69 g/L to 180 g/L. Despite this rise in hemoglobin, the change in viscosity, and the accompanying cardiovascular alterations, the Doppler remained unchanged.

of vasodilatation, second rising because of tissue and placental turgor/edema), alterations in heart rate, and, ultimately, in the electromechanical events of the cardiac cycle, perhaps due to relative coronary ischemia in turn due to decreased afterload. It is perhaps not surprising that Doppler indices correspond better with fetal status than they do with actual hemoglobin measurements in the posttransfusion patient. Although further research is required, it is likely that intracardiac Doppler evaluations will assume more significance as our understanding improves.

Physical Exam Summary

Fetal evaluation in severely alloimmunized pregnancy is complicated and not addressed merely by getting a fetal blood sample. There is much overlap between physical and functional evidence of disease, cohorts of hemoglobin measurement, RBC patterns, and fetal biochemistry. This corroborates the emphasis on gathering as much information as possible about each fetal patient before determining risks and prognosis, scheduling intrauterine management, or resorting to premature delivery and neonatal treatment.

INTRAUTERINE TRANSFUSIONS

Indications

Indications have been discussed extensively above, but are summarized as follows (Figure 6-9): hemoglobin <5th percentile for gestation, bilirubin >80 mmol/L, hemolytic crisis depicted in RBC smear, and hydrops on ultrasound. "Suggestive" signs, incipient hydrops, bilirubin >60 mmol/L, serial ΔOD 450 rising to 80% Zone 2, serial hemoglobin not rising with gestation, and sudden large rise in antibody concentration, mandate the "cordo-IVT." The cordo-IVT is set up exactly as for formal IVT, but *the infusion is not begun until the fetal hemoglobin is known* at the bedside. The gestational age limitations traditional with IPT, i.e., rarely >32 weeks, never >34 weeks, (97) reflected the *mortality* of IPT versus intensive care nursery; these are not relevant to IVT. The respiratory support, bilirubin clearance, and reduced regulatory requirements of intrauterine life combine to mean that regardless of pulmonary maturity, intrauterine treatment is just as safe and more effective than neonatal. Even as late as 36 weeks, we will begin intrauterine transfusions rather than deliver, if technical concerns, e.g., anterior placenta are satisfactory.

INTRAVASCULAR FETAL TRANSFUSION (IVT)

Technique

On surveying the literature, one finds a variety of procedural options associated with enhanced outcome in the most severely affected fetuses. Our team has achieved consistent and encouraging success with almost complete conversion from IPT to simple (bolus) IVT. While we reported some of the best results using IPT [especially beginning in 1980 when ultrasound guidance for IPT and for fetal surveillance were added (8)], our initial positive experience with IVT has been confirmed over the last seven years, attaining the success rates shown in Table 6-9. As we approach our 600th IVT, the methodology continues to evolve. What follows is an outline of how we perform intravascular fetal transfusion with highlights about specific situations in which special steps are taken.

Prerequisites

The conditions under which an intrauterine transfusion team are established have been outlined in detail (98). The team must function in an integrated fashion, with a designated team leader for policy decisions, scheduling therapies, and, most importantly, decisions of immediacy *during* the procedure. The liaisons between the team itself and the blood group serology lab, the blood banking facility, and the referring physicians, as well as the patient care facilities applicable to mother and fetus are emphasized here. Team members are as

Table 6-9 Likelihood of Intact Survival—1993 (Pre-IVT Counselling−U of M IUT Team)

	Non-Hydropic	Hydrops
First IVT <24 weeks	90%	70%
First IVT >24 weeks	98%	85%

interchangeable as possible and must be able to assemble on a moment's notice to provide comprehensive service to urgent situations, such as an accident at cordocentesis or unexpected arrival of a moribund hydrops. For such emergent situations, an intrauterine transfusion program cannot be undertaken in an outpatient facility remote from an obstetric hospital.

For the intrauterine therapy suite, sterile supplies (procedures are fairly frequently interrupted and a second set of equipment has to be used, e.g., with severe maternal supine hypotension), personnel and equipment for bedside testing of specimens, and so on must all be available. This point deserves emphasis: even in the most dire circumstances, it is better to withhold therapy a few more hours in order to have the procedure be conducted efficiently and safely than to risk the one therapeutic opportunity when the situation is not ideal. We allocate team resources to lodging, travel, and other nonmedical functions in order that the desirable cooperation between parents and the team is established.

Preparation

Establishing clear indications for proceeding to fetal transfusion is critical. We have had no deaths or serious fetal complications with simple PUBS, no matter how anemic the fetus was found to be. However, once the infusion begins, the potential for life-threatening complication is real, no matter how healthy the fetus is when the procedure starts.

The G&M specimen is sent well in advance to allow the requisite blood work. The donor unit is centrifuged to provide a hematocrit of 88%–92% (approximately 10 minutes at 4,000 rpm, vs. six to seven minutes at 4,000 rpm for standard packed cells). The unit is freshly donated, Group O, Rh-negative, HIV/HTLV-negative, CMV-negative, fully cross-matched, buffy coat poor, and irradiated immediately prior to the procedure. The last of these steps is relatively new in our practice. We have never had a case of grapt versus host disease, including our entire series of IVT, our series of IPT, and all newborn exchange transfusions. We are, however, aware of at least one certain case of grapt versus host disease caused by intravascular fetal transfusions(99) and have utilized standard irradiation procedures for the past several years. With Class 3/4 hydrops, platelet concentrate is also obtained for suspension of the packed red cells prior to infusion.

The fetal surgical suite is adjacent to the delivery suite, but we do not insist on an open maternal operating theater, anesthetic standby, or other such preparations. The procedure is done on a day-surgery basis, with morning admission and evening discharge, depending on the conduct of the procedure.

Team

We use a three-person team—an ultrasonographer and operator (both perinatologists) and an infuser (usually a neonatologist)(100). Having all three at the procedure allows some degree of discussion of therapeutic options should minor complications arise. The possibility of major complications is addressed with the patient and team before the procedure in order that decisions may be made quickly. We use the approach with the needle intersecting the ultrasound beam transversely, but others find it easier with a different number of personnel, needle approach, and choice of vascular targets. Additional preparation is required for severe hydrops—maternal oxygen and oxygen monitoring, platelet suspension, fetal monitor, and neonatal resuscitation kit. Finally, in extreme cases, the fetal heart rate is monitored continuously until the moment of the transfusion and immediately thereafter, with staff available to effect immediate delivery should fetal resuscitation fail at the appropriate gestational age.

Antibiotic Prophylaxis

Some centers have elected not to use antibiotic prophylaxis; others continue without evidence that it works. We still provide prophylaxis against likely skin pathogens and likely intrauterine pathogens, using amoxicillin 500 mg t.i.d., PO, and cloxacillin at the same dosage the evening pre-IVT for six doses each. This protocol has been followed for nearly 30 years in almost 1,500 procedures with no fetal infections, no maternal infections, and no fetal or maternal side-effects. Clearly, the incidence of such infections is quite low, and it would take an enormous number of patients to prove or disprove the benefit of such prophylaxis, unlikely given the relatively small number of current cases.

Premedication

We have not subjected this topic to a randomized trial. We use morphine sulfate 5 mg IM, and Promethazine 25 mg IM one hour pre-IVT. Maternal sedation induces maternal ease and our clear impression is that it assists in fetal quiescence. In patients where no sedation was given due to drug allergies or maternal refusal, the majority have been completed despite the continued normal fetal activity, however, maternal pain, diaphoresis, and pain-related dyspnea were all notably increased. We no longer use diazepam because of its prolonged action and interference with postprocedure monitoring.

Procedure

Preinfusion Planning

Target. The umbilical vein is larger, easier to puncture, does not go into spasm, bleeds a shorter time, and is frequently straighter at its insertion into the placenta. At this point, it is firmly anchored, and turbulence, so critical in ensuring safety, is easily documented. The umbilical vein is our target of choice, but the entire sequence of potential targets noted in Figure 6-21 are considered before we elect not to proceed with transfusion at that time. We will spend as much time as necessary, manipulating the fetus and/or altering maternal position in order to visualize an adequate target; patience in this step is the key to a high rate of first-time needle insertions and low rate of failed procedures (see Table 6-12). As term is approached, the fetus may obscure the posterior insertion or distort the anterior insertion because the cord is wrapped around him. Extreme tension on the cord when the fetus is entwined in it has led to multiple severe decelerations when the uterus contracts, a significant problem post-IVT beyond 32 weeks.

We would rather have available the full information from postprocedure monitoring, so do not automatically use pancuronium, and, therefore, would be happiest with the firmly-anchored insertion of the cord into the placenta. On unusual occasions, this site may not be firmly anchored, requiring unusual measures (Figure 6-22). The fetal end of the cord at the skin, or less commonly, intrahepatically, was once our second site of choice, but we are comfortable with the free loop and now use it more frequently, always with fetal paralysis. Conditions for elective use of intraperitoneal transfusion are discussed in a later section. On the rare occasion when fetal hydrops has supervened in previous pregnancies before 18 weeks, intracardiac transfusion may be elected at 16–17 weeks.

Maternal Prep. After 28 weeks, maternal tilt is used to avoid interruption of the procedure by severe maternal supine hypotension. The maternal abdomen is prepped in sterile fashion as for open surgery, including surgical attire. The patient's partner is not automatically excluded, but is not allowed within the surgical field. We use a small amount of 1% Xylocaine S.C., precisely over the targeted vessel, trying not to raise such a bleb that it causes acoustic shadowing.

Needle Insertion

Before 28 weeks, a 22-gauge spinal needle is used, 20-gauge thereafter. Needle length is based on the measured distance from the skin plus the possibility that uterine contractions may lengthen the distance by as much as 3 cm. Not only have uterine contractions pulled the needle out directly, they have induced maternal supine hypotension, which was not apparent prior to the onset of the contraction, and occasionally caused 90°–120° of uterine rotation. In all such cases, the end result is unintentional removal of the needle from the vessel, with the poten-

Figure 6-21 Ideal IVT targets. **6-21A** The classic anterior cord insertion.

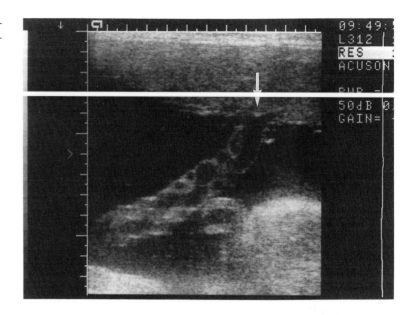

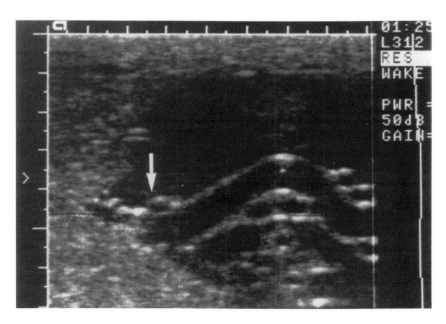

Figure 6-21B This posterior cord insertion is readily accessible, but may not be visible at all later in gestation.

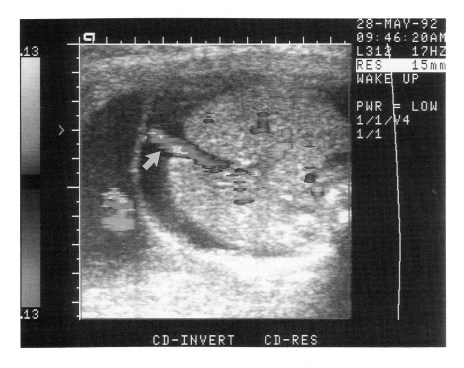

Figure 6-21C The intrahepatic portion of the umbilical vein sometimes is the only available vascular target and is the preferred site for some groups.

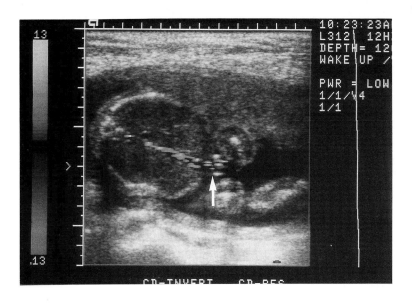

Figure 6-21D The abdominal skin cord insertion may be available for needle insertion when the fetus is facing posteriorly and the intrahepatic portion is not reachable.

Figure 6-21E We have become accustomed to the use of a free loop, pinned against the posterior wall of the uterus or against the fe-
~~tus as a secondary target. We~~
always use pancuronium when this target is selected.

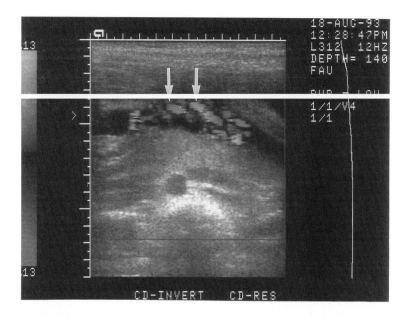

Figure 6-22 An unusually large maternal lake made approaching this anterior cord insertion an adventure. A 22-gauge needle was chosen, despite the relatively large vessel, because less resistance was encountered as the needle was inserted through the membranes. On virtually every occasion of the five IVTs undergone by this fetus, post-transfusion backbleeding in this large maternal space could be visualized.

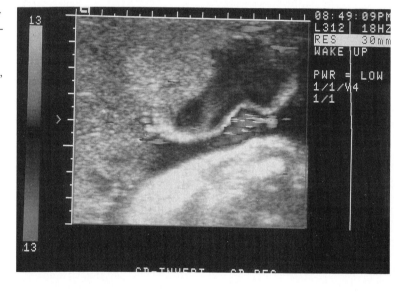

tial for increased bleeding or a shortened transfusion. The needle is visualized as it penetrates the maternal fascia, with vigorous "bouncing" (operator-controlled needle excursions of 5–8 mm) of the needle tip as near-field resolution is not adequate alone.

Once the uterus is entered, needle visualization is usually easy, regardless of placental location. The needle is moved firmly in 1-cm increments toward the target until approximately 3–5 mm above the intended vessel, where smaller increments and smaller-amplitude bouncing are used to bring the needle tip to rest against the vessel. Once the needle is against the vessel, confirmed by indentation of the vessel wall, a firm to very firm thrust (when the gestation is >32 weeks) is used to introduce the needle into the vessel.

A sequence then follows to confirm needle placement is proper within the vessel. It is possible to have the needle part way in a fetal vessel and part way within the maternal lake directly adjacent or, alternatively, part way through the vessel into the amniotic cavity. Bedside testing for fetal blood is effective at the first transfusion, but after serial IVT has replaced fetal blood completely, in a Group 0 mother especially, it will be virtually impossible to discern maternal from fetal origin based on laboratory testing, so reliance is on ultrasound methodology. The needle tip is visualized within the vessel, and blood flow should be without hesitation up the needle, noting that high pressure on the syringe barrel will draw the vessel wall against the needle and occlude it. The most important confirmation is infusion of 0.2–0.4 ml of saline, visualized as "puffs" of turbulence along the appropriate vessel. Infusion of the transfusion is not acceptable unless such vessel verification is 100% satisfactory. Even with the moribund hydrops, in the most desperate straits, absolute attention is paid to avoiding intramural infusion as there is virtually no chance to resuscitate the severe hydrops when the vessel wall is impeached by as little as 0.5 ml of densely-packed donor blood.

Fetal Paralysis

A critical step occurs between the infusion of saline to identify the vessel and the infusion of pancuronium to paralyze the fetus. This is to check the return up the needle. This is absolutely critical as there is good evidence of pancuronium having caused caustic injury to fetal vessels with a subsequent intramural hematoma and fetal demise (101).

It is at this moment that the final decision regarding fetal paralysis using pancuronium 0.25 mg per estimated kg of fetal body weight is made. Although fetal paralysis is used in about 70% of non-hydrops, and 40% of hydrops, we use pancuronium only when it is clear that fetal movement has the potential to cause vascular injury. This decision is subjective, and the vigor of fetal movements, the cord position around the fetus, relative amount of amniotic fluid, proximity of the fetus to the needle tip, uterine irritability, proposed total volume and, therefore, proposed total duration of the procedure, are all important variables.

Pancuronium has had no long-term effects in any of the hundreds of fetuses who have received it for various fetal transfusions throughout the past decade. When it is given as a bolus at the dose suggested, pancuronium induces a dense paralysis virtually immediately. In many cases, such immediacy is essential, and for this, we are prepared to sacrifice the concerns of lengthy paralysis. At dosages of 0.05–0.10 mg/kg, paralysis may take 15–60 seconds, with corresponding "vulnerability" of the vessel during that time, perhaps enhanced by frequent jittery fetal movements as paralysis begins. The reward for tolerating this movement as paralysis sets in is a very short duration of postprocedure paralysis, which reduces the anxiety of monitoring during the time when variation in fetal heart rate is abnormal as a consequence of pancuronium. The latter is clearly a dose-related phenomenon with two components. The first component is the flat trace observed with the absence of fetal movements (Figure 6-23A). The second is the presence of cyclic fetal heart rate rhythms, closely mimicking classical sinusoidal heart rate, and often a

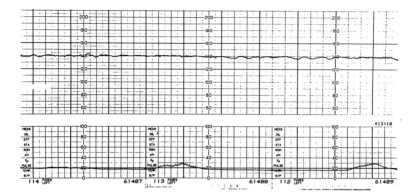

Figure 6-23 Fetal heart rate "abnormalities" provoked by pancuronium infusion. **6-23A** Abolition of all variation in association with complete fetal paralysis. It is impossible to know whether this fetus is asphyxiated.

concern to staff monitoring such patients for the first time (Figure 6-23B). In general, recovery of active fetal movement fully perceived by the mother is in the order of one and a half to two hours for each 0.1mg/kg of estimated fetal body weight, e.g., about four and a half to six hours if the maximum 0.3 mg/kg is given.

Red Cell Infusion

Irradiation is done just prior to the procedure to minimize the potential effects of he-

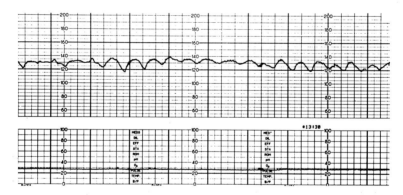

Figure 6-23B Sinusoidal heart rate typical of pancuronium paralysis after approximately 30–45 minutes, during the return to normal variation. Because a large dose of pancuronium is used, it is unclear whether this sinusoidal pattern represents the last phases of pancuronium blockade being established, or the initial phases of the blockade wearing off. The fetus is absolutely immobile during this time. This dissociated pattern, of course, does not reflect fetal anemic status as it is seen post-IVT regardless of the volume delivered and the post-IVT hemoglobin level attained.

molysis, mainly increased potassium load and reduced lifespan (102). Red cells are suspended in 10–15 ml of sterile saline and the bag gently agitated to render the mixture infusable. The aim is to maximize hemoglobin concentration, taking into account the needle length and gauge (305 g/L blood will go smoothly down a 9-cm 20-gauge needle, but only a few ml, under great pressure, are sufficient to clog a 17-cm 22-gauge needle). Infusion is carried out at a relatively rapid rate with continuous ultrasound monitoring. This is one of the strongest reasons why our team has retained the use of different individuals to maneuver the needle and operate the ultrasound. The infusion is given in 10-ml aliquots, 60 sec/10 ml, with a 60-second period before the next aliquot is started. Verbal signals between team members allow the infusion to be terminated instantaneously if adequate turbulence is not demonstrated.

Continuous intravenous turbulence is the *sine qua non* of IVT (Figure 6-24). Even in the most difficult situations, we do not allow the infusion to proceed unless turbulence is readily demonstrated, with correspondence directly to the off/on signals of the infusor. There is *some* latitude in this circumstance, where the paralyzed fetus rolls back against the cord and assumes a position that obscures the actual needle insertion. In this case, the transfusion is allowed to proceed if the needle is in the umbilical vein and if saline infusion is readily observed at a more proximal point along the course of the cord. Cessation of turbulence is the first sign of a problem in the vast majority of complicated procedures, with the fetal heart rate changing some number of seconds later. It is our feeling that we have averted most severe accidents by relying on the turbulence and stopping *immediately* if turbulence stops.

In the case of arterial infusion, turbulence may be more difficult (Figure 6-25). Because arteries are usually tortuous, along the placental surface, one usually sees only one or two cross-sections where turbulence is evident, meaning arterial transfusions tend to take longer, with many stops and starts to confirm proper needle placement.

We use visual, i.e., two-dimensional grey scale, turbulence rather than duplex pulsed Doppler evidence of turbulence (Figure 6-26) because the latter depends on exact angle of insonation, may fluctuate between one aliquot and the next, is altered by changes in uterine tone, may be obscured completely by the corresponding arterial pulse, and becomes much less pronounced as larger-volume transfusions progress. Because the vessel resolution is so poor and because the effects of turbulence range from indiscernible to completely distorting, we find color Doppler flow mapping virtually useless in this aspect of fetal transfusion.

A fetal heart rate is obtained after each 10-ml aliquot, but the ultrasonographer is able to be reassured of a normal fetal heart rate by the changes in turbulence that occur with fetal cardiac activity. In the case of an intravenous infusion, this is the continued relatively high velocity passage of the turbulence down the vessel, and in the intra-arterial infusion, this is the *pulsatile* nature of the turbulence within the vessel.

Turbulence is probably generated by many factors. The nonlaminar flow, the difference in density between the donor blood and that of the anemic fetus, the speed of the red cells under high pressure infusion, the pressure of nitrogen "bubbles," and the angle at which the needle is placed within the vessel, which determines the persistence of turbulence downstream, all contribute. With a large caliber near-term vessel, when the needle more or less cannu-

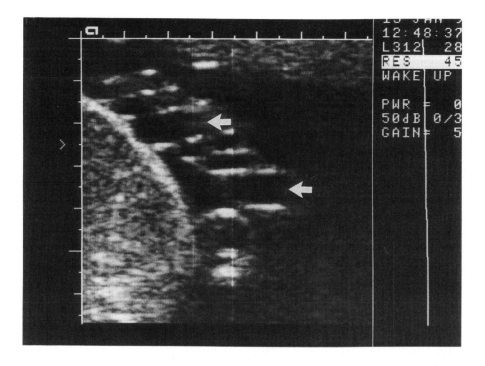

Figure 6-24 The hallmark of safe IVT, intravascular turbulence in the umbilical vein. **6-24A** Shows the cord in longitudinal section, in the interval between infusion aliquots.

Figure 6-24B Note the turbulence present in the umbilical veinwhen the infusion is resumed.

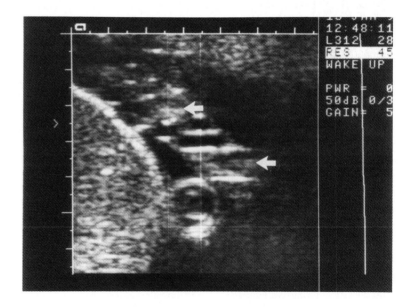

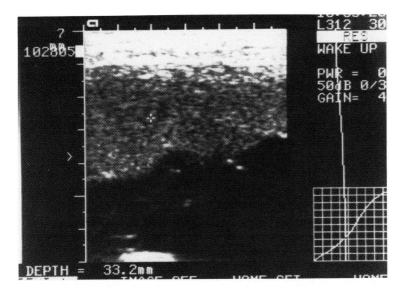

Figure 6-25 Intra-arterial turbulence is often much more difficult to visualize. Note the small area of turbulence at the placental surface where the umbilical artery has been cannulated. **6-25A** No fusion.

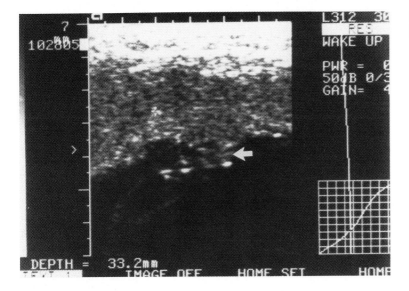

Figure 6-25B During infusion (arrow).

lates the vein, the fetus is not profoundly anemic, towards the end of the transfusion as the internal diameter of the needle decreases (by layering of the inside of the needle with red cells), which results in a lower rate of infusion, and, finally, the individual performing the infusion tires towards the end of a 120-ml procedure, turbulence may become hard to see. The ultrasonographer is the controller in this situation, and if turbulence is not adequate, infusion does not proceed.

FHR is monitored throughout. After pancuronium, a virtually constant fetal heart rate of 150 ± 6 bpm is maintained, unless a serious change in intravascu-

Figure 6-26 Doppler evidence of intravenous turbulence during infusion.

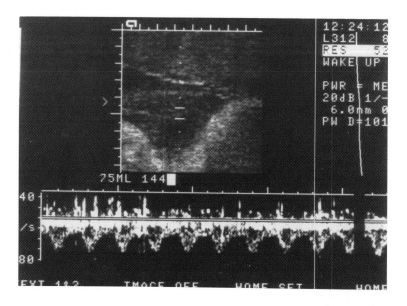

lar pressure (by intramural infusion, profound vasospasm, or induced uterine effects) occurs. In the unparalyzed fetus >30 weeks, there is often a progressive decrease in FHR (presumably as intravascular pressure rises as the target volume is achieved), about five bpm with each of the final two or three aliquots. As long as turbulence is ideal, the heart rate is stable/recovers slightly between infused aliquots, and the rate does not fall below 100 bpm, we continue infusion. In some fetuses after 34 weeks, the heart rate continues to fall slightly after transfusion. The redeeming feature of this bradycardia is that because it occurs in the absence of pancuronium, fetal heart rate variation and fetal movements are maintained, allowing assurance of ongoing fetal well-being. This feature conditions our approach to fetal paralysis. We have never made an error, either of omission or commission, in post-IVT monitoring of a fetus who was *not* paralyzed.

In addition to monitoring FHR and turbulence during IVT, there may be utility in observations of the fetal arterial velocity waveform. We have noted situations in which the waveform changes shape acutely, likely on a volume-determined basis. We interpret the square wave pattern shown in Figure 6-27A as requiring a reduction in the rate of infusion and, on occasion, have eliminated the last one or two aliquots from a large transfusion when this pattern persisted. On rare occasions, large-volume transfusions have resulted in the apparent elimination of diastolic velocities, presumably on the basis of a completely-full fetal circulation (Figure 6-27B). Restitution of normal Doppler velocities took place over four hours in this case; the course of therapy was ultimately successful, with term delivery of a healthy infant. Among transfusions carried to the complete target volume, we have seen this phenomenon in 3/480 (0.7%).

Volume/Rate Decisions

The expected pretransfusion hemoglobin is usually fairly accurately predicted based on

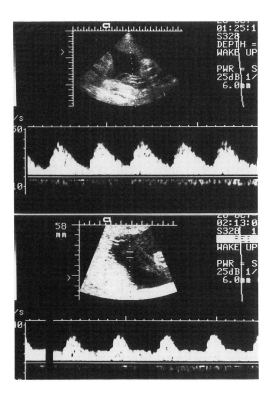

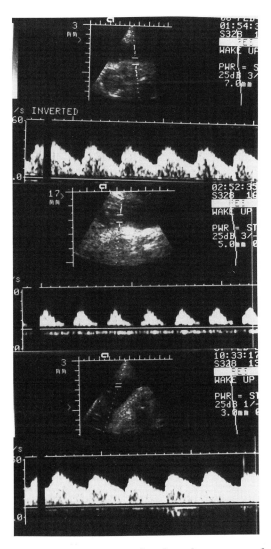

Figure 6-27 Abnormal Doppler patterns associated with high-volume IVT. **6-27A** Shows the "square wave" Doppler found in approximately 15% of large transfusions, associated with a decrease in baseline fetal heart rate unless the fetus is paralyzed with pancuronium. This pattern resolves over the four to eight hours following transfusion. Of interest, this finding also has been seen in donor fetuses during acute twin-to-twin transfusion.

knowledge of the post-transfusion hemoglobin concentration and the expected decline in fetal hemoglobin over the interval. In all cases, we determine the *volume* of the transfusion (rather than an endpoint in hemoglobin) to be reached and plan on transfusing to that volume unless one of the following occurs: significant change in the fetal heart rate, fetal Doppler or overt cord complication; maternal supine hypotension or other intractable symptoms; ≥75% of the transfusion volume has been administered and the

Figure 6-27B A more disturbing derangement of umbilical artery velocimetry is seen rarely, when diastolic velocities are abolished and maximal velocities throughout the cardiac cycle are greatly diminished. Because of persistent repetitive severe variable decelerations, repeat cordocentesis was performed on this fetus some eight hours following IVT. The post-IVT hemoglobin level was 190 g/L, the blood gas and pH values were normal, and no significant amount of blood was removed. This pattern recovered spontaneously over the next 12 hours, associated with complete resumption of normal fetal activity. Both fetuses in this figure survived and are intact with normal long-term follow-up.

needle is dislodged for any reason; there have been three punctures, even if <75% completion has been achieved; or if the bedside reporting of the pretransfusion hemoglobin is either <60 g/L or much greater than 100 g/L. (In the former situation, the fetus may not tolerate a full transfusion, owing to the altered cardiovascular status of a return to serious (and unexpected) anemia. In the latter, the full transfusion volume would raise the hemoglobin >200 g/L, where hyperviscosity could supervene.) Barring any such occurrence, the full volume of donor blood is delivered, based on gestational age (Table 6-10). (Note specific exceptions with regard to severe hydrops below. Also, see Table 6-13.)

Needle Removal

A post-transfusion sample is sought, but we never reinsert the needle to obtain this as

Table 6-10 Planned IVT Transfusion Volumes

Gestation Weeks	Estimated Fetal Blood Volume (ml)	IVT Volume (ml)
18	38	15
19	44	18
20	50	20
21	58	23
22	66	27
23	75	30
24	85	34
25	97	39
26	111	44
27	125	50
28	144	58
29	163	65
30	183	73
31	205	83
32	231	92
33	259	103
34	286	114
35	313	125
36	344	130

satisfactory results have been obtained on the basis of theoretical calculations (see "When to do the Next IVT"). The needle is removed directly in line with the insertion angle. Even if this is very tangential, care must be given not to allow the needle to straighten out during removal, thus avoiding vessel laceration. The needle is removed *slowly* until the tip is visualized clearly out of the vessel; rapidly pulling it out has occasionally been associated with vessel tearing, significant increase in the total time of bleeding, and subjective evidence of increased volume of bleeding.

Some blood loss almost always follows IVT. Parameters for "normal" bleeding after needle removal are: duration, 0–150 seconds; mean, artery 105 seconds, vein 92 seconds (p, N.S.); threshold for cardiovascular collapse in nonhydrops, 300 seconds; effect on fetal heart rate, none; effect on cardiac contractility, color flow mapping, umbilical artery velocimetry, none; effect on ascending aorta peak velocity, 10–20% reduction; effect on fetal activity, none; characteristics, sharp, narrow jet, tapering to periodic spurts, oozing, then stopping—*not* broad-based "gush" spreading in all directions or "rooster-tail" fan of turbulence (these are vessel tears) (Figure 6-28).

The underlying principles are not proven in humans, but it is likely that bleeding occurs in direct relation to fetal blood pressure and stops because a certain volume of loss produces a sufficient drop in blood pressure to allow the hole to be plugged by a combination of tissue pressure and aperture narrowing (by thrombus formation). The observations in Table 6-11 reflect these inter-related factors. There is shorter bleeding time when a free loop of cord is used owing to the thickness of the Wharton's jelly, noting that at relatively mature gestations, this is much thinner within 2 or 3 cm

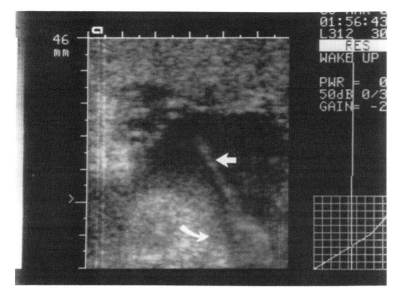

Figure 6-28A Backbleeding into the amniotic fluid following removal of the needle after a complete IVT. The jet of blood from the umbilical vein puncture (arrow) ricochets off the fetal limb beneath it (curved arrow). Although this bleeding continued as a vigorous "fountain" for 120 seconds, it then slowed to a trickle and stopped in 140 seconds. Fetal recovery was uneventful.

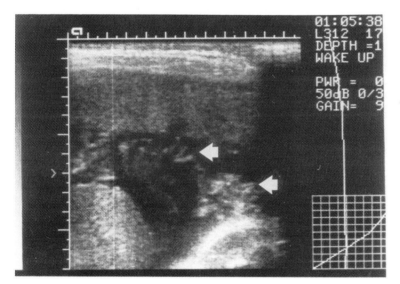

Figure 6-28B This appearance is absolutely dissimilar. This gush of blood erupted from the vessel immediately on needle removal and was associated with virtually immediate exsanguination and cardiovascular collapse. Intracardiac fetal resuscitation was attempted but was unsuccessful, as the cardiac cavity virtually disappeared. At autopsy, there was a large tear in the umbilical vein, associated with depleted Wharton's jelly at the point of needle insertion. This fetus was grossly hydropic and had a platelet count of only 8,000.

of the cord insertion (where needle insertion is usually carried out) than it is in the midpoint of the cord. At gestations under 28 weeks, this does not appear to be a factor, where the relatively lower intravascular pressures may mean bleeding is less in the very premature fetus, but then, his circulating blood volume is much smaller.

In vitro observations may be helpful in explaining the apparent "safety" of significant-looking bleeding as seen in Figure 6-28. Ultrasound is capable of illustrat-

Table 6-11 Duration of Bleeding After Needle Removal

More	Less
Thrombocytopenia	Normal hematology
Full transfusion	Incomplete IVT
Placental surface	Through Wharton's jelly
Rapid (>15 ml/min) IVT	Slow (<8 ml/min) infusion
Hydrops (vessel factors)	Non-hydrops
>32 weeks	<24 weeks
? Transamniotic	? Transplacental
? Artery	? Vein

No Difference: Needle Gauge, Post-transfusion Hemoglobin Level, Pancuronium, Maternal Oxygen

ing absolutely minimal blood loss (Figure 6-29), so watching and timing the bleeding is not in itself sufficient to estimate volume. Mean bleeding volume through a 22/20-gauge hole in a pulsatile-perfusion model using term human umbilical cords is 3.8 ml/min (103). Maximum volume is 8 ml/min (although lacerating the vessel can raise this to 30 ml/min), tolerable total volumes considering the average characteristics of post-IVT bleeding. These observations using similar pressures in both perfused arteries and perfused veins showed little or no difference in volume lost. Although the clinically-observed bleeding time is slightly longer in arterial puncture, possibly related to higher intravascular pressure, it may well be that the thicker muscular walls of the artery mean the aperture is smaller than in venipuncture, meaning the net blood loss is the same.

Backbleeding in the case of transamniotic procedures (most commonly with a posterior placenta) is not difficult to observe and is monitored until it has stopped completely. Even a small amount of oozing must be followed to cessation, as this may not stop but accelerate after a few minutes, leading to significant volume loss. Where needle insertion has been entirely transplacental, knowledge of backbleeding is usually nil. We have noted increased turbulence within the maternal venous lake directly overlying the cord insertion of an appropriate duration for normal backbleeding, but these observations are infrequent and difficult to verify as fetal bleeding. On at least two occasions of which we are aware, bleeding from the puncture site into the placenta has been delayed and, thus, unnoticed, resulting in lethal exsanguination.

Unless bleeding exceeds 300 seconds, we have not seen any significant effect on fetal cardiovascular status. However, for any backbleeding ≥ 220 seconds, hemoglobin levels at subsequent transfusion are lower than usual, so an allowance of two to five days is subtracted from the transfusion-transfusion interval.

When to Do the Next IVT

Our goal is to suppress fetal RBC production to a minimum, which is accomplished by keeping the hemoglobin concentration above 80 g/L, our target pre-IVT hemoglobin level. Based on results of our first 50 IVT-, we expect a decline in donor red cell concentration equivalent to 3–4 g/L/day. To build in a margin of safety, the interval to the next IVT is [*Post-IVT HB–TARGET HB /4*], in days.

Easier said than done. What precisely constitutes a "true" post-transfusion hemoglobin is open to question. There is rapid volume expansion during transfusion. This is partially balanced, or may even be completely compensated, by rapid flux of fluid across the placenta to the mother. The exact volume status of the human fetus at the end of transfusion is unknown. Animal models

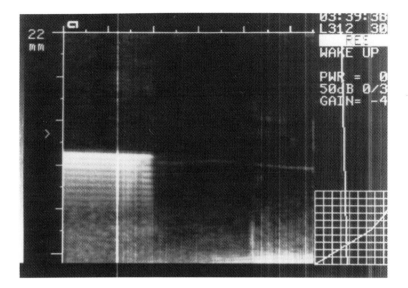

Figure 6-29 Ultrasound is able to detect the most minute amounts of blood when it streams into fluid. Shown here is a needle attached to a syringe with 2 ml of adult red cells, hemoglobin 120 g/L, and only the force of gravity on the barrel of the syringe propelling efflux, at a rate of 0.05 ml/min, clearly visible.

may or may not be helpful as it would appear that, for example, the sheep fetus is capable of massive fluid shifts virtually instantaneously, whereas circumstantial data from the human situation suggests that volume restitution may occur over hours rather than minutes (104). For example, the tracing in Figure 6-30 shows the return of

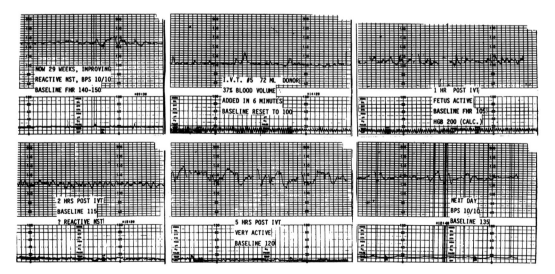

Figure 6-30 Fetal heart rate in a fetus who is not paralyzed for her large-volume IVT. Note the significant resetting of the baseline to a low level, and gradual recovery over several hours following IVT. It seemed reasonable to explain this on the basis of fetal hypervolemia, which was reconstituted during the post-IVT interval, with return to the previous baseline. Note that there are no repetitive decelerations, the fetus was active, and baseline variability was maintained.

the FHR to the pre-IVT level of 140, which took place over *six hours* following a large-volume transfusion in a near-term fetus.

Analysis of pre-/post-transfusion fetal serum bilirubin levels, which ought to remain unaffected by the red cells infused, suggests significant volume expansion in short, fast transfusions, which theoretically must be readjusted post-IVT (Figure 6-31). In the human situation, repetitive PUBS to follow the course of fetal hemoglobin after transfusion would not be ethical and might not produce reliable results, owing to the small but mandatory volumes of blood lost at each procedure. Cannulation of the fetal circulation with an in-dwelling catheter has not been attempted for the purposes of post-transfusion hemoglobin monitoring. In some cases, repeat cordocentesis and/or IVT is mandated in the 24–48 hours following the index procedure, with results depicted in Figure 6-32. Such cases provide

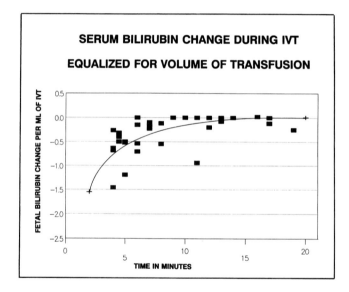

Figure 6-31 Fetal serum bilirubin levels pre- and post-IVT were analyzed to produce this plot. To neutralize the effect of volume, the change observed over the duration of the transfusion was divided by the volume of the transfusion. In only one of 40 cases did the bilirubin concentration rise. When plotted against the time between the pre- and post-bilirubin levels, the result is a highly significant reciprocal equation.

$$Bilirubin\ concentration\ change = 0.118 + \frac{-308}{TIME},$$

indicates that as time between bilirubin levels increases, the change in bilirubin concentration approaches zero. This is strong evidence that during fast, short transfusions of significant volume, there is rapid increase in circulating blood volume, which is not completely compensated. During longer infusions, despite the fact that just as much volume is given across that duration, fetal compensatory mechanisms are invoked that achieve very significant volume restitution.

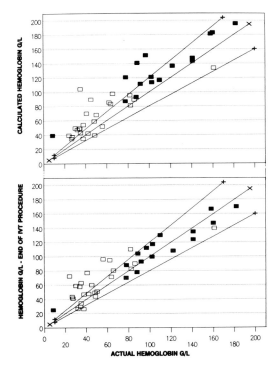

Figure 6-32 On some occasions, repeat procedures are necessary within 48 hours of previous transfusions. While a number of these were necessitated because of the severity of fetal disease (Class 3 or 4 hydrops shown as open boxes), the remainder were the result of a variety of complications, including short procedures, abnormal FHR following IVT, or prolonged periods of fetal paralysis following IVT. Results reflect the relationship between the fetal hemoglobin *calculated* on the basis of ideal fetal circulating volume and the known amount of blood administered (upper panel) and the hemoglobin *measured* at the end of the IVT procedure (lower panel), respectively, with the actual hemoglobin at the time of later procedure. The lines indicate unity (exact correspondence of prediction and actual hemoglobin measured at the later procedure), (*abscissa*) plus or minus 20%. Neither method of prediction was very accurate for hydrops, although both methods achieved statistically similar results. Prediction in non-hydropic fetuses was much better by the observed post-IVT hemoglobin than when ideal calculations were utilized. The consistent overestimation seen in the upper panel suggests that volume restitution *after* the completion of the procedure is less than anticipated by simple dilution calculations. This, in turn, suggests that previous calculations based on the concept of red cells as the "dye" in a dilution procedure to measure fetal blood volume were substantially inaccurate and *underestimated* the actual fetal blood volume.

some data on post-IVT hemoglobin values/volume status, and suggest that some non-hydropic fetuses do experience post-IVT volume restitution, but that for slow or longer IVT, most of the volume response is achieved during the procedure. In hydrops, the observation is the opposite, raising the possibility that one of the compensations of hydrops pre-IVT is preferential shunting—functional decrease in circulating volume—which is reversed after transfusion (effectively increasing circulating volume). However, in almost all these cases, there was something distinctly unusual about the fetal disease or the fetal response to transfusion, meaning these observations may not reflect the normal course of events in terms of volume restitution.

Many groups use *measured* post-transfusion hemoglobin level as representative of the maximum achieved and, therefore, infer a rate of hemoglobin concentration decline of about 3 g/L/day, corresponding to the post-transfusion hemoglobin at the next procedure (105,106). In our situation, we achieve good predictability of hemoglobin at the subsequent transfusion using *calculated* values and the 4 g/L/day decline, but this may well be a case of using two "errors" to correct one another (Figure 6-33).

Immediate Impacts of IVT

Therapeutic

> **Restoration of red cells mass.** This seems obvious, but it is interesting to see how rapidly complete mixing takes

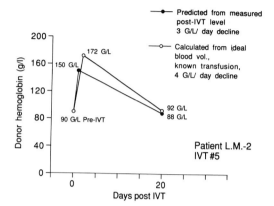

Figure 6-33 Two ways of predicting hemoglobin expected at the next transfusion. The dotted lines assume that the post-IVT hemoglobin level rises further with continued volume restitution, achieving a higher level of post-IVT hemoglobin concentration, from which there is a 4 g/L/day decline. The second, more commonly used, method assumes nothing except that the post-IVT *measured* hemoglobin level is the highest that is achieved. Decline from this peak is estimated at 3 g/L/day, with very similar results in predicting the timing of the next transfusion.

place. Although turbulence is visible for up to one complete circulation, e.g., turbulence coming along the placental surface in umbilical branch veins when the transfusion aliquot has been completely infused in the umbilical vein within the cord, this does not persist for more than a few seconds after infusion is stopped. The hemoglobin level does not change in post-IVT samples drawn at one and five minutes following complete infusion; it likely would fall if mixing were incomplete.

pH, blood gases. There are small, but consistent changes in these parameters that reflect: (a) the acidic pH (6.5–6.9) of infused blood, (b) the time needed to oxygenate the infused blood, (c) the CO_2 and lactate load of the transfusion, and (d) the respiratory effect of needle-induced contractions. Thus, the pH

falls (0.02 ± 0.002, $p < 0.001$) the pO_2 falls (4.2 ± 4.1 TORR, N.S.), and the pCO_2 rises $4.4 + 2.1$ TORR, $p < .01$). Unless there is a severe procedural complication, these changes revert in minutes (in the absence of further contractions).

Fetal behavior. In Class 4 fetuses, resuscitation is often dramatic, with fetal movement resuming during the infusion or within minutes. Failure to do so is an ominous sign, mandating continuous maternal oxygen by mask and early (four to six hours) repeat IVT.

Physiologic

Cardiac function. While this is actually improved in some Class 3/4 fetuses given oxygen and small-volume IVT, in the majority, the changes are complex. The healthy fetus given a large bolus transfusion improves myocardial shortening but may experience a net decrease in cardiac output. Small increments in viscosity, fetal vessel tone, uterine tone, as well as changes in heart rate, ANP output, and higher regulation may all work to decrease total output. Of course, much of this inferential-direct cardiac output is not measured. The fetus may simply be returning from his anemia-generated state of increased cardiac output to normal once the vasodilatation of anemia/hypoxemia is reversed.

Urinary output. This increases in the 24 hours post-IVT, in some fetuses to such an extent that there is measurable increase in amniotic fluid volume. This is balanced by decreased renal blood flow in the first few hours after transfusion, at least in some cases (107).

Other parameters. Reticulocyte release, EPO levels, and platelet count all may become *more* abnormal if the procedure is long or traumatic or involves fetal hypotension or bradycardia. One common pathway is likely adrenaline release, which is apparently independent of pancuronium blockade. These factors actually behave quite predictably, i.e., regressing to normal, when viewed on the longer term.

Post-transfusion Monitoring

Immediate. Once the needle is removed, backbleeding has been followed to cessation, and FHR is within the normal range, the sterile field is dissembled and the team leaves. The ultrasonographer, however, is left for approximately 10 minutes to complete the circulatory check, which includes verification of stable heart rate, stable Doppler indices, including umbilical, cerebral, and intracardiac flow velocity waveforms, and color Doppler flow mapping. Normal cardiac diameter and umbilical vessel diameters are verified, and the patient is transferred to the labor suite for continuous FHR monitoring until a fully reactive tracing is achieved. In cases where pancuronium has not been utilized, a minimum of two hours post-transfusion monitoring is obtained.

Short term. Provided the fetal heart rate monitoring is satisfactory, routine ultrasound is performed the next day, examining the point of needle insertion for hematoma, the fetus for Biophysical Profile Score and anatomic normality, and the amniotic cavity for excessive clot and/or particles. In the case of the latter, which we have observed on two occasions, repeat PUBS is indicated to ensure the majority of the transfusion had not been lost by delayed bleeding.

Interval Monitoring. This is carried out by the referring agency and consists of Biophysical Profile Scoring with cardiotocography on a weekly basis, including evaluation for the possible reappearance of hydropic changes (primarily early ascites).

Complications (Table 6-12)

Cord Hematoma

Two different types of cord hematoma may occur. In both, if a severe complication is going to develop, it will be obvious in seconds. The first form is a *hemorrhagic hematoma,* often visible as it forms; it may happen as the result of dislodgement of the needle or immediately following removal of the needle. In this situation, the fetal heart rate and cardiac output are monitored on an acute basis, while the needle is removed enough to be clear of the vessel but poised for reinsertion. If fetal heart rate derangement (rapidly accelerating tachycardia and marked decline in cardiac output, with little or no umbilical arterial velocities, diminished heart size/filling) does not ensue, the needle may be reinserted and further aliquots of blood transfused as indicated. On three occasions, fetal exsanguination has taken the form of a progressive subchorionic perifunic hematoma. Vascular collapse may be so rapid as to prevent reinsertion; cardiac puncture and resuscitation is our immediate choice, successful in two of three.

Acute *compressive cord hematoma* (Figure 6-34) is less often visualized, but the cessation of intravascular turbulence, and immediate severe bradycardia are dramatic. If a severe bradycardia ensues due to cord compression, attempts at aspirating hematomata have usually been successful, although we do not persist with this if blood does not return promptly up the needle.

Table 6-12 Complications of Intravascular Fetal Transfusion

Problem	N	% Fetuses	% IVT	Mortality N	Mortality %[a]	Rescue IU	Rescue NN[b]
Compressive cord hematoma	9	7.0	1.5	1	11	5[c]	3
Bradycardia—unknown cause	33	23.3[d]	5.6	1	3	31[e]	1
Moderate 100–120/>60 sec	21	16.3	3.6	0	—	21[e]	0
Serious 80–100/60–120 sec	8	3.9[a]	1.4	0	—	8[f]	0
Severe <80/>30 sec or 80–100/>129 sec	4	3.1	0.6	1	25	2[g]	1
Exsanguination bleed	16	12.4	2.7	5	3.9	9[h]	2
Rupture of membranes all >5 days post-IVT	4	3.1	0.6	2	50	N/A	N/A
Maternal/fetal supine hypotension	26	17.1	44	0	—	N/A	N/A
Abnormal monitoring[i] post-IVT, all causes	22	9.3[d]	3.7	3	30	6[j]	1
Failed procedure	17	10.9[d]	2.9	2	11.8	2[k]	1
Failed IVT, sample obtained	23	12.4[d]	3.9	3	13	1[k]	2
"Short" IVT (<50% intended volume)	17	11.6[d]	2.7	0	—	N/A	N/A

IU = Intrauterine resuscitation. NN = Neonatal.
a = Mortality per occurrence of the complication. b = "Crash" cesarean section, intensive care nursery resuscitation, intact survival. c = Successful aspiration of cord hematoma, resolution of bradycardia 5/5. d = More than one occurrence in some individuals. e = Spontaneous resolution with maternal positioning ± O$_2$. In three cases, remainder of procedure deferred (>50% intended volume given), 18 cases procedure resumed, successfully concluded. f = All had maternal repositioning, maternal oxygen by mask with ultimate resolution; four instances (two fetuses) vecuronium bromide infusion. g = One had reduction exchange, one had intracardiac adrenaline and saline. h = Six intracardiac, three umbilical vein. i = ^{i}. Sustained tachycardia (8), repetitive decelerations (6), absent variability, no fetal movement >six hours post-IVT (7), and sustained bradycardia (1). Includes mortality due to delayed exsanguination (2), heart failure due to possible overtransfusion, sustained bradycardia (1). j = Cordocentesis with minor volume reduction (2). Simple cordocentesis, normal findings (4). Remainder (12) spontaneously resolved. k = Intracardiac resuscitation/transfusion.

Bedside evaluation of the hemoglobin concentration of this aspirated blood will verify the donor origin of the hematoma as the hemoglobin concentration will be very high, usually exceeding the maximum range of the bedside instrument. The only treatment for bradycardia of this origin at a viable gestation is immediate cesarean section. It may not be accidental that this complication is very infrequent in the preterm and younger fetus. The relatively small amounts of Wharton's jelly at earlier gestations may mean that extravasation of the infused transfusion mass is more likely to cause complete dislodgement of the needle and nonfunic infusion, as opposed to the larger diameter cord with greater thickness of Wharton's jelly at later gestations, in which case, extramural infusion has been noted to track up and down the vessel, producing broadly-based cord compression.

"Bubbles"

On occasion, uncomplicated IVT results in the generation of small ultrasound "bubbles," which remain in circulation, trapped in a superior loop of the cord, swirling and producing a characteristic pulsatile artifact as shown in Figure 6-35. In no case has this been associated with any fetal or neonatal

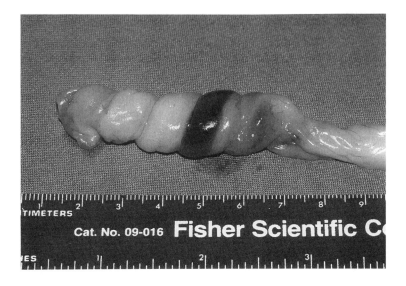

Figure 6-34A A free loop of cord was being used for this IVT at 34 weeks. The fetus jumped violently as the saline flush to confirm proper vessel insertion was given. This cord hematoma was visible within the wall of the cord and produced an immediate, profound bradycardia. Cesarean section within eight minutes resulted in a healthy infant who spent two days in the intermediate care nursery, and received one simple transfusion. Had this procedure been performed in an outpatient setting remote from the delivery suite, the outcome undoubtedly would have been significantly different.

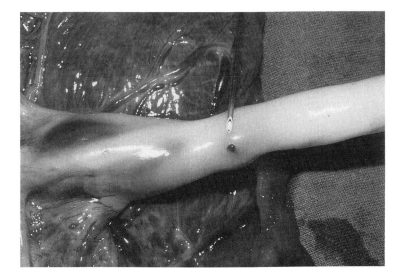

Figure 6-34B Contrast this to the appearance of a normal cord following puncture with the 20-gauge spinal needle used for IVT.

Figure 6-35 "Nitrogen bubbles." See text.

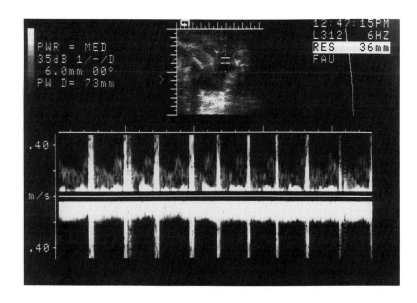

morbidity, and we are certain that this is not related to the inclusion of small bubbles of air within the transfusion setup. The combination of pressure gradient (high in the syringe, low in the fetus), temperature gradient (rapid warming in the fetus), and blood gas composition may mean altered partial pressures of dissolved gases.

Bradycardia

Persistent profound bradycardia in the absence of exsanguination or overt cord hematoma has been quite unusual in our experience (12/589, 2% of procedures, Table 6-12). Temporary moderate bradycardias certainly occur, especially when the transfusion volume intended is being approached, but this usually responds to either slowing or stopping the infusion. In such cases (21, or 3.6% of the time), it has never been progressive. When more serious bradycardia supervenes without overt hemorrhage or absent cardiac output, aspiration is attempted (for non-visualized hematoma), but if this is not productive, the needle is removed. Oxygen is started by maternal face

mask if simple repositioning does not help. In eight cases, the bradycardia reversed with these measures; four of these occurred in two fetuses given boluses of vecuronium. In another four cases, the bradycardia either persisted for >2 minutes or worsened. In these four cases, there was one intrauterine death at 20 weeks, possibly due to heart failure in a Class 4 fetus whose hemoglobin was raised from 33 to 120 g/L in a single intracardiac transfusion; one infant was delivered by urgent cesarean section when the bradycardia had incompletely resolved (fetal heart rate 115 after one hour); the other two were managed as shown in Table 6-12.

Exsanguination

This has occurred on 17 occasions in 16 fetuses. It was recognized immediately on 14 occasions as progressive enlarging perifunic subchorionic hematoma (three cases, one lethal), high volume sustained intraamniotic hemorrhage (10 cases, two lethal), or high-volume sustained intraplacental hemorrhage (one case, successfully resuscitated). In three cases, there was no post-IVT bleeding initially, but FHR monitoring was abnormal in the postprocedure period and repeat scanning (two cases, IVT #19 and IVT #116) or "crash" cesarean section for a terminal FHR (IVT #83) proved ongoing blood loss and circulatory collapse. Ultrasound findings in exsanguinating hemorrhage included empty heart, collapsed umbilical vein (the arteries usually remain visible), barely-discernible umbilical arterial velocities (pulsed/Doppler), no discernible umbilical arterial flow mapping (color Doppler), absent fetal activity, and fetal heart rate 180–220.

In nine cases, fetal rescue by intracardiac transfusion (N=6) or repeat umbilical vein cannulation (N=3) resulted in continuation of an intact fetus. Three of these fetuses were profoundly thrombocytopenic in association with their Class 3/4 hydrops fetalis (Figure 6-36).

In the remainder, four with Class 3/4 disease, two non-hydropic, normal platelet counts were present, but the bleeding was unexpectedly prolonged, and/or subchorionic hematoma developed. In another case (IVT #65), the fetus caused a 1.2 cm umbilical vein laceration when he pressed his foot against the needle and then moved it laterally by forceful extension of his leg, plowing the needle along the course of the vessel. Because the fetus was at 33 weeks, he was strong enough to cause an exsanguinating injury but also was able to tolerate a few minutes of hypotension with a "crash" cesarean section, neonatal resuscitation, and intact survival. In another case (IVT #19), surface placental vessels had been lacerated by needle insertion through the placenta, then through the amniotic cavity, to reach a fundal cord insertion in the center of a fundal placenta. Postprocedure monitoring showed sustained "oozing" lasting > two hours, and a fetus who stopped his previous vigorous movement, leading to emergency cesarean section, neonatal transfusion, and uncomplicated survival at 31 weeks. Had these injuries occurred at an earlier gestation, outcome would have been worse.

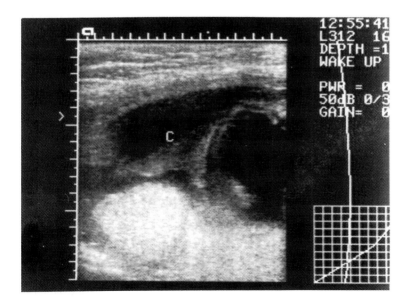

Figure 6-36 Exsanguination with large clot attached to anterior fetal abdominal wall. Despite the virtually complete absence of platelets, the blood will clot when exposed to amniotic fluid. This fetus had cardiovascular collapse and was resuscitated with repeat umbilical vein cannulation and combined platelet/red cell infusions. This fetus survived intact, but such experiences may be associated with the risk of long-term CNS compromise.

Of the remaining five cases, six occurrences of exsanguination resulted in fetal
demise. In one unfortunate fetus (IVT #107),
the first exsanguinating hemorrhage was reversed by intracardiac fetal transfusion, but
owing to the severe nature of fetal disease
(Class 4, HB 13 g/L), we did not transfuse a
very large volume (16 ml intracardiac at 22
weeks gestation). Thus, it was necessary to
return for another transfusion within four to
eight hours, at which time the umbilical
cord at the fetal insertion was utilized, but
this resulted in an apparent vessel tear and
exsanguinating fetal hemorrhage, which
did not respond to intracardiac transfusion.
In the remaining cases, exsanguination was
so vigorous in two cases and not detected in
the other two cases, so that the fetal heart
was collapsed, the vessels were collapsed,
and there was no avenue for resuscitation.
On one of these occasions, the pericardial
effusion was so large that intracavitary cardiac placement was precluded. Reflecting
this experience, our current practice includes: (1) platelet supplement in all Class
3/4 fetuses, (2) ensuring the fetal heart
is a potential emergency target before starting any IVT, (3) 17-cm 20-gauge spinal
needle for intracardiac transfusion, and
(4) *advance* decision about potential viability
and "crash" cesarean section in case of
hemorrhage.

Incomplete Procedures (Table 6-13)

About 28% of procedures do not deliver
the target volume. In 4%, more blood
is infused than planned due to hemorrhage, leaky tubing, or pretransfusion values much lower than expected (<1% of
cases). In the remaining 24% of procedures
(18% of fetuses), less blood is infused than
originally planned. Table 6-13 does not include fetuses in Class 3 or 4 where the
volume is automatically scaled down by
20–40%.

Table 6-13 Target Volume Not Achieved (N=139)

	N	% of IVT
Target Reduced (pre-IVT Hb >100 g/L)	40	6.8%
"Short" Procedures	59	10.0%
10–50% target volume given	17	2.9%
50–75%	16	2.7%
75–90%	26	4.4%
Failed Procedures (0–10% Target)	40	6.8%
Failed cordocentesis, failed IVT	17	2.9%
Cordocentesis successful, failed IVT	23	3.9%

One must consider unsatisfactory the 57
(9.7%) procedures where less than half the
volume is delivered, but in fact, most of the
cases in the "short" procedure category and
many of the "cordo successful, IVT failed"
group were procedures stopped because the
fetus was stable and the hemoglobin was
>100 g/L, but the needle was no longer in
place. In these cases, the procedure was
rescheduled (up to 16 days later depending
on the post-IVT level, bleeding, etc.), and in
>98% the subsequent procedure was suc-
cessful, with intact survival in 99%.

In patients where the IVT was difficult
but the cordocentesis proved severe
anemia, the team was obliged to persevere,
thus precluding "failed" procedure despite
worse technical problems, i.e., in most cases
"failure" or "short" procedure was an elective choice taken in mid-procedure.

In the group where no fetal sample
was obtained (16 fetuses, 17 occurrences),
there was no direct reassurance of a satisfactory hemoglobin. Thus, the procedure
was rescheduled for the next day (7/7 suc-

cessful), the route of administration was switched to intraperitoneal (3/3 successful) or intracardiac (five Class 4 fetuses; three died, two were resuscitated successfully), or exsanguinating hemorrhage occurred.

Longer-term Complications
___

On seven occasions, the pretransfusion hemoglobin at subsequent procedures has been markedly lower than predicted. In the one patient already noted (IVT #83), this occurred on two successive occasions, at the second and third intravascular fetal transfusions (24 and 27 weeks respectively), with intrauterine demise six hours following the procedure due to fetal-maternal hemorrhage within the placenta. We suspect intraplacental fetomaternal *chronic* hemorrhage on the basis of elevated maternal AFP (108).

In a second case (IVT #116), fetal movements resumed, then there were three violent fetal movements noted by the mother and recorded on the monitor, following which, there was no further fetal movement and the fetal baseline dropped from 145 to 120 and remained flat. The patient was immediately transferred back to the fetal operating suite and slow persistent intra-amniotic bleeding was noted. By that time, however, the fetal heart was empty and barely visible, the cord vessels were not visible, there was no cardiac output, and attempted intracardiac needle insertion was unsuccessful. With these two notable exceptions, we have never had a fetal loss other than at the immediate time of the procedure.

Another case of FHR monitoring led to successful neonatal rescue (IVT #19, already discussed). In several other cases, however, prolonged abnormal FHR patterns were misleading. In 12 fetuses on 18 occasions (one fetus four times, two others twice each), sustained tachycardia, persis-

tently repetitive deep variable decelerations, or prolonged absent FHR variation with no fetal movement followed pancuronium infusion. Ultimately, the abnormal patterns were so prolonged that repeat PUBS was mandated (N=6). Fortunately, there were no sequelae to these repeat procedures.

In interval monitoring, the suspicion of the referring hospital that hydrops was recurring has never been substantiated, although the patient is always returned to our center if there is any suspicion.

Fetal Brain Injury
___

There is significant information, as formal case reports or as anecdotal accounts, of serious fetal brain injury following intravascular fetal transfusion (109–112). The injuries are heterogeneous, both in brain location and in severity. They range from "total cerebral infarction" through "atrophic hydrocephalus" to more localized hemorrhagic lesions and all the way to mild hydrocephalus. Nicolaides has linked the appearance of atrophic hydrocephalus to sustained bradycardia, but this association has not been consistent (109). Morrow et al. resuscitated a severely hydropic fetus at 17 weeks gestation with two initial intracardiac transfusions and no apparent bradycardia, good recovery from the moribund state, but had progressive hydrocephalus within a few weeks, followed by termination of pregnancy, which revealed massive posterior fossa hemorrhage (113).

Because the information is still largely anecdotal, it is not possible to determine whether there is a common element, whether this is injury related to the severely compromised status of the fetus *prior* to the transfusion (i.e., an inevitable consequence of resuscitating a fetus who is near death), related to some complication, or in fact directly related to intravascular transfusion per se. Our experience with 55 fetuses who had a hemoglobin level of <60 g/L at the time of their first transfusion includes six cases of possible fetal brain effects associated with their resuscitation. In none of these six was there any bradycardia either during or after the procedure. In four of the six, hydropic changes were severe and the fetus was moribund, this group including the only two with residual CNS effects on long-term follow-up. The volumes given, the rate of transfusion, change in hematocrits, technical elements of the individual procedures, blood gases before and after the transfusion, and many other data points have been reviewed in detail, there are no consistent associations. Two children have residual effects in the form of localized ischemic/hemorrhagic cerebral palsy. The other four had transient dilation of the occipital horns of the lateral ventricles, persisting from one to four weeks, in all cases resolving during fetal life, and without residual effect. This dilatation, although transient, was definite but did not include any alteration in fetal behavior once a stable hemoglobin >100 g/L had been attained.

We have not seen these marginal CNS findings in individuals transfused whose hemoglobins were not quite so low, although two of the individuals who had transient hydrocephalus were nonhydropic but with hemoglobins at very low extremes (45 and 52 g/L, respectively).

Obviously, the possibility that this is related to straightforward therapy is real and should be noted in counselling these parents. However, at the present time, not enough is known about the preconditions to such injury to allow true counselling in this matter as the rate of brain injury is so low as to be statistically insignificant and, therefore, a distractor in considering whether or not to embark upon a life-saving course of intrauterine therapy.

Other Fetal Complications

Complications of prematurity, very common with IPT, have been reduced but not eliminated with IVT. Other problems, including lethal cases of CMV and hepatitis (114,115), graft versus host disease (99), and necrotizing enterocolitis (116) have followed both IVT and IPT. Long-term studies of development are as yet incomplete, but growth alteration is not apparent (117) and two-year old IVT survivals have no evident surplus of sensorineural deficit (12).

Maternal Complications of IVT

Each time something untoward happens during a transfusion, there is substantial maternal anxiety, especially once the patient becomes familiar with the normal conduct of a transfusion. Ultimate fetal consequences of this acute anxiety and its physiologic effects have not been measurable, but the lasting psychological effects have been noted by many of our mothers. Uterine irritability always occurs and is worse in multiparous women near term (larger and, therefore, longer IVT) or when the procedure is long due to technical problems. We have never used tocolysis and have not had a patient go into premature labor following IVT, with the exception of one mother with twins, preeclampsia, and accelerated mirror syndrome who ruptured her membranes and labored.

As noted, we have never had a maternal infection. On seven occasions, crash cesarean section and its attendant morbidity have followed fetal complications of transfusion. In a significant number of women, additional antibodies have developed, including C, E, e, FyA, FyB, KPA, S, s, N, M, and many other low-frequency antigens. This totalled development of new antibodies in 23 cases and 57 women with exacerbation by two dilutions or more of the index antibody. Because many of these sustained multiple antibody conversions/exacerbations, the total number of women affected was 63 (49%), a substantial consequence of transfusion. In three of these women, the large number of antibodies reduced the available donors such that 48 hours was required to identify suitable donors at each of the subsequent procedures. The development of these antibodies is automatically detected by the principle of re-cross-matching in detail at the occasion of each subsequent transfusion. In six such cases, the half-life of circulating donor cells was shortened by donor incompatibility with the new maternal antibodies.

Results

The results of this therapy speak for themselves, as related in disease-specific data shown in Table 6-14. The reasons for unsuccessful courses of therapy are summarized in Table 6-15 and the potential fetal surgical remedies have been explored. In our practice, although we had achieved very good results with intraperitoneal fetal transfusion, especially through the benefits of detailed ultrasound and the development of better intra- and post-operative techniques, the ability to treat the moribund hydrops with intravascular techniques was a landmark improvement.

Our first IVT involved a fetus who was deteriorating rapidly despite serial intraperitoneal transfusions. Due to maternal history and very high anti-D level (66 µg/ml, 330 IU/ml), we had begun IPT prior to the fetus becoming hydropic or the ΔOD 450 rising further. Because of worsening placental edema, hydramnios, and delay in absorption of the intraperitoneal fluid, we repeated the intraperitoneal transfusion only four days later, and the aspiration of ascites at that time showed that very little of the blood had actually been absorbed.

The fetus became moribund and we were faced with inevitable demise despite serial IPT. We had heard, but not yet read of, and had not yet seen an example of intravascular fetal transfusion. Although we had be-

Table 6-14 Summary of Results—Intrauterine Transfusion

Procedure	N	Fetuses	Deaths	Survival
IVT—All Cases	589	129	15*	88.4
Class 1	3.5**	80	2*	98
Class 2	3.6	14	2	86
Class 3	4.1	17	4	76
Class 4	6.6	18	7	61
IPT Required	11	11	1*	91
ICT Required	11	10	5	50

*Includes one neonatal death, an Intensive Care Nursery accident not related to IPT procedure, Day 6 of life.
**CLASS 1–4 mean IVT/fetus.

Table 6-15 Mortality in IVT Fetuses

Cause	N
Procedural	
IVT-exsanguination	3
Cord hematoma	1
Bradycardia	1
Delayed hemorrhage	2
Fetal Disease	
Class 4, no cardiac output	2
Abruptio placentae (9 days post-IVT)	1
Maternal Drug Abuse	2
IV cocaine between procedures, Class 4 disease, no cardiac output	
Neonatal	
Prematurity—twins 25 weeks, mat. preeclampsia	2
Neonatal accident in ICN	1

gun to do cordocentesis the year prior, as a result of Daffos' original work, we were not familiar at all with techniques for delivering blood into the fetal circulation. We were afraid of volume-overload, vessel tearing, hematoma, and the strain on the fetal heart of a baby who was clearly dying. We approached the mother with three options: repeated intraperitoneal transfusion (which we believed to be futile), intracardiac transfusion (which we, and she, believed to be too dangerous), and an attempt at intravascular transfusion, acknowledging that we did not really know how to do this. Transfusions of nine ml, 11 ml, 18 ml, and 22 ml demonstrate our temerity at using large volumes over the three weeks that fetus was transfused. Further, we believed that the only route of delivering large volumes of fetal blood was with IPT, so we performed a further intraperitoneal transfusion, which led to rupture of the membranes, precipitant labor, fetal distress, and cesarean section for a very distressed fetus.

That baby survived despite many complications of her prematurity and some complications of her alloimmune disease. The hydrops was not reversed because the interval of treatment was too short, but her hematologic parameters and cardiac performance were satisfactory.

The management of that "survivor" is contrasted with her brother, who was treated by our team 2 1/2 years later. Although severe alloimmunization was again present, resulting in the initiation of intravascular fetal transfusions at 20 weeks, ultimately requiring a total of eight procedures, he was born at term, with a normal hemoglobin and normal serum bilirubin, required no intensive care support of any kind, and was ready for discharge prior to his mother because she had her third repeat cesarean section. The transfusion volumes he received at comparable gestations were an average of five times the volume given over less than 20% of the infusion time and with about 1% of the stress and tension in the fetal surgical theater. The therapy for these siblings exemplifies the progress summarized in Table 6-16.

Table 6-16 Progress in Application of IVT

1986–89	vs	1990–93
67	Fetuses	62
287	IVT	302
41%	Hydrops	35%
30%	Class 4*	50%
37%	1st IVT <24 W	44%
75	Internal (days)M	95
34.4	Weeks at deliveryM	37.2
5	ICN daysM	1
40%	"Ideal"	60%

Ideal Outcome: Term Delivery, No "Crash" C/S, Normal Apgars, Normal pH, HB >100 g/L, No Respirator, Home with Mother

*% of all Hydrops. M = Mean

SPECIAL CASE: CLASS 4 HYDROPS

This is a fragile fetus, and usually there is but one opportunity to reverse the rapidly lethal trend. Exsanguination from inadequate coagulation, exsanguination from vessel tearing, fetal cardiac output inadequate to permit transfusion, the fragile cardiac status being overwhelmed by the transfusion, and the aberrant behavior of some of the maternal patients have all contributed to losses among these severe hydrops. We have used the following modifications to address these problems, with enhanced success.

Oxygen Administration (118)

On her arrival in the fetal surgery suite, the mother is placed on oxygen by tightly-sealed rebreathe mask, 7L/min, continuously until the fetal hemoglobin has been raised to >100 g/L (usually after the third transfusion, after approximately 36 hours). Even when the placenta is profoundly hydropic, such therapy delivers significantly increased amounts of oxygen to the fetus (Figure 6-37). On occasion, the Class 4 fetus responds to this maternal oxygen therapy with resumption of more frequent movements and assumption of a more normal cardiotocogram pattern. This is an encouraging prognostic sign, as is the assumption of normal activity following a transfusion in such fetuses. Conversely, failure of the fetus to begin moving within two hours of the first successful transfusion, while still receiving maternal hyperoxygenation, has been associated with failure to resuscitate the fetus and ultimate stillbirth.

Platelets (119,120)

Classes 3 and 4 are the only situations in which the fetal platelet count may be se-

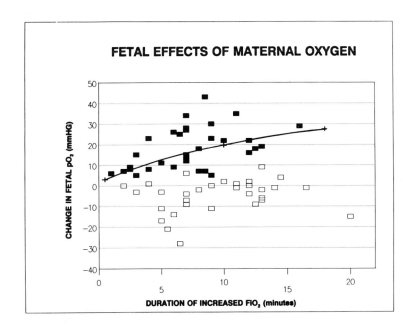

FETAL EFFECTS OF MATERNAL OXYGEN

Figure 6-37 Oxygen administration during the course of intravascular fetal transfusions in fetuses receiving serial treatment. None of these fetuses had any residual fetal hemoglobin as all were having their second or subsequent IVT. Oxygen produces a prompt and definite increase in fetal pO_2, with a curvilinear (positive decelerating) relationship over time. While the majority of fetuses whose mothers did not receive oxygen had reasonably stable pO_2 (open boxes), those whose mothers also had significant uterine hypertonicity during the procedure showed substantial decline in pO_2.

verely reduced, and such findings have been associated with (note that we cannot prove that they are the *cause* of) exsanguinating fetal hemorrhage (Figure 6-38). Since we began our policy of suspending the red cells for transfusion of such fetuses in platelet concentrate (as opposed to the small amount of saline usually used), we have not had an exsanguinating fetal hemorrhage in a Class 3/4 fetus. We use 15–20 ml platelet concentrate to suspend the average tightly-packed unit of red blood cells, and this leads to a post-transfusion fetal platelet increase of 70–90,000, a hemostatic level. Our intent and clinical impression is that such platelet infusions temporarily provide enough platelets to plug the hole left behind in the abnormally friable vessels in order that needle removal can be safely accomplished.

Volume/Rate Limitations

A number of centers have documented the decreased ability of the severe hydrops to withstand the stresses of large-volume transfusions (110,121,122). It has been our policy for a number of years to administer multiple transfusions on a highly frequent basis and to reduce the rate of these infusions. The significant procedural differences between Class 1 and Class 4 fetuses are outlined in Table 6-17. Although this results in a multitude of procedures over a short initial time span (Figure 6-39), since moving to this regime, we have not had any incidence of post-transfusion cardiac failure, reinforcing our impression that the Class 4 fetus indicates by his abnormally reduced behavior, that he does not have the same tolerances (cardiac and otherwise) as the nonhydropic fetus.

PROCEDURAL ALTERNATIVES

Our almost complete conversion from the intraperitoneal approach to the intravascular route is based on a detailed comparison

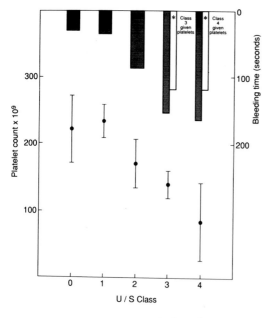

Figure 6-38 Association of thrombocytopenia with prolonged bleeding time in Class 3 and Class 4 hydropic disease.

Table 6-17 Procedural Differences-Class 1 vs. Class 4

Class 1	vs	Class 4
27.0	Start	23.4
63.7	HB	35.8
90.8	HB↑	43.3
5.7	ML/Min	3.5
38%	Vol ↑	21%
5%	Vol ↑/Min	3%

All Received Maternal Oxygen, Pre- and Post-, Platelet Suspension, Continuous Fetal Monitoring Until HB >100 g/L. IVT Smaller, Slower, More Frequent.

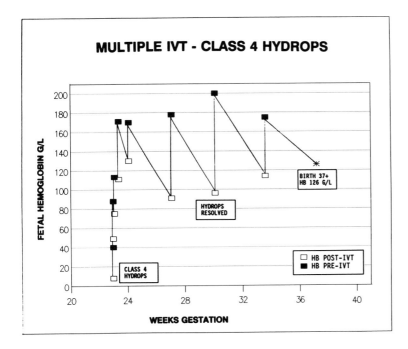

Figure 6-39 Frequent IVT in severe hydrops, with five procedures in the first 60 hours. This fetus had a pretransfusion hemoglobin of 8 g/L (0.8 g/dL), and ultimately did well after seven IVT and term delivery.

using highly-matched cases treated with either technique (Table 6-18) (29). In virtually every aspect where comparison was possible, enhancement using intravascular techniques was noted. In some cases, notably the number of procedures and the frequency of vascular complications, intraperitoneal transfusion alone is superior. In ultimate intact survival of fetuses who are non-hydropic and >24 weeks at the time the procedure was started, there was no difference in outcome. However, successful outcome was defined as intact survival with an extremely high rate of cesarean section at >34 weeks in the ITP patients, whereas the goal in IVT patients was able to be upgraded to term vaginal delivery (where obstetrical factors allowed) of a fetus requiring no time in Intensive Care Nursery and no more than one simple transfusion as neonatal therapy.

Several groups combine intravascular and intraperitoneal transfusions, per-

formed contiguously during the same procedure (105,123). Under cover of the pancuronium given as the initial intravascular aliquot is delivered, the fetus is in a stable situation, the hemoglobin is known, and the initial beneficial effect of intravascular transfusion has been attained without exposure to high volumes. The remaining transfusion mass may then be delivered intraperitoneally using a 22- or 20-gauge spinal needle (not the catheter method described above) under ultrasound control. Ultimately, a longer time period is attained before the next transfusion is required, the complications of fetal hypervolemia are avoided, and procedural liabilities were not increased. However, morbidities *are* attributable to the intraperitoneal component of such procedures, and the results of these transfusion programs are not better than our own. Although the data provided is somewhat sketchy, our conclusion is that similar total volumes may

Table 6-18 Choice of Management—IVT vs IPT [Matched Control Trial—1990 (29)]

Factor	IPT	IVT	P
Number of Procedures	2.4	3.9	0.03
Attempts/Transfusions	1.8	1.2	0.02
Procedural Complications	38%	10%	0.004
Traumatic Death	18%	3%	0.001
Delivery G.A.	31W	34W	0.011
Exchange Transfusions	1.8	0.8	0.007
ICN Days	8.2	6.1	0.044
Nonhydrops Alive	83%	98%	NS
Hydrops Alive	48%	86%	0.01
Class 4 Alive	0/6	4/6	

be delivered with safety by the exclusively intravascular route as with sequential IVT-IPT; the fetus is able to tolerate such volumes directly intravenously. Our intervals to next transfusion are quite similar so we have not moved towards combined procedures.

INTRAPERITONEAL FETAL TRANSFUSION—TECHNICAL CONSIDERATIONS

The reasons for conversion to IVT as our primary approach, the reasons why we do not use combined IVT-IPT despite our long history of success with the intraperitoneal route, have already been examined. We remain satisfied, however, to use IPT at either extreme of gestational age, when IVT is not practical due to small vessel size (<18 weeks, umbilical vein diameter <4 mm) or inaccessible vessel (>32 weeks, posterior placenta, fetus spine mostly anterior, hiding the cord). In the latter case, efforts to expose a suitable target may be successful using maternal ambulation, resting in the semi-prone position, or even with external manipulation of the fetus.

As well as the relative contraindications to IVT above, several conditions must be met to proceed to IPT: (a) nonhydropic fetus with known hemoglobin (early pregnancy, e.g., successful cordocentesis, failed IVT) or reliably predictable (late pregnancy, as the last transfusion following serial IVT); (b) ideal fetal position (Figure 6-40); (c) adequate team experience in performance and monitoring; (d) posterior placenta, i.e., transplacental IPT is not indicated except in the most unusual of circumstances <18 weeks.

Technique

Prerequisites, antibiotic prophylaxis and premedication, preparation of donor blood, and setup prior to needle insertion are all as for IVT. The volumes used are slightly larger than for IVT and are still derived by the formula: *[weeks gestation in weeks minus 20] × 10 ml*, e.g., 120 ml at 32 weeks. We will use five to eight ml weekly at 17 to 18 weeks and seven–10 ml weekly at 19 to 20 weeks.

The different extremes of age at application call for different techniques, but it happens that neither requires fetal paralysis in our approach (Table 6-19). In either case, the needle enters the fetus in one of the lower quadrants away from the midline, although penetration of the immature fetal abdomen (usually prior to skin keratinization) is very easy compared to the vigorous thrust to deliver the Tuohy into the near-term abdominal cavity.

At early gestation, small amounts of agitated saline (1–2 ml) are infused briskly, with the typical rising "bubbles" if needle placement is free, then the red cell infusion is commenced immediately. Turbulence must be visible at the needle tip through-

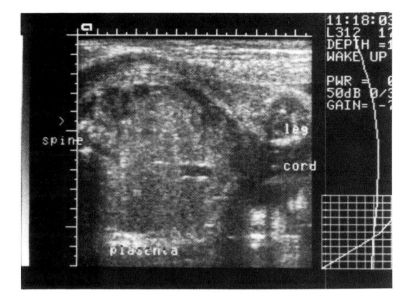

Figure 6-40 Ideal position for intraperitoneal transfusion. The fetal spine is to the left and the lower fetal flank is anterior. The umbilical cord is well visualized, not in the path of the needle. Fetal limbs are not flexed up between the fetus and the maternal skin surface. There is no placenta in this picture (it is directly posterior).

out and the FHR is an additional governor—rates <130 or the appearance of any arrhythmia call for termination of the infusion. As with later IPT, a more typical (normal) response is an increase in FHR, although tachycardia >180 is less usual. The transfusion mass in the fetal abdomen may not be as recognizable as in the late preg-

Table 6-19 Technical Aspects of IPT

Early IPT	*vs*	*Late IPT*
17–20	Gestational age range	32–36
No	Paralysis	No
22-Ga spinal	Needle	16-Ga Tuohy
Not used	Catheter	#18 epidural cath, (distal 5 cm removed)
1 ml/min	Infusion rate	10 ml/6–7 minute cycle
IVT—5 days	Next transfusion	Last before delivery

nancy IPT, and absorption has seemed complete in only 3 to 4 days. Early IPT has always been a unique procedure for each fetus followed by serial IVT.

In the late pregnancy version, we continue to utilize the Tuohy-needle-epidural catheter system, which emulates Liley's original method (91,97). Following abdominal insertion, the catheter is threaded (almost always seen coiling free in the abdomen by ultrasound), the needle is withdrawn, and free placement is confirmed with agitated saline bolus (Figure 6-41). If there is the slightest doubt, Renografin 20% five to seven ml is infused and placement confirmed on simple abdominal x-ray (Figure 6-42), showing the classic "semi-lines" of dye between adjacent bowel loops (124). The infusion is monitored ultrasonically and the abdominal transfusion mass is usually definitely visible at the 60–70 ml mark, and always by 90–100 ml (91). Since this is almost always the last in the intrauterine series, and the pre-IPT hemoglobin should be 90 ± 10 g/L, based on the previous IVT, delivery is usually carried out in three-and-a-

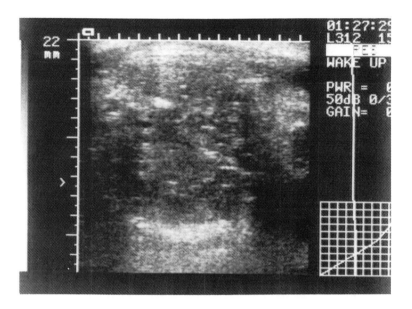

Figure 6-41 Intraperitoneal saline bolus confirms proper placement for safe intraperitoneal transfusion.

half to four weeks. Post-IPT monitoring is similar to IVT, with ultrasound evidence of complete absorption in four to six days, noting that fetal breathing movements are essential in this absorption process, another reason to avoid paralysis and heavy sedating (124). More elaborate technical detail is provided elsewhere (97).

Complications

In this restricted usage, we have not had any significant complications. The classic concerns of traumatic death or exsanguination requiring emergency premature delivery remain in theory. The exacerbation of all fetal and maternal risks by transplacental IPT *do not* remain, as this approach is no longer utilized. Ruptured membranes and premature labor, wound hematoma or superficial infection, chorioamnionitis, and other minor maternal problems are all possible with the late version but not features of the early approach. Because IPT is never indicated in the modern management of hy-

drops, the problems of nonabsorption/ failure to respond to therapy are likewise not relevant.

Our only death, in a fetus who had IPT as part of his intrauterine treatment, followed misadventure during placement of a subclavian line on Day 6 of life, almost five weeks following IPT. The other 10 of 11 fetuses to have IPT are all well, with no evidence of long-term compromise, as is the one case where IPT was infused in the fetal descending colon (124).

INTRACARDIAC FETAL
TRANSFUSION (ICT)

Putting a needle in the fetal heart is not as difficult, or as dangerous, as one might think. On the other hand, there are not many centers who have adopted this as a preferential method of transfusing the anemic fetus, so it is difficult to evaluate outside of the emergency situations in which it has been reported (126). This is true of our experience as well (127). We have used intracardiac

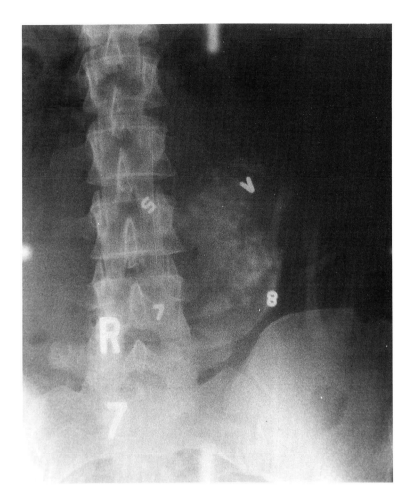

Figure 6-42A When the demonstration of proper, free needle placement is not achieved, installation of Renografin and simple flat-plate x-ray will confirm proper placement. Between the markers 8 and V, the fetal abdominal cavity is identified by crescents of dye lying between the adjacent loops of fetal small bowel. This confirmation allows confident installation of large volumes of blood.

transfusion on 11 occasions in 10 fetuses. Five of those fetuses survived solely because of the intracardiac transfusion, which was used to resuscitate them from exsanguinating hemorrhage. They then were able to complete their courses of intravascular transfusion without incident, and were all delivered at term, and remain healthy intact survivors.

Among those who did not survive intracardiac transfusion is one infant noted previously who had two such procedures as a result of exsanguinating hemorrhage from vessel tearing, the second ICT unsuccessful.

Three others had ICT in relation to apparent failure of serial IVT; the fetus died of intercurrent maternal intravenous cocaine abuse in two, and the third died approximately eight hours following partial resuscitation which had utilized intracardiac transfusion. In the final case, although an intracardiac transfusion was given, there was no improvement at all in the moribund status; the intraventricular blood pH had been 6.93, and the fetus died a few hours later. Thus, although Westgren et al. (128) have published a series that includes several intracardiac transfusions, the experience from

Figure 6-42B Instillation of intraperitoneal donor blood produces a visible fluid rim in the fetal abdomen (arrows) as total volume approaches 80 ml.

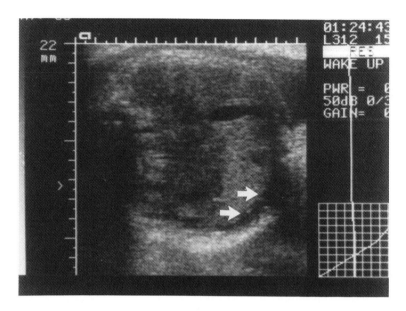

many centers is of this procedure in absolutely dire circumstances.

Technical Aspects

The fetal heart can be entered with a needle as long as the spine is not directly anterior. In that case, one needle is used to impale the fetus and turn him, and a second needle is introduced into the thorax before the first is removed. As long as fetal position is satisfactory, entry into the heart is usually straightforward. We use a 20-gauge needle because the increased stiffness enables some degree of direction once the needle is between ribs. With a more flexible 22-gauge needle, leverage on the needle frequently only moves the fetus and does not result in any change in the angle of insertion.

While physiologically one might prefer to enter the right ventricle to avoid delivering the unmixed transfusion mass directly into the cerebral circulation and to allow the blood to make as rapid a transit to the placenta as possible, this is usually not a matter of choice. The ventricles are much more sta-

ble in terms of needle placement, but our experience has been satisfactory with a few occasions of transfusing the right atrium. Turbulence in the fetal heart is demonstrated just as in the vessels, although a larger bolus of saline is usually required because of rapid efflux. Continuous turbulence within the ventricular cavity should be demonstrated, as it is not difficult to have the needle migrate outside the cavity or, indeed, into the pericardial space, where infusion of even a small amount of blood will be instantly lethal. On two of the occasions when we have attempted intracardiac transfusion, in fact, the pericardial effusions have been so large as to preclude entry through the myometrium. Turbulence is readily seen in the umbilical arteries as well (Figure 6-43) (129).

It is difficult to know how much volume to give during an intracardiac transfusion. While one does not want to waste this opportunity to restore the fetal hemoglobin to a reasonably normal level, undoubtedly the fetus who requires intracardiac transfusion as an emergency life-saving maneuver does

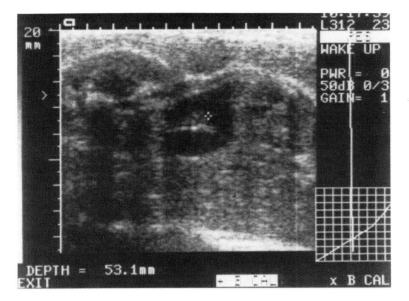

Figure 6-43 Intracradiac fetal transfusion during emergency resuscitation. **6-43A** The needle is in the right ventricle, and proper placement is identified by continuous turbulence during infusion. In this case, cardiac function returned to normal after the first 10 ml, in association with maternal oxygen administration.

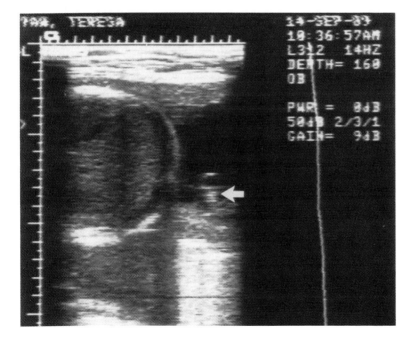

Figure 6-43B Turbulence in the umbilical artery (arrow) during the infusion phase of an intracardiac transfusion. Turbulence is also visualized in the descending aorta but could not be seen in the ascending aorta or intracranial vessels. In this case, at least, the theory of right ventricle infusion leading to preferential streaming of blood down the distal aorta to the placenta was confirmed.

not have the same tolerance to volume as his more stable counterpart. Our tendency is to give 50% of the IVT volume and to plan on repeating the transfusion in the near future. On one occasion we decided to exceed this principle because the fetus was 18 weeks, the vessels were not visible, and the fetus was already severely hydropic; we raised the hemoglobin from 19 g/L to 130 g/L, and lethal fetal cardiac failure supervened over the next eight hours.

Complications

In the five survivors, there have been no permanent complications of the therapy, and all are well at follow-up intervals of two years or more. In three of the five, there was detectable echogenicity at the point of needle entry, including substantial pericardial effusions, which resolved over two to three weeks. In no case was there any significant arrhythmia, prolonged fetal immobility, or any abnormalities of the post-ICT FHR monitoring. When effective, resuscitation by ICT appears not to carry risk of fetal brain injury.

As more experience is gained with this technique, it may become fairly routine at transfusions before 20 weeks to consider whether or not the umbilical vein or the intracardiac route offers the best safety and easiest access. At gestations beyond 20 weeks, however, we would reserve this approach to the emergency situations described.

FETAL EXCHANGE TRANSFUSION

Initially performed as routine by some groups, exchange transfusion now appears to be reserved for severe hydrops (110,130,131). The argument is that in order to achieve "normal" hemoglobin levels with one transfusion in such severely anemic fetuses, the volumes of donor blood would be prohibitive. While our approach is, therefore, to give multiple small transfusions over a relatively short period of time, another approach has been to perform exchange transfusion. No data are available on a consistent basis to allow direct comparison, and the interested reader is referred to the reports of Grannum et al. (110,131).

Technical Aspects

The procedure is virtually identical to IVT, but, of course, takes twice as long due to the withdrawal component of an exchange transfusion. The usual aliquots of 10 ml are infused with subsequent withdrawal of 10 ml. Although the procedure relies heavily on bedside testing to give immediate values, the authors describe calculations, which have been computerized, to estimate the status of transfusion when there are technical difficulties in withdrawing the blood. Exchange transfusion has been recommended in cases where there is poor myocardial contractility, and in those cases, the intraprocedure echocardiography must be exemplary. Following the procedure, monitoring is similar, most fetuses reverted to serial simple transfusion, and outcome seems indistinguishable from courses of therapy with intravascular transfusion alone.

The most recent report by this group suggests a relatively limited range of application for exchange transfusion per se. Our experience with severe hydrops has been as good or better than that cited for exchange transfusion. For example, our survival rate of 88% includes survival of 67% of moribund hydrops, whereas the combined application of exchange transfusion and simple IVT produced a survival rate of 81%, zero in three moribund hydropic fetuses. Our conclusion to date has been that while the hemoglobin can be raised faster at one procedure when exchange transfusion is used, this is not necessarily safe in view of the borderline cardiac status of severely-affected infants.

SUMMARY

Cordocentesis has provided highly-detailed data and access to many more sources than we are currently able to evaluate. Intravascular transfusion has proven a therapeutic medium of great advantage and probably has not yet been fully exploited. Thus, both monitoring and treatment of the alloimmunized fetus will likely continue to progress.

These two aligned techniques have provided the quantum leap that has made even very early, very severe disease accessible for treatment. All of the factors shown in Table 6-20 have followed the very positive experience with IVT. There should be no underestimation of the important contribution of high-resolution ultrasonography. Why a few groups may not have shared the improved experience with IVT (132,133) may be explained in part by local technical limitations. The claims of those experiencing good results with IVT are neither fleeting nor extravagant (52). They are consistent and still growing. Although the most extreme cases still require technical innovation, such innovation takes place on a background of detailed understanding of fetal transfusion and the pathophysiology of severe anemia. One can realistically offer hope for virtually every fetus who still has cardiac output. This most shining example of fetal investigation, monitoring, and treatment will undoubtedly continue to approach the goal of 100% survival.

Table 6-20 7 Years of IVT—Impacts

IVT a Routine Procedure 19 − 34+ Weeks

Nonhydrops = Intact Term Survivor

Fetal Resuscitation a Reality

Physiologic/Pathophysiologic Data

"Repeat Customers"

Technical Skill Radiates Benefit
- Nonimmune anemia, e.g., parvovirus
- Alloimmune thrombocytopenia
- Procedures, e.g., V-A shunts, T-A shunts

References

1. Harman CR, Manning FA. Alloimmune disease. In: Pauerstein CJ, ed. Clinical Obstetrics. New York: John Wiley & Sons Inc, 1987;21:441–469.
2. Le Van Kim C, Mouro I, Cherif-Zahar, C et al. Molecular cloning and primary structure of the human blood group RhD polypeptide. Proc Natl Acad Sci USA 1992; 89:10925–10929.
3. Levine P, Stetson RE. An unusual case of intra-group agglutination. JAMA 1939; 113:126–127.
4. Freda VJ, Gorman JG, Pollack W. Successful prevention of experimental Rh sensitization in man with an anti-Rh gamma²-globulin antibody preparation. Transfusion 1964; 4:26–32.
5. Bowman JM. Suppression of Rh isoimmunization. Obstet Gynecol 1978;52:385–393.
6. Albar H, Harman CR, Pollock JM, Bowman JM, Menticoglou S, Manning FA. Amniotic fluid spectrophotometry in the midtrimester. (Abstract) Presented at the Annual Meeting of the Society of Obstetricians and Gynecologists, June, 1992.
7. Weiner CP, Williamson RA, Wenstrom KD, Sipes SL, Grant SS, Widness JA. Management of fetal hemolytic disease by cordocentesis. I. Prediction of fetal anemia. Am J Obstet Gynecol 1991;165:546–553.

8. Harman CR, Manning FA, Bowman JM, Lange IR. Severe Rh disease - poor outcome is not inevitable. Am J Obstet Gynecol 1983;145:823–829.

9. deCrespigny LCh, Robinson HP, Quinn M, Doyle L, Ross A, Cauchi M. Ultrasound-guided fetal blood transfusion for severe rhesus isoimmunization. Obstet Gynecol 1985;66:529–532.

10. Nicolaides KH, Soothill PW, Clewell W, Rodeck CH, Campbell, S. Rh disease: intravascular fetal blood transfusion by cordocentesis. Fetal Ther 1986;1:185–192.

11. Harman CR, Manning FA, Bowman JM, Lange IR, Menticoglou SM. Use of intravascular transfusion to treat hydrops fetalis in a moribund fetus. Can Med Assoc J 1988;138:827–830.

12. Doyle LW, Kelly EA, Rickards AL, Ford GW, Callanan C. Sensorineural outcome at two years for survivors of erythroblastosis treated with fetal intravascular transfusions. Obstet Gynecol 1993;81:931–935.

13. Chown B, Duff AM, James J, et al. Prevention of primary Rh immunization: first report of the Western Canadian trial. Can Med Assoc J 1969;100:1021–1024.

14. Zipursky A, Israels LG. The pathogenesis and prevention of Rh immunization. Can Med Assoc J 1967;97:1245–1257.

15. Bowman JM. Efficacy of antenatal Rh prophylaxis. In: Frigoletto FD Jr, Jewett JF, Konugres AA, eds. Rh Hemolytic Disease: New Strategy for Eradication. Boston: GK Hall, 1982:143–160.

16. Friesen AD, Bowman JM, Price HW. Column ion-exchange preparation and characterization of an Rh immune globulin (WinRho) for intravenous use. J Appl Biochem 1981;3:164–175.

17. Harman CR. Hemolytic disease of the fetus and newborn. In: Rakel RE, ed. Conn's Current Therapy. Philadelphia: WB Saunders Co., 1993:361–366.

18. Bowman JM. Maternal Rh blood group immunization: past, present, future. J Soc Obstet Gynecol 1989;11:27–35.

19. Bowman JM, Pollock JM. Failures of intravenous Rh immune globulin prophylaxis: an analysis of the reasons for such failures. Transfusion Med Rev 1987;1:101–112.

20. Biggins KR, Bowman JM. Rh(D) alloimmunization in the absence of exposure to Rh(D) antigen. Vox Sang 1986;51:228–230.

21. Bowman JM. Hemolytic disease (erythroblastosis fetalis). In: Creasy RK, Resnik R, eds. Maternal Fetal Medicine: Principles and Practice, 2nd ed, Philadelphia: WB Saunders, 1989;35:613–649.

22. Bowman J, Harman C, Manning F, Menticoglou S, Pollock J. Intravenous drug abuse causes Rh immunization. Vox Sang 1991;61:96–98.

23. Bowman JM, Pollock JM, Manning FA, Harman CR, Menticoglou S. Maternal Kell blood group alloimmunization. Obstet Gynecol 1992;79:239–244.

24. Bowman JM, Harman CR, Manning FA, Pollock JM. Severe erythroblastosis fetalis produced by anti-cellano. Vox Sang 1989;56:187–189.

25. Bowman JM, Pollock JM, Manning FA, Harman CR. Severe anti-C hemolytic disease of the newborn. Am J Obstet Gynecol 1992;166:1239–1243.

26. Bowell PJ, Brown SE, Dike AE, Inskip MJ. The significance of anti-c alloimmunization in pregnancy. Br J Obstet Gynaecol 1986;93:1044–1048.

27. Bowman JM, Friesen RF. Multiple intraperitoneal transfusions of the fetus for erythroblastosis fetalis. New Engl J Med 1964;271:703–707.

28. Liley AW. Intrauterine transfusion of foetus in haemolytic disease. Br Med J 1963;2:1107–1109.

29. Harman CR, Bowman JM, Manning FA, Menticoglou SM. Intrauterine transfusion—intraperitoneal versus intravascular approach: a case-control comparison. Am J Obstet Gynecol 1990;162:1053–1059.

30. Harman CR, Bowman JM, Manning FA, Menticoglou SM. Six years of success with intravascular fetal transfusion. J Soc Obstet Gynecol Canada 1994 (in press).

31. Harman CR. Fetal monitoring in the alloimmunized pregnancy. Clinics in Perinatology 1989;16:691–733.

32. Liley AW. Liquor amnio analysis in management of pregnancy complicated by Rhesus isoimmunization. Am J Obstet Gynecol 1961;82:1359–1370.

33. Ananth U, Queenan JT. Does midtrimester ΔOD 450 of amniotic fluid reflect severity of Rh disease? Am J Obstet Gynecol 1989;161:47–49.

34. Harman CR, Albar HA, Pollock JM, Bowman JM, Menticoglou SM, Manning FA. Prospective evaluation of a curve for midtrimester amniotic fluid assessment in alloimmunized pregnancies. Am J Obstet Gynecol 1994 (in press).

35. Hauncher JD, Stolorow MD. Rh-typing on stained material—single threads. (Laboratory Protocol) State Police Scientific Laboratory, Plymouth, Michigan, 1990.

36. Fuhrman HC, Klink F, Grzejszczyk G, et al. First trimester diagnosis of RH_O (D) with an immunofluorescence technique after chorionic villus sampling. Prenat Diagn 1987;7:17–21.

37. Rodesch F, Lambermont M, Donner C, et al. Chorionic biopsy in management of severe Kell alloimmunization. Am J Obstet Gynecol 1987;156:124–125.

38. Kanhai HH, Gravenhorst JB, Gemke RJ, Overbeeke MA, Bernini LF, Beverstock GC. Fetal blood group determination in first-trimester pregnancy for the management of severe immunization. Am J Obstet Gynecol 1987;156:120–123.

39. Kickler TS, Blakemore K, Shirey RS, et al. Chorionic villus sampling for fetal Rh typing: clinical implications. Am J Obstet Gynecol 1992;166:1407–1411.

40. Nance SJ, Nelson JM, Horenstein J, Arndt PA, Platt LD, Garratty G. Monocyte monolayer assay: an efficient noninvasive technique for predicting the severity of hemolytic disease of the newborn. Am J Clin Pathol 1989;92:89–92.

41. MacKenzie I, Guest CM, Bowell PJ. Fetal blood group studies during mid-trimester pregnancy and the management of severe isoimmunization. Prenat Diagn 1983; 3:41–46.

42. Bowell PJ, Selinger M, Ferguson J, Giles J, MacKenzie IZ. Antenatal fetal blood sampling for the management of alloimmunized pregnancies: effect upon maternal anti-D potency levels. Br J Obstet Gynaecol 1988;95:759–764.

43. Bennett PR, Le Van Kim C, Colin Y, et al. Prenatal determination of fetal RhD type by DNA amplification. N Engl J Med 1993;329:607–610.

44. Moise KJ, Carpenter RJ. Increased severity of fetal hemolytic disease with known Rhesus alloimmunization after first-trimester transcervical chorionic villus biopsy. Fetal Diagn Ther 1990;5:76–78.

45. Blakemore KJ, Baumgarten A, Schoenfeld-Dimaio M, Hobbins JC, Mason EA, Mahoney MJ. Rise in maternal serum α-fetoprotein concentration after chorionic villus sampling and the possibility of isoimmunization. Am J Obstet Gynecol 1986;155:988–993.

46. Lo Y-MD, Bowell PJ, Selinger M, et al. Prenatal determination of fetal RhD status by analysis of peripheral blood of Rhesus-negative mothers. (Letter) The Lancet 1993; 341:1147–1148.

47. Price JO, Elias S, Wachtel SS, et al. Prenatal diagnosis with fetal cells isolated from maternal blood by multiparameter flow cytometry. Am J Obstet Gynecol 1991;165:1731–1737.

48. Chueh J, Golbus MS. Prenatal diagnosis using fetal cells in the maternal circulation. Sem Perinat 1990;14:471–482.

49. Mueller UW, Hawes CS, Wright AE, et al. Isolation of fetal trophoblast cells from peripheral blood of pregnant women. The Lancet 1990;336:197–200.

50. Bianchi DW, Flint AF, Pizzimenti MF, Knoll JHM, Latt SA. Isolation of fetal DNA from nucleated erythrocytes in maternal blood. Proc Natl Acad Sci 1990;87:3279–3283.

51. Kanter MH. Derivation of new mathematic formulas for determining whether a D-positive father is heterozygous or homozygous for the D antigen. Am J Obstet Gynecol 1992;166:61–63.

52. MacKenzie IZ, Selinger M, Bowell PJ. Management of red cell isoimmunization in the 1990s. In: Studd J, ed. Progress in Obstetrics and Gynaecology—vol 9. Edinburgh: Churchill Livingstone, 1991; 3:31–53.

53. Bowell P, Wainscoat JS, Peto TEA, Gunson HH. Maternal anti-D concentrations and outcome in Rhesus haemolytic disease of the newborn. Br Med J 1982;285:327–329.

54. Nicolaides KH, Rodeck CH. Maternal serum anti-D antibody concentration and assessment of rhesus isoimmunisation. Br Med J 1992;304:1155–1156.

55. Pollock JM, Bowman JM. Anti-Rh(D) IgG subclasses and severity of Rh hemolytic disease of the newborn. Vox Sang 1990;59:176–179.

56. Hadley AG, Poole GD, Fraser ID. Predicting the severity of haemolytic disease of the newborn: prospective evaluation of the chemiluminescence test. (Letter) Vox Sang 1992;63:291–292.

57. Moise KJ Jr. Monocyte monolayer assay in assessment of anti-D strength. Philadelphia: Sixth Annual Conference on Percutaneous Umbilical Blood Sampling, 1991.

58. Hadley AG, Kumpel BM, Leader KA, Poole GD, Fraser ID. Correlation of serological, quantitative and cell-mediated functional assays of maternal alloantibodies with the severity of haemolytic disease of the newborn. Br J Haemat 1991;77:221–228.

59. Spinnato JA. Hemolytic disease of the fetus. Am J Obstet Gynecol 1992;166: 1589–1590.

60. Weiner CP. Hemolytic disease of the fetus. (Letter) Am J Obstet Gynecol 1992;166:1590.

61. Spinnato JA. Hemolytic disease of the fetus: a plea for restraint. Obstet Gynecol 1992;80:873–877.

62. Bowman JM, Pollock J, Menticoglou S, Harman CR, Manning FA. Hemolytic disease of the fetus: a plea for restraint. Obstet Gynecol 1993;81:478.

63. Weiner CP. Hemolytic disease of the fetus: a plea for restraint. Obstet Gynecol 1993;81:478–479.

64. Spinnato JA. Hemolytic disease of the fetus: a plea for restraint. (Response) Obstet Gynecol 1993;81:479–480.

65. Management of isoimmunization in pregnancy. ACOG Technical Bulletin No. 148—October 1990. Int J Gynecol Obstet 1992;37:57–62.

66. Whitfield CR. A three-year assessment of an action-line method of timing intervention in Rhesus isoimmunization. Am J Obstet Gynecol 1970;108:1239–1244.

67. Nicolaides KH, Rodeck CH, Mibashan RS, Kemp JR. Have Liley charts outlived their usefulness? Am J Obstet Gynecol 1986;155:90–94.

68. Harman CR. Ultrasound in the management of the alloimmune pregnancy. In: Fleischer AC, Romero R, Manning FA, Jeanty P, James AE Jr, eds. The Principles and Practice of Ultrasonography in Obstetrics and Gynecology, 4th ed. Connecticut: Appleton & Lange 1990;24: 393–416.

69. Joshi AK, Muzio LR. Conservative management of a severely alloimmunized pregnancy: case report. Am J Obstet Gynecol 1988;158:479–480.

70. Steyn DW, Pattinson RC, Odendaal HJ. Amniocentesis—still important in the management of severe Rhesus incompatibility. S Am Med J 1992;82:321–324.

71. Reiss R, Iams JD, O'Shaughnessy R, Cordero L, Kennedy M, Strohm P. Management of isoimmunized pregnancy. New Engl J Med 1987;316:165.

72. Goodlin R, Lloyd D. Fetal tracheal excretion of bilirubin. Biol Neonat 1968;12:1–12.

73. Ananth U, Warsof SL, Coulehan JM, Wolf PH, Queenan JT. Midtrimester amniotic fluid delta optical density at 450nm in normal pregnancies. Am J Obstet Gynecol 1986;155:664–666.

74. Bowman JM, Pollock JM. Transplacental fetal hemorrhage after amniocentesis. Obstet Gynecol 1985;66:749–754.

75. Harman CR, Bowman JM, Manning FA, Menticoglou SM. Alloimmune hydrops before 20 weeks gestation. Am J Obstet Gynecol 1994 (in press).

76. Stegner H, Fischer K, Pahnke VG, Kitschke HJ, Commentz JC. There is evidence that amniotic fluid arginine vasopressin is a marker for fetal stress in Rhesus erythroblastosis. Acta Endocrinol 1986;112:267–270.

77. Harman CR, Pollock JM, Widness J, Manning FA, Bowman JM, Menticoglou S. Amniotic fluid erythropoietin levels reliably reflect fetal status. (Abstract) Presented at Meeting of the Society of Obstetricians and Gynecologists, June, 1991.

78. Finne PH. Erythropoietin levels in the amniotic fluid, particularly in Rh-immunized pregnancies. Acta Paediatr 1964;53:269–281.

79. Voutilainen PEJ, Widness JA, Clemons GK, Schwartz R, Teramo KA. Amniotic fluid erythropoietin predicts fetal distress in Rh-immunized pregnancies. Am J Obstet Gynecol 1989;160:429–434.

80. Weiner CP, Wenstrom KD, Sipes SL, Williamson RA. Risk factors for cordocentesis and fetal intravascular transfusion. Am J Obstet Gynecol 1991;165:1020–1025.

81. Nicolaides KH, Clewell WH, Mibashan RS, Soothill PW, Rodeck CH, Campbell S. Fetal haemoglobin measurement in the assessment of red cell isoimmunisation. The Lancet 1988;i:1073–1074.

82. Weiner CP. Human fetal bilirubin levels and fetal hemolytic disease. Am J Obstet Gynecol 1992;166:1149–1454.

83. Nicolaides KH. Studies on fetal physiology and pathophysiology in Rhesus disease. Sem Perinat 1989;13:328–337.

84. Copel JA, Grannum PA, Green JJ, et al. Fetal cardiac output in the isoimmunized pregnancy: a pulsed Doppler-echocardiographic study of patients undergoing intravascular intrauterine transfusion. Am J Obstet Gynecol 1989;161:361–365.

85. Lingman G, Legarth J, Rahman F, Stangenberg M. Myocardial contractility in the anemic human fetus. Ultrasound Obstet Gynaecol 1991;1:266–268.

86. Margulies M, Voto LS, Mathet E, Margulies MJ. High-dose intravenous IgG for the treatment of severe Rhesus alloimmunization. Vox Sang. 1991;61:181–189.

87. Nicolaides KH, Fontanarosa M, Gabbe SG, Rodeck CH. Failure of ultrasonographic parameters to predict the severity of fetal anemia in Rhesus isoimmunization. Am J Obstet Gynecol 1988;158:920–926.

88. Reece EA, Gabrielli S, Abdalla M, O'Connor TZ, Hobbins JC. Reassessment of the utility of fetal umbilical vein diameter in the management of isoimmunization. Am J Obstet Gynecol 1988;159:937–938.

89. Copel JA, Grannum PA, Belanger K, Green J, Hobbins JC. Pulsed Doppler flow-velocity waveforms before and after intrauterine transfusion for severe erythroblastosis fetalis. Am J Obstet Gynecol 1988;158:768–774.

90. DeVore GR, Mayden K, Tortora M, Berkowitz RL, Hobbins JC. Dilation of the fetal umbilical vein in Rhesus hemolytic anemia: a predictor of severe disease. Am J Obstet Gynecol 1981;141:464–466.

91. Harman CR. Specialized applications of obstetric ultrasound: management of the alloimmunized pregnancy. Sem Perinat 1985;9:184–197.

92. Harman CR, Widness J, Pollock JM, Bowman JM, Manning FA, Menticoglou S, Weiner C. Fetal serum erythropoietin in severe Rh disease. (Abstract) Presented at the Annual Meeting of the Society of Obstetricians and Gynecologists, June, 1990.

93. Thilaganathan B, Salvesen DR, Abbas A, Ireland RM, Nicolaides KH. Fetal plasma erythropoietin concentration in red blood cell-isoimmunized pregnancies. Am J Obstet Gynecol 1992;167:1292–1297.

94. Moise KJ, Mari G, Fisher DJ, Huhta JC, Cano LE, Carpenter RJ Jr. Acute fetal hemodynamic alterations after intrauterine transfusion for treatment of severe red blood cell alloimmunization. Am J Obstet Gynecol 1990;1963:776–784.

95. Rightmire DA, Nicolaides KH, Rodeck CH, Campbell S. Fetal blood velocities in Rh isoimmunization: relationship to gestational age and to fetal hematocrit. Obstet Gynecol 1986;68:233–236.

96. Oepkes D, Vandenbussche FP, Van Bel F, Kanhai HHH. Fetal ductus venosus blood flow velocities before and after transfusion

in red-cell alloimmunized pregnancies. Obstet Gynecol 1993;82:237–241.

97. Harman CR, Bowman JM. Intraperitoneal fetal transfusion. In: Chervenak FA, Isaacson GC, Campbell S, eds. Ultrasound in Obstetrics and Gynecology, Vol 2. Boston: Little, Brown and Company, 1993:115: 1295–1313.

98. Harman CR, Farquharson D. Standards for programs performing intrauterine fetal transfusion (Policy Statement). Journal SOGC. 1991; Feb/Mar, pp. 19–21.

99. Carmody F, Bowman JM, Pollock J. Graft versus host disease following intrauterine fetal transfusion. Aust NZ J Obstet Gynaecol 1994 (in press).

100. Manning FA, Harman CR. Fetal Transfusion. In: Iffy L, Apuzzio JJ, Vintzileos AM, eds. Operative Obstetrics, 2nd ed. New York: McGraw-Hill 1992;7:70–81.

101. Seeds JW, Chescheir NC, Bowes WA Jr, Owl-Smith FA. Fetal death as a complication of intrauterine intravascular transfusion. Obstet Gynecol 1989(SII);74:461–463.

102. Thorp JA, Plapp FV, Cohen GR, Yeast JD, O'Kell RT, Stephenson S. Hyperkalemia after irradiation of packed red blood cells: possible effects with intravascular transfusion. Am J Obstet Gynecol 1990;163:607–609.

103. Segal M, Manning FA, Harman CR, Menticoglou S. Bleeding after intravascular transfusion: experimental and clinical observations. Am J Obstet Gynecol 1991;165:1414–1418.

104. Brace RA. Ovine fetal cardiovascular responses to packed red blood cell transfusions. Am J Obstet Gynecol 1989; 161:1367–1374.

105. Nicolini U, Kochenour NK, Greco P, Letsky E, Rodeck CH. When to perform the next intrauterine transfusion in patients with Rh alloimmunization: combined intravascular and intraperitoneal transfusion allows longer intervals. Fetal Ther 1989;4:14–20.

106. MacGregor SN, Socol ML, Pielet BW, Sholl JS, Silver RK. Prediction of hematocrit decline after intravascular fetal trans-

fusion. Am J Obstet Gynecol 1989;161: 1491–1493.

107. Mari G, Moise KJ Jr, Deter RL, Carpenter RJ Jr. Doppler assessment of renal blood flow velocity waveforms in the anemic fetus before and after intravascular transfusion for severe red cell alloimmunization. J Clin Ultrasound 1991;19:15–19.

108. Nicolini U, Kochenour NK, Greco P, et al. Consequences of fetomaternal haemorrhage after intrauterine transfusion. Br Med J 1988;297:1379–1381.

109. Nicolaides KH, Thorpe-Beeston JG, Salvesen DR, Snijders RJM. Fetal blood transfusion by cordocentesis. In: Chervenak FA, Isaacson GC, Campbell S, eds. Ultrasound in Obstetrics and Gynecology, Vol 2. Boston: Little, Brown and Company, 1993;116:1315–1320.

110. Grannum PAT. In utero intravascular exchange transfusion for severe erythroblastosis fetalis. In: Chervenak FA, Isaacson GC, Campbell S, eds. Ultrasound in Obstetrics and Gynecology, Vol 2. Boston: Little, Brown and Company, 1993; 117:1321–1326.

111. Parer JT. Severe Rh isoimmunization—current methods of in utero diagnosis and treatment. Am J Obstet Gynecol 1988; 158:1323–1329.

112. Dildy GA III, Smith LG Jr, Moise KJ Jr, Cano LE, Hesketh DE. Porencephalic cyst: a complication of fetal intravascular transfusion. Am J Obstet Gynecol 1991;165:76–78.

113. Morrow RJ, Ryan G, Johnson J. Case Report. Posterior fossa hemorrhage following intrauterine fetal transfusion. Am J Obstet Gynecol 1994 (in press).

114. Evans DGR, Lyon AJ. Fatal congenital cytomegalovirus infection acquired by an intrauterine transfusion. Eur J Pediatr 1991;150:780–781.

115. Mandelbaum B, Brough AJ. Hepatitis following multiple intrauterine transfusion. Report of a case. Obstet Gynecol 1967;30:188–191.

116. Musemeche CA, Reynolds M. Necrotizing enterocolitis following intrauterine blood

transfusion. J Pediatr Surg 1991;26:
1411–1412.

117. Utter GO, Socol ML, Dooley SL, MacGregor SN, Millard DD. Is intrauterine transfusion associated with diminished fetal growth? Am J Obstet Gynecol 1990;163:
1781–1784.

118. Harman CR, Menticoglou SM, Pollock J, Manning FA, Bowman JM. Human fetal pO2 reponses to maternal oxygenation. Am J Obstet Gynecol 1994 (in press).

119. Harman CR, Bowman JM, Menticoglou S, Pollock JM, Manning FA. Profound fetal thrombocytopenia in Rhesus disease: serious hazard at intravascular transfusion. The Lancet 1988;ii:741–742.

120. Nicolaides KH, Rodeck CH, Millar DS, Mibashan RS. Fetal haematology in Rhesus isoimmunisation. Br Med J 1985; 290:661–663.

121. Hallak M, Moise KJ Jr, Hesketh DE, Cano LE, Carpenter RJ Jr. Intravascular transfusion of fetuses with Rhesus incompatibility: prediction of fetal outcome by changes in umbilical venous pressure. Obstet Gynecol 1992;80:286–290.

122. Selbing A, Stangenberg M, Westgren M, Rahman F. Intrauterine intravascular transfusions in fetal erythroblastosis: the influence of net transfusion volume on fetal survival. Acta Obstet Gynaecol Scand 1993;72:20–23.

123. Moise KJ Jr, Carpenter RJ Jr, Kirshon B, Deter RL, Sala JD, Cano LE. Comparison of four types of intrauterine transfusion: effect on fetal hematocrit. Fetal Ther 1989;4:126–137.

124. Harman CR, Menticoglou SM, Bowman J M, Manning FA. Current techniques of intra-peritoneal transfusion: do not throw away the Renografin. Fetal Ther 1989;4:
78–82.

125. Menticoglou SM, Harman CR, Manning FA, Bowman JM. Intraperitoneal fetal transfusion: paralysis inhibits red cell absorption. Fetal Ther 1987;2:154–159.

126. Nicolaides KH, Rodeck CH. In utero resuscitation after cardiac arrest in a fetus. Br Med J 1984;288:900–901.

127. Harman CR, Manning FA, Menticoglou S, Bowman J. Fetal exsanguination at intravascular transfusion. (Abstract) Presented at the 46th Annual Meeting of the Society of Obstetricians and Gynecologists, Halifax, June, 1990.

128. Westgren M, Selbing A, Stangenberg M. Fetal intracardiac transfusions in patients with severe Rhesus isoimmunisation. Br Med J 1988;296:885–886.

129. Harman CR, Menticoglou SM, Manning FA, Albar H, Bowman JM. Intracardiac fetal transfusion as an emergency recourse. Fetal Diagn Ther 1994 (in press).

130. Poissonnier M-H, Brossard Y, Demedeiros N, et al. Two hundred intrauterine exchange transfusions in severe blood incompatibilities. Am J Obstet Gynecol 1989;161:709–713.

131. Grannum PA, Copel JA, Plaxe SC, Scioscia AL, Hobbins JC. In utero exchange transfusion by direct intravascular injection in severe erythroblastosis fetalis. New Engl J Med 1986;314:1431–1434.

132. MacKenzie IZ, Bowell PJ, Ferguson J, Castle BM, Entwistle CC. In utero intravascular transfusion of the fetus for the management of severe Rhesus isoimmunization—a reappraisal. Br J Obstet Gynaecol 1987;94: 1068–1073.

133. Voto LS, Margulies M. In utero intravascular transfusion of the fetus for the management of severe Rhesus isoimmunization—a reappraisal. (Letter) Br J Obstet Gynaecol 1988;95:730–731.

PLATELET DISORDERS IN PREGNANCY

MARY PILLAI

7

Platelet disorders are sufficiently common that they will be encountered from time to time in prenatal care. A great deal of confusion exists regarding what constitutes a normal platelet count in pregnancy, and people frequently ascribe risks to mothers and/or fetuses that are not necessarily both part of the same disorder.

Maternal thrombocytopenia is the most common platelet abnormality found, and most often, this will be gestational thrombocytopenia, thrombocytopenia associated with preeclampsia, or thrombocytopenia related to recognized obstetric causes of disseminated intravascular coagulation. Previously undiagnosed maternal autoimmune thrombocytopenia will occasionally be encountered and is the most likely diagnosis when thrombocytopenia is present in early pregnancy. The most serious, but also the least common, perinatal platelet disorder as far as the fetus is concerned is alloimmune thrombocytopenia, which is usually only diagnosed after an affected fetus is born and carries a significant risk for future pregnancies.

Pregnancy-associated Thrombocytopenia

The advent of automated platelet counts has led to the recognition that during pregnancy many healthy women become thrombocytopenic by conventional criteria (platelets $< 150 \times 10^9/L$) without apparent cause.

Sejeny et al. (1) reviewed 11 early reports of small sample size and found these varied widely in their findings. The most consistent finding in subsequent reports has been a small but significant fall in platelet count as pregnancy progresses (1–3), together with evidence of a shorter platelet life span consequent upon accelerated destruction in pregnant women (4,5). A longitudinal study looking at changes occurring in individual healthy pregnant women found considerable individual variation with the apparent fall in the group accounted for by a considerable fall in a few individuals (6).

A prospective study of 6715 healthy pregnant women who delivered during a three-year period showed that 513 (7.6%) had mild thrombocytopenia at term (platelet counts 97–150 $\times 10^9/L$) (7). This had no discernible effect on the women or their infants. The frequency of thrombocytopenia in their infants was no greater than that of babies born to women with normal platelet counts. A further study of this gestational or pregnancy-associated thrombocytopenia (PAT) confirmed its benign nature concerning both mother and fetus (8) and confirmed that maternal platelet counts rose to the normal range in the postnatal period. The normal ranges for platelet counts varied with race and in Black women also varied with gestation (8). The study found that PAT may be a recurrent phenomenon.

A significant rise in platelet volume (macrothrombocytosis) has been documented, especially in late pregnancy (9). The most striking change is in the range of distribution of platelet volume, which is thought to reflect increased platele turnover with a decreased platelet survival time in normal pregnancy (10). These findings support the concept of a low-grade chronic activation of the coagulation cascade in normal pregnancy that increased toward term (5). The site for this is thought to be within the uteroplacental circulation. The differentiation of this mechanism from direct effects of pregnancy-induce prostaglandin alterations may be difficult. Because of the benign nature of PAT, it has been recommended that the incidental discovery of mild thrombocytopenia (100–150 $\times 10^9/L$) in late pregnancy does not require any intervention (11,12). There may remain a problem, however, with differentiating individual cases with autoimmune thrombocytopenia of moderately severe extent, particularly where no platelet count is available from early pregnancy.

Preeclampsia

Thrombocytopenia is the most common hemostatic problem seen in preeclampsia, but its severity is inconsistent. There is increasing evidence that preeclampsia starts in the first trimester with poor placentation, endothelial damage, and platelet dysfunction in the mother. Endothelial damage results in increased plasma levels of fibronectin and von Willebrand's factor. There is a chronic consumptive coagulopathy with reduced levels of antithrombin III. At the severe end of the spectrum it may be associated with elevated liver enzymes in the so-called HELLP syndrome (Hemolysis, Elevated Liver Enzymes, Low Platelets). This is a progressive disorder, and although the platelet count initially continues to fall postpartum, spontaneous resolution is usual

by the fifth day. Although life-threatening thrombocytopenia has been reported with preeclampsia (13), platelet transfusions are seldom indicated. Delivery is the treatment, and this succeeds because of removal of the placenta and marked decrease in platelet consumption in the involuting placental bed.

Rare Causes of Maternal Thrombocytopenia in Pregnancy

These include medical conditions, such as thrombotic thrombocytopenic purpura and hemolytic uremic syndrome. The former may be difficult to differentiate from preeclampsia. They have been well reviewed by Weiner (14) and are not discussed further in this chapter.

Chorangioma of the placenta is a rare placental tumor, which, when large, may cause maternal and/or fetal thrombocytopenia, hydrops, and increased likelihood of preeclampsia (15,16). Figure 7-1 illustrates a choriangioma that resulted in hydrops, car-

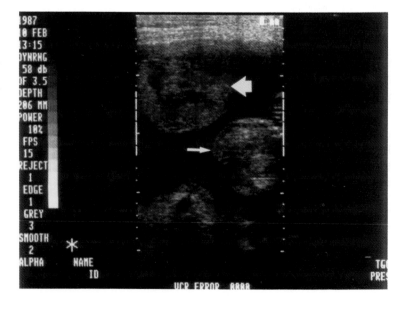

Figure 7-1A Chorioangioma (large arrow) is twice the size of fetal abdomen (small arrow) at 24 weeks gestation. Other than hydramnios, the ultrasound fetal assessment was normal.

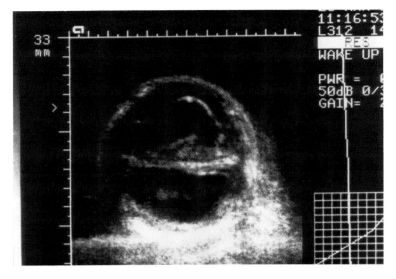

Figure 7-1B By 28 weeks gestation, striking changes had occurred, including loss of fetal breathing movement and tone and progressive hydrocephalus, shown here. At birth, thrombocytopenia (24.0 × 10⁹/L) and consumptive coagulopathy (P.T. >28 seconds) were documented. The infant was without cerebral function and died shortly after birth.

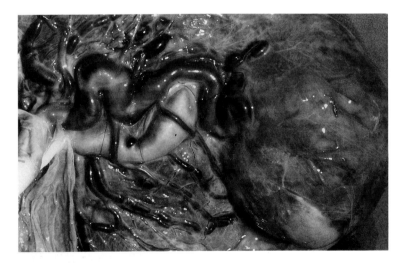

Figure 7-1C Gross morphology showing the placental tumor on right with distended fetal vessels. Compare the caliber of the right umbilical artery (large arrow) feeding the tumor to the left umbilical artery (small arrow). On Doppler ultrasound and on gross measurement in utero, these vessels were strikingly different within the fetus as well.

diomegaly and lethal fetal intracranial hemorrhage, likely caused by the severe thrombocytopenia and disseminated intravascular coagulopathy proven at birth.

Thrombocytopenia and the Fetus

Normal fetal platelet counts range from 150–250 X 10⁹/L (17,18), and counts of less than 50X10⁹/L have been associated with a perinatal death incidence in the order of 6% (19) (mostly in autoimmune and alloimmune thrombocytopenia). Indeed the majority of fetal deaths due to complications of thrombocytopenia may occur early in pregnancy (20). In the neonate, thrombocytopenia may present with symptomless thrombocytopenia, purpura, or severe hemorrhage, which most frequently is intracerebral. Until recently, it was thought that the greatest risk of intracranial hemorrhage was at the time of delivery; however, it is now apparent that the thrombocytopenic fetus is at risk of this complication antenatally, particularly when the platelet count falls below 50 X 10^9/L (21–23).

QUALITATIVE PLATELET DISORDERS

The most common cause of this is ingested medications, predominantly nonsteroidal anti-inflammatory agents. Aspirin causes covalent acetylation of the platelet cyclo-oxygenase, resulting in a storage pool defect that continues for the life of the exposed platelets (seven to ten days).

Congenital qualitative platelet defects are rare but may be associated with severe hemorrhage. They include the Bernard-Soulier syndrome (giant platelets with defective adhesion), and Glanzmann's thrombasthenia (autosomal recessive platelet aggregation defect). Severe hemorrhage resulting in fetal loss at the time of cordocentesis has been reported where the fetus was affected by Glanzmann's thrombasthenia (24).

Studies in patients with easy bruising have revealed presence of abnormal platelet function in the face of a normal platelet count in a significant percent (25). This condition is virtually the same as thrombopathia described by a number of independent groups (26). It predominantly affects females and is indistinguishable from the platelet aggregation defect seen with aspirin and in patients with systemic lupus erythematosus and autoimmune thrombocytopenia (27). In all of these conditions, antiplatelet antibodies have been found in a high percentage of affected individuals, suggesting that the antibody may contribute to or be responsible for both qualitative and quantitative platelet disorders. The incidence of qualitative platelet

disorder is said to be considerably more common than classic ITP (25,28,29), however, whether these women or their infants are at greater risk for hemorrhage than normal pregnant women has not been reported.

IMMUNE THROMBOCYTOPENIA (ITP) AND PREGNANCY

There are two clinically recognized varieties of ITP, acute and chronic. The majority of cases of the acute form of the disease affect children, are self-limiting, and are not at increased risk of developing ITP in adult life. Autoimmune thrombocytopenia, with transplacental active transport of maternal antiplatelet antibody to the fetus, is most commonly due to chronic maternal ITP but may occur secondary to maternal systemic lupus erythematosus (SLE) and lymphoproliferative disorders.

The human placenta has receptors for the Fc portion of the IgG molecule, allowing active transplacental passage of the IgG antibodies (30,31), which may mediate fetal thrombocytopenia. Autoimmune thrombocytopenia primarily affects young women in the reproductive years and is the most common immune disorder in pregnancy. It is characterized by production of an IgG autoantibody directed against specific platelet components (32–34). Antibody-coated platelets are rapidly removed from the circulation by the reticuloendothelial system, and despite a bone marrow response with increased platelet production, thrombocytopenia occurs.

Diagnosis

To satisfy this diagnosis, there should be an isolated thrombocytopenia with no other hematological abnormality and no evidence of a cause, such as splenomegaly or lymphadenopathy, no evidence of preeclampsia or history of drugs that can cause thrombocytopenia. Maternal bone marrow examination should reveal normal or increased numbers of megakaryocytes (35). Direct antiglobulin test (Coombs' test) and tests for SLE should also be done in patients presenting with ITP as thrombocytopenia may be the first manifestation of more generalized autoimmune disease.

Prognosis

Hedge (36) analyzed early reports of cases in the literature and found an overall prevalence of neonatal thrombocytopenia of 52%, with significant morbidity in 12%. Where the mother had a previous splenectomy, the incidence of neonatal thrombocytopenia and morbidity was increased further (37).

These reports are at variance with more recent studies that have found a low incidence of maternal and infant morbidity in patients with ITP (7,20,38), no correlation between fetal and maternal platelet counts (19,39), and no correlation between the presence or the level of maternal platelet antibodies and fetal platelet counts (19,20,39,40).

Platelet counts in affected infants frequently fall following delivery, and may reach a nadir of $<10 \times 10^9/L$ between two and six days of age. However, it has been noted that thrombocytopenia at or following delivery is generally not associated with significant morbidity (20,41) and recovers spontaneously within weeks.

Antenatal Management

It is possible to identify IgG antibodies that cross the placenta (33) and also to distinguish platelet-bound antibody from the more dangerous free IgG antibody in maternal plasma (40,42). However, apart from confirming the cause of thrombocytopenia, this is not useful in the management. From maternal considerations, the management of pregnant women with this disorder should be similar to that of non-pregnant individuals with the goal of treatment being remission, not cure. Prior to the availability of steroids, this condition was associated with a significant maternal mortality. However, over the past 30 years, maternal deaths due to ITP have become extremely rare. If the maternal platelet count falls below $20 \times 10^9/L$, steroids are the treatment of first choice (43). They are thought to act by suppression of antibody production and inhibition of sequestration of antibody-coated platelets. Although the efficacy of this treatment in raising the maternal platelet count is well established, there is disagreement on the effectiveness of maternal treatment in minimizing neonatal thrombocytopenia. Kaplan et al. (44) reported no improvement in platelet count of fetuses with severe thrombocytopenia with either maternal prednisone (four cases) or intravenous immunoglobulin (three cases). It has been suggested that betamethasone or dexamethasone are preferable to prednisone as better blood levels are achieved in the fetus (45) However, dexamethasone in doses of 3–5mg daily has been associated with a high incidence of oligohydramnios, although this was not associated with an adverse outcome (46).

Splenectomy is considered appropriate in nonpregnant women who fail to respond to steroids or who need long-term high dose therapy and in the past has been advocated in the middle trimester (47). However, at the present time, it is rarely, if ever, indicated in pregnancy. Immunosuppressive therapy and danazol for ITP are contraindicated with pregnancy.

Recently, there have been a number of anecdotal reports of successful intravenous administration of high-dose human immunoglobulin (0.4g/kg/day for five days every three weeks, or 1g/kg one day per week) to treat maternal ITP in pregnancy (48–53). This is thought to work by prolonging the clearance time of IgG-coated platelets by the maternal reticuloendothelial system resulting in an increase in the platelet count. A response is seen within days and lasts around three weeks. As IgG can cross the placenta, this treatment should theoretically provoke the same response in the fetus. However, this was not evident in the three fetuses reported by Kaplan et al. (44) and there is even evidence that exogenous IgG may not cross the placenta to full effect (53,54). A Canadian multicenter randomized control trial of weekly high dose (1g/kg) immunoglobulin from 36 weeks to delivery is now in progress and, hopefully, will establish the place of this treatment modality in women with established ITP (55).

Hedge et al. (36) recommend use of immuoglobulin in all patients with platelet counts below 75 X 10^9/L. However, the main drawback of immunoglobulin is its cost, and in the absence of a large prospective series, its use in moderately affected pregnant women will remain controversial. It should be appreciated that the relatively high morbidity and morality associated with this condition in the 1950s appears to have fallen even prior to the introduction of methods of assessing fetal platelet counts, maternal antibody levels, and treatment with human immunoglobulin.

The role of cordocentesis (PUBS) in the management of ITP is controversial. Its value would be to provide an additional criterion (fetal thrombocytopenia) for maternal treatment and also to monitor the effectiveness of such treatment by documenting improvement in the fetal platelet count. If severe fetal thrombocytopenia were found, intravascular fetal platelet transfusions could be given at weekly intervals, for example. However, reports of severe fetal thrombocytopenia are largely confined to alloimmune rather than autoimmune thrombocytopenia. One must set against such an unlikely occurrence the risks of the procedure, namely fetal mortality following PUBS, which is variously reported at 0.4%–2% per procedure (44,56), and serious morbidity in 5% (57). Weiner (57) found no antenatal or neonatal intracranial hemorrhage among 90 cases of maternal autoimmune thrombocytopenia in one center over 20 years. A recent study of 162 deliveries in women with ITP reported a 1.2% incidence of intracranial hemorrhage, a 3% incidence of total serious haemorrhage (58). A new prospective study of 50 consecutive pregnancies associated with maternal ITP at Grace Hospital, Vancouver, found 40% of all babies had thrombocytopenia *at birth*, with 10% having severe (<50 X 10^9/L) thrombocytopenia *at birth*. A further 18% of neonates developed severe thrombocytopenia in the one to five days postnatally. Of these, two babies suffered intracranial hemorrhage with platelet counts of <10 X 10^9/L and 50 X 10^9/L (55). The reported incidence of serious hemorrhage with autoimmune thrombocytopenia in many series over the last decade is sufficiently low that, even in the presence of efficacious treatment, the risks of PUBS may be unjustified. In reality, none of the proposed therapies has yet been demonstrated to reliably benefit the fetus, and thus, it has been argued that at present there is no clinical indication for PUBS where the mother has simple ITP (59).

In contrast, Daffos states that the rate of fetal and neonatal complications is usually underestimated in genuine autoimmune thrombocytopenia (60). This presumably underlies his recommendation of a more aggressive protocol of fetal blood sampling beginning at 20 weeks gestation to diagnose fetal thrombocytopenia, repeated at 23 weeks, if thrombocytopenic, to assess the effect of maternal treatment on the fetal platelet count, and a final sample at 37 weeks to determine mode of delivery (39).

This controversy suggests that currently the role of cordocentesis in the antenatal management of ITP, outside the context of a randomized trial in a center with appropriate experience in the procedure, would seem hard to justify.

Delivery

To minimize the risk of maternal hemorrhage, it is desirable for the maternal platelet count to be greater than 50 X 19^9/L, particularly at the time of delivery. In most cases, this can be achieved with steroids and immunoglobulin therapy. On the rare occasion that transfusion of platelets is necessary, it should be remembered that any platelet transfusion in a woman of childbearing potential carries the risk of sensitization resulting in neonatal/fetal alloimmune thrombocytopenia (NAIT) in the index or subsequent pregnancies. This risk is greatest in Pl^{A1}-negative individuals. The lack of correlation between either fetal platelet count and maternal platelet count or fetal platelet count and maternal IgG levels leaves open to question management strategies based on maternal status. It has been recommended, for example, that if (a) the maternal platelet count is less than 100 X 10^9/L (37,61), (b) the spleen is absent regardless of the platelet count (62), or (c) there is any question that vaginal delivery will be difficult (63), then cesarean section is justified by the risk of fetal intracranial hemorrhage,

theoretically preventing the head compression of vaginal delivery.

The recommendation that if reliable platelet antibody tests demonstrate no appreciable platelet-bound or free serum anti-platelet IgG, then cesarean section is unnecessary (63), would seem inappropriate; these maternal tests are not sufficiently predictive of fetal platelet count.

Although there has been no randomized study assessing the risk of intracranial bleeding in babies with low platelet counts who are born vaginally, most obstetricians are reluctant to allow vaginal delivery to proceed in the presence of a count below 50 X 10^9/L. Thus, another management protocol advocated is direct measurement of fetal platelet count by scalp sampling during labor (64–66), with delivery by cesarean section where a result of <50 X 10^9/L is found. The main drawback of this approach is that it is not practicable until there is sufficient cervical dilatation, which precludes planned delivery and total avoidance of labor. If labor does predispose to intracranial hemorrhage, it may be desirable to avoid the first four to five centimeters of dilatation. The validity of platelet counts obtained by this method also has been questioned (67,68). A more logical approach in the 1990s would seem to be direct antenatal fetal blood sampling at term (48,69), and currently, many centers advocate a single cordocente-sis in late pregnancy to determine the route of delivery.

The assumed benefit of cesarean section has recently been refuted (7,12,59,70). Indeed, in their retrospective review, Browning and James found the incidence of intracranial hemorrhage lower for vaginal delivery than for cesarean section for the whole group (0.5 vs 2.0%). Among severely affected fetuses with platelet counts below 50 X 10^9/L, the risk of intracranial bleeding was 2% with vaginal delivery and 5% for cesarean section (59). One criticism of their conclusion is that they did not divide the cesarean section group into those delivered electively and those that had labored; on review of the literature, this information is not available in most reports. In any case, however, knowledge of the fetal platelet count, which is most likely (90%) to be normal, would obviate cesarean section.

Infants of Mothers with ITP

The outcome for the majority of these infants is good, and resolution of thrombocytopenia can be anticipated as the level of maternal antibodies in newborn circulation declines. The platelet count should be monitored initially twice daily, then daily over the first two to six days, as it generally falls following delivery, reaching a nadir at two to six days (19). This probably reflects increased clearance of antibody-coated platelets by the reticuloendothelial system. As stated above, the current incidence of perinatal intracranial hemorrhage is perhaps 1–4% overall, occurring predominantly in the presence of severe thrombocytopenia. This prompts immediate treatment for neonatal levels below $50 \times 10^9/L$. High-dose intravenous immunoglobulin has been reported to produce a response in 75% of cases within 48 hours (71). A dose of 0.4g/kg/day for two days or 1g/kg as a single infusion has been recommended (72). Steroids in a dose equivalent to 2mg/kg/day may also be beneficial (72). If these fail, platelet transfusion and/or exchange transfusion may be indicated but are not appropriate for initial therapy.

Conclusions

Review of the current literature would support the following recommendations concerning the obstetrical management and delivery of women with autoimmune thrombocytopenia:

- Where antenatal monitoring of the maternal platelet count reveals severe or symptomatic thrombocytopenia, steroid administration has been shown to improve the maternal platelet count. The benefit of this to the fetus is as yet unproven.
- Women who have symptomatic or severe (pl<$50 \times 10^9/L$) steroid-unresponsive ITP may benefit from a course of human immunoglobulin commencing a few days prior to planned delivery, although the efficacy of this in influencing fetal thrombocytopenia awaits the result of a multicenter randomized trial.
- Women who have chronic severe steroid unresponsive ITP may benefit from additional courses of immunoglobulin earlier in pregnancy; however, validation of this and efficacy in the fetus must also await the outcome of the current trial.
- Fetal blood sampling offers the only means of detecting fetal thrombocytopenia and assessing its severity; however in the absence of proven benefit of treatment modalities (steroids, immunoglobulin, or fetal platelet transfusions), the appropriateness of early cordocentesis, except in the setting of a randomized trial, is questionable.
- Early reports appear to have overestimated the risk to both the mother and the fetus. For the fetus/neonate, there remains a small (1–4%), but important, risk of perinatal intracranial hemorrhage. Cesarean section has been assumed the safest mode of delivery for the thrombocytopenic fetus, although evidence for this is lacking.
- If a fetal platelet count is considered important to the decision of mode of deliv-

ery, then cordocentesis at term in an appropriate center is preferable to an intrapartum fetal scalp sample.

- The infant platelet count should be monitored at birth and for several days. Steroids have a role in severe or symptomatic neonatal thrombocytopenia. The role of neonatal immunoglobulin infusion must await the outcome of a current randomized trial.

ALLOIMMUNE THROMBOCYTOPENIA

This condition has hitherto been called Neonatal Alloimmune Thrombocytopenia (NAIT), but it is now known that the disease process begins in early fetal life. NAIT is a rare but severe thrombocytopenia, occurring in one out of every 1,000–5,000 pregnancies (46,73,74). The condition is analogous to Rhesus hemolytic disease, except that platelets are the target of the alloantibody. The fetal platelets carry a platelet-specific antigen (most frequently PlA^{-1}–Zw^a) inherited from the father but lacking in the mother (75–77). Only 2.5% of Caucasian women are PlA^1-negative, and only a small percentage of these individuals become sensitized against PlA^{-1}, either by exposure in pregnancy, or by platelet transfusion. In subsequent pregnancy, the anti-PlA^{-1} IgG alloantibody crosses the placenta and results in fetal thrombocytopenia. Unlike Rhesus disease, firstborn infants are often affected, and it is estimated that almost all subsequent PlA^{-1}-positive fetuses will be affected. (78). In Caucasians, 97.5% of fathers will be PlA^{-1}-positive and about 5% of these will be heterozygous. The likelihood of recurrent PlA^{-1} fetal-maternal incompatibility is, therefore, roughly 94% in general. In practice, determining paternal zygosity for PlA^{-1} will determine whether the recurrence risk is 50% or 100%. Platelets express

ABO, HLA, and platelet-specific antigens. Although fetomaternal incompatibility for antigens of any of these systems could theoretically cause NAIT, most cases seem to be a result of maternal antibodies directed against platelet-specific antigens. In Europe and North America, the majority of serologically proven NAIT cases are due to incompatibility for the platelet-specific antigen PlA^{-1} (also known as the ZW^a antigen) (76). In a survey of 348 cases, 78% were due to anti-Pl^{A1}, and 19% were due to anti-Br^a (79). Other platelet antigens account for a minority of cases of NAIT and include Bak^a (75), Bak^b (80), Zw^b (81), Br^b (82), Ko^a (83), and Sr^a (84). Within the Oriental population, Yuk^a is important.

Only a small percentage of PlA^{-1}-negative women become immunized (85). The HLA phenotypes DR3 and DRw52 are important predisposing factors (73,86). Other HLA types can make antibody in high titer, but a PlA^{-1}-negative woman is 76.5 times more likely to do so if she also carries HLA-DR3 (87). Conversely, more than 90% of PlA^{-1}-immunized individuals have HLA-DR3 (88).

Effects on the first child are usually unexpected, as PlA^{-1} typing is not part of routine antenatal screening, although it has been suggested that such screening might have the potential to compete with other programs if the efficacy of treatment can be proven (89). Seventy-five to 90% of subsequent pregnancies are affected (46,90), and the degree of thrombocytopenia is usually as severe or worse than in the first affected child (91). Monitoring maternal anti-PlA^{-1} antibodies does not accurately predict the severity of fetal thrombocytopenia (90). Appropriate female relatives of a mother who has delivered an affected infant should have their platelet and HLA types determined to evaluate their risk of NAIT. In our series of 11 women with NAIT, two were referred in

Figure 7-2A Decreased fetal movement in a primigravida prompted obstetric ultrasound, revealing massive intrauterine intracranial fetal hemorrhage at 36 weeks gestational age. Hydrocephalus, macrocephaly, and only a few, jerky fetal movements were present.

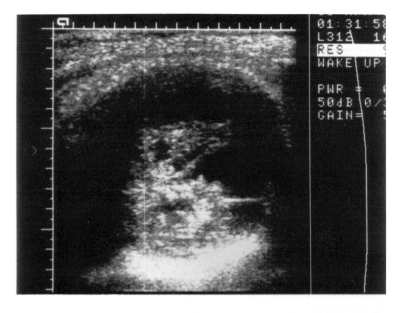

first pregnancies because their sisters were PlA^{-1} alloimmunized. Figure 7-2 illustrates the intracranial findings of an affected fetus at 36 weeks gestation. The scan was coincidental; however, on taking a history, a previous child had had neonatal thrombocytopenia attributed to sepsis and the mother's sister had also had a baby with neonatal thrombocytopenia who had suffered a GI bleed. It is likely that many cases of NAIT go unrecognized or neonatal thrombocytopenia is attributed incorrectly to a different cause.

Unlike ITP, in which the incidence of symptomatic fetal thrombocytopenia is now generally accepted to be low, the occurrence of antenatal fetal intracranial hemorrhage in this condition appears significant (22,23,92,93), although its prevalence and time of occurrence are not precisely known. Fetal platelet antigens are fully expressed by 18 weeks gestation (94), and fetal blood sampling has shown severe thrombocytopenia in affected fetuses as early as 20 weeks (90). The prognosis varies according to the severity of the bleed. When

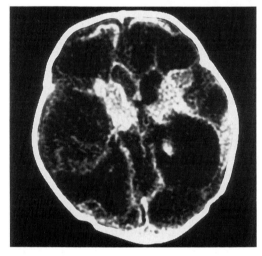

Figure 7-2B Corresponding CAT scan showing severe porencephaly. The infant survived with a platelet count of 9.0×10^9/L and continues in a vegetative state.

no complication occurs, the thrombocytopenia resolves spontaneously within weeks of birth. The frequency of neurological sequelae is difficult to estimate since deficits may not become apparent for months or years after birth, but sequelae have been found in as many as 25% (93,95) and mortality may be as high as 15% (96).

Antenatal Management

With fetal blood sampling, it has become possible to confirm the diagnosis of NAIT and its severity in the fetus. In contrast to ITP, the risks of fetal intracranial hemorrhage with NAIT appear to justify this approach. In addition to obtaining fetal platelet counts, platelet concentrates may be transfused to the fetus. This has been used just prior to delivery (90,97,98), or serially in the last trimester (23,96,99). However, Daffos et al. (100) state that in most cases, severe thrombocytopenia is already present by 20 weeks, and a spontaneous rise in platelet count in fetuses with this kind of thrombocytopenia has never been observed. The lifespan of platelets is such that the fetus would have to be transfused every four to five days to maintain a stable platelet count. Transfusing to a super-normal level (600×10^9 or more) on a weekly basis might also ensure adequate protection (96). Washed maternal platelets may be used for this purpose and avoid the risk of transfusion transmitted infection. However, this approach is not practical for repeated transfusions.

In the majority of cases of NAIT that have been treated, maternal intravenous immune serum globulin (IVIgG) has been used with or without concomitant corticosteroids. Outcome measures were neonatal morbidity and newborn platelet counts. Since successive pregnancies are expected to be more severely affected and a spontaneous rise in fetal platelet count is not expected in NAIT, serial fetal platelet counts and comparison with previous affected siblings are used to assess response to treatment. Bussel et al. reported that weekly immunoglobulin (1.0g/kg maternal weight) was effective in

elevating the fetal platelet count in all of a group of seven thrombocytopenic fetuses diagnosed and followed by cordocentesis (46). Table 7-1 details the response of nine affected fetuses treated in this way at Mount Sinai Hospital (101) and eight affected fetuses treated in Vancouver (102). While some response in some fetuses was apparent, the incomplete sucess prompted the addition of maternal steroids, as shown by the nine further cases from Mount Sinai in Table 7-2 (101). In all cases, treatment was justified by severe thrombocytopenia in untreated previous siblings. In 10 cases, that severely affected sibling had intracranial hemorrhage, which occurred antenatally in 30%. Others have reported the failure of this treatment in NAIT (90,103), and Nicolini et al. (96) reported no improvement in one such fetus despite documenting transplacental passage of maternal IVIgG by high levels of fetal immunoglobulin. While the optimal treatment is yet to be decided by a multicenter randomized trial (104), at least one positive aspect of the preliminary results (Tables 7-1, 7-2) must be that none of the infants had intracranial hemorrhage regardless of platelet count.

On the strength of this encouraging pilot data, a trial has been implemented comparing women with severe platelet alloimmunization, in groups randomized to receive either weekly IVIgG 1 gm/kg weekly or the same IVIgG with the addition of Dexamethasone 10 mg p.o. Because of the randomization, individual case data is not available, but interim review of the overall trial continues to be promising. Of the 29 fetuses randomized with platelet counts, <100 $\times 10^9$/L, 24 (83%) were treatment successes, with mean rise of platelet count by 65 $\times 10^9$/L. Three of the remaining 5 had some response with the addition of 60 mg of prednisone daily (mean platelet rise 28 $\times 10^9$/L). Of note, at least 5 fetuses have died at the

Table 7-1 Patients Treated with IVIgG Alone

Patient	Treatment	Plt. Count (GA)	Plt. Count (GA)	Plt. Count (GA)	Plt. Count (At Birth)	ICH	Untreated Sibling Plt. Count	ICH
1	IVIgG (1g)	$32 \times 10^9(23)$	—	—	38×10^9	No	30×10^9 20×10^9	Yes Yes
2	IVIgG (1g)	$1 \times 10^9(30)$	$6 \times 10^9(36)$	—	39×10^9	No	18×10^9	Yes
3	IVIgG (1g)	$150 \times 10^9(22)$	$45 \times 10^9(28)$	$140 \times 10^9(34)$	215×10^9	No	38×10^9	No
4	IVIgG (1g)	$18 \times 10^9(20)$	$51 \times 10^9(25)$	$50 \times 10^9(32)$	85×10^9	No	15×10^9	Yes (AN)
5	IVIgG (1g)	$129 \times 10^9(22)$	$28 \times 10^9(27)$	$79 \times 10^9(32)$	140×10^9	No	15×10^9	No
6	IVIgG (1g)	$65 \times 10^9(28)$	$309 \times 10^9(36)$	—	322×10^9	No	8×10^9	No
7	IVIgG (1g)	$32 \times 10^9(22)$	—	—	43×10^9	No	9×10^9	Yes (AN)
8	IVIgG (1g)	$55 \times 10^9(36)$	—	—	$57 \times 10^9(38)$	No	7×10^9	No
9	IVIgG (0.5g)	$12 \times 10^9(32)$	—	—	12×10^9	No	25×10^9	Yes
10*	IVIgG (1g)	185×10^9 (20–24)	$125\bullet \times 10^9$ (28–34)	—	$75 \times 10^9(36)$	No	$<10 \times 10^9$	No
11*	IVIgG (1g)	$15\bullet \times 10^9$ (20–24)	—	—	-(16)	Yes	$<10 \times 10^9$	Yes
12*	IVIgG (1g)	$85\bullet \times 10^9$ (20–24)	50×10^9 (28–34)	—	$70 \times 10^9(35)$	No	10×10^9	No
13*	IVIgG (1g)	—	$15\bullet \times 10^9$ (28–34)	—	$224 \times 10^9(34)$	No	$47/35 \times 10^9$ (twins)	No
14*	IVIgG (1g)	$23\bullet \times 10^9$ (20–24)	—	—	$15 \times 10^9(25)$	No	23×10^9	No
15*	IVIgG (1g)	$5\bullet \times 10^9$ (20–24)	18×10^9 (28–34)	—	$70 \times 10^9(34)$	No	5×10^9	Yes
16*	IVIgG (1g)	$25\bullet \times 10^9$ (20–24)	164×10^9 (28–34)	—	$293 \times 10^9(37)$	No	20×10^9	No
17*	IVIgG (1g)	140×10^9 (20–24)	$45\bullet \times 10^9$ (28–34)	—	$215 \times 10^9(38)$	No	38×10^9	No

IVIgG = Intravenous gammaglobulin; Dex = Dexamethasone; Predn = Prednisone; Plt = Platelet; GA = Weeks of gestational age; ICH = Intracranial hemorrhage; AN = Antenatal; • = Indicates IVIgG commenced following sampling. Kornfeld I, Ballem P, Farquharson DF, Wilson RD, Wittman BK. The use of IVIgG in the prophylaxis and treatment of severe NAIT—The British Columbia experience, 1988–92. SOGC Abstract 1992: 574.

Table 7-2 Patients Treated with IVIgG and Corticosteroids

Patient	Treatment	Plt. Count (GA)	Plt. Count (GA)	Plt. Count (GA)	Plt. Count (At Birth)	ICH	Untreated Sibling Plt. Count	ICH
1	IVIgG (1g) Dex (5mg)	—	—	—	30×10^9	No	3×10^9	Yes (AN)
2	IVIgG (1g) Dex (5mg)	$36 \times 10^9(20)$	$193 \times 10^9(25)$	$108 \times 10^9(32)$	64×10^9	No	30×10^9	No
3	IVIgG (1g) Dex (5mg)	$92 \times 10^9(31)$	$237 \times 10^9(37)$	—	235×10^9	No	10×10^9	No
4	IVIgG (1g) Dex (3mg)	$13 \times 10^9(27)$	$26 \times 10^9(32)$	—	42×10^9	No	11×10^9	No
5	IVIgG (1g) Dex (3mg)	$14 \times 10^9(22)$	—	—	50×10^9	No	2×10^9	Yes (AN)
6	IVIgG (1g) Dex (1.5mg)	$159 \times 10^9(23)$	$78 \times 10^9(32)$	—	134×10^9	No	20×10^9	No
7	IVIgG (1g) Dex (1.5mg)	$25 \times 10^9(22)$	$43 \times 10^9(28)$	—	204×10^9	No	18×10^9	No
8	IVIgG (1g) Predn (10mg)	$2 \times 10^9(28)$	$10 \times 10^9(39)$	—	17×10^9	No	40×10^9 / 14×10^9	No / Yes
9	IVIgG (1g) Predn (10mg)	$96 \times 10^9(27)$	$92 \times 10^9(32)$	—	200×10^9	No	5×10^9	No

IVIgG = Intravenous gammaglobulin; Dex = Dexamethasone; Predn = Prednisone; Plt = Platelet; GA = Weeks of gestational age; ICH = Intracranial hemorrhage; AN = Antenatal.

time of the first (pre-treatment) cordocentesis, so platelet transfusion is now advocated with *all* cordocenteses for NAIT (105).

Daffos et al. (106) reported an increase in fetal platelet count with maternal administration of prednisolone 10mg daily from the 23rd week of gestation. Use of dexamethasone in a dose of 3–5mg was associated with development of oligohydramnios in four of five fetuses (46).

There have been several published case reports of successful serial weekly in utero platelet transfusions followed by early delivery (22,90,99,107). However, the difficulties and risks inherent in this management are such that it is likely to be reserved for the exceptional case where there has been a previous infant affected by antenatal intracranial hemorrhage and failure to respond to maternal therapy. Fetal transfusion with immunoglobulin and platelets may be more practical as this approach might reduce the frequency of invasive procedures. This has been done in some centers, with mixed results. While Zimmermann and Hutch (108) achieved significant elevation in platelet count with direct fetal infusion IVIgG, our experience has been as rewarding. A single fetus treated on two occasions with high-dose intravenous immunoglobulin by PUBS in our center did not respond by an improvement in platelet count despite very high fetal IgG levels. A modest elevation in platelet count was achieved when maternal IVIgG was added.

All such invasive procedures, however, may bear significant risk. As shown by Berkowitz (105), all of the five fetal deaths were by exsanguination in fetuses with severe thrombocytopenia (4 < 9 X 10^9/L, the other 10 – 19 X 10^9/L). No cordocentesis deaths occurred once treatment had begun. All of the fetuses who died had previous affected siblings with severe disease (counts <29 X 10^9). Two further losses related to

other complications of cordocentesis occurred among the eight fetuses treated in Vancouver (102). It is now recommended that platelet in-fusion be given to the fetus at all initial procedures to cover the risk of hemorrhage before the needle is removed. Consideration should also be given to starting maternal IVIgG four weeks prior to the first planned procedure to reduce this risk. By far, the largest number of cases of NAIT have been treated with maternal IVIgG. However, no clear manage-ment protocol has been established. A North American multicenter prospective trial is currently in progress and aims to evaluate intravenous maternal immunoglobulin alone or together with dexamethasone 1.5mgPO daily.

Management of Delivery

Ideally, pre-delivery PUBS should have documented a fetal platelet count clearly above 50 X 19^9/L, and if the value is lower than, this infusion of suitable platelets at the time of cordocentesis is recommended. With this management, cesarean section should be used for obstetric indications only. Muller et al. (110) reported good results in three thrombocytopenic fetuses transfused with washed, irradiated maternal platelets prior to delivery. The fetuses showed a sustained increase in platelet counts with no recurrence of thrombocytopenia postpartum. If this is not technically possible, then antigen-negative or washed maternal platelets, if no donor is available, should be prepared prior to delivery so that they are available for immediate transfusion into the neonate, and consideration is given to delivery by cesarean section.

Most obstetricians would perform elective cesarean section unless the fetal platelet count at predelivery PUBS is > 50 X 10^9/L, despite lack of data to support that vaginal delivery is necessarily more hazardous.

The Neonate

Different modalities of postnatal treatment have been proposed, including corticosteroids, exchange transfusions, transfusion of random compatible or maternal platelets, and high dose intravenous immunoglobulins. Treatment should begin as soon as significant thrombocytopenia is diagnosed to minimize bleeding complications. Because the disease presents with unexpected neonatal thrombocytopenia, often with a bleed, on the first occasion, diagnosis is frequently delayed while more common causes of thrombocytopenia are considered (72). Severe isolated thrombocytopenia without obvious etiologic cause indicates measurement of the maternal platelet count

Table 7-3 *NAIT Protocol* (Winnipeg) (Affected Sibling, Homozygous Father)

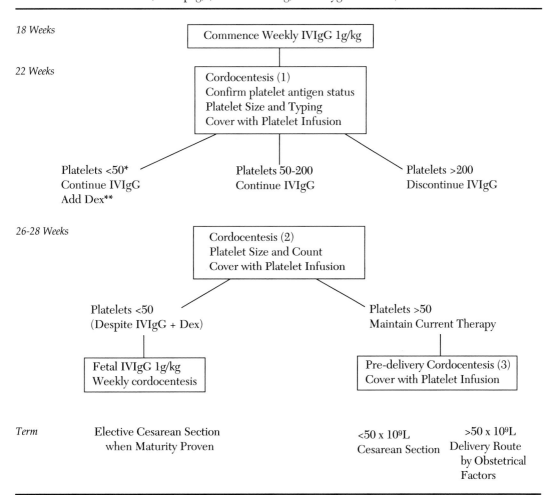

*All platelet counts expressed as N X 10^9/L.
**Dex = Dexamethasone 10 mg OD.
 If no response after maternal IVIgG, Dex, fetal IgG, consider weekly platelet transfusion.

and platelet antibodies to look for evidence of maternal ITP and alloimmune thrombocytopenia, respectively. In cases of the latter, screening the newborn will usually fail to detect platelet antibodies as they are tightly bound to platelets. Failure of the infant to respond to a random donor platelet transfusion (98% of which will be PlA^{-1} positive) also provides strong evidence of alloimmune thrombocytopenia. Initial treatment with antigen-negative platelets is most appropriate because of its rapid and consistent efficiency. Intravenous immunoglobulin has been given to infants with NAIT and has resulted in an increase in platelet count. However, the beneficial action is not as rapid as compatible platelet transfusions (111–114).

ITP and NAIT

At the outset, it seems obvious that there is no relationship between ITP (a maternal disorder with rare fetal consequences) and NAIT (a serious fetal disorder with no maternal significance). Burrows and Kelton point out, however, that the frequency of multiunit platelet transfusion in women with severe ITP is very high. In such women, repeated exposure to and serious alloimmunization against various platelet antigens would seem almost inevitable. It may be that a significant proportion of infants manifesting serious neonatal problems associated with maternal ITP are, in fact, affected with undiagnosed NAIT. While their studies have illustrated a number of such cases, further prospective evaluation is required.

Conclusions

To identify women at risk of having platelet incompatible pregnancies by platelet and HLA typing of all pregnant women is not feasible at present. However, these investigations are appropriate where there has been neonatal thrombocytopenia or a family history that puts the woman in an at-risk group.

The optimal management to prevent severe intracranial hemorrhage in NAIT is not certain. Noninvasive treatment with maternal intravenous immunoglobulin and steroids is currently being evaluated. When fetal thrombocytopenia has been diagnosed, various platelet and immunoglobulin transfusion strategies are being explored. However, further data about the natural history of NAIT and the efficacy of this treatment are also needed. The protocol currently used in our center is detailed in Table 7-3. Certainly, this disorder is sufficiently rare and serious that prenatal management should be undertaken in a center experienced in invasive fetal procedures and with the necessary hematological laboratory backup.

References

1. Sejeney SA, Eastham RD, Baker SR. Platelet counts during normal pregnancy. J Clin Path 1975;28:812–813.
2. Cairns JW, Manon A, Waters DAW, et al. Platelet levels in pregnancy. J Clin Pathol (letter) 1977;30:392.
3. Pitkin RM, Witt DL. Platelet and leucocyte counts in pregnancy. JAMA 1979;242: 2696–2699.
4. Rakoczi R, Tallian S, Bagdany G, Gati I. Platelet life span in normal pregnancy and preeclampsia as determined by a nonradioisotope technique. Thromb Res 1979; 15:553–556.
5. McKay DG. Chronic intravascular coagulation in normal pregnancy and preeclampsia. Contrib Nephrol 1981;25:108–111.
6. Sill PR, Lind T, Walker W. Platelet values during normal pregnancy. Br J Obstet Gynaecol 1985;92:480–483.

7. Burrows RF, Kelton JG. Thrombocytopenia at delivery: a prospective survey of 6715 deliveries. Am J Obstet Gynecol 1990;162:731–734.

8. Matthews JH, Benjamin S, Gill DS, Smith NA. Pregnancy-associated thrombocytopenia: definition, incidence and natural history. Acta Haematol 1990;84:24–29.

9. Fay RA, Hughes AO, Farron NT. Platelets in pregnancy: hyperdestruction in pregnancy. Obstet Gynecol 1983;61:238–240.

10. Wallenburg HCS, Van Kessel PH. Platelet lifespan in normal pregnancy as determined by a nonradioisotopic technique. Br J Obstet Gynaecol 1978;85:33–36.

11. Burrows RF, Kelton JG: Incidentally detected thrombocytopenia in healthy mothers and their infants. N Engl J Med 1988;319:142–145.

12. Aster RH. 'Gestational' thrombocytopenia. A plea for conservative management. New Engl J Med 1990;323:264–266.

13. Schwartz ML, Brenner WE. Pregnancy-induced hypertension presenting with life-threatening thrombocytopenia. Am J Obstet Gynecol 1983;146:756–759.

14. Weiner CP. Thrombotic microangiopathy in pregnancy and the postpartum period. Semin Hematol 1987;24:119–129.

15. Limay NS, Tchabo J-G. Asymptomatic thrombocytopenia with chorioangioma of placenta. Am J Obstet Gynecol 1989;161:76–77.

16. Spirit BA, Gordon LN, Cohen W, Yambao T. Antenatal diagnosis of chorangioma of the placenta. Am J Radiol 1980;135: 1273–1275.

17. Forestier F, Daffos F, Galacteros F, Bard-Akjian J, Rainaut M, Beuzard Y. Hematological values of 163 normal fetuses between 18 and 30 weeks of gestation. Pediatric Research 1986;20:342–346.

18. Ludomirski A, Weiner S, Ashmead GG, Librizzi RJ, Bolognese RJ. Percutaneous fetal umbilical blood sampling: procedure, safety and normal fetal hematologic indices. Am J Perinatol 1988;5:264–266.

19. Kelton JG. Management of the pregnant patient with idiopathic thrombocytopenia purpura. Ann Int Med 1983;99:796–800.

20. Kelton JG, Inwood MJ, Barr RM, Effer SB, Hunter D, Wilson WE, Ginsburg DA, Powers PJ. The prenatal prediction of thrombocytopenia in infants of mothers with clinically diagnosed immune thrombocytopenia. Am J Obstet Gynecol 1982;144:449–454.

21. Martin JN, Morrison JC, Files JC. Autoimmune thrombocytopenia purpura: current concepts and recommended practices. Am J Obstet Gynecol 1984;150:86–96.

22. Nicolini U, Rodeck CH, Kochenour NK, Greco P, Fisk NM, Letsky E, Lubenko A. Inutero platelet transfusion for alloimmune thrombocytopenia. The Lancet 1988;2:506.

23. Mueller-Eckhardt C, Kiefel V, Jovanovic V, Kunzel W, Becker T, Wolf H, Zeh K. Prenatal treatment of fetal alloimmune thrombocytopenia. The Lancet 1988;910.

24. Forestier F. Cordocentesis in fetal thrombocytopenia. Presented at the First Congress on Platelet Immunobiology, Paris, 1990.

25. Karpatkin S, Lackner HL. Association of antiplatelet antibody with functional platelet disorders. Am J Med 1975;59:599–604.

26. Karpatkin S. Autoimmune thrombocytopenic purpura. Blood 1980;56:329–343.

27. Regan MG, Lackner H, Karpatkin S. Platelet function and coagulation profile in lupus erythematosus. Ann Intern Med 1974;81:462–468.

28. Karpatkin S, Garg SK, Siskind GW. Autoimmune thrombocytopenic purpura and the compensated thrombocytolytic state. Am J Med 1971;51:1–4.

29. ten Cate JW, de Vries SI, Sixma JJ, Van Berkel W. Defective collagen-induced platelet aggregation in a normal population. Thromb Diath Haemorr 1971;25:234–240.

30. Schlamowith M. Membrane receptors in the specific transfer of immunoglobulins from mother to young. Immunol Commun 1976;5:481–500.

31. Kohler PF, Farr RS. Elevation of cord maternal IgG immunoglobulins: evidence for an active placental IgG transport. Nature 1966;210:1070–1071.

32. Hegde UM, Gordon-Smith EC, Worrlledge SM. Platelet antibodies in thrombocytopenic patients. Br J Haematol 1977;56: 191–197.

33. Van Leeuwen EF, Helmerhorst FM, Engelfriet CP, Von dem Borne AEGK. Maternal autoimmune thrombocytopenia in the newborn. Br Med J 1981;283:104.

34. Von dem Borne AEGK. Autoimmune thrombocytopenia. Bailliere's Clin Immunol Allerg 1987;1:269–302.

35. Difino SM, Lachant NA, Kirshner JJ, Gottlieb AJ. Adult idiopathic thrombocytopenic purpura. Clinical findings and response to therapy. Amer J Med 1980;69: 430–442.

36. Hedge UM. Immune thrombocytopenia in pregnancy and the newborn. Br J Obstet Gynaecol 1985;92:657–659.

37. Carloss HW, McMillan R, Crosby WH. Management of pregnancy in women with thrombocytopenic purpura. JAMA 1980; 144:2756–2758.

38. Burrows RF, Kelton JG. Low fetal risks in pregnancies associated with idiopathic thrombocytopenic purpura. Am J Obstet Gynecol 1990;163:1147–1150.

39. Daffos F. The fetus at risk for thrombocytopenia. In: Harrison MR, Golbus MS, Filly RA, eds. The unborn patient. Philadelphia: WB Saunders, 1990:210–214.

40. Cines DB, Dusak B, Tomaski A, Mennuti M, Schreiber AD. Immune thrombocytopenic purpura and pregnancy. N Engl J Med 1982;306:826–831.

41. Weiner C. Thrombocytopenia and cordocentesis. Clarifications requested. Am J Obstet Gynecol 1989;161:1091–1092.

42. Hedge UM, Bowes A, Powell DK, Joyner MV. Detection of platelet bound and serum antibodies in thrombocytopenia by enzyme linked assay. Vox Sang 1981;41:306–312.

43. Karpatkin S. Autoimmune thrombocytopenic purpura. Sem Haematol 1985; 22:260–288.

44. Kaplan C, Daffos F, Forestier F, Tertian G, Catherine N, Pons JC, Tchernia G. Fetal platelet counts in thrombocytopenic pregnancy. The Lancet 1990;336:979–982.

45. Christiaens GCML, Nieuwenhuis HK, Von dem Borne AEGK, Ouwehand WH, Helmerhorst FM, Van Dalen CM, Van der Tweel I. Idiopathic thrombocytopenic purpura in pregnancy: a randomized trial on the effect of antenatal low dose corticosteroids on neonatal platelet count. Br J Obstet Gynaecol 1990;97:893–898.

46. Bussel JB, Berkowitz RL, McFarland JG, Lynch L, Chitkara U. Antenatal treatment of neonatal alloimmune thrombocytopenia. N Engl J Med 1988;319:1374–1378.

47. Kagan R, Laros RK. Immune thrombocytopenia. Clin Obstet Gynecol 1983;26: 537–546.

48. Scioscia AL, Grannum PAT, Copel JA, et al. The use of percutaneous umbilical blood sampling in immune thrombocytopenia purpura. Am J Obstet Gynecol 1988; 159:1066–1068.

49. Tchernia G, Drefus M, Laurian Y, Derycke M, Mirica C, Kerbrat G. Management of immune thrombocytopenia in pregnancy: response of infusions of immunoglobulins. Am J Obstet Gynecol 1984;148: 225–226.

50. Lavery JP, Koontz WL, Liu YK, Howell R. Immunologic thrombocytopenia in pregnancy: use of antenatal immunoglobulin therapy: case report and review. Obstet Gynecol (Suppl) 1985;66:41–43.

51. Mizunuma H, Takahashi Y, Tagushi H, et al. A new approach to idiopathic thrombocytopenic purpura during pregnancy by high-dose immunoglobulinG infusion. Am J Obstet Gynecol 1984;148:218.

52. Morgenstern GR, Measday B, Hedge M. Autoimmune thrombocytopenia in pregnancy: new approach to management. Br Med J 1983;287:584.

53. Davies SV, Murray JA, Gee H, et al. Transplacental effect of high-dose immunoglobulin in idiopathic thrombocytopenia (ITP). The Lancet 1986;i:1098–1099.

54. Pappas C. Placental transfusion of immunoglobulin in immunothrombocytopenic purpura. The Lancet 1986;i:389.

55. Ballem P, Blanchette V, Andrew M. Trial design. Canadian multicentre trial of ante-

natal intravenous immune serum globulin in maternal ITP. Toronto, 1991.

56. Nicolaides KH. Cordocentesis. In: Drife JO, Donnai eds. Antenatal diagnosis of fetal anomalies. London: Springer-Verlag, 1991; 212.

57. Weiner CP. Cordocentesis. In: High risk pregnancy. Arias F, ed. Obstetrics and Gynecology Clinics of North America. Philadelphia: WB Saunders, June 1988; 15:2:283–301.

58. Samuels P, Bussel JB, Braitman LE, Tomaski A, Druzin ML, Mennuti MT, Cines DB. Estimation of the risk of thrombocytopenia in the offspring of pregnant women with presumed immune thrombocytopenic purpura. N Engl J Med 1990;323:229–235.

59. Browning J, James D. Immune thrombocytopenia in pregnancy. Fetal med rev 1990; 2:143–157.

60. Daffos F, Efficacy of management of isoimmunization with fetal umbilical blood sampling remains unproved. Am J Obstet Gynecol 1990;162:298.

61. Territo M, Finklestein J, Oh N, Hobel C, Kattlove H. Management of autoimmune thrombocytopenia in pregnancy and in the neonate. Obstet Gynecol 1973;41:579–584.

62. McMillan R. Chronic idiopathic thrombocytopenic purpura. N Engl J Med 1981; 304:1135–1147.

63. Letsky E. Hematologic disorders. In: Baron W, Lindheimer M, eds. Medical disorders during pregnancy. Chicago: Mosby, 1990: 303–306.

64. Ayromlooi J. A new approach to the management of immunologic thrombocytopenic purpura in pregnancy. Am J Obstet Gynecol 1978;130:235–236.

65. Scott JR, Cruickshank DP, Kochenou RMD, et al. Fetal platelet counts in the obstetric management of immunologic thrombocytopenia purpura. Am J Obstet Gynecol 1980;136:495–499.

66. Scott JR, Rote NS, Cruikshank DP. Anteplatelet antibodies and platelet counts in pregnancies complicated by autoimmune thrombocytopenia. Am J Obstet Gynecol 1983;145:932–939.

67. Christiaens GCML, Helmerhorst FM. Validity of intrapartum diagnosis of fetal thrombocytopenia. Am J Obstet Gynecol 1987;157:864–865.

68. Moise J, Patton DE, Cano LE. Misdiagnosis of a normal fetal platelet count after coagulation of intrapartum scalp samples in autoimmune thrombocytopenic purpura. Am J Perinatol 1991;8:295–296.

69. Moise KJ, Carpenter RJ, Cotton DB, et al. Percutaneous umbilical cord sampling in the evaluation of fetal platelet counts in pregnant patients with autoimmune thrombocytopenia purpura. Obstet Gynecol 1988;72:346–350.

70. Cook RL, Miller RC, Katz VL, Cefalo RC. Immune thrombocytopenic purpura in pregnancy: a reappraisal of management. Obstet Gynecol 1991;78:578–583.

71. Blanchette V, Andrew M, Perlman M, Ling E, Ballin A. Neonatal alloimmune thrombocytopenia: role of high-dose intravenous immunoglobulin G therapy. Blut 1988; 59:139–144.

72. Blanchette V, Sacher RA, Ballem PJ, Bussel JB, Imbach P. Commentary on the management of autoimmune thrombocytopenia during pregnancy and the neonatal period. Blut 1989;59:121–123.

73. Blanchette VS, Chen L, Salomon de Friedberg Z, Hogan VA, Trudel E, DeCary F. Alloimmunization to the PlA1 platelet antigen: results of a prospective study. Br J Haematol 1990,74:209–215.

74. Blanchette VS, Peters MA, Pegg-Fiege K. Alloimmune neonatal thrombocytopenia. Review from a neonatal intensive care unit. Curr Stud Hematol Blood Transfus 1986; 52:87–96.

75. Von dem Borne AEGK, von Reisz E, Verheugt FWA, ten Cate JW, Koppe JG, Engelfriet CP, Nijenhuis LE. Baka, a new platelet-specific antigen involved in neonatal alloimmune thrombocytopenia. Vox Sang 1980;39:113–120.

76. Von dem Borne AEGK, Van Leeuwen EF, von Riesz LE, van Boxtel CJ, Engelfriet CP. Neonatal alloimmune thrombocytopenia: detection and characterization of the re-

sponsible antibodies by the platelet immunofluorescence test. Blood 1981;57: 649–656.

77. Mueller-Eckhardt C, Marks H-J, Baur MP, Mueller-Eckhardt G. Immunogenetic studies of the platelet specific PlA1 (Zwa). Immunobiology 1982;160:375–381.

78. Shulman NR, Jordan JV. Platelet immunology. In: Colman, Hirsh, Marder, Salzmann, eds. Haemostasis and thrombosis: basic principles and clinical practise. Philadelphia: WB Saunders, 1982:274–342.

79. Mueller-Eckhardt C, Kiefel V, Grubert A, Kroll H, Weishiet M, Schmidt S, Mueller-Eckhardt G, Santoso S. 348 cases of suspected neonatal alloimmune thrombocytopenia. The Lancet 1989;i:363–366.

80. McGrath K, Minchinton R, Cunningham I, Ayberk H. Platelet anti-Bakb antibody associated with neonatal alloimmune thrombocytopenia. Vox Sang 1989;57:182–184.

81. Mueller-Eckhardt C, Becker T, Weisheit M, Witz C, Santoso S. Neonatal alloimmune thrombocytopenia due to fetomaternal Zwb incompatibility. Vox Sang 1986;50:94–96.

82. Kiefel V, Shechter Y, Atias D, Kroll H, Santoso S, Mueller-Eckhardt C. Neonatal alloimmune thrombocytopenia due to anti-Brb. Vox Sang 1991;60:244–245.

83. Grenet P, Dausset J, Dugas M, Petit D, Badoual J, Tangun Y. Purpura thrombopenique neonatal avec isoimmunisation foetomaternelle anti-Koa. Arch Fr Pediatr 1965;22:1165.

84. Kroll H, Kiefel V, Santoso S, Mueller-Eckhardt C. SRa, a private platelet antigen on glycoprotein IIIa associated with neonatal alloimmune thrombocytopenia. Blood 1990;11:2296–2302.

85. Mueller-Eckhardt C, Mueller-Eckhardt G, Willen Ohff H. Immunogenicity of an immune response to the human platelet antigen Zwa is strongly associated with HLA-B8 and DR3. Tissue antigens 1985; 26:71–76.

86. Valentin N, Vergracht A, Bignon JD, Cheneau ML, Blanchard D, Kaplan C, Reznikoff-Etievant MF, Muller JY. HLA-DRw52a is involved in alloimmunization

against PL-A1 antigen. Human immunology 1990;27:73–79.

87. Muller JY. Neonatal alloimmune thrombocytopenias. Bailliere's clinical immunology and allergy 1987;1:427–442.

88. Reznikoff-Etievant MF, Muller JY, Julien F, Paterau C. An immune response gene linked to HLA in man. Tissue antigens 1983; 22:312–313.

89. Gafni A, Blanchette VS. Screening for neonatal alloimmune thrombocytopenia: an economic perspective. Curr Stud Hematol Blood Transf 1988;54:140–147.

90. Kaplan C, Daffos F, Forestier F, Cox W, Lyon-Caen D, Dupuy-Montbrun MC, Salmon C. Management of alloimmune thrombocytopenia: antenatal diagnosis and in utero transfusion of maternal platelets. Blood 1988;72:340–343.

91. Reznikoff-Etievant MF. Management of alloimmune neonatal and antenatal thrombocytopenia. Vox Sang 1988;5:193–201.

92. Morales WJ, Stroup M. Intracranial haemorrhage due to isoimmune neonatal thrombocytopenia. Obstet Gynecol 1985;65 (Suppl):20–21.

93. Muller JY, Reznikoff-Etievant MF, Patereau C, Dangu C, Chesnel N. Thrombopenies neo-natales allo-immunes: Etude clinique et biologique de 84 cas. Presse Med 1985; 14:83–86.

94. Gruel Y, Boizard B, Daffos F. Determination of platelet antigens and glycoproteins in the human fetus. Blood 1986;68:488–492.

95. Deaver JE, Leppert PC, Zaroulis CG. Neonatal alloimmune thrombocytopenic purpura. Am J Perinat 1986;3:127–131.

96. Nicolini U, Tannirandorn Y, Gonzalez P. Continuing controversy in alloimmune thrombocytopenia: fetal hyperimmunoglobulinemia fails to prevent thrombocytopenia. Am J Obstet Gynecol 1990;163: 1144–1146.

97. Daffos F, Forestier F, Muller JY, et al. Prenatal treatment of alloimmune thrombocytopenia. The Lancet 1984;ii:632.

98. De Vries LS, Connell J, Bydder GM, Dubowitz LMS, Rodeck CH, Mibashan RS, Waters AH. Recurrent intracranial

haemorrhages in utero in an infant with alloimmune thrombocytopenia. Case report. Br J Obstet Gynaecol 1988;95: 299–302.

99. Murphy MF, Pullon HWH, Metcalfe P, et al. Management of fetal alloimmune thrombocytopenia by weekly in utero platelet transfusions. Vox Sang 1990; 58:45–49.

100. Daffos F., Forestier F. Prenatal treatment of fetal alloimmune thrombocytopenia. The Lancet 1988;1:910.

101. Lynch L, Bussel JB, McFarland JG, Chitkara U, Berkowitz RL. Antenatal treatment of alloimmune thrombocytopenia. Obstet Gynecol 1992;80:67–71.

102. Kornfeld I, Bellam P, Farquharson DF, Wilson RD, Wittman BK. The use of IVIG in the prophylaxis and treatment of severe NAIT—The British Columbia experience 1988–1991. Proc Soc Obstet Gynecol. Vancouver 1992.

103. Mir N, Samson D, House MJ, Kovar IZ. Failure of antenatal high-dose immunoglobulin to improve fetal platelet count in neonatal alloimmune thrombocytopenia. Vox Sang 1988;55:188–189.

104. Berkowitz RL, Bussel J. Interim review of the randomized trial of alloimmune fetal thrombocytopenia. Presented at the 6th annual Percutaneous Umbilical Blood Sampling Meeting, Philadelphia, 1991.

105. Berkowitz RL. Update on patients randomized in the therapeutic trial of alloimmune thrombocytopenia. Presented at the 8th annual PUBS meeting, Philadelphia, 1993.

106. Daffos F, Forestier F. Prenatal treatment of fetal alloimmune thrombocytopenia. The Lancet 1988;910.

107. Nicolaides K. Cordocentesis. In: Drife JO, Donnai D, eds. Antenatal diagnosis of fetal abnormalities. London: Springer-Verlag, 1991:210–212.

108. Zimmermann R, Huch A. In–utero fetal therapy with immunoglobulin for alloimmune thrombocytopenia. Lancet 1992; 340:606–607.

109. Bowman JM, Harmon C, Menticoglous S, Pollock J. Intravenous fetal transfusion of immunoglobulin for alloimmune thrombocytopenia. Lancet 1992;340:1034–1035.

110. Muller JY, Kaplan C, Reznikoff-Etievant MF, et al. In utero fetal sampling in neonatal alloimmune thrombocytopenia: justification and usefulness. Curr Stud Hematol Blood Transf 1988;54:127–135.

111. Sidiropoulos D, Straume B. Treatment of neonatal isoimmune thrombocytopenia with intravenous immunoglobulin. Blut 1984;48:383–386.

112. Derycke M, Dreyfus M, Ropert JC, Tchernia G. Intravenous immunoglobulin for neonatal isoimmune thrombocytopenia. Arch Dis Child 1985;60:667–669.

113. Massey GV, McWilliams NB, Mueller DG, Napolitano A, Maurer HM. Intravenous immunoglobulin in neonatal isoimmune thrombocytopenia. J Pediatr 1987;111: 133–135.

114. Suarez CR, Anderson C. High-dose intravenous gammaglobulin (IVG) in neonatal immune thrombocytopenia. Am J Hematol 1987;26:247–253.

FETAL PLEURAL EFFUSIONS

8

JANET I. VAUGHAN
NICHOLAS M. FISK
CHARLES H. RODECK

In the newborn, accumulation of lactescent chyle or lymph, chylothorax, is the most common cause of pleural effusion (1). In the fetus, pleural effusions are nonspecific collections identified by ultrasound. Establishing the underlying etiology is paramount as this will determine the prognosis and the treatment modalities offered. Idiopathic pleural effusions in utero are not chylous but serous in nature so are termed *primary fetal hydrothorax* (PFHT). PFHT occurs in about one in 15,000 pregnancies (2). The effusions may be clinically benign, but 50% will cause fetal or neonatal death, usually secondary to pulmonary hypoplasia with or without associated hydrops (2). PFTH is amenable to successful treatment in utero and is, therefore, a disease that deserves more understanding.

ULTRASONIC FEATURES

Ultrasonically, normal, nonaerated, fluid-filled fetal lungs appear solid with a uniform echogenicity. Together with the heart, which normally lies in the midline with the apex towards the left, they fill the thorax (Figure 8-1). The heart and great vessels are the only hypoechoic structures normally situated in the chest. In a longitudinal section with the transducer perpendicular to the muscle, the fetal diaphragm is seen convex towards the lung, separating thorax from abdomen. Pathognomic in the antenatal detection of fetal pleural effusions is the ultrasonic demonstration of an echo-free area lying between the lung, chest wall, and diaphragm. Effusions may be unilateral or, if bilateral, may be discrepant in size. In small effusions, the echogenic area only partially surrounds the lungs. In large effusions, the fetal lung appears echogenic with the configuration of a butterfly wing (3), particularly obvious if the lung is collapsed and

lying adjacent to the mediastinum (Figure 8-2). Polyhydramnios is common. Ultrasonic detection of mediastinal shift and subcutaneous edema indicate progressive pathology (Figure 8-2, 8-3).

Ultrasonic diagnosis is made either because of referral for clinical polyhydramnios or during routine ultrasonography (5). The first reports of antenatal diagnosis were by Carroll (6) and Defoort and Thiery (7). The fetuses they describe had large pleural effusions as well as generalized skin edema. In 1979, Thomas and Anderson (8) reported isolated pleural effusions in a 32-week fetus, which subsequently died neonatally from pulmonary hypoplasia. Ultrasonic detection at 15 weeks gestation is the earliest reported (9).

ETIOLOGY

Fetal pleural effusions are nonspecific entities. Careful and thorough investigation of the fetus is essential to establish the primary etiology for this will greatly affect the clinical course and prognosis. Primary fetal hydrothorax and/or chylothorax are ultimately diagnoses of exclusion.

Structural Malformations

Isolated fetal pleural effusions may occur secondary to structural abnormalities. Congenital diaphragmatic hernia may present ultrasonically as a fetal hydrothorax with no evidence of ascites or skin edema (5,10,11). The hernial sac, which only occurs in about 20% of all diaphragmatic hernias, fills with fluid and envelops the lung. Of the three cases reported with no associated hydrops, one neonate died of pulmonary hypoplasia (10) and two survived, although one of these babies underwent thoracoamniotic shunting at 22 weeks gestation (5).

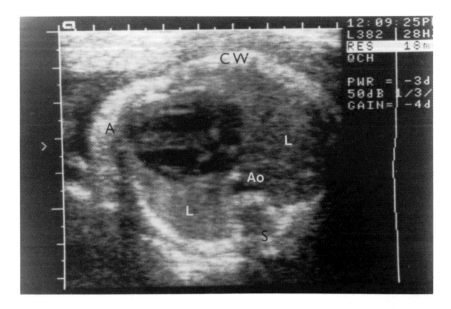

Figure 8-1 Ultrasound scan of a normal fetal thorax in transverse section
showing the four-chamber heart, with apex (A) to the left, and both lungs (L).
Ao = aorta; S = spine; CW = chest wall.

Isolated pleural effusions with no identifiable malformations may be due to congenital pulmonary lymphangiectasia. The effusions may be unilateral (12) or bilateral (13) with no distinguishing features. Congenital pulmonary lymphagiectasias are generally fatal in the neonatal period and may have a familial occurrence (14). Successful treatment in utero has been reported in a case with bilateral effusions and hydrops (15).

Observation of the lung tissue itself may reveal pathology. Extralobar sequestration of lung, which usually appears as an echogenic mass located between the lower lobe and the diaphragm, causes pleural effusions but usually in the presence of hydrops (12,16–19). Fetal mediastinal tumors may also cause pleural effusion with or without hydrops. Those reported include fetal thyroid teratoma (5) and congenital goiter (20). Cardiac abnormalities can sometimes cause hydrops with discrepantly large pleural effusions (21). Pleural effusion and hydrops has also been detected and treated in utero in the *Opitz-G* syndrome (22).

Chromosomal Abnormalities

There is a well-recognized association between congenital pleural effusions and Down's syndrome (23). In our own series, one of 11 fetuses with isolated fetal pleural effusions had Trisomy 21, while Nicolaides and Azar reported two of 17 fetuses with isolated pleural effusions (5). This gives a combined rate of 11%.

Neonatal chylothorax is a feature of Turner's syndrome (1). Pleural effusions in association with cystic hygromas and hydrops are not uncommon (24). Antenatal documentation of an isolated unilateral pleural effusion is reported with a Turner's mosaic (5).

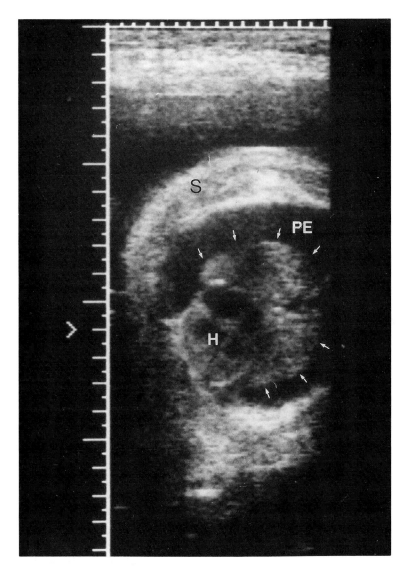

Figure 8-2 Ultrasound cross-sectional view of a fetal chest with bilateral hydrothoraces. The "butterfly wing configuration" is demonstrated with the lungs (arrows) collapsed and lying adjacent to the mediastinum. S = subcutaneous edema; PE = pleural effusion; H = heart. (Reproduced from Vaughan & Rodeck (4) with permission from Churchill Livingstone.)

Miscellaneous

Maternal adenovirus type 3 infection (25), tracheoesophageal fistula (26), Noonan's syndrome (27), and a multiple malformation complex (Diamond-Blackfan anemia, tracheoesophageal fistula, Klippel-Feil deformity and renal tubular acidosis) (28) have all been reported as causing symptomatic-isolated pleural effusions in the newborn, but have not been reported prenatally.

Nonimmune Hydrops

Nonimmune hydrops fetalis (NIHF) is defined as generalized edema of soft tissue in utero, with or without effusions in serous cavities, with no hematological evidence of

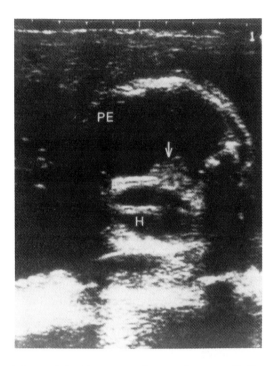

Figure 8-3 Transverse ultrasound section of a fetal chest showing a large right-sided pleural effusion with mediastinal shift, displacement of the heart, and a markedly compressed right lung (arrow). PE = pleural effusion; H = heart. (Reproduced from Rodeck et al. (50) with permission from the Massachusetts Medical Society.)

Table 8-1 Causes of Hydrops Fetalis

Disease Entity	No.	%
Cardiovascular	206	26
Chromosomal	80	10
Thoracic	74	9
Twin transfusion	64	8
Anemia	47	6
Infection	32	4
Urinary tract malformation	26	3
Cystic hygroma	17	2
Impaired fetal movement	15	2
Peritonitis	11	1
Hepatic	11	1
Genetic metabolic disease	7	1
Nephrotic syndrome	1	0
Miscellaneous	34	4
Not determined	179	22
Total	804	100

(Reproduced from Machin 1989 (30) with permission from Alan R. Liss. Inc.)

isoimmunization (29). These changes are readily identifiable by ultrasound (Figure 8-3), but they are not specific for determining the etiology, which may be due to over 100 documented factors (30). The overall mortality in NIHF remains high at 75% to 95% (29,31,32), with pulmonary hypoplasia being the most common cause of perinatal death, irrespective of underlying etiology (29,31). Saltzman et al. (33) demonstrated that 87% of fetuses without anemia as the cause of hydrops had pleural effusions compared to a 20% incidence with anemia. In 1,414 cases of NIHF reviewed by Machin (30), 63% were caused by six identifiable disease processes: cardiovascular, chromosomal, thoracic, twinning, anemia, and infection (Table 8-1).

INVESTIGATION

Ultrasound

Detailed ultrasound investigation is the key to successful etiological diagnosis. Twins and all the common structural abnormalities associated with fetal pleural effusions and hydrops can then be excluded (Table 8-1). In particular, echocardiography must be performed to exclude both structural abnormalities and arrhythmias as these can account up to 53% of nonimmune hydrops (21). More subtle abnormalities able to be detected include fixed limb deformities, tumors, including placental chorioangioma and markers suggesting genetic syndromes.

When ultrasound has been unable to determine a cause for the fetal pleural effusions, maternal and invasive fetal investigation may be required.

Maternal

Complete blood count and grouping with antibody status, investigation for syphilis, TORCH (toxoplasmosis, rubella, cytomegalovirus, and herpes simplex viruses) and Parvovirus B19 infections, diabetic evaluation and Kleihauer-Betke test should all be performed on the maternal blood. Other investigations are dependent on the specific clinical situation, but include hemoglobin electrophoresis and anticardiolipin and SS-A antibody status.

Invasive Procedures

Invasive techniques are required to determine the fetal karyotype and infection status. Although possible through amniocentesis, ultrasound-guided fetal blood sampling and chorionic villus sampling (CVS) ensure more rapid results (34–36). Using fetal blood has the advantage that the fetal hemoglobin and blood film may be assessed.

Diagnostic thoracocentesis may unmask cardiac or instrinsic thoracic pathology after decompression restores normal anatomical relationships. Pleuroamniotic shunting itself may have a diagnostic role by distinguishing hydrops subsequent to PFHT that resolves from hydrops of other etiologies that progress despite long-term drainage (5). Often, a combination of tests may be performed for more complete evaluation.

DIAGNOSIS

Definitive diagnosis may now be possible in 70–80% of nonimmune hydrops (21,30). In Machin's series, 22% had no cause deter-

mined (30). As antenatal therapy may prevent the sequelae of pulmonary hypoplasia, it has been suggested that pleural effusions in cases of unexplained NIHF should be assumed to be primary, in that the hydrops is secondary to the pressure of the effusion and not its cause (9,30).

Reports analyzing the etiology in series of isolated fetal pleural effusions are very limited. In our experience, approximately 10% (one of 11) are due to chromosomal abnormalities. Of fetuses with significant isolated effusions that underwent pleuroamniotic shunting, the incidence of chromosomal abnormality was 17.6% (three of 17) and of structural abnormality was 11.8% (two of 17) (5). Unless a specific structural abnormality is found, the remainder are diagnosed as primary fetal hydrothorax.

NATURAL HISTORY OF PRIMARY FETAL HYDROTHORAX

Fetal

The severity of primary fetal hydrothorax ranges from clinically insignificant to thoracic compression that results in lethal neonatal pulmonary hypoplasia or hydropic stillbirth. Determination of the natural history is difficult as there are very few published series that address this specific issue (2,37), and the multiple case reports vary considerably in their documentation (Table 8-2). In the largest published series, Longaker et al. had an overall mortality of 53% of 32 fetuses with PFHT (2).

Spontaneous Resolution

There are at least four case reports of fetuses with PFHT that have spontaneously resolved over three to 12 weeks (Table 8-2) (9,38–40). Furthermore, in their series examining the natural history of PFHT, Pijpers

Table 8-2 Case Reports of PFHT with No Intervention

Author	Year	GA	Hydrops	Outcome	Diagnosis
Carroll (6)	1977	36	+	IUD	PH
Defoort (7)	1978	31	+	IUD	dilated lymph ducts
Thomas (8)	1979	32	0	NND	HT,PH
Bovicelli (43)	1981	34	0	NND	PH
Lange (45)	1981	32	+	alive	HT
		39	0	alive	chylothorax
Jouppila (12)	1983	34	0	NND	CL
Peleg (44)	1985	33	+	NND	PH
		34	+	NND	PH
		33	0	NND	PH
Kerr-Wilson (13)	1985	33	0	NND	CL
Roberts (9)	1986	15	0	alive	resolved
Castillo (42)	1987	26	+	NND	PH
		26	+	NND	PH
		38	0	NND	PH
Booth (47)	1987	34	+	alive	chylothorax
Bruno (46)	1988	33	0	alive	chylothorax
Adams (39)	1988	16	0	alive	resolved
		25	0	NND	PH
		36	0	alive	chylothorax
Yaghoobian (38)	1988	25	0	alive	resolved
Lien (40)	1990	16	0	alive	resolved
Parker (41)	1991	18	0	alive	HT

IUD = intrauterine death; NND = neonatal death; PH = pulmonary hypoplasia; HT = hydrothorax; CL = congenital lymphangiectasia; 0 = absent; + = present.

et al. (37) and Longaker et al. (2) reported spontaneous resolution in two of eight and three of 29, respectively. All these fetuses survived. Spontaneous variation with resolution at 24 weeks, then recurrence at 35 weeks gestation was reported by Parker and James (41). The infant was born asymptomatic at 36 weeks gestation with an effusion that was managed conservatively (Table 8-2).

Isolated Pleural Effusions

Pijpers et al. reported 100% survival in six fetuses with bilateral pleural effusions and no associated hydrops (37). In the series of Longaker et al., there was also 100% survival in the fetuses with isolated pleural effusions, but if hydrops developed in a previously nonhydropic fetus, the survival was only 38% (2). Despite these optimistic series, the absence of hydrops is not 100% predictive of survival. Table 8-2 documents seven nonhydropic fetuses with pleural effusions diagnosed at 25–38 weeks, all of whom died neonatally from pulmonary complications after conservative management and delivery at 34–40 weeks gestation (8,12,13,39,42–44). Postmortem diagnosis of congenital lymphangiectasia was made in two cases (12,13), the remainder had PFHT.

This gives a mortality of 46.7% among non-hydropic fetuses.

Hydrops

Longaker et al. reported a mortality rate of 52% with NIHF (2). Of eight case reports that document hydropic fetuses with PFHT and no antenatal intervention, six died (75%), two in utero and four neonatally (Table 8-2) (6,7,42,44,45). Pulmonary hypoplasia contributed to at least five of these deaths (6,42,44). There is probably considerable underreporting in cases of intrauterine death in unexplained hydrops.

Neonatal

Chylothorax is the most common cause of primary pleural effusion causing respiratory distress in the neonate. In pediatric series in which the diagnoses were made postnatally, 40% of newborns were symptomatic at birth and 64% in the first 24 hours of life (48). The mortality rate was 15% despite this being a series of babies with a specific diagnosis, no associated anomalies, and no hydrops. Accurate diagnosis is made by observing the pleural fluid change from serous to opalescent after alimentation and then by demonstrating chylomicrons with light microscopy or electrophoresis (1,48–51). Treatment for congenital chylothorax consists of pleural drainage and after a period of intravenous fluids, a diet of medium-chain triglycerides to reduce lymphatic flow (49). Complications of long-term conservative management include weight loss, hypoproteinemia, hyponatremia, and lymphocytopenia (51). Spontaneous resolution is usual, but either pleurectomy or ligature of the thoracic duct is possible as definitive treatment for chronic pathology (51,52). Long-term complications are uncommon. Nineteen of 20 children had a nor-mal clinical examination at an average age of 15 months follow-up (48). One three-month-old infant is reported to have occasional sternal retraction and X-ray evidence of left upper lobe atelectasis (53).

PATHOPHYSIOLOGY

Hydrothorax

Understanding the pathophysiology of primary fetal hydrothorax is limited by our inability to make a positive diagnosis. This includes differentiating effusions destined to become "chylous" from other causes of hydrothorax. As the white cell population in chyle contains a high percentage of lymphocytes (48), several investigators have assumed that antenatal demonstration of pleural lymphocyte counts above 80% enables a specific diagnosis of fetal "chylothorax" (2,54–57). However, there are no reports that correlate antenatal pleural lymphocyte counts with definitive postnatal chylothoraces. PFHT may itself be a heterogeneous group of disorders.

Chylothorax

Accumulation of lymphatic fluid can result from overproduction or impaired reabsorption, or abnormal or damaged lymphatic vessels may leak. In pediatric series, chylothorax is more commonly unilateral and right-sided, suggesting thoracic duct pathology (48,58). In a persistent left-sided congenital chylothorax, Gates et al. elegantly demonstrated thoracic duct leakage in a patent vessel by radionuclide lymphangiography (59). Lymphography has also demonstrated a defect of the cisterna chyli in a seven-week-old with a chyloperitoneum (60). These findings suggest an anatomical defect, the level of which would determine the development of a chyloperitoneum or chylothorax. However, these abnormalities are difficult to demonstrate histopathologically on fetal autopsies, and the extent to which these events happen physiologically or secondary to other pathology is unknown (54).

Pulmonary Hypoplasia

This form of arrested lung growth is characterized by small but fully formed bronchi with failure of alveolar development (61). Compression of the developing lung by a fetal hydrothorax may inhibit lung growth to produce pulmonary hypoplasia (9,42–44), the main cause of death in neonates with isolated hydrothorax or nonimmune hydrops associated with pleural effusions (9,31,42,62).

Although most often lethal, with early neonatal death most frequent, there is a spectrum of neonatal respiratory manifestations (63). The canalicular phase, during the second trimester, is critical for lung development (64), but gestational age and severity and duration of the effusions all contribute to the development and extent of pulmonary hypoplasia (2,42,61,62).

Polyhydramnios

Alteration in amniotic fluid dynamics secondary to fetal lung collapse or interference with fetal swallowing secondary to a raised intrathoracic pressure are two mechanisms postulated to cause hydramnios (65).

Hydrops

Isolated fetal hydrothoraces may progress to generalized hydrops when the rise in intrathoracic pressure causes vena caval obstruction, which impedes venous return and causes congestive cardiac failure (7,30,50,55,65). Circulatory disturbance eventually causes tissue hypoxia and acidemia leading to fetal death (50,66,67). However, most fetuses hydropic due to PFHT, survive in utero, dying neonatally from pulmonary hypoplasia (2,Table 8-2).

TECHNIQUES TO DIAGNOSE PULMONARY HYPOPLASIA

With pulmonary hypoplasia as the main cause of mortality in PFHT, the ability to distinguish fetuses with potentially normal lung development from those with established lung hypoplasia would enable selection for prenatal treatment. Definitive diagnosis of pulmonary hypoplasia is dependent on autopsy criteria, including low lung-to-body weight ratio (67,68), low radial alveolar count (67,68), and reduced lung DNA (64). Conservative antenatal methods for detecting fetal pulmonary hypoplasia are indirect, and most lack adequate sensitivity to be clinically useful. Invasive monitoring may prove to be more informative.

Ultrasound

Thoracic Morphology

Adams et al. have suggested that hypoplastic fetal lungs appear small and rigid with an abnormal rounded contour, while normal lungs maintain the usual shape and "undulate gently within the effusions during fetal movement, suggesting pliability" (39).

Thoracic Measurement

Normograms using reproducible measurements have been established for both fetal thoracic circumference and lung lengths in relation to gestational age (70). Both measurements increase linearly throughout gestation, but the thoracic-to-abdominal circumference ratio and the lung-to-humerus ratio remained constant at 0.89 and 0.93, respectively. Numerous studies have correlated reduced thoracic measurements with the occurrence of pulmonary hypoplasia in the context of ruptured membranes or renal disease, but the measurements used are unable to assess pulmonary hypoplasia in the context of pleural effusions (71).

Castillo et al. (31) reported a lung/thoracic ratio specific to determining pulmonary hypoplasia in the presence of fetal pleural effusions. A coronal section of the fetal thorax at the level of the lung hilus enables a measurement from the hilus to the lung edge and another from the hilus to the thoracic wall. In all four cases with pulmonary hypoplasia, the lung/thoracic ratio was <0.6. Lack of reproducibility and the lungs' inherent capability for elastic recoil limit the usefulness of this measurement.

Breathing Movements

The theory that lung hypoplasia associated with oligohydramnios may be due to inhibited fetal breathing suggested an alternative ultrasound assessment to predict abnormal lung development. Conflicting results have been obtained by researchers, with Moessinger et al. demonstrating that fetal breathing movements(FBM) continue in the presence of oligohydramnios and do not correlate with pulmonary hypoplasia (72), while Blott et al. supported the hypothesis that FBM are absent in fetuses with pulmonary hypoplasia (73). FBM were defined differently by the two groups. Fisk et al. examined FBM before and after amnioinfusion in fetuses with severe oligohydramnios and found no difference in incidence (74). There are no studies correlating FBM and pulmonary hypoplasia in fetuses with PFHT.

Thoracocentesis

Pleural Pressures

Nicolini et al. described a technique for measuring pressure within fetal pleural space using subtraction manometry (75). Two saline-filled polyvinyl catheters were flushed to ensure the absence of air bubbles, then connected each at one end to a needle, one within the amniotic cavity and another within the pleural space. The other end of the catheters were connected to a silicone strain-gauge transducer (EM 750, Elcomatic Ltd, Glasgow, U.K.). The pressure scale was referenced to zero at the maternal skin surface. Pressure readings from both transducers were continuously recorded on a multichannel chart recorder. A third channel recorded the excess pressure of the intrapleural space over the intra-amniotic cavity.

Our recent data show no relationship between the initial intrapleural pressure and gestational age of 11 fetuses with hydrothoraces, seven of whom survived and four of whom had pulmonary hypoplasia confirmed at autopsy. All had raised intrapleural pressure, suggesting external compression of the fluid on the lung. In five fetuses, two with hydrops, we have intrapleural pressures obtained both before and after aspiration of the pleural fluid (Figure 8-4). In the three fetuses that survived, the intrapleural pressures remained at or above zero after complete aspiration. However, in the two that were subsequently diagnosed as having pulmonary hypoplasia at autopsy, the postaspiration pressures were negative with respect to the intra-amniotic pressure.

Rodeck et al. (50) observed a hydropic fetus whose left hemithorax partially drained following pleuroamiotic shunting and then refilled. Analysis of this fluid, aspirated sep-

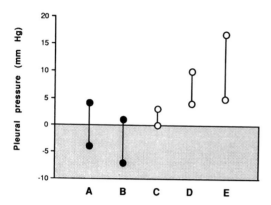

Figure 8-4 Pre- and post-aspiration pleural pressures (mm Hg) obtained by subtraction manometry in five fetuses with hydrothoraces. A and D were hydropic. The shaded area represents negative pressure with respect to the amniotic cavity. Patients A and B (closed circles) had negative post-aspiration pressures and died perinatally with autopsy-proven lung hypoplasia. Patients C, D, and E (open circles) had positive post-aspiration pressures and survived.

arately, showed fetal squames, indicating that amniotic fluid had entered the chest through the valveless shunt and confirming a negative pressure gradient. The fetus delivered at 29 weeks and died neonatally of pulmonary hypoplasia with a lung/body weight ratio of 0.0075/1.

Pleuroamniotic Shunting

Long-term drainage of the fetal chest may be a useful diagnostic procedure. Two criteria are reported to have favorable prognostic implications.

Lung Re-expansion

Rodeck et al. reported failure of lung re-expansion following pleuroamniotic shunting in two fetuses that subsequently died neonatally due to pulmonary hypoplasia (50). In this series, eight fetuses with pleural effusions, including five with hydrops, were shunted at 25–35 and delivered at

32–39 weeks of gestation. In all six infants that survived, the lungs fully expanded after treatment.

In our recent series of 16 pleuroamniotic shunts inserted at Queen Charlotte's Hospital, London, 11 lungs completely reexpanded with survival in all 11 infants. In the five infants whose lungs did not completely re-expand, all died neonatally of pulmonary complications.

Resolution of Hydrops

Nicolaides and Azar inserted pleuroamniotic shunts in 28 fetuses with pleural effusions and unexplained hydrops (5). The hydrops resolved one to three weeks after shunting in 13 fetuses, 12 of whom survived with no pulmonary complications. One neonate died of pulmonary hypoplasia secondary to congenital diaphragmatic hernia. In the 15 fetuses in whom the hydrops did not resolve, two died in utero and 11 died neonatally.

Resolution of hydrops occurred in three of the five fetuses shunted by Rodeck et al. (50). These three survived with no pulmonary complications, while the two with persistent hydrops died neonatally of pulmonary hypoplasia.

MANAGEMENT

The aim of management of fetuses with PFHT must be to prevent pulmonary hypoplasia while reaching a safe gestational age for the fetus to be delivered in a nonhydropic state. The option of pregnancy termination should be discussed for fetuses whose effusions appear during the second trimester, particularly if associated with chromosomal or other structural abnormalities.

Factors reported to be prognostically useful in determining treatment options are listed in Table 8-3. Nonhydropic fetuses, unilateral effusions without mediastinal shift, and spontaneous resolution were all associated with 100% survival. However, effusions presenting prior to 33 weeks gestation, and delivery before 35 weeks gestation both reduced the survival rates considerably. The presence or absence of polyhydramnios was not predictive of outcome (2), but its influence on preterm labor and consequent prematurity will indirectly affect outcome.

Conservative Management

With a rate of spontaneous resolution of about 12% and the relatively good prognosis of PFHT unassociated with hydrops, conservative management may have a role in non-progressive effusions, particularly if small or unilateral with no mediastinal shift (2,37). Serial ultrasonography at fortnightly intervals is necessary to monitor any changes.

The development of mediastinal shift, significant lung compression, polyhydram-

Table 8-3   Prognostic Indicators

Characteristic		% Survival
Age at diagnosis	<33 wks	43
	>33 wks	80
Age at delivery	<35 wks	30
	>35 wks	79
Spontaneous resolution	Yes	100
	No	52
Hydrops	Yes	52
	No	100
Bilateral	Yes	52
	No	100*

*Without mediastinal shift.
(Reproduced from Longaker et al. 1989(2) with permission from WB Saunders Company.)

nios or hydrops fetalis justifies prenatal intervention to prevent premature delivery and pulmonary hypoplasia.

Thoracocentesis

Antenatal

Table 8-4 summarizes the case reports of fetuses whose pleural effusions were managed by prenatal thoracocentesis. The average number of aspirations per fetus was 2.2 (range one to five). All authors reported that unless delivered, reaccumulation of the effusion(s) occurred within 10 days, with one hour being the most rapid.

Isolated pleural effusions in three fetuses at 19–22 weeks of gestation resolved in utero after multiple aspirations. The babies were born at term and had normal pulmonary development. Despite multiple aspirations, the effusions in three other cases continued to progress, and all died early neonatal deaths due to pulmonary insufficiency. The overall mortality was 46.2% in 13 fetuses. Two of seven nonhydropic fetuses (28.6%) and four of six with hydrops (66.6%) died. Except for one procedure-related intrauterine death, the deaths were neonatal and respiratory.

Thoracocentesis facilitates neonatal resuscitation if performed immediately prior to delivery. Petres et al. (65) reported a case in which pleural fluid reaccumulated within hours of aspiration at 36 weeks. An intrapartum aspiration of 152 ml enabled delivery of an infant in good condition. Similarly, Schmidt et al. (77) performed a thoracocentesis in a hydropic fetus at 35 weeks gestation, just prior to cesarian section. The baby was born in good condition, but subsequently required assisted ventilation for 20 days. A fetus with *Opitz-G* syndrome has been treated with thoracocentesis and intravascular albumen infusion (22).

Table 8-4   Management by Thoracocentesis

Author	Year	GA	Hydrops	Asp	Reacc	Outcome	Diagnosis
Petres (65)	1982	36	0	2	<1	alive	chylothorax
Redwine (76)	1983	30	+	1	del	NND	—
Elser (54)	1983	34	0	1	del	alive	HT
Benacerraf (55)	1985	19	0	3	7	alive	resolution
Schmidt (77)	1985	35	+	1	del	alive	chylothorax
Kurjak (78)	1985	22	0	2	10	alive	resolution
Benacerraf (56)	1986	17	0	5	7	alive	resolution
Longaker (2)	1989	27	+	1		IUD	cord torsion
		27	+	1	<7	NND	PH
		34	0	2	<7	NND	PH
		28	0	4	<7	NND	PH
Landy (57)	1990	24	+	5	6	NND	HMD
King (79)	1991	34	+	1	1hr	alive	chylothorax

GA = gestational age; Asp = number of aspirations; Reacc = reaccumulation in days; del = delivery; hr = hour; IUD = intrauterine death; NND = neonatal death; HT = hydrothorax; PH = pulmonary hypoplasia; CL = congenital lymphangiectasia; HMD = hyaline membrane disease; + = present; 0 = absent; — = no comment.

Postnatal

Successful postnatal thoracocentesis immediately following delivery is reported in 10 infants whose diagnosis was made prenatally (37,45,46,80). Four infants subsequently required long-term pleural drainage, but all survived. In contrast, Longaker et al. reported only a 50% survival rate in the 20 infants that were managed with postnatal drainage (2).

Technique

Using a sterile technique and local anesthesia, antenatal thoracocentesis is an ultrasound-guided procedure using a 20-gauge spinal needle. With the fetus in a transverse ultrasonic section, the best approach is anterior or lateral. Once in the amniotic cavity, the needle is thrust into the fetus with one movement as touching the body will cause it to move. The pleural fluid is completely aspirated. If the effusions are bilateral, two procedures may be required. Afterwards, the thorax is scanned to assess lung re-expansion and the presence of any residual fluid. Although the fetal heart rate and sampling sites are assessed for complications, these are rare. Serial ultrasound scans are required to assess fluid reaccumulation.

Pleuroamniotic Shunting

Because pleural fluid reaccumulates rapidly after prenatal aspiration, long-term drainage is necessary to prevent pulmonary hypoplasia and reverse hydrops and polyhydramnios.

Animal Studies

Prior to any human fetal surgical intervention, confirmation of the pathophysiology and the efficacy of therapy should be obtained from experimental animal models.

In six fetal lambs, Harrison et al. placed a balloon in the left hemithorax and dilated it progressively through the third trimester.

All six died neonatally from pulmonary hypoplasia. However, in another five fetal lambs, decompression by balloon deflation in the middle of the third trimester permitted survival at birth (81).

Clinical Experience

In 1986, Seeds and Bowes first reported the insertion of pleuroamniotic catheters into a 30-week fetus who was contracting with polyhydramnios and large pleural effusions (82). Although delivery was effected five days later, the effusions significantly reduced, the fundal height decreased, and the contractions settled after catheter placement. After delivery, the infant made good recovery after chest drainage and ventilatory support.

More definitive treatment from thoracoamniotic shunting was demonstrated in a 20-week-old fetus, grossly hydropic secondary to a large single cyst associated with Type 1 cystic adenomatoid malformation (83). Complete resolution of the hydrops occurred within three weeks of placement, and the infant delivered at 37 weeks had no respiratory complications.

Blott et al. reported the first series of fetuses treated with pleuroamniotic shunts for fetal pleural effusions (84). Eleven fetuses, five of whom were hydropic, were shunted from 22–35 weeks of gestation and delivered one to 16 weeks later. Eight infants survived, and of the three that died neonatally, two had congenital abnormalities and one developed septicemia with no autopsy evidence of lung hypoplasia.

The therapeutic efficacy of pleuroamniotic shunting is confirmed in fetuses with PFHT whose hydrops is reversed in utero (Table 8-5). The series of Nicolaides and Azar includes the cases reported by Blott et al. (5,84). Of 34 hydropic fetuses treated, 17 (50%) resolved, of which 16 (94%) survived, with no respiratory complications. Only two infants survived when the hydrops persisted(12%). The overall survival is 52.9% (18/34) in hydropic fetuses. Following thoracocentesis, there are no reported cases of reversal of hydrops and the survival rate of hydropic fetuses is poor (Table 8-4). Similarly, the survival rate of hydropic fetuses treated conservatively is about 25% (2/8) (Table 8-2).

Technique

The most popular catheter used for pleuroamniotic shunting is a double-pigtail silastic catheter (Rocket of London, UK) (Figure 8-5) with external and internal diameters of 0.21 and 0.15mm, respectively. There are lateral holes around the coils and the amniotic coil is perpendicular to the rest of the catheter so as to lie flat against the

Table 8-5 Reversal of Hydrops in Utero After Pleuroamniotic Shunting

Author	Hydropic Fetuses	Therapeutic Response		Survival	
		R	NR	R	NR
Rodeck et al. (50)	5	3	2	3	0
Longaker et al. (2)	1	1	0	1	0
Nicolaides & Azar (5)	28	13	15	12	2
Total	34	17	17	16	2
Percent		50%	50%	94%	12%

R = reversal of hydrops; NR = nonreversal of hydrops.

Figure 8-5   Double-pigtail catheter of a 6-French silastic (Rocket of London, UK) with two curves at right angles to each other. A guidewire is used to straighten the catheter for insertion into the cannula.

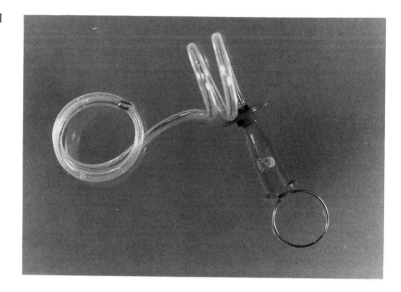

Figure 8-6   Shunt insertion set (RM Surgical Developments, UK), showing the cannula and trocar with the short and long introducers.

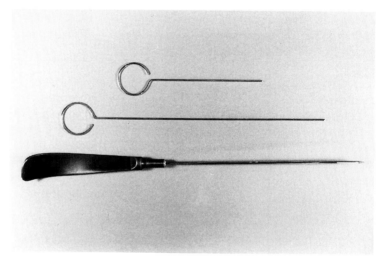

thoracic wall and minimize the risk of removal by the fetus. We have been using this equipment for vesicoamniotic shunting since 1982 (83).

Fetal shunt placement is an outpatient procedure performed under aseptic conditions with prophylactic antibiotic cover. Local anesthetic is routinely used and, occasionally, maternal sedation. Fetal paralysis is not required. As with thoracocentesis, ultrasound is used to obtain a transverse section of the fetal thorax. A 15-cm metal trocar and cannula (external diameter 3mm, RM Surgical Developments, UK) (Figure 8-6) is introduced under ultrasound visualization transabdominally into the amniotic cavity, then through the midthoracic wall into the effusion. The trocar is removed, the catheter inserted into the cannula, and one end positioned in the pleural cavity with the short introducer rod. The cannula is then withdrawn into the amniotic cavity, where the rest of the catheter is deposited with the longer introducer (Figure 8-7). For bilateral effusions, drainage of the contralateral wall is achieved either by rotating the fetal body using the tip of the cannula (5) or by a second puncture.

Once inserted, the proximal end of the catheter appears as a pair of echogenic lines within the fetal thorax, with the effusion drained and the lung re-expanded and appropriate mediastinal relationship restored (Figure 8-8). The distal end of the catheter protrudes from the thoracic wall.

In cases with gross polyhydramnios, amniocentesis may facilitate shunt insertion by decreasing the distance traversed (50) and will also improve visualization.

Follow-up

Weekly ultrasound scans should be performed to assess reaccumulation of the pleural fluid as the catheter may become blocked or dislodged. This occurred in four of 47 cases in the series of Nicolaides and Azar (5). Further shunts were inserted without complication.

Ultrasound surveillance also enables hydropic fetuses to be monitored. Resolution is a good prognostic indicator. Persistence or progression carries a poor prognosis, and termination should be considered if gestational age permits.

Complications

Apart from shunt displacement (5,50), complications appear to be rare. Drainage of amniotic fluid into the maternal peritoneal cavity causing ascites, followed by

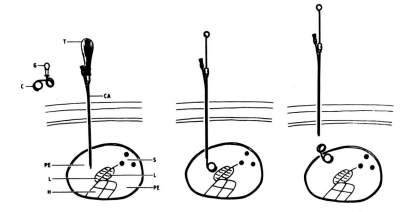

Figure 8-7 The technique of pleuroamniotic shunt insertion. The trocar (T) and cannula (CA) are inserted transabdominally and transamniotically into the pleural effusion (PE) (left panel). The trocar is removed, the catheter straigtened over the guidewire and fed into the cannula, and the wire removed. A short introducer rod is then inserted to position half the catheter in the fetal hemithorax (center panel). The cannula is then withdrawn into the amniotic cavity, and a long introducer rod is inserted to position the other half of the shunt in the amniotic cavity (right panel). H = heart; S = spine; L = lungs. (Reproduced from Rodeck et al. (50) with permission from the Massachusetts Medical Society.)

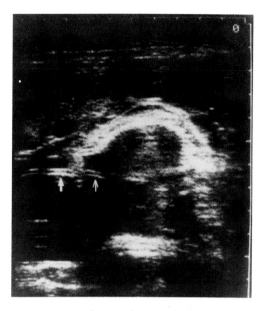

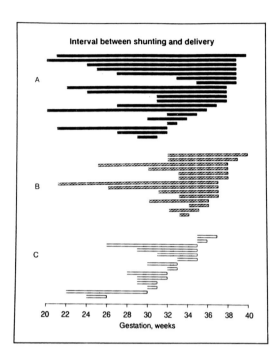

Figure 8-8 Ultrasound scan of a 32-week fetal thorax with a pleuroamniotic shunt in situ showing the intrapleural (thin arrow) and extrapleural (thick arrow) portions. The effusions have drained and the lungs re-expanded. (Reproduced from Rodeck et al. (50) with permission from the Massachusetts Medical Society.)

Figure 8-9 Interval between shunting and delivery in 47 fetuses with pericardial effusion, cystic adenomatoid malformation, and pleural effusions. The horizontal lines connect the gestation at shunting with the gestation at delivery. Group A (solid) were nonhydropic, Group B (hatched) hydropic and survived, Group C (open) hydropic and died. The shortest shunt-delivery interval was in Group C as treatment did not prevent worsening of hydrops. (Reproduced from Nicolaides and Azar (5) with permission from S. Karger AG.)

resolution, has been reported (15). Potential complications include preterm rupture of membranes, preterm labor, infection, fetal or maternal bleeding from punctured vessels, and fetal damage. Anti-D immunoglobulin prophylaxis must be given to Rhesus-negative women to prevent isoimmunization.

Preterm labor is not uncommon in these patients as the majority have clinical polyhydramnios. Tocolysis may be used during the procedure to try to prevent premature delivery, particularly if actively contracting.

Shunt-Delivery Interval

Prolongation of pregnancies treated by pleuroamniotic shunting range from one to 20 weeks (5,50). Figure 8-9 presents graphi-

cally the interval between shunting and delivery in 47 pregnancies treated at King's College Hospital, London (5). Group A represents 19 nonhydropic infants with pericardial effusion (n=1), cystic adenomatoid malformation (n=3) and pleural effusions (n=15), all of whom survived. Of the 28 hydropic fetuses, 14 infants survived (Group B) and 14 died (Group C). Although the mean gestational age at shunting was similar (A=27, B=30, C=29), the time between shunt insertion and delivery was shorter in

Group C (A=10, B=7, C=3). In this group, shunting did not halt progression of poly-hydramnios and hydrops.

Delivery

If the pregnancy continues, the insertion of a pleuroamniotic shunt does not alter the timing or route of delivery. Delivery should take place in a hospital that can appropriately resuscitate a potentially ill neonate. Following delivery, the catheters are clamped immediately to avoid the development of pneumothoraces.

Pleurocutaneous Shunting

Roberts et al. described the insertion of a pleurocutaneous catheter inserted into a fetus with a progressive unilateral hydrothorax at 25 weeks gestation (9). Drainage decreased over five days, and the catheter was removed after one week with no reaccumulation. The infant delivered at term with no complications.

CONCLUSIONS

Ultrasonic detection of fetal pleural effusions should prompt investigation to exclude underlying structural or chromosomal abnormalities. Associated fetal hydrops should be appropriately investigated. Isolated fetal pleural effusions and unexplained nonimmune hydrops fetalis may be assumed to be due to primary fetal hydrothorax. Although 12% of isolated PFHT resolve spontaneously with excellent perinatal outcome, progressive effusions with major mediastinal shift and lung compression may result in pulmonary hypoplasia with or without associated hydrops. PFHT that occurs in the second trimester carries a significant risk as critical lung development may be inhibited. The overall mortality in PFHT

is 53%. Antenatal diagnosis of pulmonary hypoplasia is unreliable, so the management of pregnancies with PFHT must rely on prognostic indicators. Conservative management is satisfactory in resolving or small nonprogressive effusions. The development of mediastinal shift, significant lung compression, or hydrops fetalis prior to 35 weeks gestation justifies prenatal shunting to prolong the pregnancy, reverse fetal hydrops, and prevent pulmonary hypoplasia. After 35 weeks gestation, pleural drainage may facilitate neonatal resuscitation if performed immediately prior to delivery.

References

1. Chernick V, Reed MH. Pneumothorax and chylothorax in the neonatal period. J Pediatr 1970;76:624–632.
2. Longaker MT, Laberge J-M, Dansereau J, et al. Primary fetal hydrothorax: natural history and management. J Pediatr Surg 1989; 24:573–576.
3. Vintzileos AM, Campbell WA, Nochimson DJ, Weinbaum PJ. Antenatal evaluation and management of ultrasonically detected fetal anomalies. Obstet Gynecol 1987;69:640–660.
4. Vaughan JI, Rodeck CH. Interventional procedures. In: Meire H, Cosgrove D, Dewbury K, eds. Clinical Ultrasound—A Comprehensive Text. Edinburgh: Churchill Livingstone (in press).
5. Nicolaides KH, Azar GB. Thoraco-amniotic shunting. Fetal Diagn Ther 1990;5:153–164.
6. Carroll B. Pulmonary hypoplasia and pleural effusions associated with fetal death in utero: ultrasonic findings. Am J Roentgenol 1977; 129:749–750.
7. Defoort P, Thiery M. Antenatal diagnosis of congenital chylothorax by gray scale sonography. J Clin Ultrasound 1978;6:47–48.
8. Thomas DB, Anderson JC. Antenatal detection of fetal pleural effusions and neonatal management. Med J Aust 1979;2:435–436.
9. Roberts AB, Clarkson PM, Pattison NS, Jamieson MG, Mok PM. Fetal hydrothorax in

the second trimester of pregnancy: success-ful intrauterine treatment at 24 weeks gestation. Fetal Therapy 1986;1:203–209.

10. Gilsanz V, Emons D, Hansmann M, et al. Hydrothorax, ascites, and right diaphragmatic hernia. Radiology 1986;158:243–246.

11. Whittle MJ, Gilmore DH, McNay MB, Turner TL, Raine PAM. Diaphragmatic hernia presenting in utero as a unilateral hydrothorax. Prenat Diagn 1989;9:115–118.

12. Jouppila P, Kirkinen P, Herva R, Koivisto M. Prenatal diagnosis of pleural effusions by ultrasound. J Clin Ultrasound 1983; 11:516–519.

13. Kerr-Wilson RHJ, Duncan A, Hume R, Bain AD. Prenatal pleural effusion associated with congenital pulmonary lymphangectasia. Prenat Diagn 1985;5:73–76.

14. Scott-Emuakpor AB, Warren ST, Kapur S, Quiachon EB, Higgins JV. Familiar occurrence of congenital pulmonary lymphangiectasias. Genetic implications. Am J Dis Child 1981;135:532–534.

15. Ronderos-Dumit D, Nicolini U, Vaughan J, Fisk NM, Chamberlain PF, Rodeck CH. Uterine-peritoneal amniotic fluid leakage: an unusual complication of intrauterine shunting. Obstet Gynecol 1991; 78:913–915.

16. Romero R, Chervenak FA, Kotzen J, Berkowitz RL, Hobbins JC. Antenatal sonographic findings of extralobar pulmonary sequestration. J Ultrasound Med 1982; 1:131–132.

17. Kristoffersen SE, Ipsen L. Ultrasonic real-time diagnosis of hydrothorax before delivery in an infant with extralobar lung sequestration. Acta Obstet Gynecol Scand 1984;63:723–725.

18. Davies PF, Shevland JE, Townley G. Antenatal diagnosis of extralobar sequestration. Aust Radiol 1989;33:290–292.

19. Weiner C, Varner M, Pringle K, Hein H, Williamson R, Smith WL. Antenatal diagnosis and palliative treatment of nonimmune hydrops fetalis secondary to pulmonary extralobar sequestration. Obstet Gynecol 1986; 68:275–280.

20. Sinniah D, Sivanesan S. Sporadic congenital goiter and pleural effusion. Amer J Dis Child 1971;122:245–246.

21. Skoll MA, Sharland GK, Allan LD. Is the ultrasound definition of fluid collections in nonimmune hydrops fetalis helpful in defining the underlying cause or predicting outcome? Ultrasound Obstet Gynecol 1991; 1:309–312.

22. Patton MA, Baraitser M, Nicolaides KH, Rodeck CH, Gamsu H. Prenatal treatment of fetal hydrops associated with the hypertelorism-dysphagia syndrome (Opitz-G syndrome). Prenat Diagn 1986;6:109–115.

23. Foote KD, Vickers DW. Congenital pleural effusion in Down's syndrome. Br J Radiol 1986;59:609–610.

24. Nicolaides KH, Rodeck CH, Lange I, et al. Fetoscopy in the assessment of unexplained fetal hydrops. Br J Obstet Gynaecol 1985; 92:671–679.

25. Meyer K, Girgis N, McGravey V. Adenovirus associated with congenital pleural effusion. J Pediatr 1985;107:433–435.

26. Harvey JG, Houlsby W, Sherman K, Gough MH. Congenital chylothorax: report of a unique case associated with 'H'-type tracheoesophageal fistula. Br J Surg 1979; 66:485–487.

27. Chan DK-L, Ho N-K. Noonan syndrome with spontaneous chylothorax at birth. Aust Paediatr J 1989;25:296–298.

28. Lazarus KH, McCurdy FA. Multiple congenital anomalies in a patient with Diamond-Blackfan syndrome. Clin Pediatr 1984;23:520–523.

29. Graves GR, Baskett TF. Nonimmune hydrops fetalis: antenatal diagnosis and management. Am J Obstet Gynecol 1984; 148:563–565.

30. Machin GA. Hydrops revisited: literature review of 1,414 cases published in the 1980s. Am J Med Genet 1989;34:366–390.

31. Castillo RA, Devoe LD, Hadi HA, Martin S, Giest D. Nonimmune hydrops fetalis: clinical experience and factors related to a poor outcome. Am J Obstet Gynecol 1986; 155:812–816.

32. Holzgreve W, Holzgreve B, Curry CJR. Nonimmune hydrops fetalis: diagnosis and management. Semin Perinatol 1985;9:52–67.

33. Saltzman DH, Frigletto FD, Harlow BL, Barss VA, Benacerraf BR. Sonographic evaluation of hydrops fetalis. Obstet Gynecol 1989;74:106–111.

34. Daffos F, Capella-Pavlovsky, Forestier F. Fetal blood sampling via the umbilical cord using a needle guided by ultrasound. Prenat Diagn 1983;3:271–277.

35. Nicolaides KH, Rodeck CH, Gosden CM. Rapid karyotyping in non-lethal fetal malformations. The Lancet 1986;i:283–286.

36. Holzgreve W, Miny P, Gerlach B, Westendorp A, Ahlert D, Horst J. Benefits of placental biopsies for rapid karyotyping in the second and third trimesters (late chorionic villus sampling) in high risk pregnancies. Am J Obstet Gynecol 1990;162: 188–192.

37. Pijpers L, Reuss A, Stewart PA, Wladimiroff JW. Noninvasive management of isolated bilateral fetal hydrothorax. Am J Obstet Gynecol 1989;161:330–332.

38. Yaghoobian J, Comrie M. Transitory bilateral isolated fetal pleural effusions. J Ultrasound Med 1988;7:231–232.

39. Adams H, Jones A, Hayward C. The sonographic features and implications of fetal pleural effusions. Clin Radiol 1988; 39:398–401.

40. Lien JM, Colmorgan GHC, Gehret JF, Evantash AB. Spontaneous resolution of fetal pleural effusion diagnosed during the second trimester. J Clin Ultrasound 1990; 18:54–56.

41. Parker M, James D. Spontaneous variation in fetal pleural effusions. Br J Obstet Gynaecol 1991;98:403–405.

42. Castillo RA, Devoe LD, Falls G, Holzman GB, Hadi HA, Fadel HE. Pleural effusions and pulmonary hypoplasia. Am J Obstet Gynecol 1987;157:1252–1255.

43. Bovicelli L, Rizzo N, Orsini LF, Calderoni P. Ultrasonic real-time diagnosis of fetal hydrothorax and lung hypoplasia. J Clin Ultrasound 1981;9:253–254.

44. Peleg D, Golichowski AM, Ragan WD. Fetal hydrothorax and bilateral pulmonary hypoplasia. Acta Obstet Gynecol Scand 1985;64:451–453.

45. Lange IR, Manning FA. Antenatal diagnosis of congenital pleural effusions. Am J Obstet Gynecol 1981;140:839–840.

46. Bruno M, Iskra L, Dolfin G, Farina D. Congenital pleural effusion: prenatal ultrasonic diagnosis and therapeutic management. Prenat Diagn 1988;8:157–159.

47. Booth P, Nicolaides KH, Greenough A, Gamsu HR. Pleuroamniotic shunting for fetal chylothorax. Early Hum Dev 1987; 15:365–367.

48. Brodman RF. Congenital hydrothorax. Recommendations for treatment. NY State J Med 1975;75:553–557.

49. Van Aerde J, Campbell AN, Smythe JA, Lloyd D, Bryan MH. Spontaneous chylothorax in newborns. Am J Dis Child 1984;138:961–964.

50. Rodeck CH, Fisk NM, Fraser DI, Nicolini U. Long-term in utero drainage of fetal hydrothorax. N Engl J Med 1988; 319:1135–1138.

51. Puntis FL, Roberts KD, Handy D. How should chylothorax be managed? Arch Dis Child 1987;62:593–596.

52. Andersen EA, Hertel J, Pedersen SA, Sorensen HR. Congenital chylothorax: management by ligature of the thoracic duct. Scand J Thorac Cardiovasc Surg 1984;18:193–194.

53. Cugell DW, Scherl S. Spontaneous pleural effusion in a newborn infant. Am J Dis Child 1949;78:569–571.

54. Elser H, Borruto F, Schneider A, Schneider K. Chylothorax in a twin pregnancy of 34 weeks—sonographically diagnosed. Eur J Obstet Reprod Biol 1983;16:205–211.

55. Benacerraf BR, Frigoletto FD. Mid-trimester fetal thoracocentesis. J Clin Ultrasound 1985;13:202–204.

56. Benacerraf BR, Frigoletto FD, Wilson M. Successful mid-trimester thoracocentesis with analysis of the lymphocyte population in the pleural effusion. Am J Obstet Gynecol 1986;155:398–399.

57. Landy HJ, Daly V, Heyl PS, Houry AN. Fetal thoracocentesis with unsuccessful outcome. J Clin Ultrasound 1990; 18:50–53.

58. Yancy WS, Spock A. Spontaneous neonatal pleural effusion. J Pediatr Surg 1967; 2:313–319.

59. Gates GF, Dore EK, Kanchanapoom V. Thoracic duct leakage in neonatal chylothorax visualized by [198]Au lymphangiography. Radiology 1972;105:619–620.

60. Craven CE, Goldman AS, Larson DL, Petterson M, Hendrich CK. Congenital chylous ascites: lymphangiographic demonstration of obstruction of the cisterna chyli and chylous reflux into the peritoneal space and small intestine. J Pediatr 1967; 70:340–341.

61. Sherer DM, Davis JM, Woods JR. Pulmonary hypoplasia: a review. Obstet Gynecol Surv 1990;45:792–803.

62. Maeda H, Shimokawa H, Yamaguchi Y, Sueishi K, Nakano H. The influence of pleural effusion on pulmonary growth in the human fetus. J Perinat Med 1989; 17:231–236.

63. Bhutani VK, Abbasi S, Weiner S. Neonatal pulmonary manifestations due to prolonged amniotic fluid leak. Am J Perinatol 1986;3:225–230.

64. Wigglesworth JS, Desai R. Use of DNA estimation for growth assessment in normal and hypoplastic fetal lung. Arch Dis Child 1981;56:601–605.

65. Petres RE, Redwine FO, Cruikshank DP. Congenital bilateral chylothorax. Antepartum diagnosis and successful intrauterine surgical management. JAMA 1982; 248:1360–1361.

66. Fisk NM, Tannirandorn Y, Nicolini U, Talbert DG, Rodeck CH. Amniotic pressure in disorders of amniotic fluid volume. Obstet Gynecol 1990;76:210–214.

67. Tannirandorn Y, Nicolini U, Nicolaides PC, Fisk NM, Arulkumaran S, Rodeck CH. Fetal demise in cystic hygroma: insights gained from fetal blood sampling. Prenat Diagn 1990;10:189–193.

68. Wigglesworth JS, Desai R, Guerrini P. Fetal lung hypoplasia: biochemical and structural variations and their possible significance. Arch Dis Child 1981;56:606–615.

69. Askenazi SS, Perlman M. Pulmonary hypoplasia: lung weight and radial alveolar count as a criteria of diagnosis. Arch Dis Child 1979;54:614–618.

70. Chitkara N, Rosenberg J, Chervenak AF, et al. Prenatal sonographic assessment of the fetal thorax. Am J Obstet Gynecol 1987; 156:1069–1074.

71. Nimrod C, Nicholson S, Davies D, Harder J, Dodd G, Sauve R. Pulmonary hypoplasia testing in clinical obstetrics. Am J Obstet Gynecol 1988;158:277–280.

72. Moessinger AC, Fox HE, Higgins A, Rey HR, Al Haideri M. Fetal breathing movements are not a reliable predictor of continued lung development in pregnancies complicated by oligohydramnios. The Lancet 1987;ii:1297–1299.

73. Blott M, Greenough A, Nicolaides KH, Moscoso G, Gibb D, Campbell S. Fetal breathing movements as a predictor of favorable pregnancy outcome after oligohydramnios due to membrane rupture in second trimester. The Lancet 1987;ii:129–131.

74. Fisk NM, Talbert DG, Nicolini U, Vaughan J, Rodeck CH. Fetal breathing movements in oligohydramnios are not increased by amnioinfusion. Br J Obstet Gynaecol 1992; 99:464–468.

75. Nicolini U, Fisk NM, Talbert DG, et al. Intrauterine manometry: technique and application to fetal pathology. Prenat Diagn 1989;9:243–254.

76. Redwine F, Petres RE. Fetal surgery: past, present and future. Clin Perinatol 1983; 10:399–409.

77. Schmidt W, Harms E, Wolf D. Successful prenatal treatment of nonimmune hydrops fetalis due to congenital chylothorax. Br J Obstet Gynaecol 1985;92:685–687.

78. Kurjak A, Rajhvajn B, Kogler A, Gogolja D. Ultrasound diagnosis and fetal malformations of surgical interest. In: Kurjak A, ed. The fetus as a patient. Amsterdam: Excerpta Medica, 1985.

79. King PA, Ghosh A, Tang MHY, Lam SK. Recurrent congenital chylothorax. Prenat Diagn 1991;11:809–811.

80. Meizner I, Carmi R, Bar-ziv J. Congenital chylothorax — prenatal ultrasonic diagnosis and successful postpartum management. Prenat Diagn 1986;6:217–221.
81. Harrison MR, Bressack MA, Churg AM, de Lorimer AA. Correction of congenital diaphragmatic hernia in utero. II. Simulated correction permits fetal lung growth with survival at birth. Surgery 1980;88:260–268.
82. Seeds JW, Bowes WA. Results of treatment of severe fetal hydrothorax with bilateral pleuroamniotic catheters. Obstet Gynecol 1986;68:577–580.
83. Clark SL, Vitale DJ, Minton SD, Stoddard RA, Sabey PL. Successful fetal therapy for cystic adenomatoid malformation associated with second-trimester hydrops. Am J Obstet Gynecol 1987;157:294–295.
84. Blott M, Nicolaides KH, Greenough A. Pleuroamniotic shunting for decompression of fetal pleural effusions. Obstet Gynecol 1987;71:798–800.
85. Rodeck CH, Nicolaides KH. Ultrasound-guided invasive procedures in obstetrics. Clin Obstet Gynecol 1983;10:515–539.

MANAGEMENT OF FETAL CARDIAC DYSRHYTHMIAS

ROBERT J. CARPENTER, Jr.
STEVEN EDMONDSON
NANCY AYRES

9

The advent of ultrasound, which has allowed prenatal diagnosis to flourish and which has provided for the reality of intervention into the fetal milieu, has progressed rapidly in the past 10 years. From an observational platform to a tool directing invasive procedures for therapy and diagnosis, ultrasound has become the mainstay of the perinatologist as well as the general obstetrician. Ultrasound technology in its various modes—two-dimensional (2-D), M-mode, and Doppler—has been applied to the fetal heart as it has to the neonate (1,2). Three-dimensional (3-D) computer imaging of the fetus using super computers to allow rotational viewing and selection of any desired plane of imaging, is now in development (3).

One area of physiology frequently heard by the expectant mother as well as by her care givers is that of fetal cardiac arrhythmias. This chapter will address in a concise way the problems and information which can be imparted to the often worried mother, who along with her obstetrician first hears these arrhythmias.

FORMS OF ARRHYTHMIA

Cardiac arrhythmias can be divided into three basic types, with different potentials for outcome, and different requirements for evaluation. These are atrial and ventricular extrasystoles, supraventricular tachycardia, and atrioventricular (AV) block. The arrhythmias can be heard commonly as either an isolated ectopic beat with infrequent recurrence, or as a regularly recurring rhythm such as a bigeminal or trigeminal pattern with long periods of intervening normal sinus rhythm.

Since it is beyond the scope of this chapter to present the methods of echocardiographic (structural) assessment, the interested reader is referred to other sources for detailed information. With utilization of either M-mode or Doppler echocardiographic techniques, accurate delineation of the source of the disturbance can be ascertained (4-13).

Extrasystoles

Extrasystoles [premature atrial contractions (PAC) or premature ventricular contractions (PVC)] appear to be the most frequent rhythm disturbance in the human fetus (Table 9-1). The most common of these are *isolated extrasystoles*. Kleinman found 85% of his 452 patients to represent this type of arrhythmia (14). Of these 452 fetuses with a rhythm disturbance evaluated at Yale University, 385 has isolated premature beats, with 87% being supra-ventricular in origin.

An extrasystole is defined as an early (premature) beat. It is supra-ventricular if it has a p wave (atrial contraction) in front, if not, it is classified as ventricular (15). From a physiologic viewpoint, isolated extrasystoles do not result in compromised cardiac function. Reed (9) demonstrated an increase in fractional shortening following a prema-

Table 9-1   Types of Arrhythmia

	Number	%
Isolated extrasystoles	385	85.0
Supraventricular tachycardia	34	7.6
Atrial flutters/fibrillation	9	2.0
Ventricular tachycardia	3	0.7
Sinus tachycardia	2	0.4
Complete heartblock	13	2.9
Second degree AV block	2	0.4
Sinus bradycardia	4	0.9
	452	99.9%

(Modified from: Kleinmann and Copel 1989 (14) with permission from WB Saunders Company.)

ture systole, with a 49% increase in the right ventricle and a 64% increase in the left ventricle. Fractional shortening is defined as the end-diastolic dimension minus the end-systolic dimension divided by the end-diastolic dimension or

$$\% = \frac{EDD\text{-}ESD}{EDD}.$$

This postextrasystolic potentiation results from the increased diastolic dimensions occurring as a consequence of a longer diastole following an extrasystole, with subsequent augmentation of ventricular volume.

Premature systoles may be noted by either M-mode or with pulsed Doppler echocardiography. When using M-mode echocardiography, the optimal image is obtained with the cursor simultaneously passing through the atrial wall and ventricular wall (Figure 9-1). By doing so, one can simultaneously visualize the mechanical results (wall motion) of the electrical event. A non-conducted PAC is reflected in M-mode sampling at the aortic outflow tract by absence of aortic flow following the premature atrial systole. Figure 9-2 reflects this phenomenon. This image is not always techni-

cally possible to obtain; however, Doppler velocities may be simpler to obtain. The Doppler sample can be obtained in the left ventricle below the atrioventricular valve annulus, maintaining the continuity of the mitral and aortic valves, and, thus, the atrioventricular contraction sequence can be determined. A Doppler velocity of an isolated premature contraction shows an early systolic flow followed by prolonged mitral inflow. No ventricular systolic flow followed the early systole (4) (Figure 9-3).

Isolated extrasystoles are generally benign and yield a favorable prognosis. The majority of fetuses with premature systoles will have spontaneous resolution before delivery and those that persist in the neonate usually resolve within the first six weeks of life (7,9). However, these premature beats are rarely harbingers of more complex arrhythmias. In an analysis of 71 fetuses with arrhythmias (7), one fetus was first noted to have supraventricular ectopic beats in a bigeminal pattern with short (three to four beat) runs of tachycardia and subsequently developed a sustained tachycardia. In another, Kleinman noted three patients to have progression to a supraventricular

Figure 9-1 A premature atrial contraction (PAC) is demonstrated by M-mode echocardiographic tracing. The atrial (black arrow) to ventricular (white arrow) sequence of contraction is demonstrated. The PAC is an early atrial contraction conducted to the ventricle. (RA=right atrium, LV=left ventricle).

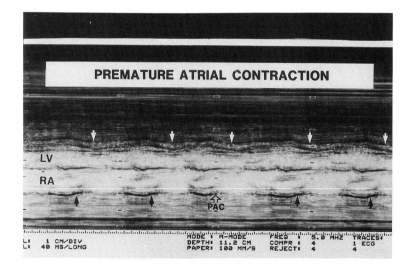

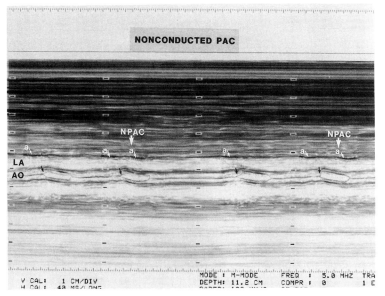

Figure 9-2 A nonconducted premature atrial contraction (NPAC) is demonstrated by M-mode. The aortic valve (AO) opening (black arrow) indicates ventricular contraction. A PAC occurs immediately following the second and fourth sinus beat but fails to conduct to the ventricle; thus, the aortic valve remains closed following an NPAC. The atrial contraction (a) is demonstrated by the white arrow. (LA = left atrium.)

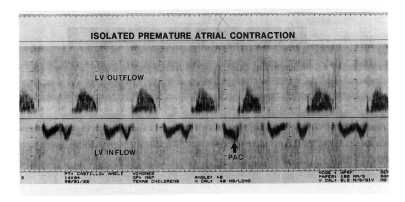

Figure 9-3 Doppler tracing demonstrates atrial systole by the left ventricular (LV) inflow and ventricular systole by LV outflow. The sample volume is in the LV outflow tract. The fourth atrial beat is a premature atrial contraction (PAC) conducted to the ventricle. The post-PAC beat demonstrates prolongation of passive atrial filling or ventricular diastole.

tachycardia (SVT). Most other reports of fetuses with premature systoles have shown that none of these patients developed tachycardia or intrauterine cardiac failure, and there were no mortalities (15,16). In our own series of over 200 patients with isolated extrasystoles, no fetus has progressed to develop SVT.

Evaluation of the fetus with suspected extrasystoles should include real-time sonography to exclude any structural cardiac defects. M-mode or pulsed Doppler can be utilized to characterize the arrhythmia. Both modalities have similar capacity for identification of the arrhythmia. Once extrasystoles are identified, the mother should be counselled to reduce/cease intake of caffeine- and nicotine-containing products, although there is no absolute evidence that these substances ingested by the mother directly contribute to fetal cardiac arrhythmias. One should consider periodic electronic fetal monitoring to uncover those rare cases that may lead to a sustained tachycardia, especially with the fetus that exhibits bigeminy or trigeminy. Optimal management of these patients can be performed by the primary obstetrical caregiver. Given the 1% potential incidence of SVT, current recommendations for surveillance are at least weekly or, preferably, twice weekly Doppler auscultation (office device) to rule out development of SVT. Since the vast majority of these are benign occurrences with an uncomplicated outcome, this information should be conveyed to the parents early in the evaluation to decrease unnecessary anxiety.

Supraventricular Tachycardia

Supraventricular tachycardia is an arrhythmia that is often seen with rates between 220 to 300 beats per minute. The sole determinant of the ventricular rate is the atrial rate (5). SVT may occur intermittently (paroxysmal) or it may be sustained. SVT most frequently arises secondary to an AV re-entry mechanism (17–18). SVT may also arise from a supraventricular ectopic focus due to abnormal automaticity of the myocardium itself. Fetal electrolyte or acid-base abnormalities may potentiate automaticity. Cardiac rhabdomyomas associated with tuberous sclerosis have resulted in cardiac tachyarrhythmias attributable to accessory conductive pathways (5). Congenital heart disease may accompany 5-10% of those with SVT (19). The most difficult fetal arrhythmias to treat are those shown postdelivery by ECG recordings to have frequent or multifocal ectopy.

The major physiologic consequence of SVT in the fetus is cardiac failure leading to nonimmune hydrops and death in utero. The ventricular compliance in the fetus is reduced (20), and when superimposed upon a rapid rate, reduction in ventricular compliance will preclude adequate ventricular

filling and, thus, contribute to cardiac failure. Wladimiroff (21) reported vascular data obtained during a fetal tachyarrhythmia and compared the findings to those found during normal sinus rhythm. He found that left ventricular stroke volume fell from 3.2±0.2 ml to 0.9±ml and that left ventricular output fell from 414±18.6 ml/min to 227±16.4 ml/min. Left ventricular ejection fraction dropped from 47% to 11%. He also noted a decline in peak flow velocity to 26.1±1.5 cm/s from 64±2.8 cm/s. Thus, a vicious cycle of increased atrial volume and increased atrial pressure allow for increased venous pressure that is transmitted to the hepatic venous bed; ascites and generalized hydrops fetalis result. We have observed both development of ascites and its resolution within 48–72 hours of sustained tachycardia. In the fetal lamb, Gest (22) and colleagues have observed the development of ascites within eight hours of artificially pacing to rates of 240 BPM. Resolution of generalized hydrops requires a much longer period. Thus, it is likely that many cases of fetal death in utero where non-immune hydrops is seen may be related to acute development of SVT that progresses to its end stage without recognition and intervention.

In 1988, Zales (23) compared electrophysiologic features in fetuses with in utero failure and neonates who developed cardiac failure postnatally. He found that the mean cycle length (beat-beat) was 243 ms (247 BPM) for fetuses with congestive heart failure (CHF) in utero compared to 208 ms (288 BPM) for those with postnatal failure. These findings imply a slower rate in those who develop in utero CHF compared to neonates who develop CHF from sustained SVT episodes with relatively short cycle lengths (fast heart rates). These findings are consistent with the parasympathetic predominance that is seen in the fetus. The most detrimental effect on cardiac function during a tachyarrhythmia will occur when atrial systole occurs superimposed on ventricular systole, i.e., when atria attempt to pump blood against a closed AV valve (24). This mechanism may account for the development of failure in utero despite the "slower" rates that occur.

Accurate characterization of SVT requires evaluation of atrial and ventricular activity. This can be accomplished with either M-mode or Doppler echocardiography. Both modalities are similar in their capacity for identifying cardiac arrhythmias. However, with Doppler echocardiography, it may be technically simpler to obtain an interpretable flow pattern and determine the sequence of atrial and ventricular contractions (Figure 9-4). M-mode image quality may be compromised by such factors as maternal obesity, polyhydramnios, and fetal movement. Further, M-mode relies on the mechanical event of wall motion, and if there is hydrops with dilated cardiac chambers, wall motion may be limited by myocardial dysfunction. Doppler echocardiography may allow for greater ease of obtaining a suitable image for evaluation with the advantage of obtaining additional information regarding valve competency and the functional state of the heart (Figures 9-5,6).

The preterm fetus is best managed with transplacental pharmacologic cardiovesion (25). Digoxin administered to the mother is the first-line drug. Appropriate maternal levels and control of arrhythmia are achieved most rapidly with intravenous (IV) loading doses (0.5–2.0 mg), achieved by an initial IV bolus of 0.5 mg and then 0.25 mg IV for two or more consecutive doses repeated every four hours. The digoxin level should be monitored with the goal of achieving a serum level of 2.0–2.2 ng/ml. Thus, the amount of drug that can be given is limited by maternal tolerance. In a series of seven fetuses with SVT (26), five mothers were given oral digoxin. These fetuses experienced a delay of three to three and a half days until a clinical response was seen. Two mothers received IV digoxin with a clinical response demonstrated in the fetus within 24 hours. In some cases, sequential fetal blood sampling with measurement of digoxin levels has been required as well as

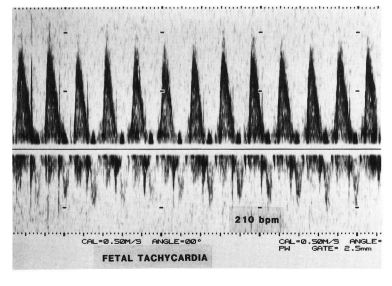

Figure 9-4 Doppler tracing of aortic flow allows accurate determination of the fetal heart rate in a fetus with supraventricular tachycardia (SVT).

Figure 9-5 Doppler aortic flow velocity demonstrates a conducted PAC that precipitates an abrupt onset of SVT at a rate of 210 BPM from the baseline fetal heart rate of 150 BPM.

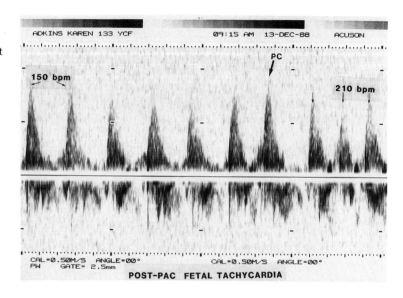

Figure 9-6 M-mode tracing of the right and left ventricles (RV, LV) demonstrates a premature contraction (PC) following a sinus beat (solid black arrow), which results in abrupt onset of tachycardia at 214 BPM.

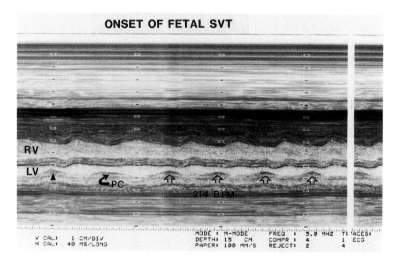

direct intravenous therapy to the fetus. Neither fetal blood sampling nor direct IV therapy to the fetus is considered routine standard of practice.

Oral maintenance therapy can be started after intravenous loading of the mother has been completed. It consists of 0.25–0.75 mg/day with monitoring of maternal serum levels as a guide for further therapy. Alternatively, although rarely required, IV therapy can be continued at a dose of 0.25mg/day. Some patients require doses up to 0.25mg TID to maintain a therapeutic level. Digoxin crosses the placenta with a fetal/maternal ratio of 0.8–1.0, and, therefore, one can anticipate fetal levels to approximate maternal levels. The presence of hydrops may significantly alter the amount of drug that actually crosses the placenta. Fetal drug concentration is directly proportional to the maternal concentration of drug and the surface area of the placenta and inversely proportional to the thickness of the placenta. With hydrops, the placental thickness is greater, and, therefore, less drug may actually cross over to the fetus. Other factors that may influence the placental crossing of a drug include factors that affect passage through membranes, such as (1) lipid solubility, (2) molecular weight of the drug, (3) ionization, and (4) protein binding. Maternal drug concentration, which also influences placental crossing of drugs, is affected by various factors, including intestinal absorption, which may be reduced in pregnancy, the larger volume of distribution that occurs with pregnancy secondary to increases in plasma volume, the decrease in plasma proteins in pregnancy, which results in decreased protein binding, and the increase in glomerular filtration rate, which may result in increased excretion of the drug. Other drugs, like flecanide and the calcium channel-blocker verapamil can increase serum digoxin levels and require a decrease in the dose of digoxin when administered concomitantly (18). Digoxin, however, frequently does not suffice as a sole agent for control of fetal SVT.

Numerous second-line drugs are available; however, verapamil appears to be the most frequently used. Verapamil is administered orally at a dose of 60–80mg TID. Verapamil does not cross the placenta as effectively as digoxin, attaining a cord blood to maternal blood ratio of 0.3–0.4 (fetal levels 30–40% of maternal levels). The effect of this drug is to impede impulse conduction across the atrioventricular node, thus preventing re-entrant supraventricular tachycardia from continuing, or slowing the ventricular rates during primary atrial tachycardia or atrial flutter. Caution must be used when administering this agent as it may result in AV block in the mother

and/or fetus (18). Dysfunctional labor or postpartum hemorrhage have not been encountered in gravidas receiving verapamil. Some centers will discontinue the use of this agent routinely prior to labor (15). However, in our center, once effective blockade has been achieved and suitable physiology restored, we maintain the mother on all drugs that have been required to control the arrhythmias.

Other agents available include propranolol, procainamide, and quinidine (13). Propranolol has had limited success alone or in combination with other agents. The potential for growth impairment and postnatal hypoglycemia have been suggested as reasons for not using this agent. Moreover, the ineffectiveness of propranolol in suppression of fetal tachycardia and the potential reduction in cardiac contractility preclude the use of this agent as a first-line drug. This is especially true in fetuses with dilated ventricles and decreased shortening fraction. Propranolol has several neonatally observed physiologic effects that are purely related to its function as a nonselective beta-receptor antagonist. These include bradycardia, hypoglycemia, hypothermia, and delayed onset of neonatal respiratory activity. Hypoglycemia occurs secondary to blockage of glycogenolysis and gluconeogenesis as well as an inhibition of normal hypoglycemia-induced counterregulatory mechanisms. Hypothermia results from interruption of interscapular brown fat metabolism, which serves as a means of calorigenesis in the immediate neonatal period. Each of these potential effects should be anticipated and the neonate observed/treated following the occurrence of these events. Many fetuses who have therapeutic levels of propranolol do not develop these physiologic changes. Therefore, the fear of this occurrence should not deter the use of propranolol in appropriate situations.

Quinidine results in elevation of serum digoxin levels when used in combination, requiring a halving of the digoxin dosage and careful monitoring of maternal serum levels. Quinidine crosses the placenta with fetal levels approaching maternal levels. Theoretical risks of quinidine use are neonatal thrombocytopenia and fetal eighth-nerve damage. In addition, quinidine may exert an oxytocic effect and potentially initiate labor (20). We have observed this in mothers when this drug has been used in fetuses with recalcitrant SVT.

Many different agents and combinations of agents have been utilized for fetuses with tachyarrhythmias after failed transplacental therapy with first-line agents. Recently, flecanide, an antiarrhythmic with electrophysiologic effects characteristic of Class 1 agents (Vaughn-Williams classification), was given orally in combination with digoxin for the treatment of refractory fetal SVT (27,28). In our center, flecanide is given 100 mg every 12 hours orally. Response is normally seen by the sixth dose, when a stable serum level should be achieved. Others consider flecainide a first-line agent for SVT (29–31). Further study is needed to confirm this experience before it is incorporated as routine therapy.

Reports of sudden death in adults being treated with Class 1C agents have slowed the routine incorporation of these agents as first- or second-line therapy. However, no deaths have been reported in fetuses or neonates being treated for tachyarrhythmias with Class 1C drugs. Most of the adverse effects of these drugs have been reported in individuals with damaged myocardium or in infants with poor ventricular function (32).

In addition to different agents and combinations, different modes of administration to the fetus have been used. Fetal intramuscular, intraperitoneal, and direct fetal vascular therapy (33–37) have been used. These modalities may be useful alternatives in the refractory case or the fetus with hydrops.

Atrial Flutter/Fibrillation

Atrial flutter is a supraventricular arrhythmia with atrial rates of 300–460 BPM and variable degrees of atrioventricular conduction block. Atrial fibrillation represents a more rapid though less organized atrial rate, often greater than 400 BPM and with ventricular rates varying between 120–200 BPM (5).

The hemodynamic consequence of atrial flutter or fibrillation is dependent upon the gestational age at which it occurs and the resulting ventricular response. Rapid ventricular rates are poorly tolerated and cardiac failure may occur. Diagnosis of either flutter or fibrillation can be accomplished with M-mode or Doppler echocardiography. Transplacental pharmacologic cardioversion is the preferred mode of therapy, utilized in the same manner as for SVT. Atrial flutter may carry a more ominous prognosis. Kleinman (18) reported a series of 18 fetuses with supraventricular tachyarrhythmia, four who had atrial flutter/fibrillation. Of three cases with atrial flutter, all had hydrops, and control of the arrhythmia was not achieved with transplacental therapy. Two of the three fetuses died, with the third requiring electrical cardioversion at birth. Atrial fibrillation/flutter may occur in the presence of a cardiomyopathy or thyrotoxicosis.

CLINICAL COURSE

Prognosis for fetuses with a supraventricular tachyarrhythmia depends upon (1) gestational age at the time of diagnosis, (2) the type and duration of the arrhythmia, (3) degree of hemodynamic compromise, (4) presence of any structural defects, and (5) fetal responses to previously attempted in utero therapies. In general, the earlier the gestational age, the more likely is an adverse prognosis. This would seem intuitive when one considers that at earlier gestational ages, ventricular compliance is reduced and there is potential for a prolonged duration for the arrhythmia. Both factors would seem to potentiate the development of in utero cardiac failure and hydrops. Any structural cardiac defects would aggravate this potential for failure by virtue of further alterations in hemodynamic response. Kleinman (7,8) reported that a sustained arrhythmia had an ominous prognosis, particularly when associated with fetal hydrops and/or structural cardiac defects associated with tricuspid or mitral regurgitation. Atrial flutter and atrial fibrillation, when contrasted to SVT, carry a poorer prognosis because of the difficulty in converting these arrhythmias to normal sinus rhythm and the adverse hemodynamics that result from sustained arrhythmias.

In the fetus with a supraventricular tachyarrhythmia, one should look for evidence of structural cardiac defects or evidence of hydrops with real-time sonography. Additionally, it would be beneficial to exclude any maternal thyroid disease and potential thyrotoxicosis. The presence of rhabdomyomas suggests tuberous sclerosis and genetic counselling would be indicated. Likewise, the discovery of structural defects may also warrant chromosomal studies and genetic counselling. Even late in pregnancy, fetal blood sampling or late chorionic villus sampling (CVS) can be used for rapid karyotyping especially if multiple malformations are observed.

The arrhythmia should be classified using M-mode or Doppler echocardiography and, once characterized, treated with transplacental pharmacologic therapy, initially, digoxin. Fetal response can be assessed with real-time sonography and M-mode or Doppler echocardiography. The addition of other agents and dosage adjustments may be necessary. The clinician needs to follow maternal drug levels and maintain a vigilant search for potential maternal toxicity. Delivery is indicated in the term fetus once diagnosed or the near-term fetus when there is worsening failure or therapeutic failure where survival would be enhanced by delivery. The preterm fetus with little potential for extrauterine survival should be aggressively treated in utero. Delivery of the fetus with a tachyarrhythmia should be at a tertiary facility with availability of neonatal and pediatric cardiology support.

CONGENITAL ATRIOVENTRICULAR BLOCK

The third major form of cardiac arrhythmia to be faced by the clinician is AV block in varying forms (12,38,39). In this abnormality, varying degrees of conduction disturbance are noted. The forms of block are divided into first, second, and third degrees.

First degree block is associated with normal heart rate and rhythm and is not identifiable by standard techniques. Therefore, recognition of this benign pattern is not reported for the human fetus. If serendipitously recognized in a fetus who is undergoing Doppler or M-mode evaluation for some other indication, no therapy is required.

Second degree block is subdivided into two distinct forms. The first is Mobitz type I (Wenckebach's phenomenon), which reflects a progressive prolongation of the PR interval until, ultimately, a ventricular response is dropped. The cycle then repeats itself and usually results in hemodynamic stability.

This type of heart block does not require treatment. It may be seen in normal newborns and children.

In Mobitz type II pattern, there is no prolongation of the PR interval preceding the dropped ventricular response. Hemodynamic stability is also present, and it may be difficult to distinguish Mobitz I from Mobitz II by sonographic technique. Advanced AV block (2/1, 3/1, etc.) may be associated with Mobitz II pattern and may imply disease of the His-Purkinje system. Because of the potential for further degree of block resulting in complete AV block, serial cardiac evaluations must be performed to detect the presence of associated cardiac abnormalities and the development of complete AV block.

Third degree (complete) A-V block is frequently seen in the fetus with development of a progressive slowing of heart rate and the potential for onset of congestive heart failure reflected as hydrops fetalis (Figure 9-7). The intrinsic rate of the ventricle is normally 60–65 BPM. We have observed that when rates ≤40 BPM develop, significant AV valve regurgitation develops. AV valve regurgitation has been observed as chamber dilatation occurs. Stretching of the valve an-

nulus results from overdistension of the cardiac chambers as in the development of hydrops in unrecognized or nonresponsive SVT; atrial pressures increase and increased pressure is transmitted to the great veins. In our affected fetuses, heart rate increases from 40 BPM to 44–46 BPM have resulted in reversal of A-V valve regurgitation.

In the largest congenital AV block series published to date, Michaelsson and Engle collected 599 cases of congenital heart block. Structurally normal hearts were seen in 418 infants (70%). Thirty-two of the normal fetuses died (7.6%), whereas 53 of 181 (29%) with structural heart disease died (40).

The incidence of the condition is rare and has been quoted to range from one in 5,000 to as low as one in 22,000 infants. Patients may be asymptomatic with ventricular rates of 50–80 BPM or symptomatic with some degree of congestive heart failure manifested as tachypnea, dyspnea, and peripheral cyanosis in the newborn period. These patients, when recognized in utero, often have associated hydrops fetalis. The degree of hydrops is variable and severity is inversely related to the ventricular rate (41).

Complete AV block has been associated most frequently with either the presence of SSA and SSB (anti-Ro and anti-La) antibod-

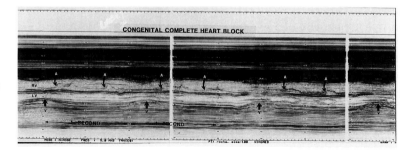

Figure 9-7 M-mode tracing of the left and right ventricles of a fetus with complete heart block. The atrial contraction is demonstrated by the opening of the tricuspid valve (A followed by curved black arrow). The ventricular rate (V black arrow) is independent of atrial contractions. The average ventricular rate is 45 BPM with an average atrial rate of 115 BPM.

ies (45%) or with structural heart disease (55%) (42–44). The antibodies are most frequently seen in patients with collagen vascular diseases, such as systemic lupus erythematosus (SLE) or Sjögren's syndrome. Varying frequencies of antibody presence have been reported (60–80%) and many patients with an affected fetus with AV block are asymptomatic for any signs of SLE or other disorders. Only two of eight patients in our own series have been identified as having some form of collagen vascular disease. This approximates the 30% incidence reported by others (45,46). One of our patients had a previous term stillbirth with hydrops probably related to AV block.

The pathology seen in the AV nodal system is damage to the bundles of His and the Purkinje system. The antibodies attach to and destroy cell nuclei containing two saline-soluble ribonucleoprotein antigens. As a result of the end-stage inflammatory response, normal progression of electrical conduction is interrupted (43). Steroids in pharmacologic amounts have been associated with the reversal of acute inflammatory change and the return to normal heart patterns.

Management of affected fetuses requires frequent auscultation or direct visualization by 2-D echocardiography or standard ultrasound imaging to exclude slow heart rates (below 40 BPM) and development of hydrops fetalis. Doppler evaluation of the AV valves can demonstrate development of trivial, as well as hemodynamically significant, AV valve regurgitation.

If a third trimester fetus is noted to develop progressive slowing of the ventricular rate, delivery in a tertiary center and immediate postnatal temporary transvenous pacing may be required for neonatal survival. These neonates have the potential for long-term, intact survival following placement of permanent pacemakers.

Although a single case of percutaneous transthoracic ventricular pacing has been reported from our center, this technology would not allow for prolonged in utero use to allow for resolution of hydrops and ultimate salvage (48).

A question frequently asked by patients who have collagen vascular diseases of some type and who are known to have SSA or SSB antibodies is, "What is my chance of having a child who develops heart block?" That question is exceedingly difficult to answer because although seen in tertiary care centers, the true denominator of all women who have lupus and who are carrying the antibody who have become pregnant in any year is difficult to acquire. However, a risk figure frequently cited, but poorly documented is approximately 1–2%.

A second question, "What are my chances of having a second child who is similarly affected?," is much easier to answer. The currently accepted recurrence rate is 20% (11).

CONCLUSION

We have tried to provide primary caregivers with information which can be of benefit to them and their patients, in a data base that will be helpful to allay fear and anxiety when physiologic or pathologic disturbances of cardiac electrophysiology occur. We strongly encourage that direct referral be made to a tertiary maternal-fetal or pediatric cardiology unit with interest and experience in dealing with significant cardiac arrhythmias. Prompt evaluation and, when required, therapy, will decrease fetal/neonatal morbidity/mortality.

References

1. Romero R, Pilu G, Jeanty P, Ghidini A, Hobbins J. The heart. In: Prenatal diagno-

sis of congenital anomalies. Connecticut: Appleton-Lange, 1988;125–194.

2. Schmidt KG, Silverman NH. The fetus with a cardiac malformation. In: Harrison MR, Golbus MS, Filly RA, eds. The unborn patient: prenatal diagnosis and treatment. 2nd ed. Philadelphia: WB Saunders, 1990;264–294.

3. Pretorius D, Nelson T. Three-dimensional imaging of the human fetus. Presented at 10th meeting of the International Fetal Medicine and Surgery Society, Phoenix, Arizona, June 8, 1991.

4. Cameron A, Nicholson S, Nimrod C, Harper J, Davies D, Fritzler M. Evaluation of fetal cardiac arrhythmias with two dimension M-mode and pulsed Doppler ultrasonography. Am J Obstet Gynecol 1988;158:286–290.

5. Strasburger J, Huhta JC, Carpenter RJ, Garson A, McNamara D. Doppler echocardiography in the diagnosis and management of persistent fetal arrhythmias. J Am Coll Cardiol 1986;7:1386–1391.

6. Morrow WR, Huhta JC. Fetal echocardiography. In: Garson A, Bricker JT, McNamara DG, eds. The science and practice of pediatric cardiology. Philadelphia: Lea & Febiger, 1990;805–827.

7. Kleinman CS, Donnerstein RL, Jaffe CC, DeVore GR, Weinstein EM, Lynch DC, Talner NS, Berkowitz RL, Hobbins JC. Fetal echocardiography a tool for evaluation of in utero cardiac arrhythmias and monitoring of in utero therapy: analysis of 71 patients. Am J Cardiol 1983;51(2):237–243.

8. Kleinman CS, Donnerstein RL, DeVore GR, et al. Fetal echocardiography for evaluation of in utero congestive heart failure. N Engl J Med 1982;306(10):568–576.

9. Reed KL, Sahn OJ, Marx FR, Anderson CF, Shenker L. Cardiac Doppler flows during fetal arrhythmias: physiologic consequences. Obstet Gynecol 1987;70(1):1–6.

10. Huhta JC, Strasburger FJ, Carpenter RJ, Reiter AA, Abinader E. Pulsed Doppler fetal echocardiography. J Clin Ultrasound 1985;13:247–254.

11. Strasburger JF. Fetal arrhythmias. In: Garson A, Bricker JT, McNamara DG, eds. The science and practice of pediatric cardiology. Philadelphia: Lea and Febiger, 1990, 1905–1911.

12. DeVore GR, Silassi B, Platt L. The fetus with cardiac arrhythmias. In: Harrison MR, Golbus MS, Filly RA, eds. The unborn patient: prenatal diagnosis and treatment. 2nd ed. Philadelphia: WB. Saunders, 1990, 249–263.

13. Allan LD, Anderson RH, Sullivan ID, Campbell S, Holt DW, Tynan H. Evaluation of fetal arrhythmias by echocardiography. Br Heart J 1983;50:240–245.

14. Kleinman CS, Copel JA. Fetal cardiac arrhythmias. In: Creasy RK, Resnik R, eds. Maternal-fetal medicine principles and practice. 2nd ed. Philadelphia: WB Saunders, 1989, 344–355.

15. Allan LD, Crawford DC, Anderson RH, Tynan M. Evaluation and treatment of fetal arrhythmias. Clin Cardiol 1984; 7:467–473.

16. Komaromy B, Gaal J, Lampe L. Fetal arrhythmia during pregnancy and labor. Br J Obstet Gynaecol 1977;84:492.

17. Romero R, Pilu G, Jeanty P, Ghidini A, Hobbins J. The heart (supraventricular tachyarrhythmias). In: Prenatal diagnosis of congenital anomalies. Connecticut: Appleton-Lange, 1988, 188–192.

18. Kleinman CS, Copel JA, Weinstein EM, Santulli TV, Hobbins JC. Treatment of fetal supraventricular tachyarrhythmias. J Clin Ultrasound 1985;13:265–273.

19. Garson A Jr. Supraventricular tachycardia. In: Gillette PC, Garson A, Jr., eds, Pediatric arrhythmia; electrophysiology and pacing. Philadelphia: WB Saunders, 1990, 383–388.

20. Reed KL, Sahn DJ, Scagnelli S, Anderson CF, Shenker L. Doppler echocardiographic studies of diastolic function in the human fetal heart: changes during gestation. J Am Coll Cardiol 1986;8:391–395.

21. Wladimiroff JW, Struyk P, Stewart PA, Clusters P, DeVilleneuve VH. Fetal cardiovascular dynamics during cardiac arrhythmia. Case report. Br J Obstet Gynaecol 1983;90:573–577.

22. Gest AL, Hansen TN, Moise AA, Hartley CJ. Atrial tachycardia causes hydrops in fe-

tal lambs. Am J Physiol 1990;258(27): H1159–1163.

23. Zales VR, Dunnigan A, Benson W Jr. Clinical and electrophysiologic features of fetal and neonatal paroxysmal atrial tachycardia resulting in congestive heart failure. Am J Cardiol 1988; 62:225–228.

24. Naito M, David D, Michelson EL, Schaffenberg M, Dreifus LA. The hemodynamic consequences of cardiac arrhythmias: evaluation of the relative roles of abnormal atrioventricular sequencing, irregularity of ventricular rhythmias, and atriofibrillation in a canine model. Am Heart J 1983; 106:284–291.

25. Shenker L. Fetal cardiac arrhythmias. Obstet Gynecol Survey 1979;34(8):561–572.

26. Wiggins JW, Bowes W, Clewell W, et al. Echocardiographic diagnosis and intravenous digoxin management of fetal tachyarrhythmias and congestive heart failure. Am J Dis Child 1986;140:202–204.

27. Perry JC, Ayres NA, Carpenter RJ Jr. Fetal supraventricular tachycardia treated with flecainide acetate. J Pediatrics 1991; 118(2):303–305.

28. Wren C, Hunter S. Maternal administration of flecainide to terminate and suppress fetal tachycardia. Br Med J 1988;296:249.

29. Maxwell DJ, Crawford DC, Curry PVM, Tynan MJ, Allan LD. Obstetric importance, diagnosis, and management of fetal tachycardias. Br Med J 1988,297:107–110.

30. Allan LD, Chita SK, Sharland GK, Maxwell D, Priestly K. Flecainide in the treatment of fetal tachycardia. Br Heart J 1991;65:46–48.

31. Macphail S, Walkinshaw SA. Fetal supraventricular tachycardia: detecting by routine auscultation and successful in utero management: case report. Br J Obstet Gynaecol 1988;95:1073–1076.

32. The Cardiac Arrhythmia Pilot Study (CAPS) Investigators. Effects of encainide, flecainide, imipramine, and moricizine on ventricular arrhythmias during the year after acute myocardial infarction: the CAPS. Am J Cardiol 1988;61:501–509.

33. Gembruch U, Hansmann M, Redel D, Bald R. Intrauterine therapy of fetal ar-

rhythmias: intraperitoneal administration of antiarrhythmic drugs to the fetus in fetal tachyarrhythmias with severe hydrops fetalis. J Perinat Med 1988;16: 39–42.

34. Weiner CP, Thompson MIB. Direct treatment of fetal supraventricular tachycardia after failed transplacental therapy. Am J Obstet Gynecol 1988;158:570–573.

35. Gembruch U, Manz M, Bald R, et al. Repeated intravascular treatment with amiodrarone in a fetus with refractory supraventricular tachycardia and hydrops fetalis. Am Heart J 1989;118(6):1335–1338.

36. Spinnato JA, Shaver DC, Flinn GS, Sibai B, Watson D, Marin-Garcia J. Fetal supraventricular tachycardia: in utero therapy with digoxin and quinidine. Obstet Gynecol 1984;65:730.

37. Gembruch U, Hansmann M, Bald R. Direct intrauterine fetal treatment of fetal tachyarrhythmia with severe hydrops fetalis by antiarrhythmic drugs. Fetal Ther 1988; 3:210–215.

38. Romero R, Pilu G, Jeanty P, Ghidini A, Hobbins J. The heart (atrioventricular block). In: Prenatal Diagnosis of Congenital Anomalies. Connecticut: Appleton-Lange, 1988, 192–194.

39. Truccone NJ, Mariona FG. Prenatal diagnosis and outcome of congenital complete heart block: the role of fetal echocardiography. Fetal Ther 1986;1:210–216.

40. Michaelsson M, Engle MA. Congenital complete heart block: an internal study of the natural history. Cardiovasc Clin 1972;4(3):85–101.

41. Rowe RD, Freedom RM, Mehrizi A, Bloom KR. The neonate with congenital heart disease. 2nd ed. Philadelphia: W.B. Saunders, 1981, 545–561.

42. Scott JS, Maddison PJ, Taylor PV, et al. Connective tissue disease, antibodies to ribonucleoprotein and congenital heart block. N Engl J Med 1983;309:209–212.

43. Taylor PV, Scott JS, Gerlis LM, et al. Maternal antibodies against fetal cardiac antigens in congenital complete heart block. N Engl J Med 1986;315:667–672.

44. McCue CM, Mantakas ME, Tingelstad JB, Ruddy S. Congenital heart block in newborns of mothers with connective tissue disease. Circulation 1977;56:82–90.

45. Kasinath BS, Katz AI. Delayed maternal lupus after delivery of offspring with congenital heart block. Arch Intern Med 1982; 142:2317.

46. Chameides L, Truex RC, Vetter V, Rashkind WJ, Galioto FM, Noonan JA. Association of maternal systemic erythematosus with congenital complete heart block. N Engl J Med 1977;297(22):1204–1207.

47. Sher MR. Rheumatic disorders. In: Taeusch HW, Ballard RA, Avery ME, eds. Diseases of the newborn. 6th ed. Philadelphia: WB. Saunders, 1990, 828–832.

48. Carpenter RJ, Strasburger JF, Garson A, Smith RT, Deter RL, Engelhardt HT. Fetal ventricular pacing for hydrops secondary to complete atrioventricular block. J Am Coll Cardiol 1986;8(6):1434–1436.

TREATMENT OF URINARY TRACT AND CNS OBSTRUCTION

10

HASSAN ALBAR
FRANK A. MANNING
C.R. HARMAN

Fetal obstructive uropathy and fetal obstructive hydrocephalus are both due to obstruction of fluid flow, leading to progressive increase in intraluminal pressure. Resulting compression will lead to destruction and atrophy of surrounding tissues, or even complete loss of organ function, with the corresponding perinatal mortality, or severe handicap with lifelong impact.

Diversion of flow around such obstructions has been tested experimentally and attempted in human subjects, in both conditions. In utero treatment of fetal obstructive uropathy has proven successful in properly selected fetuses. In utero treatment of fetal obstructive hydrocephalus, on the other hand, has been disappointing: despite technically successful in utero treatment as fetuses, these children ultimately showed intellectual and neuromuscular performance no different from untreated subjects. As a result, in utero treatment of fetal hydrocephalus is seldom proposed.

Major emphasis, therefore, will be placed on fetal obstructive uropathy, as an example of the evolution which has transpired in fetal surgery in the last decade. Careful study of the natural history of this group of disorders, the evaluation of in utero treatments and a management plan for obstructive uropathy are reviewed. The updated International Fetal Surgery Registry provides valuable multi-center reference in assessing the practice of these techniques.

RELEVANT EMBRYOLOGY

The kidney and ureter originate from the intermediate mesoderm, while the urinary bladder and urethra originate from the urogenital sinus (1). Theoretically, three different stages of kidney development could be recognized—the transient pronephros and mesonephros stages, which are replaced by the permanent metanephros early in the fifth week of gestation, by simultaneous differentiation of the metanephric diverticulum (ureteric bud), and the metanephric mesoderm (metanephric blastema) (1). The ureteric bud grows into the metanephric blastema and the two tissues induce growth and differentiation of each other (2–4).

The stalk of the ureteric bud forms the ureter, while the actively dividing ampulla forms the renal pelvis, major and minor calyces, and collective tubules. By eight weeks gestation, the ampulla extends into the metanephric mesoderm, inducing nephrogenesis and establishing communication with the new nephrons. New nephron formation continues until 34–36 weeks of gestation; by that time, each kidney contains approximately one million nephron units. With premature delivery (before the full complement of glomeruli has developed), nephrogenesis continues postnatally until the child reaches a constitutional age of 35–36 weeks. Once complete, nephrogenesis never resumes (4,5).

Urine production starts around 9–11 weeks gestation (Figure 10-1). Urine flow to the bladder through patent ureters has a low pressure profile. If there is outflow obstruction, elevated pressure will be transmitted back to the renal tubules, which are short and straight, transferring the high pressure to the renal parenchyma and damaging the newly-formed nephrons. If total obstruction of urine flow occurs before 20 weeks gestation, renal dysplasia is inevitable (6–8).

Embryology of Urinary Bladder and Urethra

From the fifth to sixth week of gestation, the cloacal septum grows caudally to fuse with the cloacal membrane, dividing the primitive cloaca into anterior urogenital sinus and posterior rectum. The anterior por-

Figure 10-1 Transverse sonogram of a male fetus at 10 weeks gestation demonstrating the penis and urinary bladder.

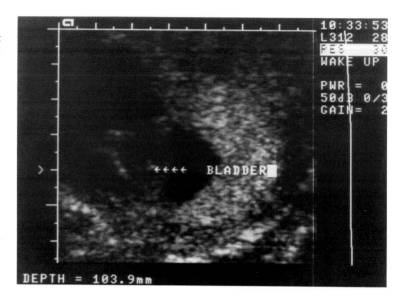

tion of the cloacal membrane becomes the urogenital membrane, which perforates; phallic growth extends this defect. Development of the distal urethra begins by formation of the urethral folds, which fuse in the midline from superior to inferior. The wolffian duct is incorporated into the urethral wall of the septum forming Müller's tubercle. In the male, the portion of the urogenital sinus proximal to Müller's tubercle becomes the prostatic urethra. The remaining distal portion of the urogenital sinus develops longitudinal ridges (the urethrovaginal folds) in its lateral walls. The cranial vestiges of the urethrovaginal folds remain as plicae colliculi, migrating laterally by lateral growth and by fusion of the bulbous and cavernous portion of the urethra (9).

There is no doubt that "valves," or tissue flaps, on the posterior urethra are congenital in origin, but the relevant embryology is still controversial (10). Young's classification in 1919 (11) was based on autopsy findings and divided posterior urethral valves (PUV) into three types (Figure 10-2).

Type I Valve

This most common PUV consists of sails or exaggerated plicae colliculi in pairs, which extend distally and laterally from either side of the verumontanum to the dorsal lateral walls of the urethra (9). Stephen et al. (12,13) suggest Type I valves result from the abnormal origin of wolffian ducts in the cloaca, leaving crescent-shaped remnants along their path of migration to the final site at the verumontanum, while King concluded that they are "probably caused by anterior fusion of the urethrovaginal folds perhaps with an abnormal insertion into the verumontanum or maybe due to failure of Cowper's gland migration" (9).

Type II Valve

According to Young's classification, Type II valves are folds that extend longitudinally from the verumontanum proximally toward the bladder neck in the floor of the posterior urethra, where they divide into fin-like membranes. Anatomical position and longitudinal orientation make it very

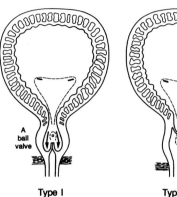
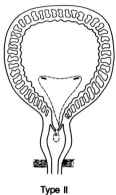
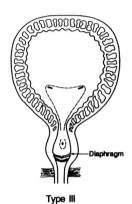

Type I   Type II   Type III

Figure 10-2 Young's classification of posterior urethral valves.

unlikely that Type II valves cause significant obstruction of urine flow (9,13). Their appearance in autopsy specimens is very rare.

Type III Valve

The type III valve is a transverse membrane that varies in consistency from thin to extremely thick, with a central perforation of varying aperture. It lies perpendicular to the long axis of the urethra, usually just distal to the verumontanum, but not attached to it. Type III valves may represent persistence of the urogenital membrane (12), i.e., perforation of the urogenital membrane is not complete, and it persists as a diaphragm-like membrane, proximal to the normally growing phallus and distal urethra (9–13).

Variation in the type and character of posterior urethral valves may explain the corresponding variety of clinical observations. Spontaneous fetal resolution of low-level obstructive uropathy; permanent correction by a single intrauterine percutaneous drainage of the fetal urinary bladder; fetuses with fixed, significant low-level obstruction, who then void spontaneously postnatally (possibly as a result of rupturing of the thin membrane valve); intermittent obstruction relieved by progressive bladder hypertrophy and the concomitant elevation

in intracystic pressures; narrowing/closure of a marginal orifice or no orifice at all in a Type III valve yielding classical PUV ultrasound findings: all reflect the embryologic variants (14–16).

Experimental Pathophysiology

Current understanding of the pathogenesis of obstructive uropathy and its sequelae, though not complete, provides a rational basis for consideration of fetal urinary diversion therapy. The evolution and development of experimental pathophysiology can be divided into four phases.

Phase One

The causal relationship between simple ureteral obstruction and the development of renal dysplasia was examined. The innovative work of the urologist David Beck (1970) demonstrated that ureteral ligation late in pregnancy in fetal sheep at >80 days gestation (22 weeks human equivalent), produced simple hydronephrosis, while earlier obstruction (60 days, 16 weeks human equivalent) produced histopathological changes highly suggestive of renal dysplasia (8).

Ureteral ligation at 70–75 days of gestation, produces renal tubular and ureteropelvic junction dilation as early as two weeks after obstruction. Changes progress until term, resulting in massive hydronephrosis with glomerular degeneration but without renal dysplasia in fetal sheep (17–19). A clear relationship between ureteral obstruction and renal dysplasia was controversial until 1983, when Harrison's group added strong support to Beck's observation. Unilateral ureteral ligation at 58–60 days gestation produced severe hydronephrosis, with histological changes resembling the dysplastic changes seen in human obstructive uropathy on the affected side (20).

Even though the fetal lamb model was more frequently used than other animal models, rabbit (21), chick embryo (22) and opossum models have also been used (23). The opossum kidney is stated to be typically mammalian, histologically resembling the human kidney. Steinhardt et al. performed unilateral ureteral ligation on a young pouch opossum at an early stage of development equivalent to a 16–18-week-old fetus. The obstructed kidneys clearly demonstrated massive hydronephrosis with histological changes typical for renal dysplasia (23). Even though there are differences between the human fetal kidney and the animal model, most of the experimental evidence, supported with our clinical observations, strongly supports a causal relationship between simple ureteral obstruction early in pregnancy and the subsequent development of renal dysplasia (24).

Phase Two

Experimental pathophysiology examined the functional and histopathologic effects of decompression of the ureter after different durations of early second-trimester ligation (25). Unilateral ureteral obstruction in early second-trimester fetal lambs (62–65 days, 16–17 weeks human equivalent) produced

unequivocal ipsilateral renal dysplasia in all controls. In the treated subjects, unilateral ureteral ligation was followed by intrauterine decompression of the obstructed kidney by cutaneous end-ureterostomy after different intervals (20, 40, and 60 days).

Both the gestation of onset and the duration of obstruction are critical in producing renal dysplasia. While early ureteral obstruction can cause renal dysplasia, subsequent ureteral decompression prior to term prevents renal dysplasia. Recovery of renal function was directly proportional to the duration of in utero decompression and inversely proportional to the duration of obstruction (26). These are landmark experiments since they provide a rational basis for consideration of in utero urinary diversion therapy in the affected human fetus (24,27).

Phase Three

The next series of experimental steps examined renal and pulmonary sequelae of bladder outlet obstruction, paralleling the clinical problems of severe posterior urethral valves (PUV). (Initially, there was difficulty in developing a satisfactory model: ligation of the urethra in fetal lambs spontaneously decompresses via urachus fistula (17–19); ligation of both urethra and urachus produces severe disease with high fetal mortality, rendering the experiment costly and inconclusive (28). A comparable fetal sheep model was eventually achieved by ligating the urachus and occluding the urethra with an aneroid constrictor.) The animal was born nonviable because of pulmonary hypoplasia and had severe bilateral hydronephrosis, hydroureter, and markedly dilated bladder. There was no evidence of renal dysplasia, but this is not surprising because urethral ligation was performed in the third trimester (28). A similar model was recently developed with urethral ligation early in the second trimester;

both renal dysplasia and immature lung hypoplasia were demonstrated (24,29).

Phase Four

These questions were addressed: (1) Are the renal pathologic changes due to bladder outlet obstruction preventable by in utero decompression? (2) How does urinary tract obstruction produce pulmonary hypoplasia? (3) Is pulmonary hypoplasia reversible by in utero decompression?

With urachal ligation and urethral occlusion at 93–107 days gestation, some of the obstructed fetuses underwent suprapubic cystostomy at a second operation about three weeks later (25). Obstructed, decompressed, and control lambs were compared. Uncorrected obstruction produced severe dilation of the urinary tract with urinary ascites as well as severe pulmonary hypoplasia, similar to severe posterior urethral valve obstruction in the human fetus. All obstructed lambs did poorly; those that did not die in utero died immediately after birth despite intensive resuscitation, due to respiratory insufficiency from pulmonary hypoplasia. Autopsy showed small hypoplastic lungs, markedly dilated urinary tract, and (as expected with such relatively late obstruction), no evidence of renal dysplasia. The decompressed lambs did far better; they had less respiratory difficulty and less urinary tract dilation and all survived (7,25).

The exact etiology of pulmonary hypoplasia is still unknown; it is most likely multifactorial (24). Simple mechanical compression of the developing lungs plays a major role in the development of lung hypoplasia. Direct lung compression may occur with space-occupying intrathoracic lesions, such as bilateral pulmonary effusions (see Chapter 8), bronchopulmonary cysts, aberrant lung development (pulmonary sequestration, hamartoma, or adenomatous hyperplasia), or intrathoracic abdominal organs via congenital diaphragmatic hernia. Indirect lung compression across intact diaphragms may produce the pulmonary hypoplasia seen with massive early ascites (usually of lymphatic obstructive nature), abdominal tumors, massive hydronephrosis, and so on.

It is widely accepted that oligohydramnios is associated with deficient pulmonary and thoracic development. Lack of fetal micturition (as in cases of severe progressive renal dysplasia), absent urine production (renal agenesis) (30), or chronic oligohydramnios (mid-trimester premature rupture of membranes) (31), are all associated with lethal pulmonary hypoplasia. The mechanism of this association is unknown. In longstanding amniotic fluid loss from early premature rupture of membranes, the principal effect is likely through restriction of growth by confinement within a small, tight intrauterine cavity—the relative contributions of "crushed chest" and pulmonary hypoplasia may vary. In renal agenesis, it has been suggested that not only the presence of restriction but also the absence of some (renal) factor necessary for lung development may be responsible. In either situation, the classical Potter's phenotype may be seen, including the flattened face, hypoplastic nose and jaw, dolichocephaly, small triangular inferior-flared rib cage, scaphoid abdomen, and severe joint restriction flexure deformities of virtually all fetal joints. Severe extrinsic chest compression may interfere with the breathing movements necessary for lung maturation (32–34) and may accelerate fetal lung fluid loss with consequent decrease in volume within the potential airway and abrogation of the growth stimulus. Replacement of amniotic fluid, whether by urinary diversion or repeated installations of normal saline, or more complex artificial amniotic fluid may prevent pulmonary hypoplasia (32). Finally, absolute obstruction by PUV would be expected to produce pulmonary hypoplasia by both mechanisms, the massive bladder pressing the diaphragm as high as the fifth ribs and the total oligohydramnios producing a crushed fetal chest.

Experimental fetal bladder outlet obstruction causing oligohydramnios in early second-trimester fetal lambs causes severe pulmonary hypoplasia very similar to that seen in the human fetus with severe posterior urethral valves. Early third-trimester urinary diversion resulted in less severe renal damage, an increase in lung size, and more mature lung morphology. While there may be interspecies differences, the reversal of oligohydramnios and improvement in the lung morphology, ultimately with survival of the animal subject, strongly support the argument for urinary diversion in the human for prevention of lethal pulmonary changes. With the availability of modern ventilators, artificial surfactant, intensive care nursery (ICN) facilities, and even neonatal ECMO (extracorporeal membrane oxygenation), the prognosis of fetuses with mild to moderate lung hypoplasia may improve dramatically.

Further work is needed in this area to clarify the etiology of lung hypoplasia.

PATHOGENESIS OF FETAL URINARY TRACT OBSTRUCTION

Low-level Obstruction

The true obstructive uropathies in this group are almost always due to one of three conditions: posterior urethral valve, urethral atresia, and persistent cloacal syndrome.

Posterior urethral valve (PUV) syndrome is a disease of the male fetus and results from mucosal fold hypertrophy (Type I) or persistent urogenital membrane (Type III)

with occlusion of the proximal portion of the posterior urethra. Obstruction may be complete or partial, sustained or transient. Failure of canalization of the urethra, in both male and female fetuses is called urethral atresia. Obstruction is always complete; oligohydramnios is the rule. Persistent cloacal syndrome is characterized by the development of a cystic pelvic mass, ambiguous genitalia, progressive hydroureter, and hydronephrosis. In our experience, urachal cyst formation is very common with this condition.

The common pathophysiology of sustained bladder neck outlet obstruction is massive bilateral hydronephrosis, hydroureter, and large, hypertrophied urinary bladder with a dilated proximal urethra.

Progressive accumulation of the urine in the bladder leads to overdistension. Vigorous and repetitive contractions lead to hypertrophy of the detrusor muscles proximal to the obstruction. As intravesicular pressure rises, progressive edema of the urethra and the obstructing valve and hypertrophy of the ureteral sphincter result, rendering the obstruction almost complete. Finally, the elevated intravesicular pressure will be transmitted to the upper urinary system and bilateral hydroureter and hydronephrosis will result.

Spontaneous decompression of the obstructed urinary system may occur at different points, most favorably by rupturing the obstructing posterior urethral valve (most likely Type III valve with a thin diaphragmatic membrane). As a result, spontaneous voiding will occur and total resolution of the obstruction will result (14–16,35). We have followed a fetus with typical features of obstructive uropathy diagnosed early in pregnancy. Repeated ultrasound follow-up showed spontaneous resolution of the obstruction, restoration of normal amniotic fluid volume, and delivery of a normal male fetus. Neonatal exam, including urethrocystoscopy and radiologic studies, failed to document a persistent anatomic cause. Spontaneous decompression through the urachus forming a urachal cyst or fistula has also been reported (14,27,36).

Less favorable is spontaneous bladder rupture with urinary ascites, which does resolve the high pressures in the urinary tract but, obviously, is not effective in restoring amniotic fluid or ameliorating lung/chest compression.

Permanent resolution of bladder outlet obstruction and oligohydramnios after bladder drainage by a single needle aspiration has been reported (15, Fetal Registry). While the exact mechanism of spontaneous resolution of the obstruction after a single needle decompression is unknown, one explanation might be the acuteness of the drop in intravesical pressure. Especially with a Type I posterior urethral valve (anatomically a longitudinal fold of mucosa extend-

ing from the verumontanum to the lateral urethral wall like a V-shaped or ball valve) (Figure 10-3), removing (once) the elevated pressure removes the aggravating factor for obstruction. As the fetus with this defect tries to void, intravesical pressure increases, forcing the urine into the pocket-like valves. The valves may be markedly distended and then become edematous, occluding the urethra. As the fetus becomes older, he may be able to develop greater intravesical pressure during voiding. As intravesical pressure increases, the valves may become more and more distended and the internal sphincter more hypertrophied. As a result, the urethra will be completely occluded. With needle aspiration, "decompression" of the bladder will lead also to decompression of the ball-like valve, resulting in collapse of the valve and loss of edema, allowing a patent urethra and spontaneous voiding.

Unfortunately, this favorable scenario happens only rarely. The usual case is in-

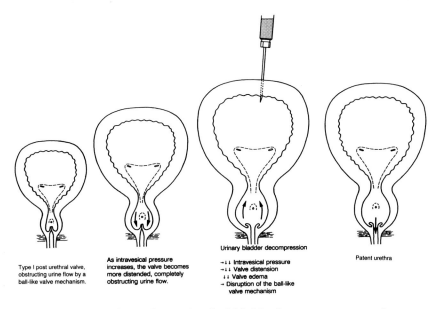

Urinary bladder decompression

Type I post urethral valve, obstructing urine flow by a ball-like valve mechanism.

As intravesical pressure increases, the valve becomes more distended, completely obstructing urine flow.

→↓↓ Intravesical pressure
→↓↓ Valve distension
↓↓ Valve edema
→ Disruption of the ball-like valve mechanism

Patent urethra

Figure 10-3 The mechanism by which bladder decompression may relieve bladder outlet obstruction due to posterior urethral valve.

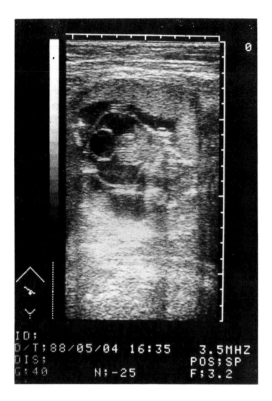

Figure 10-4 Transverse sonogram of the fetal abdomen at 14 weeks demonstrating a distended urinary bladder and urinary ascites.

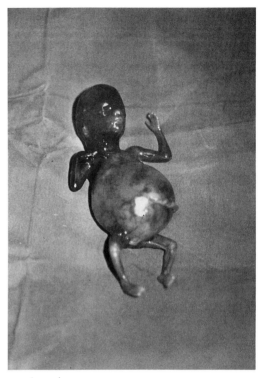

Figure 10-5 Same fetus as in Figure 10-3. The fetus has a prune belly-like syndrome and urinary ascites due to posterior urethral valve.

traperitoneal perforation of the urinary bladder, resulting in urinary ascites and massive abdominal distension (Figures 10-4,5) (37–41). In the majority of cases, the leaking point may not be identified (35,36).

If spontaneous decompression does not occur, intravesicular volume and pressure continue to rise. The urinary bladder dilates, the hypertrophied wall develops sacculation and trabeculation. Later, urinary bladder diverticulae may develop. Progressive bladder distortion leads to disruption of the ureterovesical sphincter and massive ureterovesical reflux. The ureters become tortuous and dilated, and the high back pressure will be transmitted to the kidneys

(often asymmetrically), resulting in sequential hydronephrosis and renal parenchymal atrophy. More important than the anatomic disruption is the functional effect of obstruction on the developing kidneys and lungs. The kidneys always demonstrate hydronephrosis, and the parenchyma is commonly dysplastic. Pressure-atrophy of the kidney may also be seen but probably occurs only when the obstruction becomes severe late in pregnancy (35,42–44).

Renal parenchymal damage is usually more severe on one side than the other, with relative preservation of the renal function in the contralateral kidney. This is most likely due to unequal vesicoureteric reflux favoring one kidney (35,45). This is of clinical importance in the course of urinary chemistry investigation by bladder aspiration. If admixed bladder urine is shown to be abnormal, differential urine chemistry by needle aspiration of each kidney is advisable for complete evaluation of fetal renal function (46).

Consequences of Obstructive Uropathy

The developmental deficiencies of renal and pulmonary structures and functions have been reviewed. Urethral obstruction results in a degree of oligohydramnios that reflects the extent of obstruction. A number of phenotypic changes attributable to oligohydramnios may be seen in the affected newborn. These changes vary in severity in relation to the duration and severity of oligohydramnios. These include Potter's sequelae (Potter's facies, flexion contraction of the extremities) (Figures 10-6,7) and, more importantly, pulmonary hypoplasia (16,47–51), the most common pathway to death of such infants in the neonatal period (52,53).

The natural history of the disease varies according to the onset, duration, grade, and type of urethral obstruction. Complete bladder outlet obstruction due to urethral agenesis/atresia is invariably associated with early onset urinary tract dilation, oligohydramnios, and lethal pulmonary and renal dysplasia. Posterior urethral valves, on the other hand, may produce fetal injury over an extraordinarily wide range of severity. Cases detected in utero are at the worst end of the spectrum. At the opposite end, effects may be so mild as to preclude detection until late in adult life when prostatic hypertrophy aggravates minimal urethral narrowing. The key point in determining the natural history and outcome is the time of onset of urinary tract obstruction and development of oligohydramnios. Because diagnosis and monitoring of human fetuses with obstructive uropathy by ultrasound historically were almost immediately followed by the development of invasive procedures, a detailed chronology of the natural history is not complete. This is critical, for assessment of the benefits of fetal surgery will depend

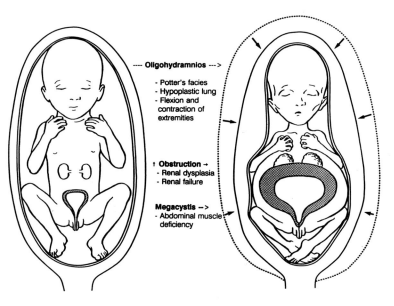

Figure 10-6 Developmental sequelae of fetal bladder outlet obstruction.

---- Oligohydramnios --->

- Potter's facies
- Hypoplastic lung
- Flexion and contraction of extremities

↑ **Obstruction →**
- Renal dysplasia
- Renal failure

Megacystis →
- Abdominal muscle deficiency

Figure 10-7 Postmortem photograph of a neonate with bilateral renal agenesis shows the typical Potter facies.

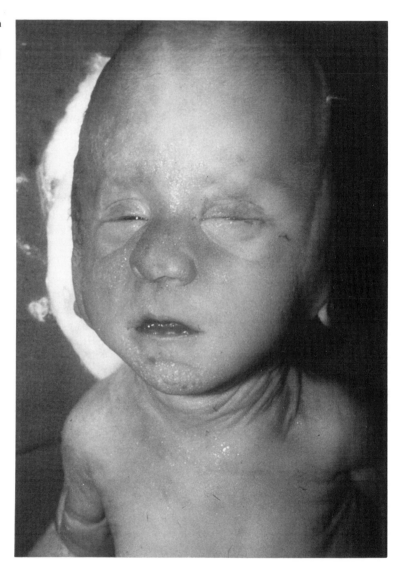

on these answers. However, at least part of the picture in humans is understood.

Persistent absence of renal function in utero as may occur with anatomical defects (renal agenesis) or functional defects (severe renal dysplasia) is frequently associated with fetal death. The mechanism of intrauterine demise has been assumed to be cord compression secondary to absolute

oligohydramnios. What proportion of fetuses present with outlet obstruction in this manner is unknown. Further, what influence, if any, absence of fetal renal function may have on other aspects of fetal homeostasis (electrolyte regulation, blood pressure regulation, erythropoietin production, and so on) is unresearched in humans. The outcome of fetuses with outlet obstruction of either later onset or less severe functional deficit appears to be highly variable. Many of these fetuses will die in utero, again, most likely as a consequence of oligohydramnios, but some will deliver liveborn, often prematurely.

A second critical natural selection process applies in the immediate postnatal period. The successful transition from fetal to neonatal life depends critically on the rapid establishment of adequate pulmonary function. Pulmonary hypoplasia prevents this vital transition in a variety of ways. Hypoxemia, absent lung inflation, high pressure ventilation, unequal lung ventilation/perfusion, difficulty with venous return into the small thoracic cavity, all will contribute to pulmonary vascular instability and the vicious cycle of persistent pulmonary hypertension of the newborn (PPHN). The proportion of liveborns with obstructive uropathy lost immediately at birth as a result of this lethal selection process is again unknown, but from many clinical observations and from reported cases, the proportion is high.

Nagayma et al. (54) described the outcome in 11 liveborn infants with obstructive uropathy (PUV) evident at birth. Five of the 11 (45%) died in the immediate neonatal period of respiratory insufficiency due to pulmonary hypoplasia. The International Fetal Surgery Registry contains 79 reported fetuses with a diagnosis of bladder outlet obstruction, mainly PUV, with severe oligohydramnios, followed by serial ultrasound examination but with no intervention predelivery (Table 10-1). Five out of 79 survived; only two of the five had normal renal function, the other three being in chronic renal failure, awaiting kidney transplants. The mortality rate in severe obstruction without antenatal treatment was 81%, with 49 (62%) neonatal deaths, all due to pulmonary hypoplasia. (In contrast, the neona-

tal mortality rate was only 35% among fetuses treated antenatally—see Table 10-7 for details.)

The prognosis for those who survived the perinatal period improved dramatically, approaching 95% for infants with PUV (55). However, most of those infants who survive the neonatal period have significant morbidity and mortality as a consequence of progressively impaired renal function despite postnatal corrective surgery. Bladder neck obstruction, especially PUV, is easy to repair postnatally; the problem is recovery of normal intra-abdominal anatomy and renal function. Most of the reported series of fetal obstructive uropathy treated in utero categorize fetal management as successful if the baby survives the first few weeks of life (56–59). On the other hand, reports detailing cases where surgical correction was postnatal describe only those who survived natural selection (stillbirth and neonatal death from pulmonary hypoplasia) and presented for surgery late in the neonatal period (60–63). As a result of this selection bias, reported outcome is good, with very low mortality, suggesting the false conclusion that bladder outlet obstruction is a benign condition that can be successfully corrected postnatally. A majority of those fetuses who survived until the time of surgery still have residual renal dysfunction, and 10–20 years later present with end-stage renal disease (64).

It is this spectrum of survival, the definition of successful outcome, and the selection bias that account for the controversy surrounding management of fetal obstructive uropathy. Ideally, in order to study the natural history of this disease and the efficacy of intrauterine treatment, a prospective randomized study should examine not only the course and outcome of the disease but also long-term outcome, end-stage renal disease, and growth and behavior pat-

Table 10-1 Natural History of Low-level Obstructive Uropathy (Bladder Outlet Obstruction with Oligohydramnios)

Author	Total # of Cases	Average GA Dx	Average GA Del.	SB	TA	NND	A&W	Live & Ren. F.	R.D. Isolated	Autopsy P. Hyp. Isolated	Both RD/PH	Chrom. Anomal	Mult. Anomal
J. Hobbins (16)	10	28.2	32.4	—	2	8	—	—	1	—	8	N/A	3
RD Pocock (47)	4	19.5	N/A	—	2	2	—	—	3	—	1	N/A	None
PW Quinlan (48)	8	25	N/A	4	0	4	—	—	2	—	6	None	3
G Noia (49)	12	24	TERM	1	2	5	1	3	6	N/A	N/A	T.21	4
Mahoney (50)	21	24–28	TERM	—	—	20	1	—	N/A	N/A	N/A	N/A	N/A
O Richards (51)	3	18.4	21≤	—	3	—	—	—	—	—	3	N/A	1
A. Reuss (51)	12	20	TERM	1	5	6	—	—	N/A	6	N/A	N/A	5
Fet. Registry (Blackmore & Crane) (52)	4	29	34.5	—	5	4	—	—	N/A	3	1	None	2
	3	18	19	—	3	—	—	—	N/A	N/A	—	1	1
	2	14	15	—	2	—	—	—	1	—	—	N/A	N/A
TOTAL	79			6	19	49	2	3	1			N/A	19

GA = gestational age. SB = stillbirth. TA = therapeutic abortion. NND = neonatal death. A&W = alive and well (variable followup). Ren. F. = renal failure. R.D. = renal dysplasia. P. Hyp. = pulmonary hypoplasia.

tern of those infants managed either way. This kind of study being unavailable, experimental and serendipitous clinical evidence must be collected carefully. Proving that intrauterine treatment of fetal urinary tract obstruction prevents renal and pulmonary sequelae will depend on careful case selection, specifically in the differentiation of those perinates who will die from disease in the fetal and immediate neonatal periods from those perinates who will survive to benefit from postnatal therapy. The secondary challenge is to devise effective therapeutic maneuvers to ensure maximum continued benefit to the selected fetus at minimal risk to the mother.

Ureteropelvic Junction Obstruction

Ureteropelvic junction obstruction (UPJ) is the most common genito-urinary tract lesion, accounting for up to 40% of recognized anomalies of this organ system (16,65). The disease is often unilateral, more commonly left-sided (66–69), and is often associated with anomalies of the contralateral kidney (67), including multicystic dysplastic kidney, renal agenesis, and ectopic kidney. Extrarenal anomalies are infrequent. The disease is more common in males (36). UPJ is of unknown etiology. Several theories have been proposed based on embryological, anatomical, histologic, and functional hypotheses (70,71). The characteristic pathophysiology includes abnormal initiation or propagation of normal peristaltic waves along the ureter, possibly due to immaturity of the pacemaker cells of ureteral smooth muscle. This is commonly associated with moderate bilateral hydronephrosis, with spontaneous resolution in utero or shortly after birth. In most cases, no anatomic narrowing of the ureter can be identified.

The degree of renal parenchymal injury varies with onset, duration, type and sever-

ity of the obstruction. At early onset, complete obstruction will lead to dysplastic changes with or without cystic formation. At later onset, partial or functional obstruction may cause progressive enlargement of the renal pelvis followed by dilation of major and minor calyces but without histological evidence of renal dysplasia. The degree of dilation does not necessarily correlate with postnatal renal functional impairment. Hydronephrosis may progress, regress, or remain the same as pregnancy continues (72–75). However, it seems to be that the degree of renal pelvis dilation (Grades IV–V, more than 1.5–2 cm) (75) and the type of renal pelvis correlate with functional impairment (76) and the necessity for corrective surgery (69).

Onset of ultrasound signs of the disease process is variable, most cases being recognized after 24 weeks gestation. Most are discovered incidentally during ultrasound for other obstetrical indications (16). Massive hydronephrosis with thinning of the renal parenchyma is unusual with this disease and signifies very severe obstruction. Marked reduction or absence of fetal urine production is not associated; amniotic fluid volume is usually normal. This is of some clinical importance since oligohydramnios with suspect UPJ implies either a second disease process (for example, dysmature IUGR with oligohydramnios due to placental insufficiency), a misdiagnosis, e.g., bilateral multicystic dysplastic kidney, or multiple congenital abnormalities, e.g., trisomy. Occasionally, *increased* amniotic fluid volume is reported, assumed to be the result of extrinsic compression of the retroperitoneal portion of the duodenum by an enlarged renal pelvis, interfering with intestinal transport. Fetal polyuria due to lack of urine concentration by the obstructed kidney (diuretic phase of renal failure) has also been proposed. In the majority of cases, hydramnios is of mild degree, with a slow and benign course. However, in rare cases, hydramnios was severe enough to cause preterm labor or maternal symptoms. Repetitive renocentesis has been used successfully to ameliorate the apparent course of the disease (77,78), but even more than in PUV, invasive fetal testing, and especially repetitive invasive "treatment," has not been shown to be necessary or efficacious in UPJ. As well, it is important to stress that these complications are extremely rare— obstetrical intervention is rarely justified (35,52,53,79–83).

The natural history of the disease is variable. In our experience, of the last 40 cases of fetal UPJ diagnosed, spontaneous resolution in utero occurred in six (15%), and in the remaining 34 cases, the disease either remained stable or progressed slowly. There were no cases in which rapid progression necessitated obstetrical intervention. The disease process was unilateral in the majority (85%). This is in agreement with most previously reported series (49,51,56,75). In a different cohort of 70 fetuses with UPJ followed without intervention in utero and prospectively postnatally for an average of 2.3 years, 56% had complete resolution of hydronephrosis at or after birth (69). Only 23% required surgery postnatally, and in the majority of these, fetal renal pelvis dilation was more than 1.5–2 cm.

One can conclude that this disease usually runs a benign course in utero and postnatally, with a small percentage requiring surgical intervention postnatally (45). Appropriate management includes serial ultrasound monitoring at a frequency of four to six weeks to follow amniotic fluid volume and progression of renal pelvis dilation. Intervention, if ever indicated, might be suggested by massive hydronephrosis appearing suddenly. Neonatal and postnatal follow-up is required for affected infants (35,36,81,84,85).

ANTENATAL ULTRASOUND DIAGNOSIS

In general obstetric populations, the incidence of fetal anomalies detected by routine ultrasound examination varies between 0.4% to 0.65%. Of these anomalies, 40–50% involve the fetal urinary system (16,36,48,52,86,87). The frequency of correct ultrasonographic diagnosis of fetal anomalies in general and fetal renal anomalies in particular (88–94) depends on many factors, such as operator experience, fetal position, and type and degree of severity of renal pathology in addition to gestational age at the time of diagnosis. While the diagnosis of congenital obstructive uropathy has been made as early as 11 weeks of gestation (88,95), less than 10% of fetal renal anomalies eventually demonstrated were diagnosed during a screening ultrasound examination done at 17 weeks gestation (86,89). This detection rate increases to 88% and 99% at 28 weeks and 33 weeks, respectively. The average gestational age at the time of diagnosis is 23 weeks (52). In North America, where routine ultrasound examination is not universal, urinary tract anomalies are usually discovered incidentally when ultrasound examination is done for other indications, such as pregnancy dating or small-for-gestational age (16). Ultrasound evidence of fetal obstructive uropathy occurs at an estimated frequency of 1/2800 cases (36,96).

Congenital obstruction of the fetal urinary tract may present across a broad spectrum of pathology, ranging from an isolated segmental lesion to diffuse, bilateral, lethal disease. Provided the glomerular unit is functioning, congenital obstruction of urine flow will always result in abnormal accumulation of urine within the collecting system and abnormal dilation of the renal tract proximal to the blockage. Ultrasound hallmarks of obstructive uropathy are fetal bladder enlargement, hydroureter, hydronephrosis (either simple or with dysplastic degeneration), and, frequently, a reduction in amniotic fluid volume. When renal involvement is bilateral, it is usually asymmetrical, one side is more severely affected than the other, or dilatation and dysplasia are featured on opposite sides. However, if the glomerular unit is nonfunctioning, characteristic features will be absence of urine production, with ultrasound findings of nondilated renal collecting system, absence of fetal bladder filling, and reduced amniotic fluid volume.

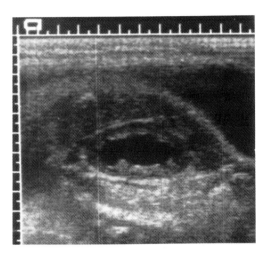

Figure 10-8   Parasagittal sonogram of the fetal abdomen demonstrating renal pelvis dilation.

High-level Obstruction

High-level obstructive uropathy is almost always due to obstruction at the junction of the renal pelvis and ureter. UPJ obstruction represents the most common cause of fetal and neonatal hydronephrosis, constituting 25–50% of all congenital urologic anomalies diagnosed in utero (36).

The diagnosis of UPJ obstruction in utero should be based on the following criteria (35,97):

1. Unequivocal dilation of the renal pelvis, with or without caliectasis (Figures 10-8,9). Maximum diameter of the renal pelvis must be at least 1 cm and/or the renal pelvis/kidney ratio >50% (97). (Dilation of the renal pelvis <10 mm is rarely associated with obstruction and may be considered a normal variant.)
2. Unequivocal calyceal dilation with or without renal pelvis dilation (35).
3. Nonvisualized ureters and normal bladder filling and emptying.

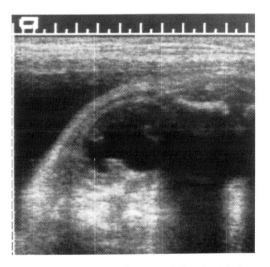

Figure 10-9   Coronal view of the fetal kidney demonstrating renal pelvis dilation due to UPJ obstruction.

The degree of hydronephrosis depends on the onset, duration, and degree of obstruction. With early onset (8–10 weeks), complete obstruction will likely result in the formation of a multicystic dysplastic kidney. Late onset UPJ obstruction results in variable hydronephrotic, i.e., dilatational, changes, but without dysplastic renal parenchymal changes. Dilation may involve the calyces and renal pelvis within the kidney (intrarenal) or be confined to the extrarenal part of the renal pelvis. Intrarenal hydronephrosis is associated with greater parenchymal damage (76). There is no ideal classification for hydronephrosis (98). Harrison suggested a semiquantitative estimate of calyceal dilation. Mild dilation would show an enlarged renal pelvis, branching infundibula, and preservation of calyces. Severe dilation would be characterized by a large single fluid collection, with thin septa representing residual connective tissue elements of the destroyed kidney.

Grignon et al. (99) suggested a morphologic classification of fetal hydronephrosis; pelvicalyceal dilation is graded according to the renal pelvis size and calyceal dilation (Table 10-2). Renal pelvis dilation <1 cm (Grade I) is considered physiological/normal and warrants no further evaluation. Dilation 1–1.5 cm suggests postnatal follow-up examination. For dilation >1.5 cm, or with calyceal dilation, most will require neonatal surgical intervention (93,99). UPJ obstruction should be differentiated from

Table 10-2 Prenatal Diagnosis of Fetal Hydronephrosis After 20 Weeks Gestation*

Grade	Calyceal Dilation	Size of Pelvis (Anterior-posterior diameter)
I	Physiological dilation	1 cm
II	Normal calyces	1–1.5 cm
III	Slight dilation	>1.5 cm
IV	Moderate dilation	>1.5 cm
V	Severe dilation atrophic cortex	>1.5 cm

*Modified from (99) Grignon et al. Urinary tract dilation in utero: classification and clinical applications. Radiology 1986;106:645.

renal cyst (single or multiple), multicystic renal dysplasia (Figures 10-10,11) and perirenal urinoma (36,98,100). Abnormal amniotic fluid volume should raise the suspicion of associated anomalies: absolute oligohydramnios suggests contralateral renal agenesis or severe dysplasia; hydramnios mandates a comprehensive examination of the fetal gastrointestinal tract and central nervous system.

Uterovesical Junction (UVJ) Obstruction and Megaureter

Ureteric dilation—megaureter—may be seen alone or associated with dilation of the renal pelvis and calyces. Megaureter may be caused by obstruction, vesicoureteral reflux, or, rarely, other conditions with neither obstruction nor reflux. Primary megaureter refers to a dilated ureter caused by an intrinsic ureteral defect, usually due to stenosis above the ureterovesical junction, whereas secondary megaureter refers to a ureter dilated by vesicoureteric reflux secondary to lower urinary tract obstruction (Figure 10-12) (98,100).

The normal ureter is not seen by ultrasound. When it is dilated >3 mm, it may appear as a tortuous, fluid-filled structure, which can be traced from the kidney down to the bladder. Megaureter should be differentiated from fluid-filled bowel, e.g., at 27–30 weeks, when liquid meconium fills the colon. The ureter is retroperitoneal, so the fluid-filled structure is seen adjacent to the fetal spine, originating from the renal pelvis and running behind the base of the bladder—dilated bowel seldom lies in this area (16,100). UVJ obstruction is diagnosed when megaureter is seen in the presence of normal bladder filling and emptying, often, but not always, associated with hydronephrosis. Initially, the ureter may be dilated and visualized segmentally and/or

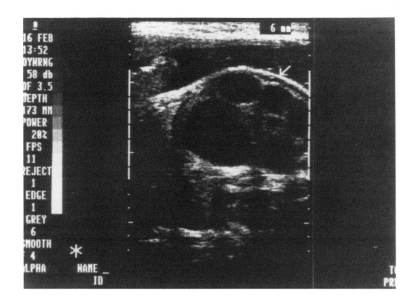

Figure 10-10 Parasagittal sonogram of the fetal abdomen demonstrating a large multicystic dysplastic kidney, causing massive abdominal distension.

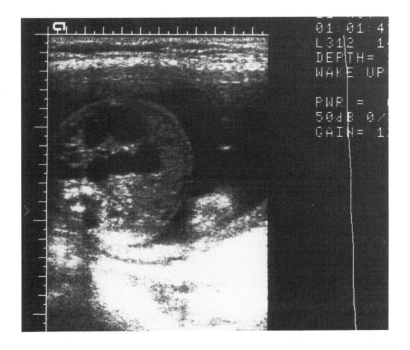

Figure 10-11 Transverse sonogram of the fetal abdomen demonstrating multicystic dysplastic left kidney. The right kidney is normal.

Figure 10-12   Transverse sonogram of the fetus demonstrating marked dilation of the distal ureters. This is a secondary obstructive megaureter due to posterior urethral valve syndrome.

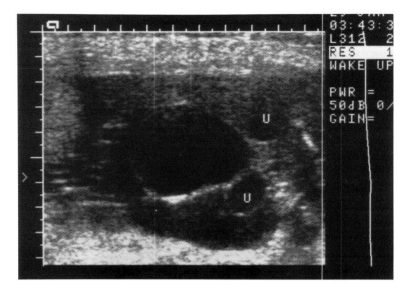

demonstrate visible (exaggerated) peristaltic waves. The diagnosis of megaureter due to primary or secondary reflux is usually difficult to make, especially since megacystis with megaureters may occur in the absence of bladder outlet obstruction. In this case, in utero retrograde pyelography (101,102) may be of value in establishing the diagnosis. Megaureter may be associated with contralateral renal agenesis, multicystic dysplastic kidney, and complete or incomplete duplication of various components (4,100,103).

Bladder Outlet Obstruction and Megacystis

Bladder outlet obstruction most commonly results from posterior urethral valve syndrome. (Table 10-3 lists other less common causes for bladder outlet obstruction or megacystis.) The cardinal signs of bladder outlet obstruction include persistent dilation of the fetal urethra proximal to the obstruction, progressive distension of the fetal bladder, and incomplete voiding—the fetal

Table 10-3   Causes of an Enlarged Fetal Urinary Bladder (Megacystis):

1. Posterior urethral valve syndrome
2. Urethral stricture
3. Urethral atresia
4. Persistent cloacal syndrome
5. Prune-belly syndrome
6. Megacystis-microcolon-intestinal hypoperistalsis syndrome

version of overflow incontinence. Chronic distension ultimately produces a bladder that is large and thin-walled (Figure 10-13).

Initially, an obstructed urinary bladder assumes a keyhole or pear-shaped appearance (Figure 10-9) with the neck of the pear representing the bladder neck and the dilated upper portion of the urethra (100). In fact, this "classical" appearance is most often demonstrated after the grossly distended bladder has been drained by needle aspiration. When the obstruction is complete and the bladder is massively dilated, it assumes a spherical shape and fills almost

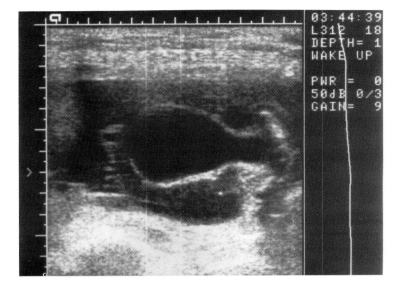

Figure 10-13 Transverse sonogram of the fetal pelvis demonstrating massive bladder distension and marked dilation of the proximal urethra, which is characteristic of posterior urethral valve syndrome.

the entire fetal abdomen. Visualization of a dilated proximal urethra is diagnostic for bladder outlet obstruction but is not always demonstrable because of fetal positioning, and it disappears when the bladder becomes markedly distended.

Other features indicative of urinary tract obstruction may assist in confirming the diagnosis of bladder outlet obstruction, but they do not occur uniformly—absence of these signs does not preclude diagnosis (16,36,48,50). Oligohydramnios occurs in 50–60% of fetuses with posterior urethral valve and in 100% of fetuses with urethral agenesis or atresia, especially after 16 weeks (60). Ureteric dilation and upper urinary tract dilatation associated with bladder outlet obstruction resemble the changes of more proximal obstruction but are always bilateral and usually symmetric. Detection of renal cortical cysts in the presence of lower urinary tract obstruction accurately indicates renal dysplasia and irreversible renal damage (104).

Hyperechogenicity of the renal parenchyma also correlates with a high probability for renal dysplasia, but is not as accurate as demonstration of renal cortical cysts (104). Assessment of renal parenchyma echogenicity is quite subjective and, therefore, less reliable (27,36). Kidney size and/or presence or absence of hydronephrotic changes do not relate to renal functional status, nor do they appear to be useful in the assessment of renal dysplasia. Dysplastic kidneys may be abnormally small or large because of asymmetric involvement. In bladder outlet obstruction, a functioning kidney is usually hydronephrotic, while a nonfunctioning kidney is small and hyperechogenic (Table 10-4). While renal vascular structures can be visualized and studied with Doppler flow velocimetry, the utility of these studies in excluding or proving renal functional impairment has not been demonstrated conclusively.

Poor prognostic indicators in bladder outlet obstruction include absolute oligo-

Table 10-4 Accuracy and Predictive Value of Sonographic Criteria in the Prediction of Renal Dysplasia with Obstructive Uropathy (104)

	Sensitivity (%)	Specificity (%)	(+) Predictive Value (%)	(−) Predictive Value (%)
Renal cyst	11	100	100	44
Increase echogenicity	73	80	89	57
Pyelocaliectasis	41	73	78	35

From (104) Mahony BS, Filly RA, Callen PW, Hricak H, Golbus MS, Harrison MR. Fetal renal dysplasia: sonographic evaluation. Radiology 1984;152:143–146.

hydramnios, a large amount of urinary ascites, dystrophic bladder wall calcification, and the presence of other congenital anomalies (104). Female fetuses tend to have a poorer prognosis than male fetuses; this is simply related to the distribution of renal anomalies. In the male fetus, posterior ureteral valve is the most common cause of bladder outlet obstruction. In the female fetus, the most common causes of bladder outlet obstruction or megacystis are urethral atresia, caudal regression anomalies, and MMIH syndrome (see below) (52), all of which have earlier and total urinary tract obstruction with concomitant renal destruction and pulmonary hypoplasia.

Megacystis-microcolon-intestinal hypoperistalsis (MMIH syndrome) a rare, uniformly lethal condition of unknown etiology primarily affecting females, is autosomal recessive and characterized by abnormalities of smooth muscle development(105). Ultrasound features include megacystis, megaureter, and massive bilateral hydronephrosis. Amniotic fluid volume is characteristically normal.

Prune-belly syndrome is a condition characterized by megacystis, megaureter, variable degree of hydronephrosis, absence of abdominal wall musculature, and bilat-

eral undescended testicles. Primary prune-belly syndrome is rare, occurring mainly in male fetuses and of unknown etiology (41,106–108). The prognosis is relatively poor, depending on the presence or absence of associated chromosomal and structural anomalies. Because of lack of abdominal wall musculature, chronic urinary tract infection and chronic constipation are common. Such individuals are azospermic and infertile in spite of corrective surgery (41).

A prune-belly-like syndrome (Figures 10-4,5) due to massive abdominal distension due to either obstructive uropathy, massive ascites, or other space-occupying lesion in the abdomen, is far more common than the primary prune-belly syndrome. The prune-belly-like syndrome may occur in either sex and has a relatively better prognosis than the primary syndrome, especially if due to posterior urethral valve in a male fetus. Ultrasound differentiation between primary prune-belly syndrome and secondary prune-belly-like syndrome is difficult. However, measuring fetal intravesicular pressure may be of value (109,110). In the case of prune-belly syndrome, the intravesicular pressure is low, while in secondary prune-belly-like syndrome, the intravesicular pressure is almost always high. Another method used is intrauterine cystography (101,102), demonstrating the site of the obstruction. Inability to demonstrate a dilated posterior urethra in a male fetus should raise the suspicion of primary prune-belly syndrome.

In summary, the ultrasound examination of a fetus suspected of having urinary tract obstruction should incorporate the following:

1. Confirmation of gestational age at the time of diagnosis.
2. Estimation of amniotic fluid volume.
3. Identification of the kidneys with assessment of the textural and architectural appearance.
4. Estimation of fetal kidney size and measurement of the kidney circumference to abdominal circumference ratio.
5. Identification of the fetal bladder and sequential observation of bladder filling and emptying.
6. Identification of the fetal genitalia (male, female, or ambiguous).
7. Comprehensive examination of fetal anatomy to rule out other congenital anomalies.

Two important points should be remembered. First, ultrasound diagnosis is not absolutely reliable in the presence of oligohydramnios. In this situation, artificial installation of normal saline into the amniotic space may improve visualization (111). Second, ultrasound diagnosis is not relied upon in isolation to select fetuses appropriate for intrauterine intervention; it is used as an initial diagnostic step to select fetuses who should then have invasive diagnostic tests, such as percutaneous umbilical cord blood sampling for karyotyping (112) or intrauterine urinary bladder aspiration for urinary chemistry and electrolyte analysis (14,15,113).

FETAL SURGERY: CASE SELECTION CRITERIA AND SURGICAL METHODS

Selection of those very few fetuses who might benefit from in utero surgical urinary tract diversion procedures may best be achieved by application of strict exclusion criteria, few of which have yet been subjected to rigorous scientific scrutiny.

Despite the optimistic enthusiasm of the fetal surgeon, there can be little doubt that repair of obstructive uropathies will almost always be a safer and more definitive procedure in neonatal subjects. Therefore, as a first principle, the fetus of sufficient age and maturity (generally ≥32 weeks gestation) to sustain extrauterine survival should never be a candidate for in utero surgery. Whereas this point may now seem obvious, the reader is reminded that within the International Fetal Surgery Registry, in utero procedures for obstructive uropathy have been done as late as 36 weeks (11). In retrospect, this would now seem quite inappropriate.

A second principle should be that the therapy would only be considered in the fetus with severe bladder outlet obstruction and progressive bilateral renal disease. The primary aim of therapy is to prevent both the renal and the pulmonary sequelae.

Obstetricians have accumulated a large experience with needle penetration of the fetal peritoneal cavity and a lesser experience with bladder puncture; for either method, the fetal death rate directly attributable to the procedure is about 5% (52,114). Therefore, the issue must not be whether therapy is possible, for it nearly always is, but rather whether such therapy will benefit the fetus and whether any potential benefit outweighs any real fetal risk against this background. The justification of perinatal therapy for unilateral disease, as has been reported (79,80), may be lacking, although in some cases, an apparent amelioration of associated maternal disease has been described (77,78).

Thirdly, the fetus with the combination of obstructive uropathy and other structural or karyotypic anomaly should not be considered a candidate for perinatal therapy. Such association is not uncommon. Of 98 treated cases reported to the International Fetal Surgery Registry, eight (8.1%) had multiple organ system anomalies and eight (8.1%) had karyotypic anomalies. Thus, 16 out of 98 (16.3%) had severe associated anomalies, a rate 15 to 30 times higher than that of the general population.

Although maternal morbidity has not been described as a complication of intrauterine fetal therapy for obstructive uropathy per se, severe maternal morbidity or death has been caused by other invasive intrauterine procedures, such as amniocentesis (115) or intrauterine transfusion (116). Serious and potentially life-threatening maternal infection (chorioamnionitis) has been reported as a consequence of diagnostic or therapeutic maternal percutaneous placement of a fetal bladder catheter (113). Therefore, it follows that a very detailed and complete ultrasound fetal organ system review should be a prerequisite to any therapeutic effort. In theory, such a review should detect all associated structural anomalies; in practice, the detection rate is about 90% (117). In selected cases, amnioinfusion not only enhances the physical examination of the fetus but also demonstrates fetal swallowing. In cases of complete obstruction, the fetus is often completely obscured in the lower or posterior aspect of the uterine cavity, with position grossly distorted by the distended bladder. In these situations, simple bladder drainage may be an essential component of fetal physical assessment by ultrasound as well as functional assessment by urine biochemistry before definitive

surgery is considered. Finally, from a procedural point of view, accurate catheter placement is very difficult in the complete absence of amniotic fluid because of restricted fetal movements, lack of space between the fetus and uterine wall, and restricted ultrasound visualization of the instrument. Preprocedure amnioinfusion improves virtually all of these problems.

Another question that needs to be answered before considering fetal therapy is whether the affected fetus has an abnormal karyotype. Choosing cordocentesis (PUBS) versus amniocentesis or vesicocentesis depends on many factors, including operator skill, placental localization, presence of amniotic fluid, and fetal position. If the cord insertion is easily accessible, PUBS is our choice for karyotyping. A total of 2–3 ml of fetal blood is adequate for karyotyping and chemistry. If the placenta is posterior or PUBS is technically difficult, amniocentesis for amniocyte culture may be considered, and is practicable within a short time after amnioinfusion. Chorionic villus sampling (CVS)/placental biopsy may be another alternative in selected cases, with rapid results from the direct prep, confirmed by long-term culture within 10 days (118–112). Fetal urine obtained by vesicocentesis may yield sufficient cells for culture, but the reliability of this method is not uniform, and some delay may be involved.

Amniotic Fluid Volume

A fixed relationship between amniotic fluid volume estimated by ultrasound and outcome in fetuses with obstructive uropathy is unclear. The use of this variable for case selection remains controversial. Since urine production is a major contributor to the dynamic amniotic fluid compartment in later pregnancy (123–125), it would follow that the most severe obstructive disease is associated with the worst oligohydramnios. The data contained in the International Fetal Registry does not support this supposition. Although the majority (77.6%) of fetuses with obstructive uropathy do have oligohydramnios (52), survival rates are similar among treated fetuses with or without oligohydramnios (40.8% and 40.9%, respectively). In addition, perinatal death due to pulmonary hypoplasia has been observed among fetuses with obstructive uropathy and apparently normal amniotic fluid volume.

This discrepancy may be due to a variety of factors. Amniotic fluid volume determination by ultrasound is generally subjective; use of objective criteria, such as largest fluid pocket measurement, has not been uniform (126). In fetuses with incomplete obstruction, there may be sufficient outflow impedance, with resulting elevation in intrarenal pressure, to cause proximal dilation and damage, while urine efflux may be enough to maintain some amniotic fluid volume. Further, it may be that the loss of connective tissue compliance, i.e., development of hydroureter and pyelectasis, preserves renal function by lowering pressures, leading to the apparent paradox of a "blown-out" upper urinary tract in the face of continued presence of amniotic fluid.

Despite opinion to the contrary (63,127), there is no evidence that oligohydramnios is a contraindication to therapy. It actually is an indication for therapy if the remainder of the investigations are normal. Chronic oligohydramnios, both in the experimental animal model and in the human, is associated with increased incidence of lethal pulmonary hypoplasia accounting for 87% of deaths among treated fetuses (31,54). It is tempting to suggest that the high incidence of pulmonary hypoplasia seen in fetuses with obstructive uropathies is, therefore, caused by this oligohydramnios.

However, the observation of lethal pulmonary hypoplasia with obstructive uropathy, even in the presence of normal amniotic fluid volume, indicates there must be more than one etiological factor for pulmonary hypoplasia. Intrinsic pulmonary compression due to bladder and urinary tract dilation may be another cause; diaphragmatic hernia, either experimental or clinical, is known to cause pulmonary hypoplasia by this method (128). An alternate explanation is that the primary insult, the nature of which remains entirely unknown, affects the endodermal lung primordia and mesodermal genitourinary primordia simultaneously.

ASSESSMENT OF FETAL RENAL FUNCTION

Evaluation of fetal renal function is becoming an integral part of individual case selection. Temporary external drainage of the fetal bladder permits direct measurement of fetal urine production rate, estimates of fetal glomerular filtration rate by creatinine or iothalamate excretion, and ongoing electrolyte composition (113). The degree of invasion and potential risks of leaving a direct connection to the fetus open at the maternal skin level means that this continuous monitoring is of limited application. The mainstay of direct evaluation of fetal renal function is transcutaneous, ultrasound-directed decompression of the fetal bladder with a single, simple needle puncture. This provides urine for analysis of electrolytes, osmolarity, protein electrophoresis (notably β2-microglobulin), amino acid concentration, as well as a potential for retrograde urography. As noted, single investigative punctures may also be therapeutic. Observation of the fetal urinary tract following drainage may be highly revealing. Indirect evidence of renal function (bladder filling and emptying, resolution of dilatation in upper collecting systems, objective changes in amniotic fluid volume) following bladder drainage is valuable in assigning prognosis. As well, successful drainage of the grossly distended urinary tract will provide an opportunity for detailed evaluation of other fetal intra-abdominal structures and review of the decompressed renal anatomy. For example, ultrasonic demonstration of renal cortical cysts, which would not resolve with drainage of the urinary tract, has a specificity of 100% and a sen-sitivity of 44% in identifying lethal renal dysplasia (104).

The aim of all these tests is selection of fetuses with an obstruction severe enough to compromise renal and pulmonary development and yet not so complete that renal function is absolutely destroyed (35). None of these tests is infallible, however. For example, monitoring bladder filling following initial drainage may lead to the erroneous conclusion that renal function has been maintained, when the bladder fills by secretion from the bladder mucosa alone.

Fetal Urinalysis

Fetal urine is produced from as early as nine weeks gestation and is an ultrafiltrate of fetal serum, made hypotonic by selective tubular reabsorption of sodium and chloride in excess of free water loss (129). In experimental urinary tract obstruction, fetal kidneys damaged by longstanding disease are "salt-wasters," producing isotonic or hypertonic urine (35).

In 20 human fetuses referred for treatment of bilateral congenital hydronephrosis. Harrison's group assessed the prognostic value of various criteria used to assess fetal renal functional potential. This evaluation included temporary placement

of fetal bladder catheters with exteriorization to measure fetal urine output and composition. Fetuses were divided retrospectively into two groups: (1) 10 cases with "poor function" based on severe renal dysplasia and pulmonary hypoplasia at autopsy or biopsy, or renal and pulmonary insufficiency at birth, and (2) 10 cases with "good function" based on nondysplastic kidney at autopsy or biopsy, or "normal" renal and pulmonary function at birth. Fetuses with "good" renal function tended to have normal amniotic fluid volume, normal kidneys on ultrasound examination, and hypotonic urine, with urinary sodium less than 100 mmol, chloride below 90, and urine osmolarity less than 210 mOsm/L. Fetuses with "poor" renal function tended to have decreased amniotic fluid volume, abnormal kidneys on ultrasound examination, and isotonic urine with urinary sodium concentration of >100, chloride >90, and osmolarity >210 mOsm/L (Table 10-5). In their retrospective study, those prognostic criteria were accurate in almost 90% of cases. However, when applied prospectively, the predictive value of those prognostic criteria suggested by Harrison's group varies between 50–100% (46,130–133). To examine the accuracy of fetal urine electrolyte prognostic criteria suggested by Harrison's

Table 10-5 Harrison's Prognostic Criteria for Urinary Electrolytes (113)

Prognosis	Na mEq/L	Cl mEq/L	Osmolarity mOsm/L
Good	<100	<90	<210
*Poor	>100	>90	>210

*Poor prognosis if one or all abnormal.
From (113) Glick PL, Harrison MR, Golbus MS, et al. Management of the fetus with congenital hydronephrosis. II. Prognostic criteria and selection for treatment. J Pediatr Surg 1985;20:376–387.

Group (113) (Table 10-6), all cases of fetal obstructive uropathy reported in the English literature and/or to the International Fetal Surgery Registry were reviewed (Table 10-7).

The following information was obtained on each fetus:

- Gestational age at time of presentation—diagnosis, treatment, and delivery.
- Amniotic fluid volume at the initial examination.
- Urine electrolytes (Na, Cl, and osmolarity).
- Predicted outcome using urine electrolyte with and without amniotic fluid volume as a predictor factor according to Harrison's prognostic criteria.
- Type of intrauterine intervention.
- The observed outcome was considered poor if there was perinatal or neonatal death due to poor renal function as a result of renal dysplasia or elective termination of pregnancy with histopathological confirmation of renal dysplasia.
- Good outcome was considered if the fetus was born alive and well for the first year of life.

Ultrasound features of the fetal kidneys as suggested by Harrison's group (104) were not included as part of formal fetal evaluation due to the subjective nature of this assessment. A total of 34 fetuses had complete information, and were included in the analysis. The results are summarized in Tables 10-8 and 10-9 and Figure 10-14.

One may accept that the prognostic criteria using fetal urine electrolyte analysis were properly based on pathophysiologic principles. These principles are that all mammalian fetuses normally have hypotonic urine, that the obstructed fetal kidney is a salt-waster producing isotonic urine, and that there is no contribution, other than by kidney function, to the liquid in the bladder. However, we, as well as other investigators (15) have been concerned that the accepted parameters for fetal urine chemistry must be inherently inaccurate in obstructive uropathy, because of the following:

1. Fetal urine aspirated from the obstructed urinary tract must, by definition, be "old" and not reflective of "cur-

Table 10-6 Prognostic Criteria for Fetuses with Bilateral Obstructive Uropathy (113,138)

Good Prognosis	Poor Prognosis*
Normal amniotic fluid volume	Severe oligohydramnios
Normal kidneys	Cystic kidneys
Sodium ≤ mEq/L	Sodium ≥100 mEq/L or >95th percentile
Chloride ≤90 mEq/L	Chloride ≥90 mEq/L or >95th percentile
Osmolarity ≤210 mOsm/L	Osmolarity ≥210 mOsm/L
Urea >4 mmol/L	Urea <4 mmol/L
Calcium <1.6 mmol/L	Calcium >1.75 mmol/L
β2-microglobulin 0 or trace	β2-microglobulin strong band

*If one or more abnormal.
[From (113) Glick PL, Harrison MR, Golbus MS, et al. Management of the fetus with congenital hydronephrosis. II. Prognostic criteria and selection for treatment. J Pediatr Surg 1985;20:376–387.
(138) Nicolaides KH, Cheng HH, Snijders RJM, Moniz CF. Fetal urine biochemistry in the assessment of obstructive uropathy. Am J Obstet Gynecol 1992;166:932–937.

Table 10-7 Reported Cases of Bladder Aspiration/Shunt

Year	Author	G.A Pres	G.A Diagn	Treatment Shunt	Treatment Aspir	G.A. Delivery	AF Normal	AF Mild	AF Mod.	AF Abs.	AF Oligo.	Na Mcg/l	Cl Mcg/l	Osm Mcg/l	Predicted Outcome	Observed Outcome	TA	SB	NND	A&W	Alive Ren Fail
1987	I. Wilkins (128)	28	28	28	28	29	-	-	-	-	+	146	117	283	Poor	Poor	-	-	+	-	-
		27	27	-	27	32	-	-	-	-	+	110	93	245	Poor	Good	-	-	+	-	-
		27	28	30	28	33	-	-	+	-	-	73	55	154	Good	Good	-	-	-	+	-
1987	A. Reuss (137)	18	20	-	20	20	+	-	-	-	-	62	55	137	Good	Poor	+	-	-	-	+
		18	24	-	32	33	-	-	+	-	-	71	57	153	Good	Good	-	-	-	-	-
		17	17	-	17	17	-	-	-	+	-	113	118	261	Poor	Poor	+	-	-	-	-
		20	22	-	22	23	+	-	-	-	-	130	100	265	Poor	Poor	+	-	-	-	-
		30	31	-	31	37	-	-	-	-	-	76	67	161	Good	Good	-	-	+	-	-
		21	21	-	21	21	+	-	-	-	-	75	61	163	Good	Good	+	-	-	-	-
		21	21	-	21	21	-	-	-	-	+	130	105	273	Poor	Poor	+	-	-	-	-
		22	22	-	22	22	-	-	-	+	-	104	82	211	Poor	Poor	+	-	-	-	-
		23	23	-	23	23	-	-	-	+	-	115	97	242	Poor	Poor	-	-	+	-	-
		30	30	-	30	30	-	-	-	-	+	130	107	273	Poor	Poor	-	-	-	-	+
		37	37	-	37	37	+	-	-	-	-	146	111	284	Poor	Good	-	-	+	-	+
1988	M. Harrison (35) Open Fetal Surgery	19	19	20	19	35	+	-	-	-	-	99	84	215	Poor	Poor	-	-	-	-	+
		22	22	-	22	33	-	-	-	+	-	88	83	255	Good	Good	-	-	+	-	-
		22	22	-	22	32	-	-	-	-	-	79	71	160	Good	Good	-	-	-	-	+
		18	18	-	18	32	-	-	-	+	-	100	91	221	Poor	Poor	-	-	+	-	-
1989	W. Holsgreve (130)	22	22	19	22	32	+	-	-	-	-	100	82	215	Poor	Poor	-	-	+	-	-
		18	18	-	18	35	-	-	-	+	-	100	94	262	Poor	Good	-	-	-	+	-
		12	14.5	14.5	14.5	35	-	-	-	-	+	90	73	197	Good	Good	-	-	-	+	-
		16	16	19	16	37	-	-	-	+	-	104	93	230	Poor	Poor	-	-	-	+	-
		19	19	19	19	32	-	-	+	-	-	83	76	180	Good	Good	-	-	-	+	-
		13	14	-	14	40	+	-	-	-	-	83	76	197	Good	Good	-	-	-	+	-
1990	Mark Evans (15)	20	20	-	20	TA	-	-	-	+	-	120	98	240	Poor	Poor	+	-	-	-	-
		32	32	-	32	40	+	-	-	-	-	35	32	107	Good	Good	-	-	-	+	-
		20	20	-	20	40	+	-	-	-	-	52	34	121	Good	Good	-	-	-	+	-
		31	31	-	31	40	+	-	-	-	-	38	35	98	Poor	Poor	-	-	-	+	-
		25	30	30	30	31	-	-	-	+	-	128	108	287	Poor	Good	-	-	-	+	-
1993	International Fetal Registry & (42,129)	18	18	-	18	18	+	-	-	-	-	100	82	217	Poor	Poor	+	-	-	-	-
		20	20	21	20	33	-	+	-	-	-	99	78	213	Good	Good	-	-	+	-	-
		11	16	18	18	20	-	-	-	+	-	111	87	233	Poor	Poor	-	+	-	-	-
		19	19	21	21	34	-	-	-	+	-	105	87	217	Poor	Poor	-	-	-	-	+
		17	17	-	17	38	+	-	-	-	-	72	64	159	Good	Good	-	-	-	+	-

GA = gestational age in weeks. TA = therapeutic abortion. SB = stillbirth. NND = neonatal death. A&W = alive and well (variable followup). Alive Ren Fail = survivor with renal failure.

Table 10-8 Accuracy of Fetal Urine Electrolyte Tests in Predicting Poor Outcome

Variable	Sensitivity	Specificity	False Positive	False Negative	P
Harrison's criteria (Abnormal urine electrolytes)	86.7	57.9	38.1	15.4	.006
When AFV is abnormal	86.7	42.1	45.1	20.0	.0595
When Na is abnormal	66.7	78.9	28.6	25.0	.0065
When CL is abnormal	46.7	68.4	46.2	38.1	.369
When Osm. is abnormal	86.9	57.9	38.1	15.4	.006
Harrison's criteria plus abnormal AFV	80.0	68.4	33.3	18.8	.015
When AFV, NA, Osm } All abnormal	66.7	78.9	28.6	25.0	.018

Table 10-9 Sensitivity and Specificity of Different Urine Electrolyte Components, with and without Amniotic Fluid Volume as a Prognostic Test, in Predicting Poor Outcome

Variables	Sensitivity	Specificity
When all (Na, Cl and osmolarity) are abnormal	46.7	78.9
When two of (Na, Cl and/or osmolarity) are abnormal	66.7	68.4
When only one of (Na or Cl or osmolarity) is abnormal	86.7	57.9
When all tests (Na, Cl, osmolarity, and AFV) are abnormal	40.0	84.2
When three of the tests (Na, Cl, osmolarity, or AFV) are abnormal	86.7	68.4
When either (Na, Cl, osmolarity, or AFV) is abnormal	86.7	63.2
When only one (Na, Cl, osmolarity, or AFV) is abnormal	93.3	31.6

rent" fetal renal function. Stagnant urine in the fetal bladder may undergo biochemical change as a result of equilibrium with fetal serum through the bladder mucosa. On this basis, normal results might represent previous normal function that has now been lost. Similarly, the finding of abnormal results might represent normal urine produced in response to normal renal function, which has undergone abnormal change in the obstructed bladder.

2. Fetal urine electrolyte excretion changes with gestational age. If the obstruction has been longstanding or incomplete for a long period of time, fetal urine electrolyte results may represent either "historic" evaluations or reflect a degree of immaturity of renal function, rather than speaking directly to abnormal kidney function.

3. Aspiration of fetal urine from the urinary bladder represents the output of urine from both kidneys. Both experi-

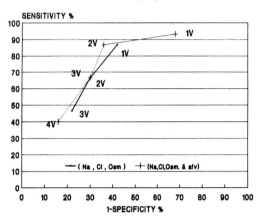

ROC for fetal urinary electrolytes based on Harrison's prognostic criteria

1V = Only one urine electrolyte is abnormal.

2V = Two urine electrolytes are abnormal.

3V = All abnormal (Na, Cl, and osmolarity)

4V = All abnormal (Na, Cl, osmolarity and oligohydramnios)

Figure 10-14 ROC for fetal urinary electrolytes and/or amniotic fluid volume (AFV) based on Harrison's prognostic criteria.

mentally and in clinical experience, it has been shown that the degree of renal damage is often not symmetrical, with one kidney being more severely damaged than the other. As a result, abnormalities in the electrolytes, osmolarity and/or protein or amino acid content of a urine sample obtained from the fetal urinary bladder can suggest two possibilities: (A) both kidneys are damaged or (B) one kidney is severely damaged while the other kidney has normal function.   Nicolini et al. reported a fetus with lower urinary tract obstruction and absolute oligohydramnios at 23 weeks, with urine chemistry obtained on a sample obtained from the fetal bladder. The results were suggestive of poor renal function. However, when samples were obtained from the right and left re-

nal pelves separately, the left kidney had normal function. As a result, a catheter shunt was placed in the urinary bladder; a male fetus was delivered at 36 weeks gestation. The diagnosis of posterior urethral valve with asymmetrical reflux was confirmed postnatally. The baby had corrective surgery and is doing well.

4. The predictive value of fetal urine electrolyte concentration and osmolarity may be more accurate when multiple urinary bladder aspirations are carried out and the trend is followed (15). It is certainly our clinical experience that the initial (stagnant) sample may suggest severe functional derangement, while a repeat puncture one or two days later shows much more normal values.

Because of the variably predictive value of urinary electrolyte concentration and osmolarity, several investigators have suggested different urine tests. Neutral amino acids in fetal urine at concentrations similar to plasma values are predictive of irreversibly destroyed kidneys because they reflect poor tubular capacity (134). Unfortunately, only a very small number of fetuses have been evaluated by this method, and it is very difficult to draw a conclusion from only five cases reported in the literature. Secondly, the pattern of plasma proteins excreted in the urine is often a reflection of the type of disease affecting the kidney. With glomerular damage, plasma proteins excreted in the urine include a high proportion of albumin and varying quantities of other plasma proteins of a molecular size larger than albumin (macromolecular proteinuria with molecular weight >70,000 daltons). With tubular damage, the proteins excreted include a significant proportion of albumin and a relatively large amount of plasma proteins of molecular size smaller than albumin (micromolecular proteinuria,

M.W. <70,000 daltons). The site and degree of underlying lesions in the kidney with pathological proteinuria can be identified by separating urinary proteins on polyacrylamide gel electrophoresis with sodium dodoecyl sulfate as detergent (SDS-PAGE) (135,136).

Beta-2-microglobulin, ammonia, and creatinine in fetal urine might be more sensitive indicators of renal function and long-term outcome (137). From our experience and that of others using Harrison's criteria, the addition of β_2-microglobulin results in higher sensitivity in predicting fetal renal function and long-term outcome. Larger studies are now available, clarifying some issues, such as the importance of gestational-age correlation in the interpretation of urine values (138). "Normal" values are established by sorting results of bladder aspiration retrospectively (i.e., ultimate outcome was normal renal function, therefore, the results belong in the normal range) in cases of urinary tract obstruction. While this methodology may not yield "normal" results, it certainly provides prognostic guidance among obstructed fetuses (Table 10-6). Overall, no parameter or combination of factors is presently satisfactory for evidence of long-term renal competence (15,27,35).

Intravesicular Pressure

Several investigators have demonstrated high intravesical pressure in fetuses with ultrasound features of obstructive uropathy due to bladder outlet obstruction, such as posterior urethral valves or urethral atresia (110 and C. Weiner, as reported to the Fetal Surgery Registry). This is contrary to what was reported by Nicolini (109), who demonstrated low intravesical pressure. Differences may exist in technique, calibration methods or patient population with different underlying etiology. Another important

possibility is that these measurements were done on fetuses at different gestational ages with variable stages of renal pathology and renal function. While functioning kidneys continue urine production leading to further urine accumulation in the bladder and further increment in intravesical pressure; nonfunctioning kidneys produce small amounts or no urine at all. As a result, low intravesical pressure may be associated with long-standing disease (110). Further clinical experience is necessary to verify this.

Urinary bladder manometry has potential value in differentiating between obstructive and nonobstructive causes of megacystis, especially in fetuses with prune-belly or MMIH syndromes, which cannot easily be differentiated from partial obstructive uropathy. Intravesical pressure is expected to be high in obstructive uropathy due to posterior urethral valve or urethral atresia, but low or normal in MMIH syndrome and in cases of prune-belly syndrome, due to their nonobstructive causes. Those with nonobstructive disease will not likely benefit from urinary diversion and should be excluded.

FETAL OBSTRUCTIVE UROPATHY: TREATMENT OPTIONS

1. Expectant Management

Expectant management with close observation and delivery at term is the treatment of choice in case of unilateral urinary tract obstruction with a normal contralateral kidney and adequate amniotic fluid volume maintained on serial observation. Expectant management may also be considered in fetuses with proven but incomplete urinary tract obstruction with normal amniotic fluid volume, with evaluation at regular intervals of the risks and benefits of early delivery.

2. Preterm Delivery

This may be elected for the fetus with bladder outlet obstruction complicated by oligohydramnios but with preserved renal function. If the gestational age is 32 weeks or more, these fetuses may benefit from preterm delivery and neonatal surgical treatment. This option recognizes the potential risks of invasive intrauterine procedures but is, in fact, infrequently used—mild disease does not require early delivery; severe disease usually presents earlier.

Termination of pregnancy is always an option for parents to consider if the diagnosis is made before fetal viability.

3. Intermittent Bladder Aspiration

Intermittent aspiration of the obstructed urinary bladder is technically simple and offers some relief from chronic overdistension of the urinary tract. Intermittent aspiration of the obstructed urinary bladder may be curative in some cases of Type I posterior urethral valve (Figure 10-3). Intermittent aspiration of urinary bladder may be considered as a temporary measure for decompressing the overdistended urinary system in fetuses who are too small to have a percutaneous vesicoamniotic shunt (Figure 10-15). Bladder aspiration is of great diagnostic value in following a fetus whose initial urinary electrolyte analysis is abnormal. Serial fetal urinary bladder aspiration showing improving urinary chemistry values suggests good potential for intrauterine vesicoamniotic shunt insertion, while fetuses with persistently abnormal urine electrolytes may be considered poor candidates for shunting. The potential risks of infection and preterm labor should be considered when the procedure is carried out.

Normal urinary tract pressures may exist for several days after each decompression,

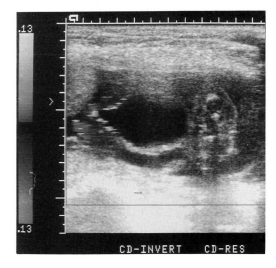

Figure 10-15A Transverse scan of the fetal pelvis demonstrating marked distension of the urinary bladder and urinary ascites. Note the umbilical arteries running on each side of the urinary bladder.

but eventually the puncture site closes, the obstruction resumes, and the potential for further injury recurs. How often, how many individual punctures, what factors balance simple decompression against shunt placement, all are unknown due to limited data.

4. Intrauterine Vesicoamniotic Shunt

Percutaneous placement of an indwelling diversion catheter from the obstructed fetal bladder to the amniotic cavity should be limited to those fetuses with proven obstructive uropathy of a persistent and progressive nature and with known immaturity. In our center, in addition to informed parental consent, case review and approval by a fetal therapy committee (composed of a neonatologist, obstetrician, ultrasonographer, and appropriate nonmedical members) are required before the procedure is attempted.

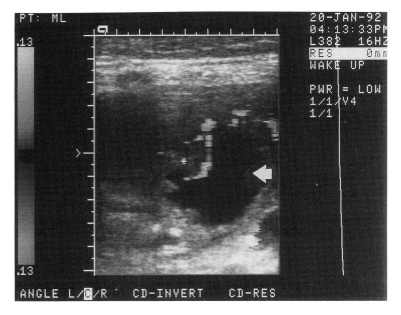

Figure 10-15B Transverse scan of the same fetus after single-needle bladder aspiration completely decompressing the urinary bladder(*). Puncture of the bladder allows fluid to leak out into the peritoneal cavity, seen as the new appearance of urinary ascites (arrow).

Preoperative medications are based on a protocol tested extensively in patients requiring intrauterine fetal transfusion (138). Prophylactic antibiotics are begun the day prior to surgery and are continued for 24 hours. Maternal and fetal sedation and analgesia are facilitated by narcotic premedication. The procedure is done in a fetal operating theater with full aseptic technique. Using a sterile ultrasound scan head, fetal lie and bladder position are confirmed, a target in the fetal lower abdomen is identified and the maternal surface fetal coordinates are noted and marked. Under local anesthetic cover, a small skin incision is made to avoid extreme downward pressure, which can rotate the fetus, the uterus, or both.

Two different catheters are available. First, the Denver fetal bladder shunt, is not widely used. Second, a double pigtail polyethylene catheter of different sizes (Figure 10-16) has become the standard catheter for vesicoamniotic shunt. Two different methods for catheter placement are available: an

overload system in which the catheter is loaded over a trochar and a hollow-needle system in which the catheter is threaded down the inside of the needle. In this center, we have abandoned the overload system—off-loading of the catheter may be very difficult; the catheter may fail to slide past the firm surface of the uterus; the catheter may "accordion" along the trochar shaft with attempts to off-load.

The system used in our center is the "Rodeck Loading System" (Figure 10-17). It consists of a 20-cm, 14-gauge cannula with an irrigation side-channel. The needle is advanced under continuous ultrasound guidance to enter the fetal bladder and the position is confirmed by the flow of urine through the side-channel, usually under some pressure. Urine is crystal clear (unless bleeding was caused by previous puncture—another reason for waiting several days after puncture before performing permanent shunt placement). The trochar is removed. Confirmation that the cannula tip is free in the bladder is confirmed by brisk in-

Figure 10-16 Double pigtail polyethylene catheter.

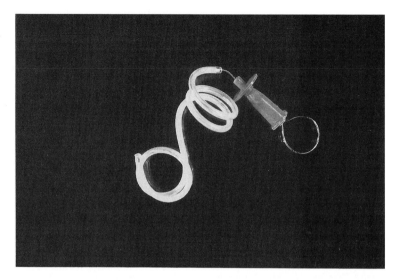

Figure 10-17 "Rodeck Loading System," consisting of a 20-cm cannula with an irrigation channel and two pushers—a short and a long one, for advancing the catheter through the cannula.

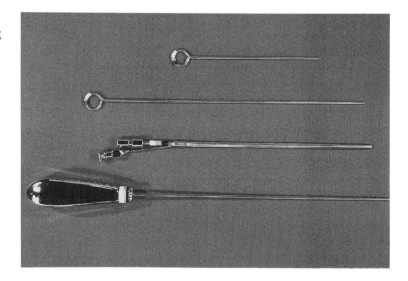

jection of one to two ml normal saline down the needle, with the resulting ultrasound observation of fluid turbulence seen within the bladder. The double pigtail catheter with "memory" (Rocket of London Ltd, London, England), threaded on a wire guide, is straightened and advanced through the needle. The catheter is manu-factured so that at least five cm of catheter will protrude from the fetal abdomen into the amniotic space. Once ultrasound evidence of the "memory" of the catheter, i.e., coiling, is clear, the needle is withdrawn into the amniotic fluid. Confirmation of withdrawal from the fetal abdomen back into the amniotic space is by aspiration of the pigmented, turbid amniotic fluid. If necessary, further infusions of saline to confirm placement, or even of 100–300 ml sterile warm saline to create an amniotic fluid pocket for withdrawal/visualization, are utilized as necessary. The latter can sometimes be accomplished via the side-channel; alternatively, second puncture and instillation via 20-gauge spinal needle at a separate appropriate site. The distal coils of the catheter lie free in the amniotic cavity (Figure 10-18). The design of the catheter favors adequate flow and retention of the catheter in the fetal bladder. The proximal end of the catheter is the most difficult to place, and care must be taken not to place the entire catheter within the fetal bladder or the proximal end within the fetal abdomen, thereby creating a (useless) vesicoperitoneal shunt and fetal urinary ascites. Alternatively, it may be reasonable to leave the proximal end of the catheter in the myometrium, allowing for fetal movement to draw the end into the amniotic space. On occasion, the distal end fails to be completely dislodged and "follows" the needle out through the skin. We have preferred to pull out the catheter and try again rather than trying to push it in from skin level.

Ultrasound is used to confirm successful catheter placement, and the changes observed are usually immediate and dramatic. Rapid bladder decompression and an increase in amniotic fluid volume or, in the case of preoperative oligohydramnios, the appearance of amniotic fluid is expected within minutes of shunt placement. The proximal and distal ends of the catheter should be visible and the areas of transabdominal passage should be noted (Figure 10-19). Failure to note those characteristics within the first 15 minutes after shunt procedure indicates improper placement and is an indication to repeat the procedure. Once

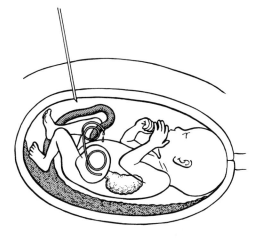

Figure 10-18   The ideal placement of vesicoamniotic shunt. The distal end of the catheter is in the bladder while the proximal end of the catheter is in the amniotic cavity.

a shunt is placed properly, it is essential to monitor the shunt function frequently (twice per week for two to three weeks, then once a week to delivery) because with fetal growth and movement, the proximal end may become dislodged or blocked. We have also observed one instance in which the fetus pulled the shunt from his abdomen. In the ideal case, vesicoamniotic shunt placement is a single short procedure. In our experience, however, the procedure may be very difficult and in one case was impossible, despite several attempts. The number of separate attempts at shunt placement before the procedure is abandoned will vary among operators; at this center, we agreed that no more than four attempts in the individual patient would occur. Of course, if the procedure is transplacental, even one attempt may be lethal for the fetus, although color Doppler flow mapping is helpful in avoiding large fetal blood vessels on the placental surface.

Figure 10-19 Vesico-amniotic shunt placement in a fetus with (PUV) syndrome at 25 weeks gestation.
10-19A Transverse section of the fetal abdomen just before shunt placement demonstrating markedly distended urinary bladder (arrow) and ureters(U). In addition, there is urinary ascites.

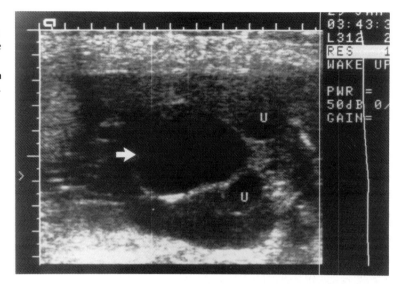

Figure 10-19B Transverse sonogram of the fetal abdomen demonstrating the position of the proximal end of the catheter (C) in the urinary bladder (B).

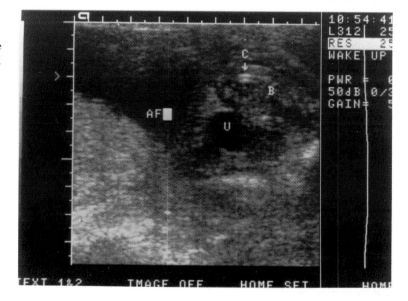

Complications

Percutaneous vesicoamniotic shunt catheter placement, even though technically straightforward, carries definite risk to the mother and her fetus. Insufficient experience and differences between institutions prevent a complete catalogue of risks associated with either single- or multiple-needle aspiration of the dilated urinary system or vesicoamniotic shunt catheter placement. Most of the complications mentioned stem either from the reported cases to the International Fetal Registry or collected from the literature. Each patient should be aware of the following possibilities:

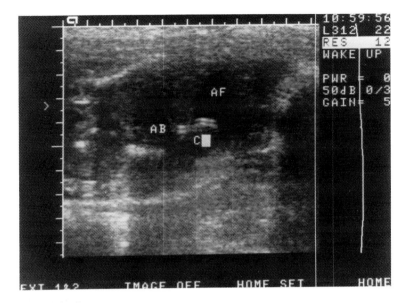

Figure 10-19C The proximal end of the catheter (C) traversing from abdominal cavity (AB) to amniotic cavity (AF).

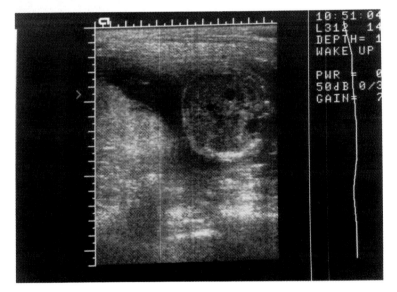

Figure 10-19D The shunt is fully functional; within a few days the urinary tract is completely decompressed (normal abdominal circumference across level of the kidneys); normal amniotic fluid volume is maintained.

1. Even the strict exclusion criteria outlined, used to select only fetuses with preserved renal function, are not absolutely reliable. As a result, irreversible, lethal damage to the lungs or kidneys may have already occurred before treatment.

2. Offering perinatal therapy does not currently guarantee that the treated fetus will not have significant and permanent morbidity postnatally, such as requiring a kidney transplant.

3. Technical failure: sometimes it is technically impossible to place the catheter

properly, due to severe oligohydramnios, fetal position, or, occasionally, massive maternal obesity. Significant uterine contractions or fibroids may also interfere.

4. Functional failure: even though the catheter is properly placed, it may fail to drain the urinary bladder. This could be due to kinking of the catheter or blockage by epithelial debris. This might occur immediately after insertion or some time later. If it occurs shortly after insertion, reinsertion of another catheter might be necessary; if it occurs later, intermittent aspiration of the urinary bladder might be a reasonable option.

5. Catheter displacement: a functioning catheter may be displaced either into the fetal abdomen (resulting in vesicoperitoneal urine leakage and the formation of urinary ascites), or the catheter might be displaced out of the urinary bladder or out of the fe-tus altogether and cease functioning. Catheter displacement might occur anytime; hence, it is mandatory to follow the fetus at least once a week to check catheter position, amniotic fluid volume, and urinary bladder size.

6. Fetal trauma: needle insertion into the fetal abdomen may damage fetal viscera, such as bowel, liver, or intraperitoneal blood vessels (35).

7. Gastroschisis: herniation of the fetal bowel or other abdominal organ might occur through the abdominal defect caused by catheter insertion (15).

8. Fetal, umbilical, or placental hemorrhage (113).

9. Premature rupture of membranes.

10. Preterm delivery of a nonviable or extremely premature fetus.

11. Intrauterine infection.

In addition to these detailed concerns, the goals and likely outcome of therapy need to be reviewed with the parents. Because of the general uncertainty about single or short-term serial urine evaluation, we usually proceed with shunt placement after the first tap has allowed demonstration of otherwise normal fetal anatomy and function. Shunt placement is done for two primary goals, at present:

1. To prevent, or reverse, lethal pulmonary hypoplasia;

2. To maintain, and hopefully to recover, as much renal function as possible. More recently, consideration has been given to shunting less severe cases with the purpose of improving long-term pediatric renal function, to avoid dialysis and ultimate transplantation in such cases.

Shunt placement is ideally performed as soon as the diagnosis is virtually certain, although the trauma of this procedure on the 15–16 week fetus has suggested to some simple bladder taps for several weeks until the fetus is larger (10–22 weeks).

Evaluation of the necessity, benefits, complications, and long-term problems of these procedures is beyond the clinical scope of any one center. The establishment of an international collaborative effort answered these concerns. What follows is a detailed and updated review of the Fetal Surgery Registry.

THERAPEUTIC RESPONSES IN FETAL OBSTRUCTIVE UROPATHY: THE FETAL SURGERY REGISTRY 1993

The establishment of a voluntary fetal surgery registry was widely publicized in the form of written notification to all North American university perinatal centers and selected British, European, Australian, and New Zealand centers and also by direct contact with members of the Fetal Medicine and Surgery Society. In addition, an ongoing literature search was established to identify all published cases of fetal surgery; the authors were contacted and requested to submit their cases to this registry. From its inception, the registry served two main functions: to provide updated information of cumulative results to members of all centers who are contemplating fetal surgery and to report periodically on the outcome of all known treated cases. The registry accepted all cases in which invasive therapy was attempted for congenital fetal disease, but this report specifically addresses cases of obstructive fetal uropathy treated in utero.

Data are presented by observational groupings only and, when appropriate, by mean ± 1 standard deviation. Because case-matched controls are not available, comparative statistical analysis of data was not possible.

More than 300 requests for registry data have been received. Twenty-eight centers have contributed 149 cases to the Registry; 139 of these cases involved treatment of either obstructive uropathy (98 cases) or hydrocephalus (41 cases) and formed the basis of this report; contributors were from the United States (12 centers), Canada (three centers), Great Britain (two centers), and a single center each in Australia, Israel, Chile, Italy, Germany, and Denmark.

Ninety-eight cases of fetal obstructive uropathy treated by in utero placement of a chronic vesicoamniotic shunt have been reported (Table 10-10). The number of cases from any single center are from one to 30, and 10 of the 23 centers reported experience with a single case only. The mean age at diagnosis of obstructive uropathy was 23 ± 4.6 weeks (range of 14.5–36 weeks) and the mean age at "in utero" therapy was 24.2 ± five weeks (range of 14.5–36 weeks). No uniformity in shunt design, construction material, or method of shunt placement is recorded. In 17 of the 98 cases (17.3%), the shunt was placed in the initial attempt; in the remaining 81 cases, two to seven attempts were required before the shunt was considered to be adequately placed.

The survival rate for 98 cases of fetal obstructive uropathy was 40.8% (40 survivors), and the oldest survivor is now 11 years of age and appears to be developing normally.

In 15 of 98 cases (25.9%), the pregnancy was electively terminated some time after shunt placement (Table 10-11). In seven of these, pregnancy was terminated because of an abnormal karyotype [trisomy 13 (three cases), trisomy 18 (two cases), tetraploidy (92,XXXX), and deletion of the large arm of chromosome 2], results which became available after treatment. Seven pregnancies were terminated because of suspected major renal dysfunction (ultrasound demonstration of renal dysplasia) apparent in the postprocedural interval. In the remaining 83 cases, pregnancy was ongoing after shunt placement, with survival in forty (48.2%).

Perinatal survival was strongly related to the primary etiology of obstructive uropathy (Table 10-11). In 31 cases, a primary diagnosis of urethral obstruction due to posterior urethral valve was confirmed; 22 of these treated fetuses survived (70.9%). In five fetuses, a primary diagnosis of prune-belly syndrome without associated anatomical structures was confirmed; four of five fetuses with this condition survived (80%). In eight cases, urethral atresia, either isolated (three cases) or in combination with persistent cloacal syndrome, was confirmed; six of them were female; only one

Table 10-10 Fetal Obstructive Uropathy: Primary Diagnosis* and Outcome in 98 Cases

Primary Diagnosis	No. of Cases	% of Total	No. of Survivors	% Survival by Diagnosis
Posterior urethral valve syndrome	31	31.6	22	70.96
Karyotype abnormality	7	7.14	0	0
Renal dysplasia by ultrasound	6	6.12	0	0
Urethral atresia	8	8.2	1	12.5
"Prune-belly" syndrome	5	5.10	4	80
?	1	1.00	1	100
Cloacal anomalies	1	1.00	0	0
Ureteropelvic function obstruction	2	2.04	2	100
Unknown etiology	37	37.8	10	27
Total	98	100.0	40	40.8

Table 10-11 Fetal Obstructive Uropathy: Outcome Related to Gestational Age at Diagnosis and Treatment

Gestational Age (weeks)	No.	At Initial Diagnosis Survivors	% Surv.	No.	At Treatment Survivors	% Surv.
<20	36	12	33.3	27	8	37.8
>20–<22	10	5	50.0	9	3	33.3
>22–<24	15	5	33.3	15	3	20.0
>24–<26	10	4	40.0	13	4	30.8
>26–<28	8	5	62.5	11	9	81.8
>28–<30	5	2	20.0	8	5	62.5
>30–<32	6	4	66.7	7	3	66.7
>32	8	3	37.5	8	5	62.5
Total	98	40	40.8	98	40	40.81

survived (12.5%); there were two males with no survivor. (In 37 cases, the primary etiology of obstructive uropathy was not confirmed; 10 of these fetuses survived (27%).) Survival was also related to fetal sex. The survival rate for male fetuses was 46.9% (39 out of 83 continuing pregnancies) but was only 16.7% for female fetuses (one of six continuing pregnancies). Survival was not related to fetal age at either the time of the initial diagnosis or the time of treatment (Table 10-12). The relationship between sur-

vival and duration of treatment could not be determined with certainty because the duration of shunt function could not be clearly established from submitted data.

Survival was not related to subjective evaluation of the amniotic fluid volume. The survival rate in cases in which amniotic fluid was judged as normal was 40.9% (nine of 22 cases), and survival with subjective oligohydramnios was 40.8% (31 of 76 cases). In one case, subjective evaluation of amniotic fluid volume was not recorded before treatment.

Table 10-12 Fetal Obstructive Uropathy: Classification of the 58 Deaths by Primary Etiology

Etiology of Death	Time of Death Stillbirth	Postnatal	Total Number	% of all Deaths
Elective termination	15	0	15	25.9
Associated anomalies	1	0	1	1.7
Procedure-related	3	2	5	8.6
Pulmonary hypoplasia	0	34	34	58.6
Renal disease	0	3	3	5.2
Total	19	39	58	100.0

Chronic morbidity in survivors was infrequent and occurred in three of 40 survivors (7.5%). One child with PUV syndrome has developed chronic renal failure that requires treatment with hemodialysis, and this child is waiting for a renal transplant. Another survivor has borderline renal function and chronic pulmonary insufficiency evident at two years of age. A third child, a female, has persistent cloacal syndrome.

Perinatal death occurred in 58 of 98 (59.2%) of treated cases [19 (32.8%) were stillbirths, and 39 (67.2%) were neonatal or infant deaths] (Table 10-12). Fifteen of the 19 stillbirths resulted from elective termination done for indications cited. Four deaths occurred proximate to the time of shunt placement and are presumed to be a direct result of fetal trauma. The remaining stillbirths occurred six weeks after shunt placement, and at autopsy, major central nervous system (CNS) abnormalities, including absent cerebellum, were discovered. These associated anomalies were not recognized prenatally.

Thirty-nine neonatal deaths were recorded (Table 10-12). In 34 of these 39 cases (87.2%), the cause of death was pulmonary hypoplasia with resultant respiratory insufficiency; all of these deaths occurred within six hours of life. One neonatal death was attributed to

premature delivery and respiratory distress syndrome; hyaline membrane disease without evidence of pulmonary hypoplasia was confirmed at autopsy. In this case, premature labor began within 48 hours of shunt placement, presumably procedure-related. Considered collectively, five perinatal deaths may be a direct consequence of fetal therapy (three stillbirths and two neonatal deaths), giving a procedure-related death rate of 5.1% (five of 98 cases). The death of one infant at two months of age was the result of chronic renal failure.

Sixteen of 98 cases exhibited developmental anomalies that were not confined to the urinary tract (16.3%). These anomalies include eight cases of karyotype abnormalities, two cases of multiple system anomalies (CNS, cardiac, gastrointestinal); and two cases of CNS abnormality (absence of cerebellum, neural tube defect).

Analysis of Registry Data

The first cases of successful transcutaneous vesicoamniotic shunting were more than 10 years ago (14,139). The Registry represents an imperfect vehicle for review of a group of fetuses treated for a variety of supposed problems with a variety of approaches since that time.

Whether these therapies were technically feasible has been settled without doubt. It is evident, however, that they are not without fetal risk.

The most important question yet unanswered is whether prenatal surgical therapy improves survival rates and reduces morbidity among affected perinates. A second critical unanswered question centers on case selection and timing and method of therapy. Data in the Registry offer some insight here. However, case report data submitted voluntarily to a central registry from multiple centers may contain inherent biases and require careful interpretation. These inaccuracies include incomplete reporting of individual cases (despite the use of a standardized form), lack of uniform criteria between centers in assessing severity, pathophysiology, and progression of disease, and lack of uniformity regarding the procedure, the type of shunt, and the gestational age at treatment. The possibility that not all cases are reported and that registry cases may be biased toward reports of successful outcome cannot be excluded. In this context, the results from the Registry should be considered as representing the best-case scenario of treated cases. Finally, the lack of a comparable untreated series of affected perinates and especially the absence of randomized controls limits the interpretation of therapeutic benefits.

The reasons for therapy are well-founded in animal experiments and in incidental human observation, which show that surgical decompression prevents accelerated renal damage, restores lung growth, and improves perinatal survival. The results of treatment with human fetuses, particularly those with PUV, are encouraging and suggest that benefit of undetermined magnitude results from therapy. Further improvement in the selection of appropriate cases for fetal therapy and in the timing of

this therapy will follow definition of several areas that remain unsolved.

The exact etiologic connection between obstructive uropathy and pulmonary hypoplasia is still unclear. As well, the precise relationships between time of onset, extent and duration of obstruction, and perinatal outcome are still unknown. (In Registry cases, as in the animal model, the earlier the obstruction is produced, the more severe are the renal and pulmonary consequences.) Variation in response suggests precise diagnosis is important: urethral atresia causes total obstruction from the onset and is associated with the poorest survival of treated cases; only the fetus treated in utero at 21 weeks gestation survived with this diagnosis. PUV produces later onset obstruction that may be partial or complete; the best survival rate for the treated fetuses occurred in this group (22 out of 31 fetuses—71%). Thus, it seems that later obstruction in the human fetus produces less damage to the kidneys and lungs and that the damage is more reversible in these cases.

Direct proof that in utero surgery for obstructive uropathy improves perinatal outcome cannot be determined from the Registry cases per se, because matched controls are lacking. The outcome of the 79 reported fetuses with untreated bladder outlet obstruction reviewed earlier (mortality 81%) suggests that a true benefit of therapy (29% for PUV-treated in utero) is present. Comparison of these two groups suggests fetal therapy for PUV improves both survival and serious morbidity in survivors. On the other hand, whereas most in utero treated fetuses with prune-belly-like syndrome survived, a high survival rate in nontreated fetuses is also reported (38,40).

There are no published series of the outcome of fetuses with urethral atresia, but a benefit of fetal surgery for this condition is likely because prolonged and sustained obstruction in fetal lambs is usually fatal (25,26,28). In the Registry, many fetuses (37.8%) had obstructive uropathy of unknown etiology not due to a proven anatomic block of the urinary outflow tract. The question of whether fetal therapy was of any benefit in these cases cannot be determined. Overall, a comparison of the results of treatment in the Registry cases with unmatched historical controls suggests that fetal therapy is beneficial.

Recognition of fetuses who cannot benefit from in utero therapy is an important step in case selection. In Registry cases, the incidence of chromosomal abnormalities in fetuses with obstructive uropathy was relatively high (8.2%), confirming the need for fetal karyotype. The ongoing development of accurate, reliable tests of fetal renal function will have considerable value in case selection. Unfortunately, at present, prenatal determination of pulmonary hypoplasia by ultrasound or another method, such as MRI (140), has not been well developed. The same applies for fetal renal dysplasia. Advances in these areas may also be expected to enhance case selection considerably.

A prospective randomized trial of this new therapy seems to be essential to address the current array of concerns. Widespread implementation of any new therapy must be based on three fundamental tenets: that (1) the therapy is possible; (2) the risks are known, and (3) tangible benefits outweigh the risks of therapy and clearly enhance survival and the quality of life. The Registry data answer the first. Perinatal therapy for fetal obstructive uropathy with either placement of a permanent vesicoamniotic shunt or, in selected cases, intermittent needle aspiration is a practical reality. The second basis for action, definition of the liabilities of these techniques, is also addressed by the Registry, but this is likely a major underestimation of the dangers of therapy.

The answer to the third question, regarding the benefits outweighing the risks, cannot be determined with certainty.

Even though it is technically simple to insert a catheter into the fetal abdomen, it is still challenging to select the fetus who will benefit from it, with minimal pre- and postnatal mortality and morbidity. Evaluating fetal renal function, following the fetal urine chemistry and electrolyte changes trend over a period of time by serial fetal urine analysis, improvements in fetal imaging, and ongoing pathophysiologic data, all may enhance our approach. Because of limitations in selecting the fetus who benefits from prenatal therapy and because of the high possibility of selecting a fetus who already has a lethal renal or pulmonary dysplasia, in our opinion, open fetal surgery has no place in modern management of fetuses with urinary tract obstruction. However, other innovative techniques, including development of fetoscopic surgery and laser therapy, will help in selecting and treating those fetuses without exposing the mother to the risk of hysterotomy and classical cesarean section.

From our review of accumulated experience, fetuses with urinary tract obstruction may be divided into four groups according to their perinatal long-term outcome.

Group I

Fetuses with urinary tract obstruction who will have a good outcome with minimal neonatal morbidity, if managed conservatively without perinatal intrauterine intervention. These include fetuses who have unilateral urinary tract obstruction with a normal contralateral functioning kidney, fetuses with lower urinary tract obstruction, but who continue to have good urine output and adequate amniotic fluid volume and minimal or slowly-progressive dilatation of the upper urinary tract. Expectant observation is all that is required.

Group II

Fetuses with urinary tract obstruction who will have a poor neonatal outcome or significant morbidity in spite of perinatal intrauterine intervention and postnatal treatment. These include fetuses who have associated lethal anomalies, multiple nonlethal anomalies, abnormal karyotype, renal or pulmonary dysplasia, or MMIH syndrome. The management of these fetuses should be conservative at most; fetal therapy is considered inappropriate; pregnancy termination may be offered.

Group III

These fetuses with uncommon forms of urinary tract obstruction may benefit from perinatal intrauterine intervention but will have permanent significant morbidity in spite of pre- and postnatal treatment. These include urethral atresia, primary prune-belly syndrome, and persistent cloacal syndrome. In view of the desperate fetal situation and the poor long-term prognosis despite surgery, randomization in a therapeutic trial would not be appropriate.

Group IV

Fetuses with urinary tract obstruction due to PUV syndrome probably will benefit from intrauterine vesicoamniotic shunt with minimal postnatal morbidity. These benefits must be well established before universal acceptance is warranted. The issue cannot be easily or accurately solved by comparison with nonmatched historical data. A properly designed, prospective multi-center randomized trial is required to answer these questions.

ANTENATAL MANAGEMENT OF FETAL HYDROCEPHALUS

Context

Unlike urinary tract obstruction, for which many further steps are indicated and for which the Fetal Surgery Registry suggests such promise, fetal hydrocephalus and antenatal therapy do not have a clearly defined, positive connection. Analysis of this relationship will illustrate clearly why careful study is necessary before any revolutionary therapy is applied to everyone.

Fetal hydrocephalus, defined as the accumulation of abnormal volumes of cerebrospinal fluid within the ventricular system of the brain, is among the more common of the fetal abnormalities, affecting between 5.3 per 1000 liveborns (141). It occurs as either an isolated finding or in association with anomalies of other organ systems. As is true with all perinatal anomalies, surveys of liveborn infants underestimate the true incidence of disease; this is especially true in the case of hydrocephalus, given the high rate of fetal death that accompanies this condition. Further, as ultrasound evaluation of the fetal ventricular system is generally done under conditions of high resolution and since dilation of the ventricular system is recognized relatively easily, more cases of fetal disease are recognized before delivery (Figure 10-20). The true incidence of fetal disease is therefore known to be higher than the neonatal estimates and is in the range of eight to 10 cases per 1000 fetuses.

Hydrocephalus is a sign of an underlying fetal disease process but is not a disease in its own right. The etiologies of hydrocephalus in the fetus are many, and the peri-

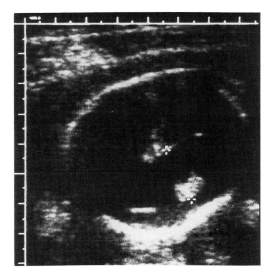

Figure 10-20   Axial sonograms of the fetal head, demonstrating: **10-20A**   mild hydrocephalus

natal prognosis will vary directly with the underlying etiology. This point is stressed at the outset since it is as clear in diseases of the fetus as it is in diseases affecting the extrauterine patient that the therapeutic aim is to treat the primary pathological process. Treatment of the signs (and symptoms) is a secondary goal. As the efficacy of therapies for the treatment of fetal hydrocephalus, both immediate and long-term, have been subjected to scrutiny, it has become evident that treatment of the sign of disease (ventriculomegaly), however successful, cannot be taken as evidence of a therapeutic triumph. It is rather the long-term outcome that is the critical endpoint.

In many ways, the advances in the detection and treatment of fetal hydrocephalus have served as a microcosm of the complexities of fetal anomaly diagnosis and in utero treatment (Table 10-13). Firstly, for this condition, it is clear that despite a common etiology, there are clear and important differences in prognosis between the affected fetus and the affected neonate. Powerful *natural selection processes*, by which fetal death is common, either in the antepartum period due to causes poorly understood or in the intrapartum period as a result of pro-

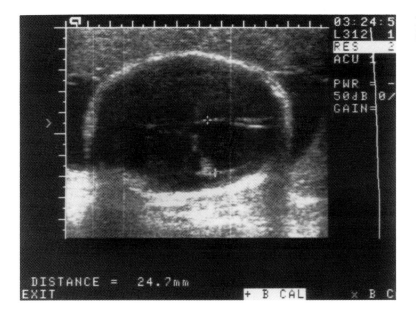

Figure 10-20B   moderate hydrocephalus

Figure 10-20C severe hydrocephalus

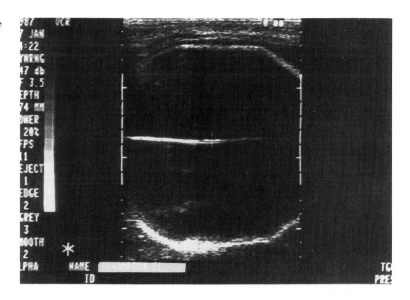

Figure 10-20D parasagittal scan of the same fetus (C) demonstrating macrocephaly and severe hydrocephalus.

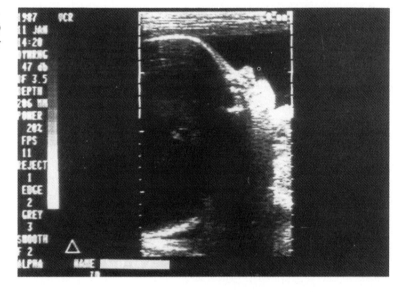

found dystocia, ensure that spontaneous delivery occurs only in the least severely affected neonate. The immediate period of transition from the intrauterine fetal environment to the air-breathing environment of the neonate is also a time of selection. The more compromised affected neonate is less able to effect this transition and, therefore,

at risk for very early neonatal death. The perinate that can survive the antepartum, intrapartum, and immediate neonatal risks is generally the one with the least severe disease but is still not immune to the development of long-term neurological disability associated with the underlying disruption of cerebrospinal fluid circulation and is

Table 10-13 Fetal Hydrocephalus: Factors
Affecting Assessment of Treatment

(A) **Natural selection process: the fetal loss rate
always exceeds the neonatal rate**
(B) **Perinatal prognosis is determined more by
disease etiology than the physical
manifestations of the disease process**
(C) **Assessment of the therapeutic efficacy must
include both structural and functional effects**
(D) **The treatment itself can cause fetal mortality
and morbidity**

prone to premature death in infancy or childhood. Antenatal diagnosis and treatment in utero alters the perinatal history but may not alter the longer-term prognosis: treated fetuses that might otherwise have died in the antenatal period as a consequence of the disease progression or might have died in labor are less likely to suffer this complication. Thus, fetal treatment may be expected to bypass the natural selection processes.

Secondly, the experience with fetal hydrocephalus demonstrates that *perinatal prognosis is more determined by disease etiology than by the physical manifestations*. Hydrocephalus will complicate most conditions that cause obstruction to free circulation of cerebrospinal fluid. Perinatal outcome, as measured by both mortality and immediate and long-term morbidity, may be expected to vary with the underlying etiology. Thus, for example, ventriculomegaly associated with simple isolated obstruction of the third ventricle might respond readily to a chronic decompression procedure and result in preservation of normal brain tissue and function, whereas ventriculomegaly secondary to primary defect in brain cell migration and organization might also respond to chronic decompression but without beneficial impact on future brain development or function.

Thirdly, clinical observations among fetuses with hydrocephalus underscore the fundamental of fetal therapy, that is the *assessment of the therapeutic efficacy of fetal treatment in the prevention or amelioration of disease must include functional as well as structural evaluation*. This latter principle is at the core of the ethical controversies that surround the concept of fetal therapy in general and hydrocephalus in particular. Outcome with hydrocephalus does not conform to a binary distribution, where the affected fetus either dies of its disease or recovers. Prognosis with this condition varies from one extreme, of death or survival with hopeless loss of cognitive, sensory, and motor function, to the other extreme, intact long-term survival without evidence or consequence of damage. Were prognosis related in some precise manner to the physical (ultrasound) manifestations of the disease process, then case selection for therapy would be simple and direct. Unfortunately, except in cases of extremes or in those conditions in which the underlying etiology is known with certainty, the relationship between physical manifestations and long-term prognosis is far from certain. In these cases, the use of immediate measures of therapeutic success, such as the resolution or amelioration of the ventriculomegaly or the gross perinatal mortality rate, may present a biased account of the overall impact of the treatment to the patient.

Whether a fetus might choose or have society choose for it, a life complicated by cortical blindness, spastic quadriplegia, or near absence of any cognitive function remains a key and unanswered question. Such questions need to be addressed by the medical community and society at large before any therapeutic success can be attributed to fetal surgery for ventriculomegaly.

Finally, the experiences with fetal therapy for ventriculomegaly illuminate the point that *intervention can result in iatrogenic fetal mortality and morbidity and also carries the small, but nonetheless real, risk of maternal complications.* Any operative procedure has risk, and the selection of a given procedure generally rests on a comparison of risk to benefit. Placing a needle into the fetal ventricle requires traversing the fetal brain tissue, incurring the risk of hemorrhage and brain injury. Unlike the extrauterine patient, the fetus cannot be physically restrained and reactions to the pain of the needle penetration enhance the risk of the procedure. The perinatal death rate associated with attempted fetal therapy for hydrocephalus (9.75%) is the *highest* reported for any percutaneous invasive fetal procedure (142).

The development of means for treatment of fetal ventriculomegaly arose simultaneously in several centers throughout the world and led to an initial flurry of activity that was steeped in optimism. As experience was gained, there was a wane in enthusiasm fuelled by the observation of a disparity between immediate and longer-term prognosis. Recognition of the important distinction became possible in a short period of time because of an agreement among clinical investigators to pool their collective experience in a Fetal Surgery Registry. This registry has been held at the University of Manitoba since its inception in 1982. The purpose of this chapter is to review the clinical results of fetal therapy for hydrocephalus as contained in this registry of international cases.

The Fetal Surgery Registry:
Obstructive Hydrocephalus

At the time of writing, there are 41 cases of fetal obstructive hydrocephalus treated by chronic ventriculoamniotic shunt placement (39 cases) or by repeated cephalocen-tesis (two cases) contained in this registry. This number of cases has not changed appreciably over the last five years, a reflection of the effect of a voluntary moratorium placed on this type of surgery by the International Fetal Medicine and Surgery Society in 1988. This moratorium was reached by consensus after consideration of the cumulative experience with the method. It is based on the premise that fetal therapy for hydrocephalus, while technically possible and often associated with an appreciable decline in either absolute ventricular size or the rate of increase, and associated with a significant improvement in the perinatal survival rate, is also associated with a high probability of severe long-term functional impairment. A codicil to the moratorium was the statement that attempts should continue to try to identify the structural and pathophysiological markers that might aid in fixing prognosis with greater precision. By this moratorium, fetal surgery for hydrocephalus was considered to be highly experimental.

These cases were submitted from 11 American centers and from a single Italian center. Unlike the experience for obstructive uropathy, no Canadian or English centers have reported an experience with treatment of obstructive hydrocephalus. In most cases, the treatment has been by placement under continuous dynamic ultrasound guidance of a Silastic shunt, usually valved, into the posterior horn of the lateral ventricle and then leaving the other end free in the amniotic cavity so that cerebral spinal fluid may egress freely from the ventricle. The method assumes that the ventricular pressure in the presence of obstruction will exceed amniotic fluid pressure. However, this observation is not always the case, and the presence of the valve prevents reflux of amniotic fluid and debris into the ventricular system,

Table 10-14   Fetal Hydrocephalus: Duration of Treatment and Outcome

Duration of Treatment	No. of Cases	% Total Cases	Outcome					
			Mortality		Normal		Handicapped	
			No.	%	No.	%	No.	%
1 day–2 wks	6	14.6	4	66.7	0	0	2	100
>2–<4 wks	11	26.8	2	18.2	3	33.3	6	66.7
>4–<8 wks	10	24.4	1	10	5	55	4	45
>8 weeks	14	32.4	0	0	4	28.6	10	71.4
Total	41	100	7	17.1	12	42.8	22	57.2

a complication that could result in a chemical ventriculitis that may further compound fetal brain development and function.

The mean gestational age at diagnosis of hydrocephalus was 25 ± 2.73 weeks (range 18–31 weeks) and at therapy was 27 ± 2.6 weeks (range 23–33 weeks). Perinatal mortality rate appeared inversely related to the duration of treatment, but there was no apparent relationship between the presence and severity of long-term neurological morbidity and the duration of therapy (Table 10-14). The assumed etiology of the ventriculomegaly varied widely; aqueductal stenosis was the most commonly cited cause

(Table 10-15). In retrospect, most of the conditions other than aqueductal stenosis were not likely to have benefitted from intervention, and inclusion of the results of these cases tends to bias the results towards an even gloomier picture. Four perinates died as a direct consequence of the attempts at therapy; one stillbirth occurred as a result of direct trauma to the brain stem and three neonatal deaths occurred as a result of chorioamnionitis that may be reasonably attributed to bacterial contamination of the intrauterine environment at the time of the procedure (procedural death rate 9.75%). At last report, the survivors had been followed

Table 10-15   Fetal Hydrocephalus: Etiology and Mortality

Primary Etiology (postnatal)	No. of Cases	% Total Cases	Mortality	
			No.	%
Aqueductal stenosis	32	76.9	4	13.3
Associated anomalies	5	12.7	2	40
Holoprosencephaly	1	2.6	1	100
Dandy-Walker cyst	1	2.6	0	0
Porencephalic cyst	1	2.6	0	0
Arnold-Chiari syndrome	1	2.6	0	0
Total	41	—	7	17

Table 10-16   Fetal Hydrocephalus: Neurological Outcome by Diagnosis

Primary Diagnosis (postnatal) %	No. of Survivors	Normal		Mild/Moderate Handicap		Severe Handicap	
		No.	*%*	*No.*	*%*	*No.*	*%*
Aqueductal stenosis	28	12	42.8	2	7.2	14	50
Associated anomalies	3	0	0	0	0	3	100
Dandy-Walker	1	0	0	1	100	0	0
Porencephalic cyst	1	0	0	0	0	1	100
Arnold-Chiari	1	0	0	1	100	0	0
Total	34	12	35.3	4	11.8	18	52.9

for intervals as short as one month and as long as 18 months. (A more detailed appraisal of long-term outcome of survivors, some of whom are now more than 8 years old, is underway at present.) Overall, about a third of survivors (35.3%) were normal at follow-up, and among fetuses treated for obstructive hydrocephalus, the results were slightly better (42.8%) (Table 10-16). Morbidity among survivors ranged from moderate developmental delay and minor motor disabilities to severe developmental delay, cortical blindness, and spastic diplegia. Prognosis was best for hydrocephalus secondary to aqueductal stenosis and the only intact survivors occurred in this group (Table 10-16).

Fetal Hydrocephalus—Is In Utero Decompression Indicated?

When viewed from the perspective of perinatal mortality, the application of in utero chronic decompression would appear to be quite efficacious and, therefore, indicated. Using aqueductal stenosis as the model, being the only condition at present for which a rational argument for attempted

treatment can be supported, in utero treatment yields a perinatal mortality of 12.5% (four of 32 cases). As there are no concurrent controlled studies, information regarding the expected outcome of fetuses with a diagnosis of aqueductal stenosis must be derived from the literature (historical controls) and is, therefore, subject to selection bias. There are three relatively large studies directed toward determining the natural history of fetal ventriculomegaly due to aqueductal stenosis (143–145). Combined, these three studies gave a perinatal survival rate of 31% (range per study 23–42%), a rate significantly lower than that reported for the treated group (87.5%). The survival rate for neonates born with overt hydrocephalus is reported at 86% (146), a rate not significantly different from that reported for fetuses treated for hydrocephalus in utero. Neonatal outcome cannot equate to fetal outcome, however, since there is powerful selection bias in operation (the fetus must live long enough in utero, and then survive labor, to appear in the neonatal group). If perinatal survival were the key endpoint used to judge treatment efficacy, then there is evidence that in utero therapy is beneficial.

The picture is quite different when long-term morbidity is used as the outcome endpoint. Considered collectively, the natural history series for fetal hydrocephalus indicate while fewer of the untreated fetuses survive, those that do (27 cases) have a normal outcome in 51.5% (14 of 27 cases). Treated cases of aqueductal stenosis have a better survival rate (28 of 32 cases), but the prospect of a normal long-term outcome (12 of 28 survivors, 42.8%) does not differ from the rate reported for the untreated cases. These differences create a difficult problem: *treatment of hydrocephalus will result in a larger number of both normal survivors and abnormal survivors.* The nut of the problem centers around the quality of life of the treated, but damaged survivors. It is unclear whether the advantages that are gained by treatment in some is justified by the serious long-term morbidity visited upon others. The problem is made even more difficult in the realization that it is not possible at the present time to predict with an acceptable degree of accuracy which fetus will have which outcome. This clinical conundrum is the primary reason for the voluntary moratorium. Unfortunately, there has been no appreciable progress in resolving this challenging clinical dilemma, and until such an advance occurs, it seems reasonable to continue to consider that fetal treatment for hydrocephalus should remain an experimental treatment and should not be endorsed as a routine or accepted treatment of fetal hydrocephalus.

Fetal Treatment For Hydrocephalus:
Future Considerations

Since the first reports of treatment of fetal hydrocephalus by chronic ventriculoamniotic shunting in 1982 (146–148), there have been remarkable improvements in the ability to visualize fetal intracranial anatomy by ultrasound. New methods for assessing cerebral blood flow velocity and distribution have become available. At the least, it is now far less likely that conditions, such as holoprosencephaly or hydrocephalus associated with other anomalies, will be subjected to treatment since such attempts are doomed to failure, and at best, it is becoming ever more possible to determine the presence, extent, and progression of cerebral damage. However, there persists a major deficit in the correlation of physical damage to the fetal brain with long-term neurological function of the perinate. The observed, but inconsistent successes with in utero therapy for fetal hydrocephalus are the promise that in some cases therapy is of benefit. What is needed now for the field to advance is a reliable means of identifying these fetuses prospectively. Such a test is likely to be difficult to develop since it must predict the ability of the fetal brain to adapt and recover from loss. It would seem almost certain that this test cannot rely on measurement of anatomical variables, but must rather be based on a survey of fetal functional activities, either as observed passively or in response to an applied perturbation. Tests that evoke and measure fetal cerebral responses to applied stimuli, such as vibroacoustic stimulation, have been reported (149). While not implying that this particular test is of value in case selection for treatment of fetal hydrocephalus, the concept raised in this work, that is, that fetal brain functional responses to an applied stimulus provide insight into its integrity, seems the most fruitful area in which to begin the search for the critical prognostic variables. Until such variables are found, the continuation of the voluntary moratorium of fetal therapy for hydrocephalus seems reasonable.

CONCLUSION

Fetal surgery is here to stay. Especially for PUV, the results are rewarding and will likely improve even further. At the other extreme are many cases of hydrocephalus and some cases of fetal urinary tract obstruction, where therapy is of no measurable benefit in most and has definitely produced harm in some. Continued diligence in a scientific, research-oriented approach is our obligation. The technical challenge of placing a shunt catheter in a small human fetus is exciting. However, the real challenge lies in selecting the fetus who will unequivocally benefit from the adventure.

References

1. Moore KL. The developing human. In: The Developing Human, Clinically Oriented Embryology. 3rd ed. Philadelphia: WB Saunders, 1982, 255–297.
2. Temple JK, Shapira E. Genetic determinants of renal disease in neonates. Clin Perinatol 1981;8(2):361–373.
3. McCrory W. Developmental nephrology. Cambridge: Harvard University Press, 1972;51–78.
4. Potter E. Normal and Abnormal Development of the Kidney. Chicago: Year Book Medical Publisher, 1972.
5. Yard A, Barakat AY, Ichikawa L. Assessment and care of the fetus. Physiological, clinical, and medicolegal principles. In: Eden RD, Boehm FH, eds. Fetal Nephrology. Appleton & Lange, Norwalk, Connecticut, 1990;5:69–92.
6. Potter EL. Kidneys, ureters, urinary bladder, and urethra. In: Potter EL, Craig JM, eds. Pathology of the fetus and the infant. 3rd ed. Chicago: Year Book Medical Publisher, 1976;22:434–473.
7. Adzick NS, Harrison MR, Glick PL, Flake AW. Fetal urinary tract obstruction: experimental pathophysiology. Sem in Perinatol, 1985;9:79–90.
8. Beck AD. The effect of intrauterine urinary obstruction upon the development of the fetal kidney. J Urol 1971;105:784–789.
9. King LR. Posterior urethra. In: Kelalis PP, King LR, Belman AB, eds. Philadelphia: WB Saunders, 1985;(1):527–558.
10. Bernstein J. The morphogenesis of renal parenchymal maldevelopment (renal dysplasia). Pediatr Clin of NA 1971;18:395–407.
11. Young HH, Frontz WA, Baldwin JC. Congenital obstruction of posterior urethra. J Urol 1919;3:289–354.
12. Stephen FD. Urethral obstruction in childhood: the use of urethrography in diagnosis. In: Douglas SF, ed. Congenital malformation of the rectum, anus, and genitourinary tracts. Edinburgh: Livingstone, 1963;209–245.
13. Henneberry MO, Stephens FD. Renal hypoplasia and dysplasia in infants with posterior urethral valves. J Urol 1980; 123:912–195.
14. Manning FA, Harman CR, Lange IR, Brown R, Decter A, MacDonald N. Antepartum chronic fetal vesicoamniotic shunts for obstructive uropathy: a report of two cases. Am J Obstet Gynecol 1983;145:819–822.
15. Evans MI, Sacks AJ, Johnson MP, Robichaux AG, May M, Moghissi KS. Sequential invasive assessment of fetal renal function and the intrauterine treatment of fetal obstructive uropathies. Obstet Gynecol 1991;77:545–550.
16. Hobbins JC, Romero R, Grannum P, Berkowitz RL, Cullen M, Mahoney M. Antenatal diagnosis of renal anomalies with ultrasound. I. Obstructive uropathy. Am J Obstet Gynecol 1984;148:868–877.
17. Tanagho EA. Surgically induced partial urinary obstruction in the fetal lamb. I. Technique. Investig Urol 1972;10(1):19–24.
18. Tanagho EA. Surgically induced partial urinary obstruction in the fetal lamb. II. Urethral obstruction. Investig Urol 1972; 10(1):25–34.
19. Tanagho EA. Surgically induced partial urinary obstruction in the fetal lamb. III. Urethral obstruction. Investig Urol 1972; 10(1):35–52.

20. Glick PL, Harrison MR, Noall RA, Villa RL: Correction of congenital hydronephrosis in utero. III. Early mid-trimester ureteral obstruction produces renal dysplasia. J Pediatr Surg 1983;18(6):681–687.
21. McVary K, Maizels M. Urinary obstruction reduces glomerulogenesis in the developing kidney: a model of the rabbit. J Urol 1989;142:646–651.
22. Berman DJ, Maizels M. The role of urinary obstruction in the genesis of renal dysplasia. A model in the chick embryo. J Urol 1982;128:1091–1096.
23. Steinhardt GF, Vogler G, Salinas-Madrigal L, LaRegina M. Induced renal dysplasia in the young pouch opossum. J Pediatr Surg 1988;23(12):1127–1130.
24. Peters CA, Mandell J. Experimental congenital obstructive uropathy. Urol Clin of NA 1990;17:437–447.
25. Glick PL, Harrison MR, Adzick NS, Noall RA, Villa RL. Correction of congenital hydronephrosis in utero. IV: in utero decompression prevents renal dysplasia. J Pediatr Surg 1984;19:649–657.
26. Harrison MR, Nakayama DK, Noall R, de Lorimier AA. Correction of congenital hydronephrosis in utero. II. Decompression reverses the effects of obstruction on the fetal lung and urinary tract. J Pediatr Surg 1982;17:965–974.
27. Manning FA. Fetal surgery for obstructive uropathy: rational considerations. Am J Kidney Dis 1987;10:259–267.
28. Harrison MR, Ross N, Noall R, de Lorimier AA. Correction of congenital hydronephrosis in utero. I. The model: fetal urethral obstruction produces hydronephrosis and pulmonary hypoplasia in fetal lambs. J Pediatr Surg 1983;18:247–256.
29. Docimo SG, Luetic T, Crone RK, et al. Pulmonary development in the fetal lamb with severe bladder outlet obstruction and oligohydramnios: a morphometric study. J Urol 1989;142:657–660.
30. Hislop A, Hey E, Reid L. The lungs in congenital bilateral renal agenesis and dysplasia. Arch Dis Child 1979;54:32–38.
31. Nimrod C, Varela-Gittings F, Machin G, Campbell D, Wesenberg R. The effect of very prolonged membrane rupture on fetal development. Am J Obstet Gynecol 1984;148:540–543.
32. Nakayama DK, Glick PL, Harrison MR, Villa RL, Noall R. Experimental pulmonary hypoplasia due to oligohydramnios and its reversal by relieving thoracic compression. J Pediatr Surg 1983;18:347–353.
33. Wigglesworth JS, Desai R, Guerrini P. Fetal lung hypoplasia; biochemical and structural variations and their possible significance. Arch Dis Child 1981;56:606–615.
34. Adzick NS, Harrison MR, Glick PL, Villa RL, Finkbeiner W. Experimental pulmonary hypoplasia and oligohydramnios: relative contributions of lung fluid and fetal breathing movements. J Pediatr Surg 1984;19:658–665.
35. Harrison MR, Filly RA. The fetus with obstructive uropathy: pathophysiology, natural history, selection, and treatment. In: Harrison MR, Golbus MS, Filly FA, eds. The Unborn Patient. 2nd ed. Philadelphia: WB Saunders, 1990;328–393.
36. Manning, FA. Common fetal urinary tract anomalies. In: Hobbins JC, Benacerraf B (eds). Diagnosis and Management of Fetal Anomalies. New York: Churchill-Livingstone, 1989, 139–161.
37. Bulic M, Podobnik M, Korenic B, Bistricki J. First-trimester diagnosis of low obstructive uropathy: an indicator of initial renal function in the fetus. J Clin Ultrasound 1987;15:537–541.
38. Smythe AR, Major MC. Ultrasonic detection of fetal ascites and bladder dilation with resulting prune belly. J Pediatr 1981;98:978–980.
39. Shweni PM, Kambaran SR, Ramdial K. Fetal ascites. A report of 6 cases. S Afr Med J 1984;66:616–618.
40. Pagon RA, Smith DW, Shepard TH. Urethral obstruction malformation complex: a cause of abdominal muscle deficiency and the "prune belly." J Pediatr 1979; 94:900–906.

41. Greskovich FJ, Nyberg LM. The prune belly syndrome: a review of its etiology, defects, treatment, and prognosis. J Urol 1988; 140:707–712.

42. Harrison MR, Golbus MS, Filly RA, et al. Management of the fetus with congenital hydronephrosis. J Pediatr Surg 1982; 17:728–742.

43. Hoover DL, Duckett JW. Posterior urethral valves, unilateral reflux, and renal dysplasia: a syndrome. J Urol 1982;128: 944–997.

44. Bellinger MF, Comstock CH, Grosso D, et al. Fetal posterior urethral valves and renal dysplasia at 15 weeks gestational age. J Urol 1983;130:1238–1239.

45. Gonzales ET. Alternatives in the management of posterior urethral valves. Urol Clin NA 1990;17:335–342.

46. Nicolini M, Rodeck CH, Fisk NM. Shunt treatment for fetal obstructive uropathy. The Lancet (Letter) 1987;ii:1338–1339.

47. Pocock RD, Witcombe JB, Andrews HS, Berry PJ, Frank JD. The outcome of antenatally diagnosed urological abnormalities. Br J Urol 1985;57:788–792.

48. Quinlan RW, Cruz AC, Huddleston JF. Sonographic detection of fetal urinary tract anomalies. Obstet Gynecol 1986; 67:558–565.

49. Noia G, Masini L, Caruso A, et al. Prenatal diagnosis of congenital uropathies. Fetal Ther 1989;4(Suppl 1):40–51.

50. Mahony BS, Callen PW, Filly RA. Fetal urethral obstruction: US evaluation. Radiol 1985;157:221–224.

51. Reuss A, Wladimiroff JW, Scholtmeijer RJ, Stewart PA, Sauer PJJ, Niermeijer MF. Prenatal evaluation and outcome of fetal obstructive uropathies. Prenatal Diag 1988; 8:93–102.

52. Manning FA. The fetus with obstructive uropathy: the Fetal Surgery Registry. In: Harrison MR, Golbus MS, Filly FA, eds. The Unborn Patient. 2nd ed. Philadelphia: WB Saunders, 1990: Chapter 32:394–398.

53. Evans MI, Drugan A, Manning FA, Harrison MR. Fetal surgery in the 1990s. Am J Dis Child 1989;143:1431–1436.

54. Nakayama DK, Harrison MR, de Lorimier AA. Prognosis of posterior urethral valves presenting at birth. J Pediatr Surgery 1986;21:43–45.

55. Williams DI. Urethral valves; a hundred cases with hydronephrosis. Birth Defects 1977;13:55–78.

56. Reznik VM, Murphy JL, Mendoza SA, Griswold WR, Packer MG, Kaplan GW. Follow-up of infants with obstructive uropathy detected in utero and treated surgically postnatally. J Pediatr Surg 1989;24: 1289–1292.

57. Steele BT, De Maria J, Toi A, Stafford A, Hunter D, Caco C. Neonatal outcome of fetuses with urinary tract abnormalities diagnosed by prenatal ultrasonography. Can Med Assoc J 1987;137:117–120.

58. McFadyen IR. Obstruction of the fetal urinary tract: a role for surgical intervention in utero? Br Med J 1984;288:459–462.

59. Diament MJ, Fine RN, Ehrlich R, Kangarloo H. Fetal hydronephrosis: problems in diagnosis and management. J Pediatr 1983; 103:435–439.

60. Callan NA, Blakemore K, Park J, Sanders RC, Jeffs RD, Gearhart JP. Fetal genitourinary tract anomalies: evaluation, operative correction, and follow-up. Obstet Gynecol 1990;75:67–74.

61. Woodard JR. The impact of fetal diagnosis on the management of obstructive uropathy. Postgrad Med J 1990;66(Suppl 1): S37–S43.

62. Arthur RJ, Irving HC, Thomas DFM, Watters JK. Bilateral fetal uropathy: what is the outlook? Br Med J 1989;298:1419–1421.

63. Thomas DFM, Irving HC, Arthur RJ. Prenatal diagnosis: how useful is it? Br Med J Urol 1985;57:784–787.

64. Warshaw BL, Edelbrock HH, Ettenger RB, Malekzadeh MH, Pennisi AJ, Uittenbogaart CH, Fine RN. Progressive to end-stage renal disease in children with obstructive uropathy. J Pediatr 1982;100:183–187.

65. Duval JM, Milon J, Coadou Y, et al. Ultrasonographic anatomy and diagnosis of fetal uropathies affecting the upper urinary tract. I. Obstructive uropathies. Anat Clin 1985;7:301–336.

66. Drake DP, Stevens PS, Eckstein HB. Hydronephrosis secondary to ureteropelvic obstruction in children: a review of 14 years of experiences: J Urol 1978;119:649–651.

67. Johnston JH, Evans JP, Glassberg KI, et al. Pelvic hydronephrosis in children: a review of 219 personal cases. J Urol 1977;117: 97–101.

68. Robson WJ, Rudy SM, Johnston JH. Pelviureteric obstruction in infancy. J Pediatr Surg 1976;11:57.

69. Ghidini A, Sirtori M, Vergani P, Orsenigo E, Tagliabue P, Parravicini E. Ureteropelvic junction obstruction in utero and ex utero. Obstet Gynecol 1990:75:805–808.

70. Antonakopoulos GN, Fuggle WJ, Newman J, et al. Idiopathic hydronephrosis. Arch Pathol Lab Med 1985;109:1097–1101.

71. Hanna MK, Jeffs RD, Sturgess JM, et al. Ureteral structure and ultrastructure. Part II: Congenital ureteropelvic junction obstruction and primary obstructive megaureter. J Urol 1976;116:725–730.

72. Arnold AJ, Rickwood AMK. Natural history of pelviureteric obstruction detected by prenatal sonography. Br J Urol 1990; 65:91–96.

73. Bernstein GT, Mandell J, Lebowitz RL, Bauer SB, Colodny AH, Retik AB. Ureteropelvic junction obstruction in the neonate. J Urol 1988;140:1216–1221.

74. Kleiner B, Callen PW, Filly RA. Sonographic analysis of the fetus with ureteropelvic junction obstruction. AJR 1987;148:359–363.

75. Grignon A, Filiatrault D, Homsy Y, et al. Ureteropelvic junction stenosis: antenatal ultrasonographic diagnosis, postnatal investigation, and follow-up. Radiology 1986;160:649–651.

76. Ryynanen M, Martikainen A, Saarikoski S. Antenatally diagnosed fetal hydronephrosis. Five years' follow-up. J Perinat Med 1990:18:313–316.

77. Seeds JW, Cefalo RC, Herbert WNP, Bowes WA Jr. Hydramnios and maternal renal failure: relief with fetal therapy. Obstet Gynecol 1984;64(S#3):26S–29S.

78. Kirkinen P, Jouppila P, Tuononen S, Paavilainen T. Repeated transabdominal renocenteses in a case of fetal hydronephrotic kidney. Am J Obstet Gynecol 1982; 142:1049–1052.

79. Vintzileos AM, Nochimson DJ, Walzak MP, Conard FU, Lillo NL. Unilateral fetal hydronephrosis: successful in utero surgical management. Am J Obstet Gynecol 1983; 145:885–886.

80. Schaaps JP, Thoumsin H, Lambotte R. Intrauterine unilateral nephrostomy. Am J Obstet Gynecol 1983;146(1):105–106.

81. Seeds JW, Mandell J. Congenital obstructive uropathies. Pre- and postnatal treatment. Urol Clin of NA 1986;13:155–165.

82. Pringle KC. Fetal diagnosis and fetal surgery. Clin in Perinatol 1989;16:13–28.

83. Bond SJ, Harrison MR. Obstructive uropathy—when to intervene. Contemp Ob/Gyn Spec. Issue Update on Surgery. 1987; 64–74.

84. Smith D, Egginton JA, Brookfield DSK. Detection of abnormality of fetal urinary tract as a predictor of renal tract disease. Br Med J 1987;294:27–28.

85. Laing FC, Burke VD, Wing VW, Jeffrey RB Jr, Hashimoto B. Postpartum evaluation of fetal hydronephrosis: optimal timing for follow-up sonography. Radiology 1984; 152:423–424.

86. Helin I, Persson P-H. Prenatal diagnosis of urinary tract abnormalities by ultrasound. Pediatr 1986;78:879–883.

87. Livera LN, Brookfield DSK, Egginton JA, Hawnaur JM. Antenatal ultrasonography to detect fetal renal abnormalities: a prospective screening programme. Br Med J 1989;298:1421–1423.

88. Drugan A, Zador IE, Bhatia R, Sacks AJ, Evans MI. Case Report. First trimester diagnosis and early in utero treatment of obstructive uropathy. Acta Obstet Gynecol Scand 1989;68:645–649.

89. Wladimiroff JW, Beemer FA, Scholtmeyer RJ, Stewart PA, Spritzer R, Wolff ED. Failure to detect fetal obstructive uropathy by second trimester ultrasound. Prenat Diag 1985;5:41–46.

90. Manchester DK, Pretorius DH, Avery C, et al. Accuracy of ultrasound diagnoses in

pregnancies complicated by suspected fetal anomalies. Prenat Diag 1988;8:109–117.

91. Rottem S, Chervenak FA. Ultrasound diagnosis of fetal anomalies. Obstet Gynecol Clin NA 1990;17:17–40.

92. Colodny AH. Antenatal diagnosis and management of urinary abnormalities. Pediatr Clin NA 1987;34:1365–1381.

93. Avni EF, Rodesch F, Schulman CC. Fetal uropathies: diagnostic pitfalls and management. J Urol 1985;134:921–925.

94. Seeds JW, Mittelstaedt CA, Mandell J. Pre- and postnatal ultrasonographic diagnosis of congenital obstructive uropathies. Urol Clin NA 1986;13:131–154.

95. Stiller RJ. Early ultrasonic appearance of fetal bladder outlet obstruction. Am J Obstet Gynecol 1989;160:584–585.

96. Manning FA, Harman CR. In utero diversion shunts for urethral obstruction. In: Sabbagha RE, ed. Diagnostic ultrasound applied to obstetrics and gynecology, 2nd ed. Philadelphia: JP Lippincott, 1987;34: 431–437.

97. Arger PH, Coleman BG, Mintz MC, et al. Routine fetal genitourinary tract screening. Radiology 1985;156:485.

98. Romero R, Pilu G, Jeanty P, Ghidini A, Hobbins JC. The urinary tract and adrenal glands. In: Prenatal diagnosis of congenital anomalies. Connecticut: Appleton & Lange, 1988;8:255–299.

99. Grignon A, Filion R, Filiatrault D, Robitaille P, Homsy Y, Boutin H, Leblond R. Urinary tract dilatation in utero: classification and clinical applications. Radiology 1986;160:645–647.

100. Grannum PA. Urinary tract anomalies. In: Nyberg DA, Mahony BS, Pretorius DH, eds. Diagnostic Ultrasound of Fetal Anomalies: Text and Atlas. Chicago: Year Book Medical Publishers 1990;433–491.

101. Gore RM, Callen PW, Filly RA, Harrison MR, Golbus MS. Prenatal percutaneous antegrade pyelography in posterior urethral valves: sonographic guidance. AJR 1982;139:994–996.

102. Stoutenbeek PH, de Jong TPVM, van Gool JD, Drogtrop AP. Intrauterine cystography for evaluation of prenatal obstructive uropathy. Pediatr Radiol 1989;19:247–249.

103. Richards DS, Seeds JW, Katz VL, Lingley LH, Albright SG, Cefalo RC. Elevated maternal serum alpha-fetoprotein with oligohydramnios: ultrasound evaluation and outcome. Obstet Gynecol 1988;72:337–341.

104. Mahony BS, Filly RA, Callen PW, Hricak H, Golbus MS, Harrison MR. Fetal renal dysplasia: sonographic evaluation. Radiology 1984;152:143–146.

105. Winter RM, Knowles SAS. Megacystis-microcolon-intestinal hypoperistalsis syndrome: confirmation of autosomal recessive inheritance. J Med Genet 1986;23:360–362.

106. Scarbrough PR, Files B, Carroll AJ, Quinlan RW, Finley SC, Finley WH. Interstitial deletion of chromosome 1 [del(1)(q25q32)] in an infant with prune belly sequence. Prenat Diag 1988;8:169–174.

107. Rabinowitz R, Schillinger JF. Prune belly syndrome in the female subject. J Urol 1977;118:454–456.

108. Short KL, Groff DB, Cook. L The concomitant presence of gastroschisis and prune belly syndrome in a twin. J Ped Surg 1985;20:186–187.

109. Nicolini U, Fisk NM, Talbert DG, et al. Intrauterine manometry: technique and application to fetal pathology. Prenat Diagn 1989;9:243–254.

110. Cullen MT, Athanassiadis AP, Grannum P, Green JJ, Hobbins JC. In utero intravesicular pressure and the prune belly syndrome. Fetal Ther 1989;4:73–77.

111. Gembruch U, Hansmann M. Artificial instillation of amniotic fluid as a new technique for the diagnostic evaluation of cases of oligohydramnios. Prenat Diagn 1988;8:33–45.

112. Nicolaides KH, Rodeck CH, Gosden CM. Rapid karyotyping in nonlethal fetal malformations. The Lancet 1986; i:283–287.

113. Glick PL, Harrison MR, Golbus MS, et al. Management of the fetus with congenital hydronephrosis II: Prognostic criteria and selection for treatment. J Pediatr Surg 1985;20:376–387.

114. Bowman JM, Manning FA. Intrauterine transfusion: Winnipeg 1982. Obstet Gynecol 1983;61:203–209.

115. Hasaart TA, Essed GG. Amniotic fluid embolism after transabdominal amniocentesis. Eur J Obstet Gynecol Reprod Biol 1983;16:25–30.

116. Bowman JM. Rh erythroblastosis foetalis 1975. Semin Hematol 1975;12:189–193.

117. Manning FA, Morrison I, Lange IR, Harman CR, Chamberlain PF. Fetal assessment based on fetal biophysical profile scoring: experience in 12,620 referred high-risk pregnancies. I. Perinatal mortality by frequency and etiology. Am J Obstet Gynecol 1985;151:343–350.

118. Gatz G, Rauskolb R, Werner L, et al. Simultaneous placentesis and amniocentesis for prenatal karyotyping: report on 250 cases. Prenat Diagn 1990;10:365–375.

119. Cameron AD, Mathers AM, Wisdom S, et al. Second-trimester placental biopsy for rapid fetal karyotyping. Am J Obstet Gynecol 1990;163:931–934.

120. Saura R, Longy M, Horovitz J, et al. Direct chromosome analysis in the second and third trimesters by placental biopsy in 30 pregnancies. Br J Obstet Gynaecol 1989;96:1215–1218.

121. Hogdall DK, Doran TA, Shime J, et al. Transabdominal chorionic villus sampling in the second trimester. Am J Obstet Gynecol 1988;158:345–349.

122. Wolstenholme J, Hoogwerf AM, Sheridan H, et al. Practical experience using transabdominal chorionic villus biopsies taken after 16 weeks gestation for rapid prenatal diagnosis of chromosome abnormalities. Prenat Diagn 1989;9:357–359.

123. Rabinowitz R, Peters MT, Vyas S, Campbell S, Nicolaides KH. Measurement of fetal urine production in normal pregnancy by real-time ultrasonography. AM J Obstet Gynecol 1989;161:1264–1266.

124. Wladimiroff JW, Campbell S. Fetal urine-production rates in normal and complicated pregnancy. The Lancet 1974;i:151–154.

125. Smith FG, Robillard JE. Pathophysiology of fetal renal disease. Semin Perinat 1989;13:305–319.

126. Chamberlain PF, Manning FA, Morrison I, Harman CR, Lange IR: Ultrasound evaluation of amniotic fluid volume. I. The relationship of marginal and decreased amniotic fluid volumes to perinatal outcome. Am J Obstet Gynecol 1984;150:245–249.

127. Elder JS, Duckett JW Jr, Snyder HM. Intervention for fetal obstructive uropathy: has it been effective? The Lancet 1987;ii:1007–1009.

128. Harrison MR, Adzick NS, Nakayama DK. Fetal diaphragmatic hernia: pathophysiology, natural history, and outcome. Clin Obstet Gynecol 1986;29:490–495.

129. Lumbers ER. A brief review of fetal renal function. J Develop Physiol 1983;6:1–10.

130. Grannum PA, Ghidini A, Scioscia A, Copel JA, Romero R, Hobbins JC. Assessment of fetal renal reserve in low level obstructive uropathy. The Lancet (letter) 1989;i:281–282.

131. Wilkins IA, Chitkara U, Lynch L, Goldberg JD, Mehalek KE, Berkowitz RL. The nonpredictive value of fetal urinary electrolytes: preliminary report of outcomes and correlations with pathologic diagnosis. Am J Obstet Gynecol 1987;157:694–698.

132. Weiner C, Williamson R, Bonsib SM, et al. In utero bladder diversion—problems with patient selection. Fetal Ther 1986;1:196–202.

133. Watson AR, Readett D, Nelson CS, Kapila L, Mayell MJ. Dilemmas associated with antenatally detected urinary tract abnormalities. Arch Dis Child 1988;63:719–722.

134. Lenz S, Lund-Hansen T, Bang J, Christensen E. A possible prenatal evaluation of renal function by amino acid analysis on fetal urine. Prenat Diagn 1985;5:259–267.

135. Pesce AJ, Boreisha I, Pollak VE. Rapid differentiation of glomerular and tubular proteinuria by sodium dodecyl sulfate polyacrylamide gel electrophoresis. Clin Chim Acta 1972;40:27–34.

136. Holzgreve W, Lison A, Bulla M. SDS-PAGE as an additional test to determine fetal kidney function prior to intrauterine diversion of urinary tract obstruction. Fetal Ther 1989;4:93–96.
137. Dumez Y, Revillon Y, Dommergues M, et al. Long-term predictive value of fetal renal function. Presented at the Fifth Meeting of the International Fetal Medicine and Surgery Society, Bonn, June, 1988.
138. Nicolaides KH, Cheng HH, Snijders RJM, Moniz CF. Fetal urine biochemistry in the assessment of obstructive uropathy. Am J Obstet Gynecol 1992;166:932–937.
139. Harrison MR, Golbus MS, Filly RA, et al. Fetal surgery for congenital hydronephrosis. N Engl J Med 1982;306:591–593.
140. Weinreb JC, Lowe T, Cohoen JM, Kutler M. Human fetal anatomy: MR imaging. Radiology 1985;157:715–720.
141. Speilberg SP, Koren G. Drugs, chemicals, and CNS malformations. In: Hoffman HJ, Epstein F, eds. Disorders of the developing nervous system: diagnosis and treatment. Oxford: Blackwell Scientific Publications, 1986;301–312.
142. Manning FA: The fetus with ventriculomegaly: the Fetal Surgery Registry. In: The unborn patient: prenatal diagnosis and treatment. Harrison MR, Golbus MS, Filly RA, eds. Philadelphia: WB Saunders, 1990:394–396.
143. Glick PL, Harrison MR, Nakayama DK, et al. Management of ventriculomegaly in the fetus. J Pediatr 1984;105:97–105.
144. Chervenak FA, Duncan C, Mert LR, et al. Outcome of fetal ventriculomegaly. The Lancet 1984;2:179–181.
145. Clewell WH, Meier PR, Manchester DK, et al. Ventriculomegaly: evaluation and management. Semin Perinatol 1985;9:98–102.
146. McCullough DC, Balzer-Martin LA: Current prognosis in overt neonatal hydrocephalus. J Neurosurg 1982;57:378–383.
147. Frigoletto FD, Birnholz JC, Greene MF: Antenatal treatment of hydrocephalus by ventriculoamniotic shunting. JAMA 1982;248:2496–2497.
148. Clewell WH, Johnson MD, Meier PR, et al. A surgical approach to the treatment of fetal hydrocephalus. N Engl J Med 1982;306:1320–1325.
149. Divon MY, Platt LD, Cantrell CJ, et al. Evoked fetal startle response: a possible intrauterine neurological examination. Am J Obstet Gynecol 1988;153:454–456.

INVASIVE TESTING AND OPPORTUNITIES FOR THERAPY IN MULTIPLE GESTATION

11

UMBERTO NICOLINI

Since the mid-19th century, twins have been classified as monozygotic or dizygotic. Dizygotic twins result from independently released ova being fertilized by different sperm, whereas monozygotic twins, arising from the division of a single fertilized ovum, share the same genotype. Overall, the frequency of twin pregnancies varies from one in 30 to one in 150 and is related to hereditary and environmental factors. Dizygotic twinning varies greatly with race, maternal age, and the use of infertility treatment. The frequency of monozygotic twins is relatively constant around three to five/1,000.

A decrease in the rate of twin pregnancies was reported from the mid-1950s until the late 1970s in both European and American countries. Many factors have been implicated in this trend: reductions in advanced maternal age and high parity at conception, improved nutrition and socioeconomic conditions, increased use of oral contraception, higher rates of miscarriages, and declining fertility rates and sperm counts. More recently, however, this secular decline has been reversed. Between 1978 and 1988, twin births increased in the United States by 33% compared to an increase of only 17% in singletons (1). Similar trends have been observed in the U.K. (2) and Italy (3). This can be attributed partly to a near doubling of pregnancies in women aged 35 years and older and to a wider use of fertility enhancing drugs. The latter factor is certainly implicated in the increasing rate of higher order multiple gestations.

The impact of twinning in terms of mortality, handicaps among survivors, and medical costs far outweighs its incidence. Perinatal morbidity and mortality are four to ten times higher in twin pregnancies than with singletons, related mainly to increased incidence of prematurity and fetal hypoxia. Although improving outcome of triplet pregnancies has recently been reported (4,5), it is common knowledge that as the number of fetuses increases, the duration of gestation and birthweight decrease. In triplet pregnancies matched against twin gestations, premature labor occurs twice as frequently. Intrauterine growth retardation (IUGR) of one or more fetuses is diagnosed in more than 50% of cases, and discordancy in birthweight complicates 67% of patients, compared to only 13% in twin pregnancies (6).

Whether multiple gestations carry an increased risk of fetal anomalies is disputed. An extensive review of the literature by Little and Bryan (7) underlined the inconsistencies of most studies. Possible biases include: (1) entry criteria: since the frequency of intrauterine deaths is increased in twins, studies including only live births may underestimate the true frequency of anomalies; (2) range of specific anomalies: some malformations occur specifically in twins, hence increased reported risks might be relevant only to these anomalies; (3) bias of ascertainment: due to the generally long stay in hospital of twins, detection of anomalies might be favored, and the diagnosis of an anomaly might lead to active search for previously undetected defects in the co-twin. Despite these limitations, out of 30 studies carried out after 1961, 20 gave a relative risk of congenital anomalies in twins >1.0, with the highest estimated value being 3.2 (8). Thus, congenital anomalies are almost certainly more common among twins than singletons. However, the increased risk is probably confined to monozygotic twins, although this has been proven only indirectly by comparing rates in like and unlike sex pairs. The twin reversed arterial perfusion sequence (TRAP), or acardiac twin malformation, and the conjoined twins phenomenon are, although rare, specific to monozygotic twin pregnancies.

Since most trisomies occur during meiosis, each twin has a theoretical risk of having an aneuploid karyotype that is comparable to singletons from mothers of the same age. Hence, an additional problem of twinning is the increased risk, per pregnancy, of chromosomal abnormalities in at least one fetus. Based on these assumptions and given a percentage of dizygotic twins equal to 80% of all twin pregnancies, Rodis et al. (9) have estimated that a woman at 33 years of age with a twin gestation has a risk of Down's syndrome equivalent to that of a 35-year-old with a singleton pregnancy. On the other hand, monozygotic twins are not necessarily genetically identical. Heterokaryotypes, or cytogenetically discordant monozygotic twins, may result from postzygotic nondysjunctional or mutational events. Van Allen et al. (10) have reported up to 50% karyotype discordancies in acardiac/normal monozygotic twin sets, but heterokaryotypes have been described in a variety of other normal/dysmorphic twin pairs, with the abnormality being an autosomal trisomy or monosomy for the chromosome X (11,12,13). To complicate the matter further, blood chimerism in sex-discordant monozygotic twins has also been reported (14).

Conventional tests aimed at assessing the risk of fetal abnormalities need evaluation criteria specific to multiple gestations. Maternal serum levels of both alpha-fetoprotein (AFP) and beta-HCG are increased in twin pregnancies when compared to singletons (15,16). The normal median of AFP for twins is two point zero to 2.5 multiples of the median at 14 to 20 weeks gestation, reflecting the double source of AFP and the greater potential for transfer across the large areas of placenta and membranes. In the amniotic fluid, AFP is, in fact, comparable to singletons of similar gestational age (17). Despite the need for a differ-

ent threshold, the finding of high levels of maternal serum AFP maintains its value in the de-tection of neural tube defects and pregnancy complications. Cuckle et al. (18) have reported 83% and 39% detection rate of anencephaly and open spina bifida, respectively, in 46 twin pregnancies with open neural tube defects using a 5.0 multiples of the median cut-off level. When not associated with neural tube defects, values in excess of 4.0 multiples of the median correlate significantly with increasing incidence of fetal and neonatal death, premature delivery, and twin-to-twin birth-weight discordance >20% (15). In cases with discordancy for anomalies associated with elevation of amniotic fluid AFP, the unaffected twin has been shown to have levels that depend on the characteristics of the septum, being normal values with dichorionic-diamniotic placentas and increased levels in monochorionic-diamniotic twin pairs (17).

Invasive techniques for prenatal diagnosis or antenatal assessment pose specific problems in multiple pregnancy. Each fetus needs to be tested separately and with confidence that the sample obtained pertains to that individual fetus. Subsequent recognition should be guaranteed by recording at the time of the procedure as many markers of identification as possible. The consequence of a mistake is obvious, when selective termination of pregnancy is requested following diagnosis of a congenital defect in only one fetus. Zygosity, or at least chorionicity, should also be diagnosed. Though possible, vascular communications that allow passage of blood between fetuses are exceptional in dichorionic fused placentas, whereas these occur in up to 98% of monochorionic placentas (19). When vascular communications are demonstrated, the intrauterine death of one fetus is associated with increased mortality or long-term morbidity of the survivor (20). *Whatever the responsible mechanism*, this poor outcome has been associated with antenatal necrosis of the cerebral white matter (21), intestinal atresia (22), renal failure (23), and pulmonary infarction (24), in the affected co-twin.

Thus, the role of invasive testing in multiple gestations includes situations with established statistical risks, e.g., aneuploidy in advanced maternal age, cases of discordance for anomalies, acquired differences, usually related to unbalanced conjoined circulation, and a large heterogeneous group where extreme prematurity threatens.

MULTIFETAL PREGNANCY REDUCTION

Reduction of the number of fetuses has emerged in recent years as a controversial option in the management of high order multiple pregnancies. The medical, financial, and social problems related to pregnancies involving three or more fetuses are innumerable. Maternal problems include increased incidence of anemia, preeclampsia, and postpartum hemorrhage (25). Due to the high incidence of prematurity, IUGR, and congenital malformations, the cost of each set of triplets to the National Health System in the U.K. has been calculated at £12,000 and of quadruplets, £25,000 (27). Selective reduction in the first trimester per se raises legal and ethical issues (28). However, this may be a more desirable alternative to terminating the entire pregnancy or taking the slim chances of a successful outcome without intervention in an iatrogenic multiple pregnancy. Dumez and Oury were the first to perform selective reduction in the first trimester using a transcervical aspiration technique (29). This approach had the theoretical risk of introducing vaginal bacteria into the uterine cavity, required dilatation of the cervix, and, by emptying the lowest sac first, increased the chances of PROM, due to devitalization of the membranes in the sac over the internal os.

A transabdominal technique, as originally described by Berkowitz et al. (30), is now the accepted method of multifetal pregnancy reduction. A 20–22-gauge needle is introduced into the thorax of a fetus, usually the most accessible, under continuous ultrasonic guidance. Potassium chloride is then injected, either directly into the fetal heart or into the pericardial region. The amount of potassium chloride required to achieve fetal asystole ranges from 0.4–7 mmol (30–32). The needle is reinserted as many times as the number of fetuses that need to be reduced, and the absence of fetal cardiac activity is confirmed 20–30 minutes later, in order to avoid the substantial risks to an injected surviving embryo. The gestational age at which most procedures are currently performed ranges from 10–12 weeks. Successful selective reduction prior to nine weeks gestation has been reported (33). Data on the high rate of spontaneous fetal loss in early pregnancy (34), however, support the view that the procedure should be delayed until the 10th–11th week, when the risk of background loss of the remaining fetus/es is falling.

In a large collaborative study, which combined data from 310 delivered patients, total loss rate was 17% (35). Both early (<2 weeks from the procedure, 6%) and late fetal losses appeared to be directly related to both the starting and the final numbers of fetuses: total loss rate was 0% for two embryos reduced to one, 18% for three to two, 21% for four to two, 31% for five to nine to two (35). A similar, but inverse, relationship was found with gestational age at delivery. A loss rate of 9.5% has recently been reported by a single group in 200 multifetal reductions mostly performed at 11–12 weeks gestation (36). The same author has observed that the maternal serum alpha-fetoprotein is increased compared to non-reduced twin pregnancies (mean level = 12 multiples of the mean), when tested a few weeks after the procedure of selective reduction, with the increase proportional to the initial number of fetuses. Although screening for neural tube defects is thus impossible by evaluation of maternal serum alpha-fetoprotein, published series do not suggest an increased risk of congenital malformations.

Similarly, clinical and hematological studies seem to rule out the risk of coagulation disorders in the mother following multifetal pregnancy reduction: out of 17 patients undergoing serial coagulation studies following the procedure, only one showed transitory elevation of fibrin degradation products, and no evidence of DIC was ever demonstrated (36). On the other hand, the procedure of selective reduction poses the theoretical risk of death or embolic damage to the surviving fetus/fetuses. Passage of potassium chloride through placental anastomoses may indeed occur in monozygotic twins. However, this risk is small in multiple pregnancies >two. Although the rate of monozygotic twins appears to be increased after infertility treatment, when compared to spontaneous conceptions, the respective frequencies are only 1.2 and 0.45%, i.e., a low frequency of vascular anastomoses would be expected (37).

When selecting the fetus/es for selective reduction, three criteria are widely accepted: (1) ease of access, (2) site of the sac in relation to the internal os, with the lower sac the least preferred due to the possible increased risk of PROM and ascending infection, and (3) relative fetal sizes. In multiple pregnancies, interfetal size variability is

larger than in singletons, and the wider variance in fetal size is already statistically significant at 11 weeks gestation (38). Thus, the finding of markedly different sizes among twins in the first trimester is not unexpected; however, given the reported association between a small-for-dates crown-rump length and pregnancy loss (39), the choice of the smaller fetuses for selective reduction seems appropriate.

There is little doubt that for pregnancies with more than four fetuses, selective fetal reduction substantially increases the chances of successful outcome. There are pure ethical concerns in all cases proposed for selective fetal reduction but perhaps most controversial is the issue of whether triplet pregnancy per se should be considered an indication. Due to earlier diagnosis, improvement in antenatal surveillance, and, especially, better neonatal care, survival in triplet pregnancies appears to have increased, when compared to historical series. A recent paper has shown comparable outcomes in reduced and nonreduced triplet pregnancies (40), but another hospital-based series, which assessed perinatal mortality in triplet pregnancies, triplets reduced to twins, and spontaneous twin pregnancies, found rates of 24%, 3%, and 4%, respectively (41). Larger prospective studies are, therefore, needed to solve the controversy of whether triplet pregnancies managed expectantly hold a worse prognosis and warrant selective reduction.

CHORIONIC VILLUS SAMPLING (CVS)

To date, the efficacy and safety of CVS in multiple pregnancies has been evaluated in only one large series (42). This study involving four centers, 126 sets of twins, and two sets of triplets reported a success rate in obtaining adequate amounts of chorionic tissue of 99.2% and a 3.9% fetal loss rate. There were two cases (0.8%) in which fetal sex was incorrectly diagnosed, presumably due to maternal cell contamination or one twin being mistakenly sampled twice. In addition, only one sample was done in 11.7% of cases because of uncertainty in differentiating separate placentas or impossibility in ensuring that each chorion was sampled individually. These results, while reassuring about the safety of CVS, underline potential pitfalls in the specificity of early prenatal diagnosis in multiple pregnancies.

The experience with CVS in singleton pregnancies shows that whether transcervical or transabdominal technique is utilized, it is the number of samplings that relates to the frequency of postprocedure pregnancy loss. Therefore, an increase in the fetal loss rate might be expected with multiple pregnancies. Although small, the available data do not support a substantial increase in the procedure-related risk. Moreover, when compared to amniocentesis, CVS appears to be a safer procedure. The main concern of CVS in multiple pregnancies is thus related not to safety, but rather to accuracy in sampling each fetus. Diagnosis of chorionicity may be facilitated in early pregnancy, relying on ultrasound assessment of placental location (separate or fused), septal thickness ($>$ or <2 mm) (43), and septal attachment to the placenta (presence or absence of a wedge-shaped area of trophoblast) (44). Monochorionic pregnancies can be regarded as monozygotic, and only one placenta needs to be sampled. On the other hand, 30% of monozygotic twins have dichorionic placentas; in these cases, the study of chromosome polymorphism, or the use of minisatellite DNA probes would not show any differences between the samples obtained, and uncertainty may arise as to whether both fetuses were sampled. Thus,

with dichorionic placentas, it is crucial that each placenta is sampled individually without reciprocal contamination. A combined transcervical and transabdominal approach, aimed at sampling near each umbilical cord insertion while avoiding passage through the placenta of the co-twin, may minimize mistakes. Despite these precautions, diagnostic errors have been made in up to 5.5% of cases (44), which may be an underestimate of the true rate. Although no firm policy has been established so far, it may, therefore, be advisable that amniocentesis is performed when like-sex dichorionic twins cannot be differentiated by cytogenetic or DNA polymorphism studies (44).

AMNIOCENTESIS

Testing each fetus by amniocentesis is easier than by CVS, due to a greater number of variables that allow distinct identification of each twin (order of presentation, laterality, site of placental insertion, size, and sex of the fetuses). Practical difficulties, however, have prompted development of at least four techniques to ensure the goal of sampling each sac individually.

When ultrasound resolution was poorer than present standards and continuous ultrasound control was not adopted routinely, needles had to be inserted into each amniotic sac and a dye injected into the first sac sampled. Two series published in 1991 and 1992 still reported more than 95% of amniocenteses being performed using this classical technique (45,46). Recently, Jeanty et al. (47) suggested the use of a single needle inserted into the first sac and then advanced through the dividing membrane into the second one. This technique has the additional advantage of avoiding the injection of a dye, provided that accurate visualization of the needle is maintained throughout the procedure. As an alternate approach, which similarly does not require the use of a dye, needles are introduced into adjacent pockets of amniotic fluid on either side of the membrane, and the first needle is left in place while the second is inserted, allowing simultaneous visualization of both needles on ultrasound (48). Finally, accurate ultrasonic assessment of the topography of each sac and the dividing membrane may allow avoidance of instillation of a dye, even when using two separate needle insertions. This approach, however, has the disadvantage of relying entirely on the confidence of the operator having sampled each individual sac, and it does not provide a permanent record for subsequent analysis.

As with CVS, only one sac needs to be sampled if a monozygotic twin pregnancy is diagnosed. When a membrane cannot be seen on ultrasound, the placenta is likely to be monoamniotic. Exceptions are the "stuck twin" syndrome and the inability to visualize a thin membrane. In both of these instances, however, the twin pregnancy is monozygotic and the error would be without consequence. Monozygotic, diamniotic-monochorionic pregnancies are more difficult to differentiate from diamniotic-dichorionic ones if the adjacent placentas appear fused on ultrasound. Counting the individual layers of the membranes as they appear on sonography has been reported to allow diagnosis of chorionicity in 68 of 69 twin pregnancies, two layers pointing to a monochorionic placenta, and three or four layers suggesting a dichorionic gestation (49). Possible source of errors include oligohydramnios, the wall of the umbilical cord being misinterpreted as a dividing membrane, and chorioamniotic separation.

The safety of amniocentesis in twin pregnancies has been the object of nine studies published after 1980, with a total of 499 pregnancies (45,50–57). There were 42 (8.4%)

pregnancy losses prior to 28 weeks gestation. This abortion rate compares unfavorably with the generally estimated risk of 0.5–1% in singletons. A controlled study would assess more properly the risk of amniocentesis in twin pregnancy, given the higher abortion rate related to twinning itself. Unfortunately, such a study is difficult to perform due to the relative rarity of twin pregnancies. If one relies on the 4.5% abortion rate found by Prompeler et al. up to the 28th week in sonographically normal twin pregnancies which did not undergo prenatal diagnosis (58), the procedure-related risk appears to be approximately twice the background rate.

Early amniocentesis (<14 weeks), by allowing easier identification of each individual fetus tested, might overcome some of the difficulties related to CVS in patients with a twin pregnancy at high genetic risk or wishing to undergo prenatal diagnosis during the first trimester. Only one small series, however, has reported six twin pregnancies investigated by amniocentesis at 10–13 weeks, and the results cannot yet be extrapolated to provide meaningful conclusions about the safety of the procedure (59). Two ml of indigo carmine were used in this series as a diagnostic dye to rule out sampling twice from the same amniotic sac. This compound has not been associated with untoward fetal effects. Indigo carmine, however, has a vasoconstrictor effect like methylene blue. The latter dye, still widely used (45) despite its known association with hemolytic anemia in the third trimester, has been suggested to cause fetal intestinal atresia when used in second trimester amniocentesis (60). The initial report of seven affected twins after intra-amniotic injection of methylene blue has recently been confirmed on a larger series of 89 twin sets, 17 of the neonates (9.5%) having atresia of the jejunum (46). The mechanism involved might be a spasm of the mesenteric artery, possibly associated with hemolytic anemia, causing ischemia of the fetal bowel. Indigo carmine may have similar effects, and its use at amniocentesis has been associated with the birth of a twin infant with jejunal atresia in one of twenty pregnancies samples (46). In view of this evidence and the present sophistication of ultrasound equipment, which only rarely does not allow identification of each sac, avoiding the use of any dye seems presently not only feasible, but also the safest option.

FETAL BLOOD SAMPLING

Fetal blood sampling in twin pregnancies has been reported specifically for a variety of indications: genetic diagnosis (61,62), twin-twin transfusion syndrome (63–65), and autoimmune thrombocytopenia (66). The list, however, is certainly incomplete. All the accepted indications to fetal blood sampling in singletons pertain to multiple pregnancies as well. An additional reason to sample fetal blood in twin pregnancies is the need to confirm an abnormal karyotype detected by CVS or amniocentesis prior to selective termination if uncertainties exist as to which twin is affected.

No data are presently available on the efficacy, accuracy, and safety of fetal blood sampling in twin pregnancies, probably due to the heterogeneity of the indications and the small number of patients investigated by individual groups. Occasional failures in sampling both twins have been reported (30), and cord entanglement following disruption of the dividing membrane has been described as an unusual complication of funipuncture (67). Blood sampling may indeed present difficulties that are unusual in singletons or are specific to twin pregnancies: (1) the placental cord insertion of one or both twins may be a long distance from the abdominal wall (as in the case of polyhydramnios with a posterior placenta); (2) use of a longer needle may be compromised by the poor ultrasound resolution in the far field; (3) if the placental cord insertions are in close proximity, the sample obtained may be wrongly attributed to the other twin; (4) dislodgement of the needle occurs more frequently, due to the double number of moving limbs; (5) because of severe oligohydramnios, sampling the "stuck twin" is impeded by poor visualization of the cord. When the placental cord insertion cannot be attributed with certainty or is inaccessible, sampling from the intrahepatic vein has been shown to constitute a safe alternate approach to cordocentesis (68). Using this technique, no failures have occurred in a series of 20 twin pregnancies undergoing fetal blood sampling (Nicolini et al: unpublished).

Perinatal deaths or major handicaps occur in one in 10 twin pregnancies with discordant birthweight, and in these, perinatal mortality shows a significant inverse correlation with birthweight (69). With growth-discordant twins, expectant management, while advantageous to the larger fetus, might raise concerns about worsening hypoxemia in the smaller co-twin. Timing of the delivery in such cases is often a difficult dilemma. Although the role of fetal blood sampling to assess acid-base balance in singleton pregnancies complicated by IUGR has been questioned (70), exclusion of hypoxemia/acidemia would be of great value in allowing continuation of the pregnancy, despite severe size discrepancy, in twin gestation. As yet, there are no published series reporting the use of blood sampling in the evaluation of fetal well-being in twins. In addition, available reference ranges of fetal acid-base balance throughout gestation may not be appropriate in the evaluation of

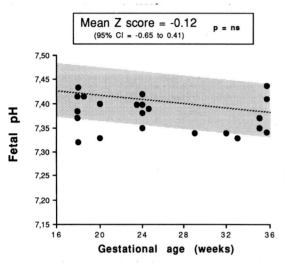

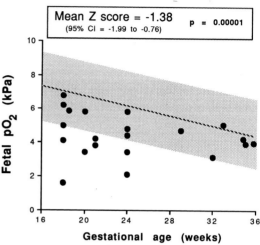

Figure 11-1   Values of venous pH at fetal blood sampling in 22 normal twins, plotted against the reference range for singletons (shaded area).

Figure 11-2   Values of venous pO_2 at fetal blood sampling in 22 normal twins, plotted against the reference range for singletons (shaded area).

twin fetuses. Figures 11-1, 11-2 and 11-3 support this hypothesis: in 22 normally grown, non-malformed twins who underwent fetal blood sampling for various indications, pH was not significantly different from the mean for singletons (Figure 11-1), whereas fetal pO_2 was on average 1.38 SDs below the mean gestation, as determined in normal singletons (Figure 11-2). Though only two twins were found to be acidemic and hypoxemic, all but three had a value of pO_2 below the singleton mean (Figure 11-3). These preliminary data support the concept that acid-base balance in twin fetuses needs to be evaluated with different criteria from those currently used and suggest that intrauterine hypoxemia may have a role in determining the smaller size of twins compared to singletons.

Individual access to the fetal circulation is of paramount importance when twins may be discordant for the condition for which they are investigated. This eventuality applies to congenital infections, autoimmune thrombocytopenia (66), and maternal allo-

immunization, in which case a twin may be antigen-negative, the co-twin being positive, or the disease may affect each twin with different severity. In the three twin pregnancies with Rh-alloimmunization we have treated so far, however, both twins had identical values of hematocrit at the first blood sampling, and very similar rates of decrease of hematocrit were observed between transfusions. This does not imply that individual assessment of each twin can be avoided prior to intravascular transfusion. The only reported exception to this rule would be the case of monozygotic twins, when intravascular access to only one twin may be sufficient, with the co-twin being transfused indirectly through the placental anastomoses (71).

SELECTIVE FETICIDE

Since 1978, when the first case of selective birth was described in a twin pregnancy discordant for Hurler syndrome (72), a woman

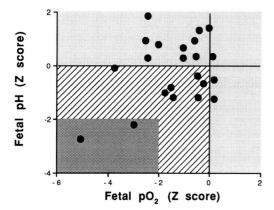

Figure 11-3 Z scores (number of standard deviations from the singleton means) for venous pH and pO_2 at fetal blood sampling in 22 normal twins. 0 = means for singletons. Shaded area = hypoxemic and acidemic. Crosshatch area = below the mean for both pO_2 and pH, but not >two SD below either singleton mean.

with a diagnosis of a chromosomal or structural abnormality in one twin can be offered the option to terminate the affected fetus and to continue successfully with the normal fetus.

During the last 14 years, several methods of selective feticide have been devised. The first attempts aimed at achieving fetal exsanguination by cardiac puncture (72), but repeated procedures were often necessary to produce fetal asystole (73). An early alternate approach was the removal of the affected fetus at hysterotomy (74). Consistent results were only described in a series of six patients using air embolization of the umbilical vein via fetoscopy (75). Other compounds injected into the fetal circulation were formaldehyde (75) and calcium gluconate (76).

The most widely used technique is now the intravascular administration of potassium chloride either via the umbilical vein or into the fetal heart (77). The recommended concentration is 2 mEq/ml, and

one to two ml are generally sufficient to cause immediate fetal asystole, without the need for preliminary withdrawal of large amounts of blood. Premature labor has been consistently reported as a definite problem of selective feticide in the second trimester (77). There are no clear explanations of this complication, which seems to be more frequent the later the gestational age at which the procedure is performed. A 7% loss rate in the surviving twin has recently been described in a series including 37 patients with dichorionic placentas (36). Higher rates are expected in monozygotic twins, due to the possible presence of vascular anastomoses. Although selective feticide using cardiac tamponade has been successfully achieved in two or three pregnancies with fetofetal transfusion syndrome (63,78,79), anecdotal experience from different groups supports the view that this is a high-risk procedure, which may result in immediate death or long-term sequelae of the co-twin.

A reliable method of ruling out placental vascular anastomoses is needed. Besides the ultrasonographic criteria that have already been discussed, invasive testing has been suggested. Injection into one fetus of a readily detectable and safe marker, with subsequent demonstration of its passage in measurable quantities in the co-twin has been the approach proposed. To test passage from one circulation to the other, adult red cells, which are easily demonstrable in the fetal circulation by the Kleihauer-Betke test, have been used (64). More recently, intravascular administration of pancuronium bromide, a neuromuscular blocking agent, caused paralysis of both twins in one twin pregnancy with proven vascular communications and allowed exclusion of correct transplacental communications in another case (80). False-negative results, however, may occur. In like-sex twins, discordancy for the presence of structural abnormalities and even different karyo-types (10–13) do not guarantee that the placenta is dichorionic. In some situations, the flow through vascular anastomoses may be markedly intermittent, or interfered with by the infusion of the marker, altering test outcome. In doubtful cases, the risk to the unaffected fetus must be weighed against the likelihood that feticide of the affected twin prevents the birth of a surviving handicapped child. With this perspective, a lethal congenital malformation may not warrant the risks of the procedure. On the other hand, selective feticide may reduce the risks of prematurity in the presence of an abnormality known to be associated with polyhydramnios. In such instances, it is difficult to give guidelines that are applicable to all different ranges of clinical situations, and a flexible approach needs to be entertained.

TWIN-TWIN TRANSFUSION SYNDROME

Vascular anastomoses are apparent in virtually all monozygous-monochorionic placentas (81). These anastomoses may be superficial, deep, or a combination of the two. Most commonly, superficial anastomoses are of the artery-artery type alone or are a combination of artery-artery and artery-vein anastomoses. In contrast, in deep anastomoses, an artery from one twin is generally found to supply a cotyledon that is drained by a venous system to the co-twin. Twin-twin transfusion syndrome, however, no matter what criteria are adopted for its definition, complicates only a minority of monozygotic-monochorionic twin pregnancies; the single presence of vascular connections is clearly not sufficient to create twin-twin transfusion. A recent review of 97 pathologically-proven monochorionic placentas, delivered at >20 weeks

gestation in a tertiary care institution during one decade, showed that only 35% of twin pairs had weight discordancy >15%, and only 40% had differences in cord hemoglobin or hematocrit >5g/dl or >15%, respectively (82). In 12 of the 34 weight-discordant monochorionic twins, antenatal infection or congenital anomalies had been diagnosed, which might have been the cause of growth discrepancy. Moreover, in a survey of mono- and dichorionic twin pregnancies, it has been shown that discordance in weight or in hematological indices at birth both occur frequently in both groups independent of each other and without other evidence of twin-twin transfusion (83). The confusion that surrounds the twin-twin transfusion syndrome is not surprising. Pathologically, vascular anastomoses need to be demonstrated, but their presence is the rule in monochorionic placentas. Findings at birth, which have been used traditionally for the clinical definition of the syndrome (84,85), are uncommon and non-specific.

Provided that using the label "twin-twin transfusion syndrome" implies that the two circulations are connected in an unbalanced fashion, the demonstration of unidirectional net flow of blood from one twin to the other should be required for its definition. However, this would be a necessary and sufficient condition only if such an imbalance is persistent throughout gestation. This does not seem always to be the case: a placental anastomosis may, indeed, lead to chronic twin-twin transfusion, but ceases to function after the death of one twin; it may become functional acutely following sudden changes in the intrauterine pressure (as when it occurs in labor) or because of increased blood pressure in one of the twins above a certain threshold (which seems to occur throughout gestation); a deep anastomosis, the "third circulation" as described by Schatz in 1882 (86), may be balanced by superficial ones that act in the opposite direction; and so on, an infinite combination of balanced and unbalanced vascular communications may occur.

Accepted antenatal criteria to define the syndrome are heterogeneous. They include estimated size of the fetuses, amniotic fluid volume, cord size, ultrasonic appearance of the placenta, fetal bladder volume, echocardiographic and Doppler studies, fetal heart rate monitoring, and fetal blood sampling. An intertwin difference in the abdominal circumference of 18–20 mm has been recommended as the best cut-off to predict birthweight differences >15% (87,88). The combination of polyhydramnios in one sac and severe oligohydramnios in the other (the "stuck twin" sign) is probably the most typical feature of both acute and chronic twin-twin transfusion syndrome (Figure 11-4) (79), the pathophysiology of both phenomena being abnormality of fetal urine production. Chronic fluid overload in the recipient twin causes enhanced release of atrial natriuretic peptide, which, in turn, leads to increased fetal diuresis (89,90); in contrast, in the smaller fetus, urine output is

markedly decreased (90). Consequently, the bladder of the larger twin is often persistently enlarged, and that of the donor twin is consistently small on serial ultrasound scans. Differences in the S/D ratio of the umbilical artery blood flow, as assessed by Doppler velocimetry, have been reported to be diagnostic of twin-twin transfusion syndrome by some authors (91–93), but denied by others (94). Differences in cord size, placental echogenicity (Figure 11-5), and echocardiographic studies have been described in some cases but do not provide a consistent key to diagnosis. Similarly, a sinusoidal heart rate pattern has been reported (95), but being related to intrauterine anemia, such an abnormality is expected to occur only in few donor twins.

In summary, all available tests aimed at diagnosing twin-twin transfusion syndrome rely on indirect evidence of the two dichotomies: decreased/increased blood volume and anemia/polycythemia. Fetal blood sampling has allowed direct access to the fetal circulation, but given the heterogeneity of the syndrome, it is not surprising that the few studies published so far have under-

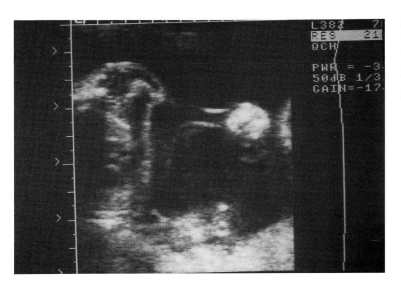

Figure 11-4 Polyhydramnios/oligohydramnios in twin-twin transfusion syndrome: the dividing membrane is adherent to the donor twin.

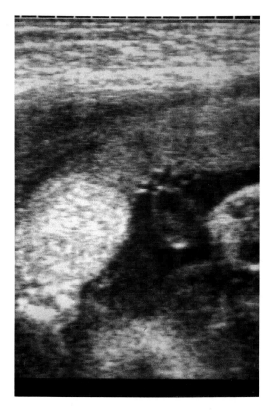

Figure 11-5 Different echogenicity of the placenta in twin-twin transfusion syndrome: the hyperechogenic portion pertains to the donor twin.

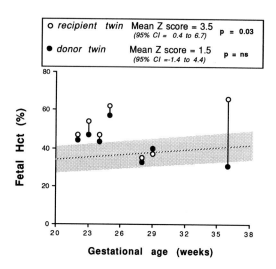

Figure 11-6 Values of fetal hematocrit (Hct) in seven pairs of twins with proven twin-twin transfusion syndrome. Shaded area = reference range for singletons.

		RECIPIENT	p	DONOR
pO₂	Mean Z score	-1.4		-2.6
	95% C.I.	-3.1 to 0.3	ns	-4.5 to -0.8
	p	ns		0.01
pH	Mean Z score	-1.3		-3.5
	95% C.I.	-3.3 to 0.6	0.04	-5.1 to -2.0
	p	ns		0.001

Figure 11-7 Number of SDs from the mean for gestation in singletons (Z score) of venous pH and pO₂ at fetal blood sampling in seven pairs of twins with proven twin-twin transfusion syndrome.

lined the inconsistencies of the acid-base balance and hematological findings (64,65). Though in one study the assessment of fetal blood viscosity was found to correlate with survival (96), most reported series of twins investigated by blood sampling have shown similar values for hemoglobin/hematocrit, and a variable distribution of hypoxemia/acidemia between donor and recipient twins. Figure 11-6 shows values of hematocrit in seven pairs of twins with suspected twin-twin transfusion syndrome, with documented passage of significant amounts of adult red cells from the smaller to the larger co-twin (64); mean hematocrit was significantly higher in the recipient than in the donor twin, but four of seven pairs did not show appreciable differences. Donor twins were hypoxemic and acidemic when compared to normal singletons, whereas the larger/recipient twins had normal values of pH and pO₂ (Figure 11-7). In agreement with the abnormal acid-base balance is the finding of increased nucleated red cell counts in all donor twins investigated (64).

However, evidence of erythroblastosis was documented in recipient twins as well (64). Whether this is related to fetofetal transfusion of donor erythroblasts, or to the effect of the donor twin's elevated serum erythropoietin levels on the recipient twin's bone marrow is not certain (97).

Discrepancies between the classical postnatal stigmata in twin-twin transfusion syndrome and the emerging evidence arising from observations made in utero may be related to several factors. Gestational age is generally lower at fetal blood sampling than that at which most studies at birth have been performed. Antenatal observations are more likely to have recruited chronic cases rather than acute cases of twin-twin transfusion syndrome. The effect of labor on circulation shunting is excluded. Finally, the selection of cases for serial detailed ultrasound examination and fetal blood sampling by cordocentesis has been on antenatal (prospective) parameters rather than on the post-hoc findings of other studies.

Survival with twin-twin transfusion syndrome is poor when diagnosis is made prior to 29 weeks (98–100). Causes of fetal/pregnancy losses include premature delivery prior to fetal viability (mainly related to uterine overdistension due to polyhydramnios) and intrauterine death of one or both twins. As already mentioned, in monozygous twins, single fetal death may cause immediate death or significant long-term morbidity of the co-twin (21,101,102). On the other hand, antenatal improvement of hydrops has been reported following the death of the co-twin in twin-twin transfusion syndrome (104), and selective feticide has been claimed to be a therapeutic solution in some, although not all, attempted cases (63,78–79).

It has been postulated that the mechanism leading to damage to the surviving twin is intravascular coagulation confined to the shared circulation, which, in turn, may cause transfer of thromboplastin-rich blood from the dead to the living twin (20). Indeed, maternal DIC has been described in a few cases of intrauterine death of one twin (104,105). In at least one patient, however, the characteristic cystic lesions of brain and kidneys of the surviving twin were found not to be associated with any derangement of fetal coagulation (106). Transfer of blood through the anastomosis into the hypotensive dying twin, with consequent acute hypovolemia in the "normal" twin, might be the alternate mechanism.

At 22 weeks gestation in a pregnancy complicated by the classical ultrasonic and clinical findings of twin-twin transfusion syndrome, we have observed the development of sustained bradycardia in the larger twin simultaneous with the smaller co-twin becoming moribund with poor heart contractility and undetectable blood flow in the umbilical artery. For a few days prior to this, the smaller twin had had reverse flow in the umbilical artery during diastole. Intracardiac puncture of the dying twin revealed severe acidemia—injection of 10 ml of maternal blood into the left ventricle, though unsuccessful in resuscitating the smaller twin, had the effect of restoring a normal heart rate in the larger one. After death of the smaller twin, the pregnancy continued uneventfully and the neonate did not show any parenchymal damage. The most likely effect of the intracardiac transfusion in this case was of raising temporarily the blood pressure of the dying twin, which probably stopped the passage of blood from the larger hypervolemic twin, and "buying time" before the supervening clotting in the dead fetus's circulation created a permanent impediment to fetofetal hemorrhage.

Based on these observations, it may be speculated that expectant management or selective feticide could be an option at the moment of the intrauterine death of the donor fetus, if only a small amount of blood is expected to pass from the recipient to the donor twin. In order to evaluate prospectively whether a large or small functional anastomosis is involved, we performed blood sampling and injection of adult red cells into the small/donor twin in five pregnancies complicated by twin-twin transfusion syndrome. Four of five pregnancies were less than 28 weeks gestation, and the final percentage of adult blood was >20% in the donor circulation. At blood sampling of the recipient/larger twin, the Kleihauer-Betke test revealed adult cells in a percentage ranging from 1–14%. The two pregnancies in which the amount of shunting appeared limited (1% only of adult cells in the recipient's blood) were managed conservatively. In both pregnancies, the donor fetus showed signs of impending death. In one, following intrauterine demise of the smaller twin, there were no consequences to the surviving co-twin. In the second, a few hours after the death of the donor twin, the recipient twin showed an ominous nonreactive heart rate tracing, and intrauterine death later supervened. At birth, it was obvious that a reversal of blood flow had occurred in utero: the smaller twin, originally the donor, now appeared plethoric, whereas the "recipient" twin was extremely pale (Figure 11-8).

Hence, there does not seem to be any test, either invasive or noninvasive, that allows prediction of which pregnancies can be managed conservatively, when intrauterine death is likely to occur in a twin-twin transfusion syndrome.

A number of alternate therapeutic options have been proposed to treat the syndrome. Decompression amniocentesis has been advocated by several authors as a means to prolong gestation by reducing the polyhydramnios. An effect of amelioration of placental blood flow has also been postulated (107). Survival rate in patients treated by single or serial decompression amniocenteses ranges from 37–79% (100,107–109), which compares favorably with <10% in untreated patients [quoted from Saunders et al, (108)]. The cumulative experience

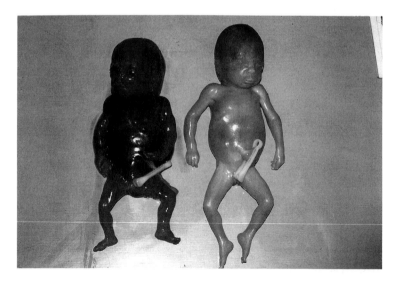

Figure 11-8 Postabortion appearance of a twin pair of proven twin-twin transfusion syndrome. The left smaller twin, originally determined to be the donor, died in utero first. The right larger twin died 24 hours later, apparently after reversal of twin-twin shunt caused exsanguination (note extreme pallor).

shows that the amount of fluid to be removed far exceeds what is commonly believed to be a safe volume to avoid the risks of placenta abruptio and premature labor. In some instances, up to five liters on one occasion have been aspirated without complications. Poor prognosis is associated with uterine hypercontractility and fetal hydrops. Still unclear is the mechanism by which only one therapeutic amniocentesis may be effective in some cases; persistent normalization of amniotic fluid volume in the recipient twin's sac and reappearance of fluid in the donor's sac does, in fact, occur at times. Increased amniotic fluid pressure has been found in polyhydramnios (110). Thus, relief of the pressure exerted over the donor twin's placental portion may decrease the pressure gradient between the two circulations and restore a balanced anastomosis. Alternatively, some anastomoses might collapse under excessive intra-amniotic pressure and reopen with its normalization.

DeLia et al. (111) pioneered a novel therapeutic approach that goes directly to the roots of the pathophysiology of twin-twin transfusion syndrome. They used the neodynium-YAG laser to obliterate superficial anastomoses under fetoscopic control and reported a survival rate of 63% (10/16 twins) (112,113). Although this seems to be a promising option, it is technically impossible with an anterior placenta, and it leaves unsolved the problem of the deep anastomoses, which cannot be occluded this way.

Successful treatment of twin-twin transfusion syndrome has been obtained in two patients by causing inadvertent puncture of a placental vessel of the recipient twin (114). In both instances, severe bleeding was recorded, and polyhydramnios subsequently resolved. This experience led some groups to attempt exchange transfusions or controlled blood aspiration from the recipient twin, but results were discouraging (115). Although selective feticide causes a minimum of 50% loss rate a priori, attempts at causing a controlled intrauterine death are currently under way. A safe method should guarantee that reverse transfusion into the dying twin does not occur. Dumez has recently reported on the use of histoacryl injected into the umbilical vein, which causes vascular obliteration while fetal asystole occurs (116). In seven patients with severe twin-twin transfusion syndrome, there were four surviving neonates, one neonatal death, and two (+7) intrauterine deaths, an overall survival rate of 29%. Although this is lower than that achieved in some series with decompression amniocentesis, the procedure warrants further evaluation in otherwise uncontrollable cases. If feticide needs to be entertained as the extreme solution, it is unclear whether better results are expected if the donor or the recipient twin is terminated. The finding of more common hypoxemia/acidemia in donor twins should support the smaller twin as the ideal candidate, but worse cardiac function, even at long-term follow-up, of the recipient twin (Nicolini U. unpublished observations) might tip the balance towards the latter.

ACARDIAC TWIN MALFORMATION

The acardiac twin malformation, first described by Benedetti in 1553 (117), has since been reported under different names, which refer either to the anatomical abnormality (holoacardius, hemiacardius, acardiac monster) or to what is reputed to be its pathophysiological basis (twin reversed arterial perfusion sequence, TRAP). This rare anomaly (one in 34,000 pregnancies or one in 100 monozygotic twins) probably develops during the early stages of embryogenesis as a result of extensive artery-to-artery and vein-to-vein anastomoses within a monochorionic placenta (118). Secondary atrophy of the heart and other tissues occurs in the perfused twin, whereas the "pumping" normal co-twin may be susceptible to cardiac failure. Perinatal mortality in the normal twin is as high as 55%, primarily related to prematurity (119). Survivors may experience congestive heart failure with right ventricular hypertrophy and relative pulmonary stenosis, poor liver function, and hypoalbuminemia, which are often corollaries of ascites and hydramnios.

When ultrasonography reveals signs of cardiac decompensation in the "pumping" twin, early delivery remains the mainstay of perinatal care, if fetal viability has been reached. In a review of 49 pregnancies complicated by acardiac twinning, however, the mean gestational age at delivery was only 29 weeks (119).

Removal of the perfused twin by laparotomy has been performed successfully in one case (120). A less invasive treatment has involved the obliteration of the umbilical artery, which supplies the acardiac fetus, by transabdominal ultrasound-guided insertion of a thrombogenic coil (121,122).

Control of polyhydramnios with indomethacin has been described (123), but concerns about potential deleterious effects on fetal renal function, and constriction of the ductus arteriosus, though reversible, limit this therapeutic option to selected cases, in which administration of the drug can be discontinued after a short course.

As usual, prospective evaluation of risks and benefits of the available treatments needs to be entertained. Intrauterine "death" of an acardiac fetus has been diagnosed by demonstrating cessation of flow in the umbilical artery, which was preceded by worsening indices of vascular impedance (125). This suggests that umbilical artery blood flow studies may identify those patients in whom spontaneous resolution of the vascular challenge to the normal twin is likely to occur. Moore et al. (120) have noted that with a high (>70%) birthweight ratio between the acardiac and the normal twin, prematurity, polyhydramnios, and congestive heart failure were significantly more frequent and accounted for 90%, 40%, and 30% of cases, respectively. This is the challenge for the future: Is there a reliable way to predict weight in an acardiac twin?

CONCLUSION

Although there may be natural population trends towards decreased frequency of twin pregnancy, the overall incidence of multiple gestations seems relatively constant when one considers increasing diagnosis at earlier gestations and the effect of assisted-fertility programs. There is no doubt that multiple gestations continue to be a major component in perinatal mortality, neonatal morbidity, and long-term developmental handicap. Invasive techniques in multiple gestation, some of them well established, some of them in their infancy, enable improvements in both diagnosis and management. Many useful steps have been made, but many cases remain frustrating, given our inability to substantially alter poor outcomes. This applies most of all to twin-twin transfusion syndrome, where it seems likely that multiple different modalities must be applied on an individual basis to achieve the best outcomes. There seems little doubt that further progress in these areas is forthcoming and that this will have widespread effect on other instances of poor outcome in multiple gestations, where exact pathophysiology is as yet unclear. Prematurity remains the most significant problem of multiple gestation. It may well be that information gained from the most pathologic cases (namely, twin-twin transfusion syndrome) will result in improvement in the management of all twin gestations.

References

1. National Center for Health Statistics. Vital statistics of the United States. 1988, Vol 1, Natality. Washington, DC: US Govt Printing Office, 1990.
2. Chamberlain G. Multiple pregnancy. Br Med J 1991; 303:111–115.
3. Parazzini F, Tozzi L, Mezzanotte G, et al. Trends in multiple births in Italy: 1955–1983. Br J Obstet Gynaecol 1991;98:535–539.
4. Newman RB, Hamer C, Miller MC. Outpatient triplet management: a contemporary review. Am J Obstet Gynecol 1989; 161:547–555.
5. Lipitz S, Reichman B, Paret G, et al. The improving outcome of triplet pregnancies. Am J Obstet Gynecol 1989;161:1279–1284.
6. Sassoon DA, Castro LC, Davis JL, Hobel CJ. Perinatal outcome in triplet versus twin gestations. Obstet Gynecol 1990;75:817–820.
7. Little J, Bryan E. Congenital anomalies in twins. Semin Perinatol 1986;10:50–64.
8. Hendricks CH. Twinning in relation to birthweight, mortality, and congenital anomalies. Obstet Gynecol 1966;27:47–53.
9. Rodis JF, Egan JFX, Craffey A, Ciarleglio L, Greenstein RM, Scorza WE. Calculated risk of chromosomal abnormalities in twin gestations. Obstet Gynecol 1990; 76:1037–1041.
10. Van Allen MI, Smith DW, Shepard TH. Twin reversed arterial perfusion (TRAP) sequence: a study of 14 twin pregnancies with acardius. Semin Perinatol 1983;7:285–293.
11. Turpin R. Monozygotisme heterocaryote. Acta Genet Med Gemellol 1970;19:188–198.
12. Rogers JG, Voullaire L, Gold H. Monozygotic twins discordant for trisomy 21. Am J Med Gemellol 1982;11:143–146.
13. Watson WJ, Katz VL, Albright SG, Rao KW, Aylsworth AS. Monozygotic twins discordant for partial trisomy 1. Obstet Gynecol 1990;76:949–951.
14. Gonsoulin W, Copeland KL, Carpenter RJ, Hughes MR, Elder FFB. Fetal blood sampling demonstrating chimerism in monozygotic twins discordant for sex and tissue karyotype (46,XY and 45,X). Prenat Diagn 1990;10:25–28.
15. Johnson JM, Harman CR, Evans JA, MacDonald K, Manning FA. Maternal serum alpha-fetoprotein in twin pregnancy. Am J Obstet Gynecol 1990;162:1020–1025.
16. Nebiolo LM, Adams WB, Miller SL, Milunsky A. Maternal serum human chorionic gonadotropin levels in twin pregnancies. Prenat Diagn 1991;11:463–466.
17. Stiller RJ, Lockwood CJ, Belanger K, Baumgarten A, Hobbins JC, Mahoney MJ. Amniotic fluid alpha-fetoprotein concentrations in twin gestations: dependence on placental membrane anatomy. Am J Obstet Gynecol 1988;158:1088–1092.
18. Cuckle H, Wald N, Stevenson JD, et al. Maternal serum alpha-fetoprotein screening for open neural tube defects in twin pregnancies. Prenat Diagn 1990;10:71–77.
19. Robertson EG, Neer KJ. Placental injection studies in twin gestation. Am J Obstet Gynecol 1983;147:170–173.
20. Benirschke K. Twin placentas in perinatal mortality. N Y State J Med 1974;61:1499–1508.
21. Bejar R, Vigliocco G, Gramajo H, et al. Antenatal origin of neurologic damage in newborn infants. Il. Multiple gestations. Am J Obstet Gynecol 1990;162:1230–1236.
22. Saier F, Burden L, Cavanagh D. Fetus papyraceus: an unusual case with congenital anomaly of the surviving fetus. Obstet Gynecol 1975;45:217–220.
23. Reisman LE, Pathak A. Bilateral renal cortical necrosis in the newborn. Am J Dis Child 1966;111:541–543.
24. Szymonowicz W, Preston H, Yu VYH. The surviving monozygotic twin. Arch Dis Child 1986;61:454–458.

25. Syrop CH, Varner MW. Triplet gestation: maternal and neonatal implications. Acta Genet Med Gemellol 1985;34:81–88.

26. Botting BJ, MacFarlane AJ, Price FV, eds. Three, four, and more. A study of triplet and higher order births. London: HMSO, 1990.

27. Campbell DM. Multiple births: too often a disaster. Br Med J 1991;302:741–742.

28. Howie PW. Selective reduction in multiple pregnancy. Legal confusion and ethical dilemmas. Br Med J 1988;297:433–434.

29. Dumez Y, Oury JF. Method for first trimester selective abortion in multiple pregnancy. Contrib Gynecol Obstet 1986; 15:50–53.

30. Berkowitz RL, Lynch L, Chitkara U, Wilkins IA, Mehalek KE, Alvarez E. Selective reduction of multifetal pregnancies in the first trimester. N Engl J Med 1988;318:1043–1047.

31. Wapner RJ, Davis GH, Johnson A, et al. Selective reduction of multifetal pregnancies. The Lancet 1990;335:90–93.

32. Tabsh KM. Transabdominal multifetal pregnancy reduction: report of 40 cases. Obstet Gynecol 1990;75:739–741.

33. Itskovitz J, Boldes R, Thaler I, et al. Transvaginal ultrasonography-guided aspiration of gestational sacs for selective abortion in multiple pregnancy. Am J Obstet Gynecol 1989;160:215–217.

34. Landy H, Weiner S, Corson SL, et al. The vanishing twin: ultrasonic assessment of fetal disappearance in the first trimester. Am J Obstet Gynecol 1986;155:14–19.

35. Dumez Y, Evans ML, Wagner RJ, et al. Efficacy of multifetal pregnancy reduction (MFPR): collaborative experience of the world's largest centers. Am J Obstet Gynecol 1991;164:255.

36. Lynch L. Embryo reduction. Presented at the Fetoscopy Working Group. XIV Annual Meeting. Istanbul 1992.

37. Derom C, Vlietinck R, Derom R, Van den Berghe H, Thiery M. Increased monozygotic twinning rate after ovulation induction. The Lancet 1987;1:1236–1238.

38. Isada NB, Sorokin Y, Drugan A, Johnson MP, Zador I, Evans MI. First trimester interfetal size variation in well-dated multifetal pregnancies. Fetal Diagn Ther 1992; 7:82–86.

39. Nazari A, Check JH, Epstein RH, et al. Relationship of small-for-dates sac size to crown-rump length and spontaneous abortion in patients with a known date of ovulation. Obstet Gynecol 1991;78:369–373.

40. Porreco RP, Burke S, Hendrix ML. Multifetal reduction of triplets and pregnancy outcome. Obstet Gynecol 1991;78:335–338.

41. Wapner RJ. Multiple gestation. Presented at the Fetoscopy Working Group. XIV Annual Meeting. Istanbul 1992.

42. Pergament E, Schulman JD, Copeland K, et al. The risk and efficacy of chorionic villus sampling in multiple gestations. Prenat Diagn 1992;12:337–384.

43. Winn HN, Gabrielli S, Reece A, Roberts JA, Salafia C, Hobbins J. Ultrasonographic criteria for the prenatal diagnosis of placental chorionicity in twin gestations. Am J Obstet Gynecol 1989;161:1540–1542.

44. Brambati B, Tului L, Lanzani A, Simoni G, Travi M. First-trimester genetic diagnosis in multiple pregnancy: principles and potential pitfalls. Prenat Diagn 1991;11: 767–774.

45. Pruggmayer M, Baumann P, Schutte H, et al. Incidence of abortion after genetic amniocentesis in twin pregnancies. Prenat Diagn 1991;11:637–640.

46. van der Pol JG, Wolf H, Boer K et al. Jejunal atresia related to the use of methylene blue in genetic amniocentesis in twins. Br J Obstet Gynaecol 1992;99:141–143.

47. Jeanty P, Shah D, Roussis P. Single-needle insertion in twin amniocentesis. J Ultrasound Med 1990;9:511–517.

48. Bahado-Singh R, Schmitt R, Hobbins JC. New technique for genetic amniocentesis in twins. Obstet Gynecol 1992;79:304–307.

49. D'Alton ME, Dudley DK. The ultrasound prediction of chorionicity in twin gestation. Am J Obstet Gynecol 1989;160:557–561.

50. Elias S, Gerbie AB, Simpson JL, Nadler HL, Sabbagha RE, Shkolnik A. Genetic amniocentesis in twin gestations. Am J Obstet Gynecol 1980;138:169–174.

51. Bovicelli L, Michelacci L, Rizzo N et al. Genetic amniocentesis in twin pregnancy. Prenat Diagn 1983;3:101–106.
52. Palle C, Andersen JW, Tabor A, Lauritsen JG, Bang J, Philip J. Increased risk of abortion after genetic amniocentesis in twin pregnancies. Prenat Diagn 1983;3:83–89.
53. Librach CL, Doran TA, Benzie RJ, Jones JM. Genetic amniocentesis in seventy twin pregnancies. Am J Obstet Gynecol 1984;148: 585–591.
54. Tabsch KM, Crandall B, Lenherz TB, Howard J. Genetic amniocentesis in twin pregnancy. Obstet Gynecol 1985; 65:843–845.
55. Kappel B, Nielsen J, Brogaard-Hansen K, Mikkelsen M, Therkelsen AJ. Spontaneous abortion following mid-trimester amniocentesis. Clinical significance of placental perforation and blood-stained amniotic fluid. Br J Obstet Gynaecol 1987; 94:50–54.
56. Brandmaier R. Nachuntersuchungen von Schwangerschaften nach Amniozentese zure pranatalen Diagnostik im zweiten Schwangerschaftsdrittel, thesis. Muchen, 1988.
57. Pijpers L, Jahoda MG, Vosters RP, Niermeijer MF, Sachs ES. Genetic amniocentesis in twin pregnancies. Br J Obstet Gynaecol 1988;95:323–326.
58. Prompeler HJ, Wilhelm C, Madjar H, Prem C, Schillinger H. Prognose von sonographisch fruh diagnostizierten Zwillingsschwangerschaften. Geburtsh Frauenheilk 1989;49:715–719.
59. Schulman LP, Elias S, Phillips OP, Dungan JS, Grevengood C, Simpson JL. Early twin amniocentesis prior to 14 weeks' gestation. Prenat Diagn 1992;12:625–629.
60. Nicolini U, Monni G. Intestinal obstruction in babies exposed in utero to methylene blue. The Lancet 1990;336:1258–1259.
61. Shah DM, Jeanty P, Dev VG, Ulm IE, Phillips J. Diagnosis of trisomy 18 in monozygotic twins by cordocentesis. Am J Obstet Gynecol 1989;160:214–215.
62. Nicolini U, Hubinont C, Santalaya J, Fisk NM, Rodeck CH, Johnson RD. Fetal serum alpha-fetoprotein in fetuses with chromosomal abnormalities. The Lancet 1988;2: 1316–1317.
63. Weiner CP. Diagnosis and treatment of twin-to-twin transfusion in the mid-second trimester of pregnancy. Fetal Ther 1987; 2:71–74.
64. Fisk NM, Borrell A, Hubinont C, Letsky EA, Nicolini U, Rodeck CH. Fetofetal transfusion syndrome: do the neonatal criteria apply in utero? Arch Dis Child 1990; 65:657–661.
65. Saunders NJ, Snijders RJM, Nicolaides KH. Twin-twin transfusion syndrome during the second trimester is associated with small intertwin hemoglobin differences. Fetal Diagn Ther 1991;6:34–36.
66. Moise KJ, Cotton DB. Discordant fetal platelet counts in a twin gestation complicated by idiopathic thrombocytopenia purpura. Am J Obstet Gynecol 1987;156: 1141–1142.
67. Megory E, Weiner E, Shalev E, Ohel G. Pseudoamniotic twins with cord entanglement following genetic funipuncture. Obstet Gynecol 1991;78:915–917.
68. Nicolini U, Nicolaidis P, Fisk NM, Tannirandorn Y, Rodeck CH. Fetal blood sampling from the intrahepatic vein: analysis of safety and clinical experience with 214 procedures. Obstet Gynecol 1990;76: 47–53.
69. Rydhstrom H. Prognosis for twins discordant in birth weight of 1.0 Kg or more: the impact of cesarean section. J Perinat Med 1990;18:31–37.
70. Nicolini U, Nicolaidis P, Fisk NM, et al. Limited role of fetal blood sampling in prediction of outcome in intrauterine growth retardation. The Lancet 1990;336: 768–772.
71. Poissonnier MH. Anastomosis in twin pregnancies with severe blood incompatibilities. International Fetal Medicine and Surgery Society Meeting, Phoenix, 1991.
72. Aberg A, Miterian F, Cantz M, Geliler J. Cardiac puncture of fetus with Hurler's disease avoiding abortion of unaffected cotwin. The Lancet 1978;2:990–991.

73. Petres R, Redwine F. Selective birth in twin pregnancy. N Engl J Med 1981;305:1218–1219.

74. Beck L, Terinde R, Dolff M. Zwillingsschwangershaft mit freier trisomie 21 eines kindes; sectio parva mit entfernung des kranken und spatere gubert des gesunden kindes. Geburtsh Frauenheilk 1980;40:397–400.

75. Rodeck CH, Mibashan R, Abramowitz J, Campbell S. Selective feticide of the affected twin by fetoscopic air embolization. Prenat Diagn 1982;2:189–194.

76. Antsaklis A, Politis J, Karagiannopoulos C, et al. Selective survival of only the healthy fetus following prenatal diagnosis of thalassemia major in binovular twin gestation. Prenat Diagn 1984;4:289–296.

77. Golbus MS. Selective termination. In: Harrison MR, Golbus MS, Filly RA, eds. The unborn patient. Chapter 18. Philadelphia: WB Saunders, 1991;166–171.

78. Wittman BK, Farquharson DF, Thomas WDS, Baldwin VJ, Wadsworth L. The role of feticide in the management of severe twin transfusion syndrome. Am J Obstet Gynecol 1986;155:1023–1026.

79. Chescheir NC, Seeds JW. Polyhydramnios and oligohydramnios in twin gestations. Obstet Gynecol 1988;71:882–884.

80. Tanaka M, Natori M, Ishimoto H, Kohno H, Kobayashi T, Nozawa S. Intravascular pancuronium bromide infusion for prenatal diagnosis of twin-twin transfusion syndrome. Fetal Diagn Ther 1992;7:36–40.

81. Robertson EG, Neer KJ. Placental injection studies in twin gestation. Am J Obstet Gynecol 1983;147:170–173.

82. Wenstrom KD, Tessen JA, Zlatnik FJ, Sipes SL. Frequency, distribution, and theoretical mechanisms of hematologic and weight discordance in monochorionic twins. Obstet Gynecol 1992;80:257–261.

83. Danskin FH, Neilson JP. Twin to twin transfusion syndrome: what are appropriate diagnostic criteria? Am J Obstet Gynecol 1989;161:365–369.

84. Tan KL, Tan R, Tan SH, Tan AM. The twin transfusion syndrome. Clinical observations on 35 affected pairs. Clin Pediatr 1979;18:111–114.

85. Rausen AR, Seki M, Strauss L. Twin transfusion syndrome. J Pediatr 1965;66:613–628.

86. Schatz F. Eine besonder Art von einseitiger Polyhydramnie mit anderseitiger Oligohydramnie bei eineiigen Zwillingen. Arch Gynaekol 1882;19:329–369.

87. Storlazzi E, Vintzileos AM, Campbell WA, Nochimson DJ, Weinbaum PJ. Ultrasonic diagnosis of discordant fetal growth in twin gestations. Obstet Gynecol 1987;69:363–367.

88. Blickstein I, Friedman A, Caspi B, Lancet M. Ultrasonic prediction of growth discordancy by intertwin difference in abdominal circumference. Int J Gynecol Obstet 1989;29:121–124.

89. Wieacker P, Wilhelm C, Prompeler H, Petersen KG, Schillinger H, Breckwoldt M. Pathophysiology of polyhydramnios in twin transfusion syndrome. Fetal Diagn Ther 1992;7:87–92.

90. Rosen DJD, Rabinowitz R, Beyth Y, Fejgin MD, Nicolaides KH. Fetal urine production in normal twins and in twins with acute polyhydramnios. Fetal Diagn Ther 1990;5:57–60.

91. Farmakides G, Schulman H, Saldana L, Bracero LA, Fleischer A, Rochelson B. Surveillance of twin pregnancy with umbilical artery velocimetry. Am J Obstet Gynecol 1985;153:789–792.

92. Pretorius DH, Manchester D, Barkin S, Parker S, Nelson TR. Doppler ultrasound of twin transfusion syndrome. J Ultrasound Med 1988;7:117–124.

93. Yamada A, Kasugai M, Ohno Y, Ishizuka T, Mizutani S, Tomoda Y. Antenatal diagnosis of twin-twin transfusion syndrome by Doppler ultrasound. Obstet Gynecol 1991;78:1058–1061.

94. Giles W, Trudinger BJ, Cook CM, Connelly AJ. Doppler umbilical artery studies in the twin-twin transfusion syndrome. Obstet Gynecol 1990;76:1097–1099.

95. Sherer DM, Ezra Y, Beyth Y, Sadovsky E. Sinusoidal heart rate pattern associated

with the twin to twin transfusion syndrome. Int J Gynecol Obstet 1990;31: 71–74.

96. Ludomirsky A, Weiner S, Capraro F, Bhutani V. Twin to twin transfusion syndrome: role at Doppler flow and fetal hyperviscosity in predicting outcome. Am J Obstet Gynecol 1991;164 (SPO abstract 5): 243.

97. Dudley DKL, D'Alton ME. Single fetal death in twin gestation. Semin Perinatol 1986;10:65–72.

98. Weir PE, Ratten GJ, Beischer NA. Acute polyhydramnios—a complication of monozygous twins. Br J Obstet Gynaecol 1979; 86:849–853.

99. Gonsoulin W, Moise KJ, Kirshon B, Cotton DB, Wheeler JM, Carpenter RJ. Outcome of twin-twin transfusion diagnosed before 28 weeks of gestation. Obstet Gynecol 1990; 75:214–216.

100. Blickstein I. The twin-twin transfusion syndrome. Obstet Gynecol 1990;76:714–722.

101. Landy HL, Weingold AB. Management of a multiple gestation complicated by an antepartum fetal demise. Obstet Gynecol Surv 1989;44:171–176.

102. Fusi L, Gordon H. Twin pregnancy complicated by single intrauterine death. Problems and outcome with conservative management. Br J Obstet Gynaecol 1990; 97:511–516.

103. Kirshon B, Moise KJ, Mari G, Rothchild S, Wasserstrum N. In utero resolution of hydrops fetalis following the death of one twin in twin-twin transfusion. Am J Perinatol 1990;7:107–109.

104. Skelly H, Marivate M, Norman R, et al. Consumptive coagulopathy following fetal death in a triplet pregnancy. Am J Obstet Gynecol 1982;142:595–596.

105. Romero R, Duffy TP, Berkowitz RL, et al. Prolongation of a preterm pregnancy complicated by death of a single twin in utero and disseminated intravascular coagulation: effects of treatment with heparin. N Engl J Med 1984;310:772–774.

106. Fusi L, McParland P, Fisk NM, Nicolini U, Wigglesworth J. Acute twin-twin trans-

fusion: a possible mechanism for brain damaged survivors after in utero death of a monochorionic twin. Obstet Gynecol 1991;78:517–520.

107. Elliott JP, Urig MA, Clewell WH. Aggressive therapeutic amniocentesis for treatment of twin-twin transfusion syndrome. Obstet Gynecol 1991;77:537–544.

108. Saunders NJ, Snijders RJM, Nicolaides KH. Therapeutic amniocentesis in twin-twin transfusion syndrome appearing in the second trimester of pregnancy. Am J Obstet Gynecol 1992;166:820–824.

109. Mahony BS, Petty CN, Nyberg DA, Luthy DA, Hickok DE, Hirsh JH. The "stuck twin" phenomenon: ultrasonographic findings, pregnancy outcome, and management with serial amniocenteses. Am J Obstet Gynecol 1990;163:1513–1522.

110. Nicolini U, Fisk NM, Talbert DG, et al. Intrauterine manometry: technique and application to fetal pathology. Prenat Diagn 1989;9:243–254.

111. DeLia JE, Rogers JG, Dixon JA. Treatment of placental vasculature with neodymium-yttrium-aluminium-garnet laser via fetoscopy. Am J Obstet Gynecol 1985;151: 1126–1127.

112. DeLia JE, Cruikshank DP, Keye WR. Fetoscopic neodymium: YAG laser occlusion of placental vessels in severe twin-twin transfusion syndrome. Obstet Gynecol 1990;75: 1046–1053.

113. DeLia JE. International Fetal Medicine and Surgery Society Meeting, Evian, 1992.

114. Vetter K, Schneider KTM. Iatrogenous remission of twin transfusion syndrome. Am J Obstet Gynecol 1988;158:221.

115. Pilu GL. Phlebotomy in twin-twin transfusion syndrome. Presented at the Fetoscopy Working Group. XII Annual Meeting. Bologna 1990.

116. Dumez Y. Twin-twin transfusion syndrome. Presented at the Fetoscopy Working Group. XIV Annual Meeting. Istanbul 1992.

117. Benedetti A. De singulis corpori humani morbis a capite ad pedem. Venezia, 1553.

118. Nicolaidis P, Nasrat H, Tannirandorn Y. Fetal acardia: aetiology, pathology and management. Br J Obstet Gynaecol 1990; 10:518–525.

119. Moore TR, Gale S, Benirschke K. Perinatal outcome of 49 pregnancies complicated by acardiac twinning. Am J Obstet Gynecol 1990;163:907–912.

120. Robie GF, Payne GG, Morgan MA. Selective delivery of an acardiac acephalic twin. N Engl J Med 1989;320:512–513.

121. Hamada H, Okane M, Koresawa M, Kubo T, Iwasaki H. Fetal therapy in utero by blockage of the umbilical blood flow of acardiac monster in twin pregnancy. Nippon Sanka Fujinka Gakkai Zasshi 1989;41: 1803–1809.

122. Porreco RP, Barton SM, Haverkamp AD. Occlusion of umbilical artery in acardiac, acephalic twin. The Lancet 1991;337: 326–327.

123. Ash K, Harman CR, Gritter H. TRAP sequence—successful outcome with indomethacin treatment. Obstet Gynecol 1990;76:960–962.

124. Cox M, Murphy K, Ryan G, Kingdom M, Whittle M, McNay M. Spontaneous cessation of umbilical blood flow in the acardiac fetus of a twin pregnancy. Prenat Diagn 1992;12:689–693.

INVASIVE PROCEDURES IN EVOLUTION

12

PHILLIPA KYLE
C. R. HARMAN

INVASIVE PROCEDURES IN EVOLUTION

The common goal of the diverse collection of procedures discussed in this chapter is *direct fetal evaluation*. The common feature of these procedures is that their application is in an unstable state of evolution. Some are coming, some are going; some have been in practice for many years, others are in their infancy. Many are virtually experimental in nature and their use is difficult to evaluate. None of these is likely to be applied on a very broad scale, but their availability in selected tertiary care centers, for specific fetal or maternal indications, will complement the detailed interventions now in more generalized application.

EMBRYOSCOPY

Early in pregnancy, the cervical canal is patent and a narrow diameter scope may be passed transvaginally to rest against the membranes.

Such a procedure—embryoscopy—even in its simplest sense, *is* an invasive procedure, by definition. The membranes are not a single unit until well on in pregnancy (1). While the amnion and chorion are usually well apposed fairly early (usually by 12–13 weeks gestational age), they are not freely transparent at that stage. Only at 22 weeks or so, when the decidua capsularis degenerates, are the membranes solely fetal and fairly transparent. Before then, the amnion and chorion laeve are separated by a space— the chorionic cavity, or extracoelomic cavity or extraembryonic space, and the chorion laeve and decidua capsularis are perfectly opaque. Thus, only after perforation of the chorion can the embryo be visualized directly (Figure 12-1).

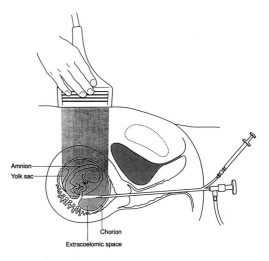

Figure 12-1 Schematic diagram of embryoscopy under ultrasound guidance. Note clearly separate chorion and amnion, separated by the extracoelomic space.

Among the earliest attempts at transvaginal direct fetal visualization were those of Westin (2), who used a large diameter (10 mm) hysteroscope to visualize fetal parts, assess fetal movement, and evaluate oxygenation in pregnancies destined for immediate termination. These observations were performed at 16–20 weeks gestation, so chorionic or chorioamnionic rupture were not obligatory. There is now no reasonable role for such a procedure at such gestational ages.

A number of authors utilized a "fetoscope," which was an inclusive term, encompassing cystoscopes, arthroscopes, hysteroscopes, bronchoscopes, and panendoscopes, of diameters from 2–12 mm—for transcervical embryo/fetal visualization (3–6). Such studies included serial observations from as early as five weeks gestation. In the large majority, termination of the pregnancy was intended, and completed, after visualization, so assessment of complications, benefits, cost, or comparative roles is not possible from the earlier studies. Further, these reports often included pregnancies beyond 14–16 weeks, where ultrasound would clearly be the modality of current choice.

Transcervical visualization techniques were advocated for assistance with invasive techniques such as transcervical chorion villus sampling (CVS), simple observation of the embryo and developing pregnancy, or even embryonic blood sampling. Therapeutic possibilities utilizing the yolk sac, e.g., for stem-cell transfusion, were also suggested by the concept of direct access to the embryo. On the other hand, the rapid evolution of endovaginal ultrasound has meant that direct visualization of the embryo and other structures in the gestational sac using embryoscopy has extremely limited application. CVS under ultrasound guidance is almost always technically successful in any case. Yolk sac therapy may be more practicable using the larger angle of approach offered transabdominally, and so on.

The more recent attempts at transvaginal *embryo* visualization at much earlier gestation, described by Ghirardini (6) and Cullen and colleagues (7–9) have used 2–4 mm diameter rigid endoscopes with fiberoptic light sources. No anesthetic other than the premedication used for the pregnancy termination procedure was added for embryoscopy. The scope is introduced through a vaginal speculum into the external cervical os, then guided ultrasonically to rest against the chorion. Chorionic puncture is done using a sharp stab, trying to avoid the placenta. The combination of wide-angle lens and small embryo size means that total body visualization is possible in most (75–90%) procedures.

A number of embryonic abnormalities have been visualized using this technique, and recent review by the group developing modern embryoscopy suggests "its potential for first-trimester diagnosis and therapy

is promising" (10). Clear and interesting illustrations are shown, and access to the embryonic (yolk sac) circulation is referenced. Embryoscopic visualization has been used to show skin hemorrhages on the surface of embryos following CVS or deliberate placental trauma, and, as such, the technique has provided useful scientific data (11). It is notable, however, that the majority of these cases have also been done in patients scheduled for termination of pregnancy immediately after the procedure. Thus, the incidence of placental separation (5%) and immediate fetal demise (1%) noted in these situations (8) may not reflect the long-term consequences of application in a large population of women wanting to continue their pregnancies. Several of the illustrative cases are greater than eight weeks gestation, most have been done after ultrasound had shown an embryonic defect, and overall numbers are small. Finally, even this most skilled and experienced team, reporting results including >200 embryoscopic procedures, showed an incidence of amniotic rupture in >20% of their most recent series (11). Comparison of these techniques with early high-resolution endovaginal ultrasound, e.g., in detecting early yolk sac abnormalities at five to ten weeks gestation (12) (Figure 12-2), has not yet been done.

There may be marginal indications for this procedure in ongoing pregnancy and for evaluation of failed pregnancies, but it is less likely that embryonic blood sampling, which is possible because the vessels on the yolk sac are accessible in the extraembryonic space, will achieve wide acceptance (10). Actual embryo "biopsy" using this technique is not possible, as it would involve overt rupture of the amnion as well as the obligatory rupture of the chorion.

The "embryoscope" and the skill to use it, are not widely disseminated.

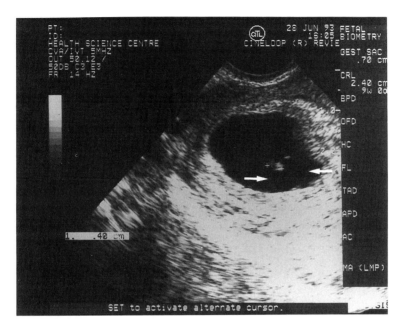

Figure 12-2 Seven-week gestation with abnormally large, irregular yolk sac (arrows). Although cardiac activity was apparent on this occasion, pregnancy loss followed within two weeks.

FETOSCOPY

Fetoscopy shares the same roots as embryoscopy, i.e., the transcervical amnioscopy of Westin (2,13). Mandelbaum et al. then described a two-puncture transabdominal technique, one for the scope, a second for the rigid fiberoptic light source. Although some photographs were published and intravascular fetal transfusion using placental surface vessels was proposed, clinical application was not clear (14). Valenti was able to perform fetal skin biopsy and fetal blood sampling using a 6 mm oval scope encompassing telescope, light source, and biopsy forceps (15). His technique was developed in pre-abortion (hysterotomy) patients during laparotomy. Scrimgeour (16) provided an initial stimulus to clinical application followed by the fundamental conversion to an ultrasound-guided procedure by Hobbins et al. (17). This report demonstrated the advantages of ultrasound guidance in correct positioning of the scope and is responsible for dissemination of a technique that was safe and practicable, followed by reports from several groups on both sides of the Atlantic of fetoscopy in ongoing pregnancy (18–22).

Patrick et al. described successful transabdominal percutaneous fetoscopy in ongoing pregnancies and not requiring general anesthetic (23). By the late 1970s, the current format of the fetoscopy procedure was established, and a wide variety of fetal data became available for the first time. Some examples (there were over 500 papers with data derived from "fetoscopy" in the English literature between 1970 and 1994) are shown in Table 12-1. References 24–33 provide a survey of representative reports.

Technique (Figure 12-3)

The technique described has changed little since the description by Hobbins

Table 12-1   Reported Applications of Fetoscopy

Fetal Structural Evaluation
  Risk of anomaly/confirmation of ultrasound
    findings (Hundreds of cases for >50 struc-
    tural disorders)
  Fetal sex determination

Fetal Blood Sampling—Diagnosis
  Blood type
  Hemoglobinopathy (>5 disorders)
  Coagulopathy (>5)
  Congenital anemias (>5)
  Thrombocytopenia
  Immunodeficiency (>10)
  Karyotype
  Fetal/maternal infection (>5)
  Hereditary metabolic disorders (>20)
  Nonimmune hydrops

Fetal Blood Sampling—Diagnosis and Treatment
  Alloimmune erythroblastosis
  Alloimmune thrombocytopenia
  Fetal-maternal hemorrhage

Fetal Biopsy
  Liver, skin, kidney, muscle

Selective Feticide (Umbilical Air Embolism)

Drainage Procedures
  Bladder, kidney, ascites, thorax

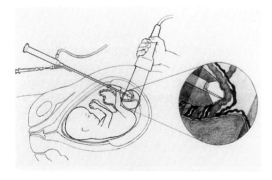

Figure 12-3   Schematic diagram of fetal blood sampling by ultrasound-directed fetoscopy. Inset: 27-gauge needle tip is introduced into the umbilical vein at the base of the cord.

and Mahoney of the ultrasound-guided approach (17). The capabilities of modern high-resolution ultrasound instruments, however, have made this a reasonably-refined process and not as tentative as in previous decades. Detailed ultrasound investigation must always precede the procedure, confirming fetal orientation, viability, and anatomic integrity, and so on. A defined indication for the procedure, specific to fetoscopy and withstanding the comparison to other ultrasound-guided techniques, is required. This criterion and its role in determining informed consent mean that few procedures are now performed and only by a select group of centers with ongoing expertise. Further prerequisites include expert placental ultrasonography, a fetal surgical suite, bedside testing for analysis of samples, and, frequently, the presence of the appropriate specialist (geneticist, pathologist, biochemistry staff).

In summary, the procedure is performed in sterile fashion, with full surgical preparation and draping. The patient is usually sedated and receives antibiotic prophylaxis. The critical step is identification of a placenta-free approach that will offer access to the required aspect (usually of the fetus) for sampling. For example, for fetal skin sampling, the back, extremities, or scalp are preferable, whereas for liver biopsy, the scope should be oriented towards the anterior abdominal surface, and muscle biopsy, kidney biopsy, and so on, would require different approaches.

With identification of the target, local anesthetic and a small skin incision down to the fascia provide access to the uterine surface.

A number of instruments remain in current use. The most frequently reported, used in many centers during the zenith of the application of fetoscopy, was the 1.7 mm diameter Needlescope manufactured by

Dyonics Inc., but this is no longer available. A variety of endoscopes, including pediatric cystoscopes and arthroscopes, and including instruments manufactured by Storz, Olympus, and Wolf, continue to be utilized. Uterine penetration requires the same (significant) force as inserting a 14-gauge needle. Many instruments have a small (26 or 27-gauge) side port, utilized for fetal blood sampling in early gestations. A fetoscope that allows concurrent insertion of biopsy forceps and continued visualization of the target would be most preferable (noting that this instrument is usually oval, and has a maximum diameter of nearly 3 mm). In older models, when biopsy was to be performed, the optical element was removed and the biopsy forceps inserted in a blind fashion. Obviously, movement of the fetus at that point in time would necessitate revisualization, and this problem contributed significantly to the daunting length of many fetoscopic procedures. Once safe insertion into the amniotic cavity has been confirmed, the operator then searches for a fetal landmark. When the fetus is large, this landmark is basically a horizon, where the amniotic fluid ends and the fetus begins. The suitability of this horizon is continuously referenced using real-time ultrasound.

For skin sampling, the scope is then pressed against the fetal surface, sometimes necessitating pinning the fetus against the opposite side of the uterus (34–35). The biopsy forceps are then introduced and samples are obtained under direct visualization. For fetal blood sampling, the 20-cm-long blood sampling needle is passed down the side port, and fetal vessels along the surface of the placenta, at the cord insertion, or at the umbilicus are utilized for fetal blood sampling. As noted in detail below, however, before several technical factors were modified, initial experience showed that

fetoscopic fetal blood sampling was often liable to be unsuccessful or contaminated (24–34,36).

Tocolytics are not utilized, and a short period of maternal and fetal monitoring follows the procedure. Bedside affirmation of a fetal source for the tissue samples is followed up by detailed confirmation of correct samples by the reference laboratory.

If intraperitoneal fetal transfusion initiated the revolution in attitudes to fetal therapy, fetoscopy provided the stimulus for exponential growth of those attitudes. Fetoscopy grew rapidly in application through the 1970s and early 1980s and was an important clinical tool in many centers. The beginnings of direct fetal testing are the foundation of the scientific approach to fetal diagnosis and therapy that we practice today. The fundamental appeal of fetoscopy was this: once you can see what you are doing, many things are possible!

Does this sound like a eulogy? Fetoscopy has not quite died, and its specialized applications may linger, but many factors have contributed to its decline.

Limitations (Table 12-2)

While fetoscopy did provide access on a reliable basis to fetal blood and tissue, this was not without condition. Vessels in the free cord are hard to hit, and placental surface vessels are usually approached at a perpendicular angle, so vessel entry was tenuous. Before 18–19 weeks, small vessel caliber makes blood sampling difficult with any technique—further handicapped with fetoscopy by the 20-cm length of the needle, the small gauge and the lack of depth perception. Later in pregnancy, the large size of the fetus interfered, and placental access may be limited by the rigid scope, round contours and relative paucity of fluid versus baby.

Table 12-2   Limitations of Fetoscopy

Technical Problems
   Long, small-gauge needle
   Limited gestational age range (16–24 weeks)
   Limited access with anterior placenta*
   Poor maneuverability if AF reduced
   Reduced depth perception
   Very difficult with bloody or very turbid fluid
   Backbleeding from puncture site*
   Fetomaternal hemorrhage*
   Large entry hole
   Fetal movement/fetal size may interfere
   Narrow field of view (55°)
   Long procedure (mean = 25 minutes)

Sample Problems
   Small samples
   Maternal blood/maternal blood
      contamination*
   Amniotic fluid contamination
   Microagglutination
   No sample obtained

AF = amniotic fluid.
*worse with placental surface vessels than cord placental insertion

Some of these hurdles were overcome with modifications in technique (37–38). An approach parallel to the fetal surface of the placenta is now used. Thus, the scope is perpendicular to the primary target (the placental cord insertion) and, at the same time, can be pointed at the secondary target—the fetal cord insertion (Figure 12-3). As well, some of these difficulties are relative rather than absolute. For example, amniotic fluid turbidity, which generally increases with advancing gestation, may or may not preclude fetoscopic visualization beyond 24 weeks. Finally, increased experience and equipment modifications have reduced the frequency of inadequate, contaminated, or failed samples, especially in assays of fetal coagulation; even the smallest amount of amniotic fluid induces erroneous results

at fetal blood sampling—this deficit was not overcome by technical improvements. While large series found encouragement in the progress to 60% or more of fetoscopies yielding pure fetal blood, 96–98% would be the norm for current ultrasound-guided percutaneous cordocentesis (PUBS).

Complications (39–41 and previous references)

Complications are listed in Table 12-3. It is difficult to be sure that representative statistics are indeed available. Few institutions have published experience with more than 200–300 procedures. Large registry reports from the regular meetings of the International Fetoscopy Group tabulated over 4000 cases, but over 20 institutions contributed, with highly disparate findings. On the other hand, it is likely that the very encouraging results of two groups (42), each with more than 1200 procedures, represent the gold standard and might not be applicable in the average situation. Thus, total loss rates range from 3–9.1%, and procedure-attributable losses from one in 150 procedures to one in 12 procedures (Table 12-3).

Several generalizations are possible from the published data.

1. Fetoscopy underwent many technical modifications in a short period of time. The authors with the largest (and longest, it turns out) experience also have the best experience. In other words, discounting the technique because of technical problems, failures, or complications may be unwarranted.
2. There is limited current indication for fetoscopy, but within the small group of applicable circumstances, the complications in Table 12-3 may not be very likely, and, of course, other complica-

Table 12-3 Fetoscopy Complications—% of Procedures

Complication	Overall*	Range*
Technical		
Blood-stained amniotic fluid	10%	5–25%
Sample contamination	7%	0–39%
Maternal sample only	0.5%	0–5%
No result	12%	8–20%
Fetal		
Mortality	3–5%	0.5–9.1%
Nonlethal fetal bleeding	3%	3–9%
Fetal distress/tachycardia	2%	0–4%
Maternal		
Premature labor and delivery	10%	3–14%
Rupture of membranes only	2%	1–5%
Membranes tented/dissected	5%	5–12%
Clinical chorioamnionitis	0.5%	0.5–2%
Alloimmunization**	0**	0.8%
Entry wound complications	1%	3–18%
Rare, but Reported, Complications		
Fetal laceration	Undetected anomalies	
Misdiagnosed deficits	Maternal hemorrhage	
Maternal visceral injury	Fetal optic (light) injury?	

*Overall is consensus, weighted to large studies; range includes many
early reports whose findings were not persistent.
**Fully preventable for D, by Rh-immuneglobulin administration.

tions may occur that are peculiar to the new applications.

3. Within the context of applications in the published surveys, an overall *attributable loss* [immediate abortion + stillbirth + procedure-related (premature) neonatal death] is three to five per 100 procedures. *Premature labor* and delivery is significantly related to the procedure. *Contamination, error or absent samples* will complicate at least 20% of cases selected for fetoscopy. The majority of *technical complications* in blood sampling are avoidable by ultrasound-directed PUBS. Most fetal complications are much worse with fetoscopy than with PUBS. The maternal complications of fetoscopy are worse as well.

Present Status of Fetoscopy

Fetoscopy is indicated for fetal visualization during biopsy procedures when fetal imaging by high-resolution ultrasound is not ideal. This would include muscle biopsy, soft tissue biopsy, and lesion-specific skin biopsy, in many cases. The need for these tests is highly specific and very uncommon. As an adjunct to difficult visualization in the obese patient or in some centers with an unusual balance of expertise, fetoscopy may have an ongoing role in general skin biopsy and very early fetal blood sampling, although such cases are also rare.

More and more centers have converted skin, liver, and other organ biopsy procedures to ultrasound-controlled techniques, and fewer and fewer subspecialty graduates are receiving training in fetoscopic procedures.

Future Applications

As suggested above, there are situations when ultrasound-directed procedures may be inadequate or impaired by difficulty in discriminating layers of soft tissue. Ultrasound technology continues to advance, so it may be that such difficulties are not enduring ones. Fetoscopic technology is not the direct focus of much technological innovation but is likely to benefit from the current surge in development of endoscopic techniques. Although limited intrauterine endoscopic surgery has been reported to date, it is entirely feasible that disorders such as shown in Table 12-4 can be treated with intrauterine surgery through single- or even multiple-entry endoscopic techniques, with ultrasound guidance and monitoring. For example, most centers where vesicoamniotic shunting is performed have developed many adjunctive maneuvers, i.e., tricks, but still have difficulty with the distal pigtail being properly placed in the amniotic space. With instillation of artificial amniotic fluid and endoscopic manipulation of the distal loop of the shunt, proper placement and function might be guaranteed.

A new generation of fetal surgical procedures may arise in difficult situations, such as diaphragmatic hernia. Endoscopic alternatives might include simply incising the fetal abdomen in the left upper quadrant and pulling the herniated contents from the chest (repairing this "gastroschisis" after birth), or performing a tracheotomy and inserting an occluding balloon to block efflux of pulmonary fluid (using the normal right lung's fluid production to "inflate" the left lung and reverse the hypo-

Table 12-4 Potential Fetal Endoscopic Surgical Procedures

Manipulation/Ultrasound Aided
  Shunt placement/correction—vesicoamniotic, pleuroamniotic, etc.
  Umbilical venous catheterization

Fetal/Placental Vessel Ligation
  Selective feticide
  Selective umbilical artery ligation, e.g., choriohemangioma
  Twin-to-twin transfusion
  Acardiac twin

Lesion-specific Biopsy
  e.g., bullae for skin biopsy

Incision and Drainage
  e.g., renal cyst

Complex Procedures
  e.g., create abdominal defect and reduce congenital diaphragmatic hernia, abrade cleft lip and suture, fetal tracheotomy and obstruction in pulmonary hypoplasia

plasia). Elimination of the hysterotomy incision might well be directly analogous to the laparotomy/laparoscopy revolution—decreased morbidity and mortality without (in the long run) reduced capability. It may well be that the hard lessons learned in the largely disappointing experience with externalization of the fetus will prove valuable in an endoscopic approach to those same fetal problems.

SPECIFIC TISSUE BIOPSIES

Prenatal diagnosis is now available for many metabolic, genetic, and chromosomal disorders on samples and their cultures obtained at CVS, amniocentesis, and PUBS. Unfortunately, some of these disorders do not express the specific defect in any of the easily available tissues (fibroblasts, chorionic villi, or blood cells), and so, a specific tissue biopsy is required.

FETAL LIVER BIOPSY

Fetal liver biopsy has been performed to diagnose or exclude specific enzyme deficiencies, predominantly those involved in the urea cycle (Table 12-5). Some of these enzymes are expressed in leukocytes, but the volume of blood required for analysis of these cells precludes their use.

Specific Enzyme Deficiencies

Ornithine Carbamyl Transferase Deficiency

This is the most frequent enzyme deficiency in the urea cycle. The enzyme is expressed in hepatocytes, intestinal cells, and leukocytes, and usually is active by 16 weeks gestation. The disorder is inherited by an X-linked trait, and males, most severely affected, usually die in the first week of life from ammonia intoxication. Female carriers are typically normal but often prefer a low protein diet. Occasionally, clinical manifestations, such as mental retardation, may appear. This variable expression may be explained by variation in the

Table 12-5 Reported Fetal Liver Biopsies

Defect Sought	Cases
Ornithine carbamyl transferase	15 (33,34,43,44)
Carbamyl phosphate synthetase	2 (45,46)
Glucose-6-phosphatase	3 (34,47)
Nonketotic hyperglycemia	1 (34)
Aromatic L-amino acid decarboxylase	1 (50)
Alanine:glyoxylate aminotransferase*	1 (48,49)

*Suggested (48), referenced (49) by different groups.

number of liver cells carrying the genetic abnormality. Fetal liver biopsy around 19 weeks gestation has diagnosed or excluded the abnormality correctly in several reports (33,34,43,44).

Carbamyl Phosphate Synthetase Deficiency (CPS-1)

This is another mitochondrial liver enzyme in the urea cycle. Deficiency, which is an autosomal recessive condition, leads to ammonia intoxication and neonatal death. Two reports of diagnosis by examination of fetal liver tissue are available (45,46).

Glucose-6-Phosphatase Deficiency

Glucose-6-phosphate is present in liver, kidney, and intestinal tissue. Deficiency of the enzyme, an autosomal recessive disorder of glucose metabolism, is termed glycogen storage disease Ia or von Gierke's disease. Clinical manifestations include hypoglycemia, lactic acidemia, hyperuricemia, hyperlipidemia, and platelet dysfunction. Mental impairment and death can occur if the metabolic abnormalities are not controlled.

Examination of fetal liver tissue has been reported in three cases (34,47). In two cases, the defect was excluded and the infants were normal at follow-up, while the defect was proven in the third, leading to therapeutic abortion.

Other Enzyme Deficiencies Diagnosed By Fetal Liver Biopsy

Diagnosis of nonketotic hyperglycemia has been attempted but was apparently unsuccessful (34). The autosomal recessive disorder of alanine:glyoxylate aminotransferase responsible for primary hyperoxaluria Type I can be diagnosed by fetal liver biopsy (48) as referenced (49), but no case details are available. Neurotransmitter amine synthesis deficiencies may produce profound central hypotonia in homozygous infants and have led to early death in un-treated children. In such rare disorders, de-tailed analysis of the family led to the identification of specific parameters for pre-natal diagnosis, carried out by fetal liver biopsy (50). As with many other hereditary disorders, absence of gene probes and non-expression by fetal blood, chorion villi, or amniocytes mean only direct biopsy can achieve diagnosis.

Technique of Fetal Liver Biopsy

Before fetal liver biopsy is performed to diagnose these metabolic abnormalities, laboratory facilities for the measurement of the specific enzyme, including suitable fetal control ranges, must be available, and absence confirmed of a reliable test on fibroblasts, etc., derived from amniotic fluid. The genetic history of the parents and affected pregnancies need to be known, and, in addition, the exact enzyme defect must be documented from a previ-ous pregnancy.

Fetoscopy

Fetal liver biopsy using fetoscopy was first described by Rodeck et al. in 1982 (43). Following insertion of the fetoscope as de-scribed previously, the fetal umbilicus and right nipple are identified. Midway be-tween these two points, immediately be-neath the right costal margin (felt as a soft sponginess beneath the firm rib), the biopsy needle is pushed into the abdomen. Several small movements within the liver tissue are made to obtain the specimen and then the needle is withdrawn into the trocar and out of the abdomen. The fetal heart rate and any other signs of bleeding are observed throughout and following the procedure.

Percutaneous Needle Biopsy

Subsequent reports have described fetal liver biopsy by the ultrasound-guided per-cutaneous approach. Using an aseptic technique, a biopsy or soft tissue sampling needle (16.5–20 gauge) is inserted through an anesthetized area of the maternal ab-domen, avoiding the placenta, into the amniotic cavity. Once the fetal right hypochondrium and liver are identified, the needle is pushed quickly into the fetal abdomen. Several small "in and out" movements along the needle pathway may be required to obtain the specimen. Once the needle is removed from the abdomen, the specimen is sent to the laboratory in the appropriate form (usually on ice, but not frozen). The fetus is then observed as for the previous procedure.

Equipment

The Tru-cut liver biopsy needle used in adults is less effective for obtaining fetal liver tissue. Most reports have described us-ing soft tissue biopsy needles, or 16.5–19-gauge two-needle sampling systems (needle and guide) with negative suction applied from an attached syringe.

Complications

Because of the small number of fetal liver biopsies reported, the risk of the procedure cannot be quantified. However, this most likely is similar to the risk associated with PUBS performed in experienced hands. Po-tential complications include failure of the procedure, fetal injury, and subcapsular liver hemorrhage, the latter particularly, be-cause fetal clotting factors are lower at this gestation (51). In the cases reported so far, none of these complications have occurred. Specifically, there have been no fetal losses and no incorrect diagnoses. From the available reports, it appears that biopsy is successful on the first attempt in two-thirds of cases, but in about 10%, no result is ever obtained. Bleeding is considered unlikely if the major vessels are avoided from correct localization of the insertion site; the fetal liver is not extremely vascular since the majority of portal blood is diverted from it. While fetal liver biopsy causes apparently lower increases in maternal serum AFP than does fetal blood sampling (both by fetoscopy), the possibility of sensitizing fetomaternal transfusion remains and requires detailed prophylaxis (52).

Accuracy

The diagnosis was accurate in the cases reported (verified in the terminated fetuses or the surviving infants), and the survivors showed no damage attributable to the procedure itself.

The Future

Fetal liver biopsy has been limited to a few cases in highly specialized centers. With the identification of specific restriction-fragment polymorphisms at the DNA locus of these enzymes, DNA probes and diagnosis will be possible if family linkage patterns are available. DNA analysis is now available for some potential cases of ornithine carbamyl transferase deficiency, for example (53,54). In fact, in one family where the OCT deficiency was proven (and therapeutic abortion carried out) on the basis of fetal liver biopsy (44), two subsequent pregnancies were successfully evaluated by CVS and DNA analysis (54). Thus, DNA analysis (from readily available tissues, such as chorionic villi, amniocytes, fetal blood, or even nucleated fetal cells extracted from the maternal circulation) becomes more practical. The requirement for fetal liver biopsy may become even less.

FETAL SKIN BIOPSY

Certain inheritable skin disorders associated with high rates of morbidity and mortality are only available for prenatal diagnosis by direct analysis of the fetal skin. Diagnosis is made following electron microscopy of the skin structure and immunohistochemical studies. Some of these disorders are listed in Table 12-6 (31,55–66). It is hoped that many of these disorders will eventually be diagnosed by DNA analysis.

Table 12-6   Fetal Skin Biopsy

Diagnosis Has Been Made with Fetal Skin Biopsy*

Epidermolysis Bullosa
  Letalis (junctional) (55)
  Dystrophica, recessive (56)
  Dystrophica, dominant (57)
  Herpetiformis (58)

Icthyosis Congenita
  Non-bullous congenital icthyosiform
    erythroderma (59)
  Lamellar icthyosis
    Bullous C.I.E. (epidermolytic
      hyperkeratosis) (60)
    Harlequin icthyosis (61)
    Sjögren-Larsson syndrome (62)

X-linked ("Anhidrotic") Ectodermal Dysplasia (63)

Oculocutaneous Albinism (64)

**Chondrodysplasia Punctata Calcificans
  (Rhizomelic) (65)**

Juvenile Neuronal Ceroid Lipofuscinosis (66)

Ehlers-Danlos Syndrome (31)

*First published report

While this list may not be complete, it is interesting that it is far shorter than the long assortments predicted for fetal skin biopsy when the technique was first developed (67).

Method

Fetal skin biopsy has been performed by two routes. Initially, fetoscopically-directed biopsy samples were obtained between 17 and 20 weeks gestation (55,61). Blind procedures, where the optical fetoscope was removed and the biopsy forceps inserted and the sample obtained without visualization, were most common initially. Only one in three of the samples obtained were actually skin: membranes, trophoblast, or myometrium were also sampled (68). An excellent recent report details the further progress in conversion to a nonfetoscopic technique by the same group of investigators—they were five times more likely to obtain useful skin samples by ultrasound-controlled techniques (69).

The part of the body for which the skin condition is commonly localized, or moreover, where an actual lesion is identified, is chosen for biopsy (33). In practice, however, it is often limited to a stationary part of the anatomy against which the fetoscope can be positioned—thorax, back, or buttocks. Four to six biopsy specimens are taken, trying to sample different sites (although, again, this distinction may be difficult, especially ultrasonically) before the fetoscope is withdrawn.

Percutaneously, skin samples have been obtained under ultrasound guidance by many groups (35,69–71). As with the previous method, the procedure is performed around 17–20 weeks gestation. A 14-gauge (35) or 16-gauge (71) angiocath with stylet is inserted into the amniotic cavity, the stylet is removed, and biopsy forceps are inserted through the angiocath. The biopsy forceps

are directed against the fetal skin, and four to six biopsies are taken.

As with all these procedures, once the instruments have been removed from the uterus, the fetus is assessed for signs of hemorrhage. With both methods, maternal sedation is used simultaneously to limit fetal activity.

Accuracy

The biopsy specimens obtained from the percutaneous route are smaller but have been considered sufficient for diagnosis (35,71). We have attempted taking skin biopsies through a 20-gauge biopsy needle under ultrasound guidance, but the size and quality of the specimen has been inadequate for tissue diagnosis. The percutaneous needle method provides more flexibility than the rigid fetoscope, but the latter offers the advantage of directly visualizing the surface aspects of the skin and, hence, possibly providing a more accurate result.

Most studies have reported perfect (100%) concordance between fetal skin biopsies and autopsy specimens following abortion of positive cases. On occasion, the diagnosis has not been confirmed specifically due to the condition of the specimen (72). In no case has a normal fetus been aborted on the basis of a false-positive prenatal skin biopsy. Ideal timing of biopsy will vary, and in at least one disorder, taking biopsies at 20 weeks resulted in the false-negative conclusion that the fetus was normal—in fact the severely-affected infant died a few hours after birth (73,74).

Most microscopic features, ultrastructural elements and antigenic markers, e.g., for immunofluorescence, are present in fetal skin by 18–20 weeks, including the hemidesmosomes critical in evaluation of epidermolysis bullosa. Complete keratinization, however, is not accomplished until after 24 weeks, and non-hair-follicle skin organelles may be absent in 26–28 week neonates (1,75), while some skin cell types are far more frequent in (normal) fetal biopsies than in newborns (76).

The disease-specific issues of proper timing in gestation, volume of sample required, immediate processing requirements, definitive diagnostic pathology, and rates of diagnostic accuracy are critical. They are also highly variable and change with each wave of new reports. Technological advances in less invasive approaches (and usually in smaller samples) have been met by a series of advances in dermatopathology (77–79), which allow for very rapid processing and a definitive diagnosis within hours. As these ultrastructural markers are evaluated further, it becomes apparent that they are expressed on nonfetal tissues (80) or in areas of normal fetal skin, remote from visible lesions. Development of biochemical or histological studies using cultured amniocytes (skin fibroblasts) has eliminated the need for direct skin biopsy. More recently, gene linkage analysis, using restriction-fragment length polymorphism techniques on standard chorion villus biopsy specimens has enabled provisional diagnosis of ectodermal dysplasia at nine weeks gestation. Fetoscopic skin biopsy, then, is subject to the same conditions as have made liver biopsy a dwindling procedure. What is necessary today may well be replaced by straightforward CVS–or amnio-based tests tomorrow.

Safety

An assessment of procedure-related problems is difficult because so few cases of sampling have been reported. Most likely, the risks are similar as for fetoscopy (2–5%) or any percutaneous needling technique (1–2%) performed in experienced hands,

supported by trends in centers that have converted from fetoscopy to percutaneous skin biopsy (67). In those fetuses that have undergone skin biopsy and progressed to term, some infants have shown a definite scar over the biopsy area, but the extent of this risk is unknown, and in most cases, scars cannot be found (31,35,81). The risk of maternal exposure to sensitizing doses of fetomaternal hemorrhage is small (82), but Rh-prophylaxis is indicated in susceptible mothers.

OTHER FETAL BIOPSIES

Given the fluctuating indications and replacement by molecular/cellular techniques for liver and skin biopsies, it is not surprising that the total of biopsies of all other fetal organs is less than 100 reported cases. Again, it is not possible to be certain that all cases done are reported, but what is certain is that the safety, efficacy, accuracy, and antenatal significance of such procedures are not established. An exception to this general statement is a small group of hereditary disorders that are serious and can be diagnosed by direct tissue evaluation but vary enough from the usual form of the disorder that current methodology using chorionic villi or cultured amniocytes is inadequate. Such exceptions include: a new mutation at the suspect locus; an extremely rare disorder where DNA probes, etc., have not yet been developed; disorders with absolutely no extrafetal expression; a "new" disorder, confined to one family without informative samples from previous affected offspring; the (heterozygous) carrier state cannot be proven and the (homozygous) affected offspring are not known in detail; or, finally, the disorder in question cannot accurately be classified. This is a list of extremely unusual exceptions.

The following is a brief mention, in order of likelihood, of the importance of these procedures to perinatal medicine.

Fetal Muscle Biopsy

Muscle biopsy specimens can be obtained from fetal thigh or calf with apparent safety, although the peroneal nerve may be injured. Fetoscopic muscle biopsy utilizing a two-instrument approach (at 16–20 weeks) obtains adequate samples that would be amenable to the detailed studies of muscle dystrophin (83).

More recently, ultrasound-directed percutaneous techniques using a Klear Kut renal biopsy gun, have excluded (84,85) or confirmed (85) the diagnosis of Duchenne's muscular dystrophy in at-risk male fetuses for whom a deletion mutation was not identifiable on DNA analysis. The procedure has theoretical risks of nerve damage, hemorrhage, infection, and so on, but in the detailed reports, no obvious problems occurred and the scars were not significant in the three survivors.

Lung Biopsies

Ultrasound recognition of abnormal lung morphology is reliable as early as 18 weeks gestation (Figure 12-4). If the lesion is uniformly lethal, specific tissue diagnosis would avert futile therapy and offer the possible route of pregnancy termination. On the other hand, if the lesion is proven to be benign or amenable to therapy, biopsy would provide a rational basis for intervention. This reasoning resulted in successful biopsy procedures following ultrasound recognition of pulmonary masses by fetoscopy (86) and by percutaneous ultrasound-directed means (87). In the latter, a 16-gauge Tuohy needle was directed toward the lateral chest, and a core of tissue

was successfully aspirated. In both cases, cystic adenomatoid malformation Type 3 (the suspected ultrasound abnormality) was confirmed, and pregnancy termination was elected.

Current ultrasound diagnosis is often more certain about this particular disorder. Further, biopsy-abnormality of one lung does not prove lethality, while apparent normality of one lung does not guarantee viability (88). Finally, as experience with lung tumors expands, it becomes apparent that such disorders are not invariably progressive and lethal; they may regress spontaneously or respond to drainage of the associated hydrothorax (89). For all these reasons, fetal lung biopsy has not seen an expanding role. It may have value, however, when no lung pathology is seen in situations where it may be likely. In prolonged rupture of membranes, for example, chest size is an imperfect means of assessing the likelihood of lethal pulmonary hypoplasia (90). With the advent of pathological criteria of more precision than simple lung weights (91), there may be a role for lung biopsy to evaluate pulmonary hypoplasia, or more likely, to demonstrate reasonably adequate parenchymal development, and provide important clinical information.

Tumor Biopsy

The majority of these reports are not tumors at all—a variety of cysts, loculated ascites, and so on have been reported under this heading, as have the lung masses above (87). Although this topic receives notice in most reviews of invasive fetal therapy, few referenced cases exist. In one report, six cystic hygromas, three sacrococcygeal teratomas, and two ovarian cysts were biopsied (70). The rationales for these procedures, done as late as 39 weeks gestation,

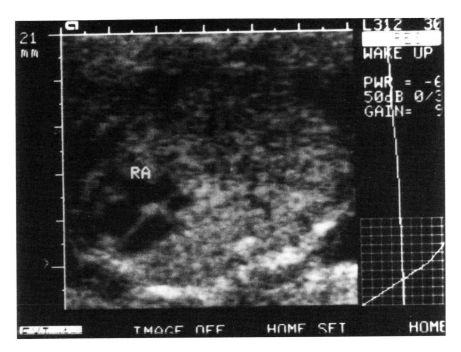

Figure 12-4 Fetal lungs almost completely replaced by (R) pulmonary hamartoma. Heart is rotated severely to (L) (counterclockwise here), with spine at 5 o'clock position in this transverse image. No hydrops was evident at 18+ weeks (this scan) but progression to hydrops was rapid, lethal by 22 weeks. (RA=right atrium.)

simply would not suffice with high-resolution ultrasonography now. In the first nine of these cases, exclusion of "possible CNS malformation" was done by aspirating liquid from the mass and finding it was not "CNS fluid." Improved ultrasound is likely to replace such procedures in many cases (92), noting, however, that (a) cystic hygroma fluid usually cultures well in the cytogenetics lab and is often the only fluid available, and (b) there may well be a significant role for reduction of large-volume masses, such as sacrococcygeal teratomas antenatally (see below). Within tumors that might be targets for sampling, color Doppler delineation of vessels often demonstrates the potential danger and persuades in favor of direct neonatal evaluation instead (Figure 12-5).

Renal Biopsy

At annual meetings of the Fetal Medicine and Surgery Society, data have been discussed, but as yet, no human cases have been published. While experimental work is ongoing as to optimal technique (93), it seems likely that the excellent correlation between antenatal ultrasound and renal pathology, fortified by the detailed pathophysiologic studies carried out by Harrison's group (94), mean that truly unknown renal pathology is unusual. The need for intrauterine contrast studies, such as infusing dye up the ureters in clear cases of posterior urethral valves (PUV) (95), is limited, but on occasion, valuable when anomalous anatomy is more complicated (Figure 12-6).

Figure 12-5A Transverse section of part of a large fetal hepatic tumor. Color flow mapping illustrated high velocity A-V malformations and nests of vessels (at arrows). Development of fetal high-output failure led to emergent delivery and neonatal (L) hepatic lobectomy, with intact survival.

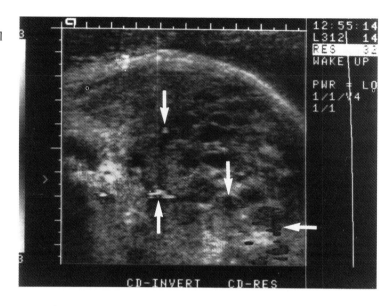

Figure 12-5B Surgical specimen shows variegated tumor occupying almost all of (L) hepatic lobe.

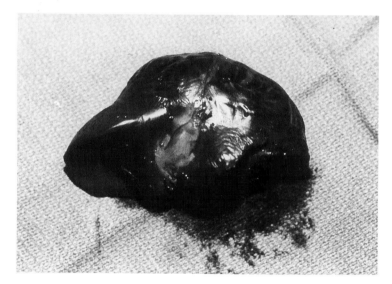

CAVITY DRAINAGE

Under this unlikely heading is a general commentary on miscellaneous procedures, reported and possible, to empty things that should not be full or to find out what is inside things we have not seen before. This significant degree of cynicism is appropriate—few of these procedure reports allow any evaluation of the postulated benefits; none feature control groups matched or not. One has no idea how many unsuccessful or even lethal versions never reach publication; follow-up reports are seldom seen.

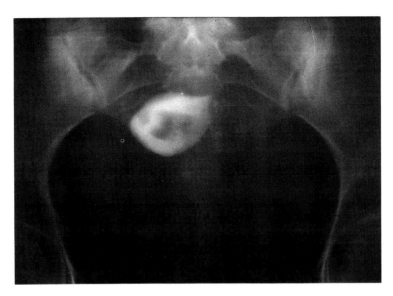

Figure 12-6 Fetal cystogram (radiogram) obtained during successful vesicoamniotic shunt placement at 28 weeks gestation.

The opposite side of the topic is that many fetal problems can be addressed if novel approaches are fortified with detailed knowledge. Invasive attempts at therapy often produce unexpected benefits. Not only does the procedure work, but also a variety of new data/samples/effects become available to allow more complete understanding of the disorder.

"There is no body cavity that cannot be reached if the needle and the courage of the operator is long enough" is an adage that applies succinctly. Some of the examples shown here, such as draining a kidney, renocentesis, have legitimate roles in very unusual circumstances, where suspicion exists of bilateral obstruction with unilateral preservation of function, for example. On the other hand, drainage of a unilateral dilated renal pelvis is probably of no therapeutic or diagnostic benefit, despite unique reports to the contrary (96,97).

It is unclear whether drainage of large fetal bronchopulmonary cysts will produce measurable benefits in reparative development of the adjacent (normal but com-

pressed) lung (Figure 12-7). In at least one case, serial drainage in fetal life allowed reexpansion of the lung, and evidence of ongoing repair confirmed histologically after neonatal lung resection (98).

These and other *cystic lung lesions*, such as cystic adenomatous hyperplasia Type I, may be amenable to drainage and might be expected to have good results compared to noncystic lung lesions, which have associated hydrothorax. In the former, the cyst is intrinsic and is compressing normal lung; decompression allows resumption of normal development (97,99,100). In the latter, drainage of hydrothorax associated with disseminated microcystic adenomatous disease will not succeed; the underlying lung is not normal and normal development is not a potential regardless of drainage (88). Pleural effusions (much more common than cystic lung lesions, often demanding urgent fetal therapy, with diverse and completely different pathophysiology) are discussed in detail elsewhere in this text. In the successful application of those principles to pulmonary tumors with hydrothorax, for

Figure 12-7 Large bronchopulmonary cyst pushes
heart to right, deforms left
lung. Cyst contents, 100 ml
straw-colored exudate,
drained on two occasions,
allowing re-expansion of
lung (98).

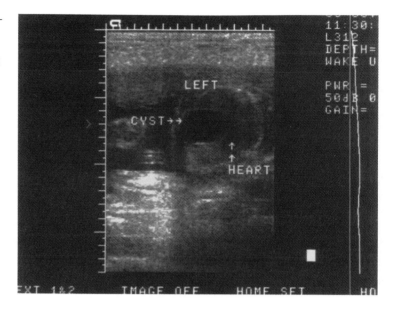

example, detailed expert ultrasonography is
key (101).

Aspiration of ovarian cysts, cystic small
bowel, mesenteric cysts, loculated or overt
ascites, cystic hygromas, and other lymphatic collections, and so on, have been
done, but most do not stand up to critical
appraisal in search of defined benefit. In
the case of large cysts of the ovary (Figure
12-8) (70,102), for example, dystocia is *not*
a problem, neonatal surgery is seldom
needed in any case (so it is not averted by
this procedure), and the cyst itself will almost always regress spontaneously in a few
weeks (103).

Massive ascites with prune belly distension and thoracic/pulmonary compromise
is usually the result of a critical, usually
lethal developmental disorder; drainage is
unnecessary, unhelpful meddling. This is
clearly in contrast to, a) the moderate ascites
related to massive pleural effusion, in which
case chest drainage solves the ascites, or, b) to
inflammatory ascites in peritonitis (Figure
12-9), in which case there is no pulmonary

compromise and no drainage is indicated,
but there may be useful diagnostic information in determining etiology, prognosis, and
newborn management, or, finally, c) tense
ascites in accelerated alloimmune erythroblastosis fetalis, which may, in fact, benefit
hemodynamic status by drainage at the time
of intravascular transfusion.

The apparently well-established role of
bladder puncture in cases of fetal urinary
tract obstruction for analysis of fetal urine is
not an open-and-shut case, as examined in
detail elsewhere. The more information that
becomes available, the less reliance is placed
on the values obtained from the admixed,
old, stagnant output of two usually differ-
ent-looking kidneys in assigning prognosis
or determining appropriateness of diversion procedures. Clearly, the trend in many
centers is now to place the shunt catheter
first, rather than ruminate (and frequently
postpone in favor of a second or third fetal
urinalysis) as to the meaning of fetal urine
values. Thus, these correlations between
understanding and application substantiate

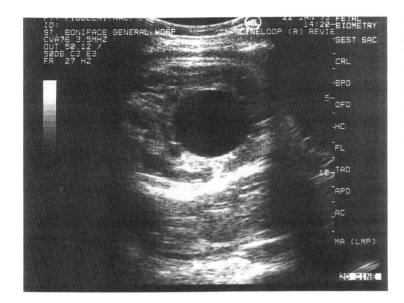

Figure 12-8 Unilateral simple ovarian cyst. Although the cyst measured up to 5 cm in cross-section, no drainage was advised. Normal vaginal delivery followed at term, neonatal surgery was not necessary, and the cyst regressed spontaneously.

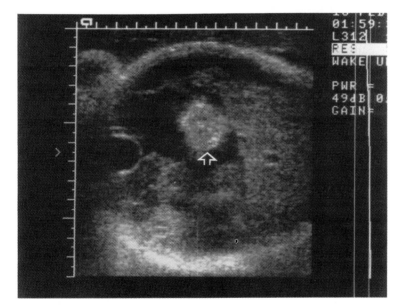

Figure 12-9 Fetal abdominal ultrasound scan showing ascites surrounding a very bright inflammatory bowel lesion (cystic fibrosis, in this case) at the hepatic flexure of the large colon (arrow). The liver is seen on the right, the bladder on the left.

the need for cautious acceptance of fetal aspiration procedures.

Technical Considerations

Detailed ultrasound examination prior and continuous high-resolution ultrasound guidance during such procedures is mandatory. Color and grey-scale Doppler may be critical in averting disaster by illustrating the vascular aspects of fetal masses. A clear and fully-explained set of objectives and an uncompromising explanation of the procedural hazards form essential components of informed consent. Laboratory capabilities, adequate personnel to assist and attend to the samples retrieved, and collaborating investigators must all be arranged in advance. Facilities for intrauterine resuscitation, emergency blood, emergency obstetric surgery, and neonatology/intensive care nursery and a highly-experienced multidisciplinary team are all prerequisites.

Once this demanding list of absolute requirements is met in entirety, aspiration procedures are usually quite straightforward. We use a 22-gauge spinal needle (or a 20-gauge needle for thoracic sampling) in most instances. Generally, an etched needle tip for sonoenhancement is not required. The same maneuvers as for PUBS, including frequent Doppler survey of vessel location, are used in establishing the precise location to be punctured. We do not use maternal antibiotic prophylaxis for such procedures. Cyst aspiration does not usually require maternal premedication or fetal paralysis, but if it seems essential for safety reasons, intravenous fetal pancuronium 0.2 mg/kg estimated fetal weight is given at the same sitting via the cord insertion. At least one route, i.e., umbilical vessels or intracardiac approach, must be clearly visualized and technically accessible to provide emergency fetal resuscitation in the event of unexpected hemorrhage, profound bradycardia, or cardiac arrest during the aspiration procedure. The procedure should not be entertained at all if such a route is prevented by oligohydramnios, fetal position, maternal/uterine anatomy, placental anomaly, and so on.

Conclusion

Incision and drainage, fetal style, is possible in almost every situation. Proof that it will be beneficial is lacking in many cases.

The explicit requirements of a clear indication and detailed informed consent should mean a very cautious and highly selective application of these techniques.

PARENTERAL ACCESS FOR FETAL TESTING

While blood sampling and several therapeutic roles for PUBS are well established, other possibilities and other approaches remain under investigation (Table 12-7). On occasion, arterial sampling may be considered advantageous, but in general, the combination of many sites of venipuncture and occasional intracardiac samples provide adequate access for obtaining blood samples. What may be required, however, is longer access. If fetal testing, e.g., response to maternal oxygen, or fetal therapy, e.g., intravenous feeding, is desired over one to two hours, placement of indwelling catheters has been carried out successfully (104). Monitoring of fetal intravenous pressure has been done with simple needles during intrauterine transfusion (105) and in the context of hepatomegaly,

Table 12-7   Fetal Functional Testing

Have Been Done:
   Indwelling catheter placement
   Intravascular pressure monitoring
   Angiography
   Intravenous pyelography, etc.
   Fluid/diuretic challenges
   Oxygen uptake test
   Fetal glucose challenge

Not Yet Reported*
   Intravenous ultrasound contrast studies
   Endocrine conversion tests
   Substrate utilization tests

congestive heart failure (106), and overt nonimmune hydrops (107).

Fetal angiography is a somewhat grandiose term for the identification of fetal vessels with a puff of saline, but in some situations, this has proven very valuable (Figure 12-10). We have used saline flushes to illustrate vessel anatomy in membranous cord insertions, placental tumors, and vasa previa. Similar observation of turbulence with rapid saline infusion may identify large-volume vein-vein anastomoses in twins. As discussed by Professor Nicolini, infusion of maternal red blood cells, i.e., adult hemoglobin, and measuring passage to the recipient, or infusing pancuronium and assessing effect, i.e., paralysis or not, on the other twin, are extensions of this vascular investigation. Note that detailed grey-scale, Doppler, and color Doppler mapping provided 99% of the data in these cases and that fetal blood sampling was the reason, not the "angiography" itself, for vessel entry. It may be, however, that the advent of contrast media (see below) will make more critical angiography (e.g., pulmonary vessels in diaphragmatic hernia, renal vessels in dysplastic disease, cerebral vessels in hydrocephalus) more practical for the fetal subject.

Fetal *dye infusion* has been performed for retrograde and intravenous pyelography and gastrointestinal patency and to outline intra-abdominal abnormal structures with immediate and follow-up X-rays (see Figure 12-6). Once again, the indications for amniography, fetal GI series, and so on may disappear with successful intrauterine application of ultrasound contrast media.

As an illustration of novel testing techniques, consider third-trimester absolute oligohydramnios. Where previous ultrasound is not available or too early, many explanations are possible. In many cases, direct testing provides valuable information:

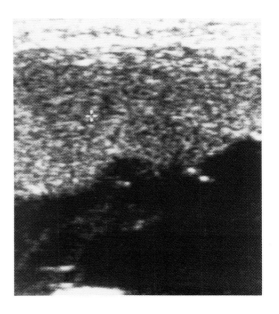

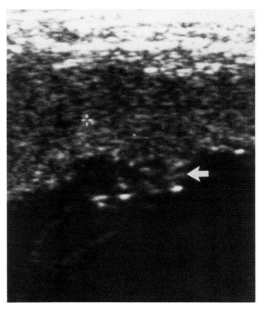

Figure 12-10 A flush of saline is invaluable to identify fetal vessels when return of blood up the needle is good, but the needle tip cannot be visualized adequately. (A) No infusion. (B) Saline infusion identifies umbilical artery on placental surface (arrow).

1. Undiagnosed rupture of membranes, i.e., normal production, external loss. Instillation of 200–300 ml amniotic fluid (see Amnioinfusion) will not only help visualization for ultrasound examination but is also enough to be certain of membrane integrity when the patient monitors drainage postprocedure.

2. Reduced production, normal swallowing, i.e., preasphyxial oliguria. In the post-term fetus, where this is most common or even in the pre-term fetus after 32 weeks, biophysical profile scoring (108) will determine fetal status accurately, and the timing and route of delivery can be ascertained. In the grossly premature or seriously growth-retarded fetus, fetal respiratory data may be desirable via cordocentesis, as discussed by Dr. Weiner in chapter five.

3. Absent production, no hypoxemia, e.g., possible Potter's syndrome. When biophysical profile score and/or fetal biochemical parameters prove hypoxemia/acidosis are absent, fetal renal function is in doubt. Intra-amniotic or fetal intraperitoneal saline may be helpful in visualization, but when fetal renal structures are apparent, the diagnosis becomes uncertain. In this unusual circumstance, we have used fetal *intravenous fluid challenges* of normal saline 50 ml over five minutes followed by furosemide intravenously on a weight-adjusted basis. In one fetus, this produced modest bladder filling and classical cesarean section was felt worthwhile (by the parents) despite estimated weight <600 gm. That 27-week infant survived intact. In two fetuses, saline/saline plus furosemide produced no response. Although both had renal structures, neither had normal neonatal renal function; one died of renal failure while the other continues on intensive dialysis (109).

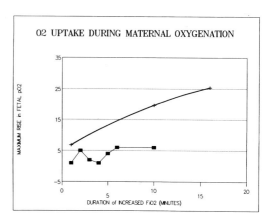

Figure 12-11 Graph of oxygen uptake during intravascular fetal transfusion of normal fetuses (curved line = regression, $p = <0.001$, $N = 35$), who show progressive pO_2 increase, contrasted with a severely growth-retarded, acidotic fetus, who showed a much reduced change in pO_2 (filled squares). Serial samples were obtained over the time indicated while mothers breathed continuous oxygen by face mask, $FiO_2 = 0.50$.

Short-term fetal responses to maternal oxygenation may offer prognostic information about intrauterine treatment of severe, immature IUGR. The fetal *oxygen uptake test* may demonstrate normal increments or varying degrees of impairment in uptake, possibly based on placental functional ability. While fetal pO_2 rises promptly when normal mothers breathe 45–55% humidified oxygen (110), in various pathologic situations, this rise may be altered (111). Clinical application of this test is just beginning, so objective evaluation is not yet possible. Examples are shown in Figure 12-11.

As suggested above, the development of *ultrasound contrast media* (112) may prove highly beneficial in the area of fetal diagnosis. The apparent enhancement of highly-vascular organs, such as liver, kidneys, and heart, and demonstrable improvement in edge-resolution between structures of similar density have not yet been duplicated in utero. These will require intravenous access and, perhaps, even regional perfusion capability to be fully exploited, but the possibilities are exciting.

As discussed in "Fetal Alimentation," fetal responses to nutrients have not been impressive to date. Fetal short-term studies in incorporation of metabolites, enzyme activation, and mobilization of substrate, and so on will undoubtedly be part of the next decade's research and therapy in IUGR. One novel way to provide long-term fetal access, and serial direct fetal monitoring, might be achieved by *intraosseous implants*. In pilot studies in fetal sheep, perfusion, medication, and telemetric biochemical monitoring have all been done via intramedullary needles (113). There is no doubt that such innovation will have profound effects on our attitudes to fetal testing. It is much more than playing with blood samples!

INTRACARDIAC PROCEDURES

A number of transcutaneous ultrasound-directed procedures feature fetal intracardiac approaches (Table 12-8). Again, none of these is a first-choice, primary procedure; the relative scarcity in the literature suggests special application based on individual expertise with these procedures. On occasion, however, these procedures prove absolutely

Table 12-8 Fetal Intracardiac Procedures

Cardiocentesis

Intracardiac Transfusion

Pericardiocentesis

Catheterization/Transvenous Pacing

Balloon Dilatation

Selective Feticide

life-saving, retrieving an otherwise potentially normal fetus from a lethal emergency. Taken in context, the role of various fetal intracardiac procedures will be clear.

Cardiocentesis

When fetal blood sampling is the only way to perform an urgently required fetal test, the heart is a potential target at earlier gestational ages (14 weeks or sooner) than the cord or individual umbilical vessels at either end. Some groups have utilized the heart as a routine secondary source for fetal blood-typing and, subsequently, for transfusion in severe maternal (historical) alloimmune hemolytic disease (114–115). Although a large series is available from only one source in the literature (116), long-term sequelae appear unusual and test results are, if anything, superior to PUBS later because the chance of amniotic fluid or maternal blood contamination are less when the needle is intrathoracic. On the other hand, overall loss rate (2–17%) among various reports, including both ultrasound-fetoscopic and ultrasound-percutaneous (114–116), is probably unsatisfactory within the context of routine testing for advanced maternal age/karyotype, low-frequency abnormalities, fetal blood typing with mild to moderate previous disease, and so on. A number of these losses have been associated with proven fetal hemophilia; this may not be a serious drawback, therefore, but the numbers of tests, subjects, and losses are all too small to speculate on a cause/effect relationship (51). Between the routine and the extreme risk, cardiac puncture has more recently been used in situations where very early testing is advantageous and by groups familiar with its use (116–119). In these reports, few, if any, fetal losses were directly attributable to the technique, evidence of yet another impact of improved ultrasound visualization.

Technique

If the fetus is active, getting the needle in the chest may be a challenge. Thus, descriptions starting with "the right ventricle is the preferred target" are probably unrealistic. Because the needle is more stable once inserted, the ventricles are preferred. We use a transthoracic approach as the transdiaphragmatic route often leads to undesirable liver/liver vessel trauma. We have been unable to needle the heart successfully when the fetus is completely spine anterior but have been successful in rolling the fetus over to an acceptable position with the needle tip. Especially for this type of problem, a 20-gauge needle is preferred over a thinner needle for improved rigidity/leverage.

Once the tip has passed into the thorax (usually the ribs will part around the needle), the angle of insertion can be adjusted to allow the needle tip to rest against the right ventricle. Insertion into the heart requires only a little force, but a sharp jabbing motion of 3–5 mm amplitude is key. If there is a large pericardial effusion, drainage prior to intracardiac insertion may be possible: in many cases, the pericardial effusion (especially if there are associated pleural effusions) makes the heart so mobile, the procedure is impossible (Figure 12-12).

If the approach and fetal status make it possible to choose, we prefer the right ventricle for sampling and/or infusion. It is generally more accessible, the heart rotates less to the left (i.e., when pressing on the right ventricle), there is some mixing prior to the infusate (either saline or blood) reaching the systemic circulation, and the cerebral circulation is bypassed via the ductus arteriosus. Once the needle is visualized against the myocardium and inserted briskly, the needle tip may or may not be visible within the chamber. Heart rates does not usually change, but the normal rolling action of the heart is abbreviated when it is punctured. Frank blood comes up without slightest resistance if position is free. A puff of saline (Figure 12-13) confirms placement. We believe fetal paralysis with pancuronium 0.2 mg/kg estimated fetal weight is

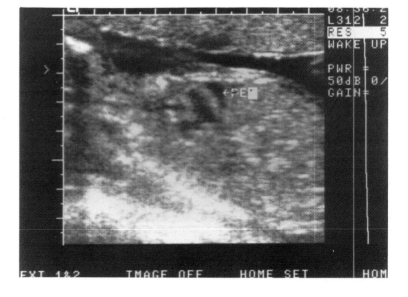

Figure 12-12 Pericardial effusion in 19-week fetus with hydropic Rh disease, fetal hemoglobin 12g/L. Fetal hemorrhage from a torn umbilical vein necessitated intracardiac transfusion, which was hampered by the effusion.

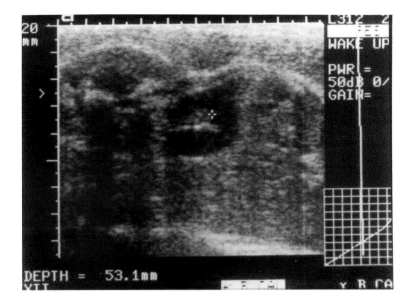

Figure 12-13 Intracardiac needle tip with saline flush (asterisk) confirming placement in right ventricle.

required for this procedure. We do not use vecuronium intracardiac. Once the necessary samples have been obtained, the needle is withdrawn swiftly along the line of insertion, with a small tug to initiate withdrawal without tenting the pericardium or stretching the perforation. If the procedure is performed for selective feticide (see pgs. 386–387) at <16 weeks, it does not appear to be essential to inject the KCl intraventricularly—anywhere in the heart appears to be effective, and even intrathoracic injection adjacent to the heart produces cardiac arrest at early gestation.

Complications

If cardiac tamponade occurs, fetal demise is usually virtually immediate. Other causes of fetal loss, e.g., infection, are likely similar to PUBS, although the small number of reports makes such an estimate difficult. Our experience is that pericardial effusions are universal, usually take several days to weeks to resolve completely but are not functionally significant following cardiac

puncture. Since our use of this procedure for fetal blood sampling is restricted to urgent/critical situations, the parents are aware preprocedure of our inability to reverse lethal complications; thus, postprocedure monitoring is brief (<15 minutes).

Intracardiac Transfusion (ICT)

We use ICT as a backup procedure for exsanguinating complications of intravascular transfusion, as a primary approach to the very early hydropic fetus where umbilical vessels are <2 mm in cross-sectional diameter, and as third alternative to transfusing the 17–20 week nonhydropic alloimmunized fetus. In the majority, however, ICT has been an emergency procedure meant to rescue a fetus in a terminal situation (120–121). This is described in detail in the chapter on alloimmune hemolytic disease, but this situation also applies to hemorrhagic complications of fetal investigation for alloimmune thrombocytopenia, qualitative (familial) platelet disorders, hemophilia, non-immune hydrops and even severe early IUGR, all of which may be associated with acute fetal shock.

Of course, intracardiac procedures should be included in the repertoire of teams doing early PUBS for the types of disorders suggested above. In addition to having the equipment, personnel, and laboratory capabilities available, checking that the fetal position is potentially accessible is a useful safeguard. Although it is fairly easy to prod the active fetus around into an acceptable position, if the fetus in shock is spine anterior, it is often impossible to attain an approach to the heart by any means.

Fetal Heart Disease

Fetal viral infection causing pericarditis and serious pericardial effusions has been considered for drainage. In rare cases, this may be a life-threatening situation for the fetus, as judged by deficient myocardial action, markedly reduced cardiac output, and altered peripheral perfusion, and confirmed by absent fetal behavior. Reported cases of successful fetal pericardiocentesis do not all provide a level of information to be clear that the procedure was absolutely necessary or to evaluate the risks or benefits of this technique. In alloimmune or nonimmune hydrops with large pericardial effusions, successful management does not require any direct treatment or drainage. Similarly, medical fetal treatment, anti-inflammatory agents including corticosteroids, seems a more likely first-line approach for viral causes, e.g., Coxsackie B, or cytomegalovirus. An expanding pericardial effusion and apparently dramatic flow deterioration (in the absence of hydrops) indicated high risk for cardiac tamponade in a 34-week fetus with a large intrapericardial teratoma; in this case, pericardiocentesis may well have been life-saving and produced a three-week remission leading to safe, term delivery (122).

The fetal heart can be paced by maternal percutaneous fetal transthoracic placement of wire leads (123), but the ultimate benefits of such a procedure are yet to be shown. While restoring an effective baseline heart rate, i.e., >60, in cases of complete heart block is associated with restoration of normal-range cardiac output, reversal of hydrops or maintenance in utero for a significant period to allow for improved maturity have not been demonstrated. Allan has suggested that transvascular pacing wires might be threaded up the umbilical vein, eliminating major interference by the fetus (124). This approach presumes the wires could be made to negotiate the intrahepatic curves of the umbilical vein and that such wires would not be thrombogenic. The umbilical artery might be usable (because there are two), but, again, the radical angles of the skin insertion/abdominal wall and abdominal wall/paravesicular turns of these vessels would probably defeat transit all the way to the heart. One potential approach would be the transthoracic placement of direct ventricular pacing wires with anchoring of the wires by endoscopic fetal skin ligatures.

Before the reader concludes that this is all science fiction, consider the possibility of intrauterine surgery for congenital heart disease. Balloon dilatation of deficient aortic valve orifices has been effective in the pediatric and neonatal management of critical aortic stenosis, leading to its application in the fetus (125). The introducing needle was advanced percutaneously through the fetal chest wall, entering the fetal heart at the apex, lying in the left ventricle. A guide wire was passed to demonstrate the angle and direction required to cross the aortic valve, then the balloon catheter itself was positioned in the valve orifice. Serial inflations of the balloon within the aortic valve orifice were associated with reduced peak velocities in aortic flow, indirect proof of therapeutic success in increasing valvular cross-sectional area and reducing the pressure gradient across the valve.

There are many issues raised by this adventure, but the primary point is that surgical therapeutic procedures that are effective in neonates may very well have a role in fetal treatment of the same lesions. The perfect incubator, the uteroplacental unit, provides ideal critical care support; the fetus, lacking the massive difficulties of his air-breathing neonatal counterpart, is in a sense the perfect cardiovascular patient; the opportunity to intervene at an earlier point in a group of diseases that are developmental in nature makes this combination all the more appealing. Undoubtedly, there will be many more examples of such very invasive fetal therapy.

A balancing consideration, however, suggests a more rigorous, scientific, pathophysiologic approach. Even in the infant in whom the balloon dilatation procedure was successful, the underlying left ventricular deficiencies proved lethal. It is likely that a clearer understanding of the origins of fetal cardiac defects is required before proper selection of cases and effective application of procedures is possible.

AMNIOINFUSION

Amnioinfusion is used for prenatal diagnosis and therapy in severe oligohydramnios presenting at early gestation, or later, when labor is established, to prevent and reduce the incidence of variable decelerations and meconium aspiration syndrome. Some of the procedures have not been fully evaluated, and so, further evidence, particularly from controlled randomized trials, is re-

quired to confirm their efficacy. In this discussion, most emphasis will be placed on the antenatal procedures.

PRENATAL AMNIOINFUSION

Diagnostic

Severe oligohydramnios, particularly in the second trimester, is associated with poor pregnancy outcome. The finding may be secondary to renal agenesis or dysplasia, posterior urethral valves, severe IUGR and, occasionally, early rupture of membranes. The underlying cause needs to be identified to enable appropriate management and counselling to ensue, and yet, an ultrasound diagnosis is limited or almost impossible with the absence of the amniotic acoustic window and the curled-up fetal position. Infusion of approximately 200 ml transabdominally will facilitate visualization of the fetus enough to make a more definitive assessment (126). Indigo carmine can be added to the infusate to help diagnose early PROM as the underlying cause of the oligohydramnios (126,127), although recently, this dye has been associated with intestinal atresia syndromes (128,129). In all reported studies, the original diagnoses were altered with improved visualization of the fetus.

Therapeutic

Pulmonary Hypoplasia

If no lethal congenital abnormalities are associated with severe oligohydramnios presenting before 24 weeks gestation, neonatal death almost inevitably occurs secondary to pulmonary hypoplasia. Despite the association of early oligohydramnios and pulmonary hypoplasia, the underlying pathophysiology of abnormal lung development is unknown. Compression limiting growth is unlikely because amniotic pressures are low in oligohydramnios (130). However, leakage of lung fluid towards the amniotic cavity, secondary to this reversal of pressures, may be contributory. It has been suggested that by maintaining normal amniotic fluid volume artificially, pulmonary hypoplasia may be prevented (130). Two uncontrolled studies using repeated amnioinfusion during the second trimester in cases of severe oligohydramnios with an overtly normal fetus have been reported. In one, only three of nine neonates survived, but of the six perinatal deaths, five showed a normal lung/body weight ratio (127). In the other, seven of nine neonates survived, and none of these demonstrated compression abnormalities (131). Thus, this procedure may have potential to prevent pulmonary hypoplasia associated with oligohydramnios, but in view of the small numbers involved in these uncontrolled studies, further evidence is required. Furthermore, multiple amnioinfusions commencing at 16 weeks gestation did not prevent pulmonary hypoplasia in a case of Potter's syndrome recently reported in the lay press (132).

Chorioamnionitis

Chorioamnionitis is a risk for women with PROM. In such cases, antibiotics have been added to a saline infusion performed transcervically with a cervical plug to prevent fluid leakage (133). Fluid levels were apparently maintained, but the evaluation of outcome is difficult due to the absence of controls. Antibiotic levels are increased in the amniotic cavity following direct administration compared to maternal oral or intravenous routes (134), but an improved perinatal outcome would need to be shown before this intervention is accepted.

Procedure (Only the transabdominal route is described) (Figure 12-14)

Following cleaning of the abdomen, local anesthetic is injected into the skin overlying a small pocket of amniotic fluid identified on ultrasound scan. If the latter is not identifiable, a potential pool is chosen, frequently around the fetal limbs or directly among loops of umbilical cord, which is continuously identified using Doppler and color Doppler ultrasound. A 22- or 20-gauge needle is inserted through the uterus, just immediately into the uterine cavity, gently, under ultrasound guidance. If no amniotic fluid or fetal blood can be aspirated, 1–2 ml of 0.9% NaCl is injected to test resistance and fluid dispersion. If this test dose is satisfactory (or more likely, not visible), a further 5–10 ml of cold saline is given as a push—the turbulence is visible on the screen, and the cold fluid on the fetus's skin usually produces a definite startle. If acceptable, warmed saline is infused to a level that allows adequate visualization on ultrasound. Indigo carmine (5 ml, diluted 1:20) can be added to the saline before infusing at a rate of 25–50 ml/min with a 50-ml syringe and plastic tubing. Amniotic fluid measurements before and after the procedure may be helpful to avoid excessive intrauterine pressures. A sanitary pad, which has been in place during the procedure, is checked for evidence of ruptured membranes and the patient is requested to document vaginal leakage of dye-stained fluid subsequently. If fetal karyotypic determination is required, PUBS or amniocentesis may be performed following amnioinfusion. The former can be performed immediately if cord access is available, whereas amniocentesis must be performed one to two days later, when mixing of fetal cells has occurred. For repeated amnioinfusion, the procedure is

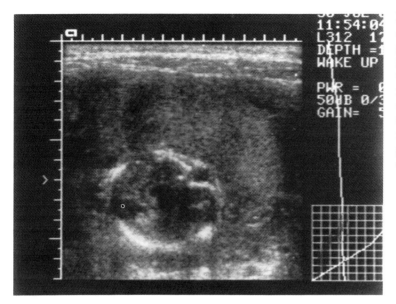

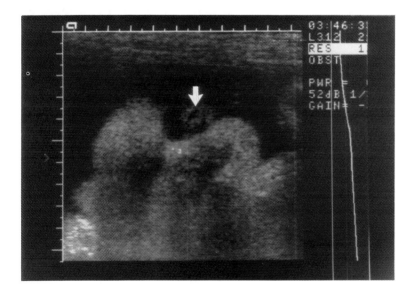

Figure 12-14 (A) Severe oligohydramnios at 27 weeks gestation. Amnio infusion of 250 ml warmed saline via ultrasound-guided 20-gauge needle allowed detailed fetal examination, demonstrating unilateral (L) cryptophthalmos (note prominent right globe, arrow) and midline facial cleft in (B).

similar, but no indigo carmine is added. Prophylactic antibiotics are advised.

Complications

Risks of the procedure include chorioamnionitis, membrane rupture, and preterm labor. In the largest series reviewed, chorioamnionitis occurred in only 2% of 61 cases (127). Whether this low incidence is explained by the use of antibiotic prophylaxis is unknown. Rupture of the membranes appears to be a small risk; most cases are considered to be diagnosed by the infusion rather than caused by it. Amnioinfusion does not appear to precipitate preterm labor if intrauterine pressure is not increased excessively.

INTRAPARTUM AMNIOINFUSION

Variable Decelerations

Repetitive decelerations are secondary to compression of the umbilical cord, placenta, and fetal head during labor and are increased with oligohydramnios. The decelerations, if persistent, can lead to fetal acidosis and increased operative delivery for presumed fetal distress. The aim of amnioinfusion is to prevent this scenario, especially when the traditional maneuvers of changing maternal position and giving maternal oxygen fail. Repetitive decelerations can be treated by amnioinfusion and may result in fewer cesarean sections performed for fetal distress (135,136). They have been shown to be prevented in cases of PROM associated with oligohydramnios (137), but less so with oligohydramnios associated with IUGR in term or post-term pregnancies (138). The reasons for these discrepancies are not clear. Although in most of the published trials, the umbilical pH at delivery is higher in the amnioinfusion group compared to controls, both of the levels are in the normal range. In addition, the criteria for operative intervention, i.e., the diagnosis of fetal distress, are not always described. Therefore, the clinical significance of the procedure is unclear, and the concern arises that the procedure may relieve "physician distress" predominantly. Therapeutic amnioinfusion may be useful for correcting abrupt fetal heart changes associated with a sudden loss of fluid at membrane rupture (139).

Meconium

Meconium aspiration syndrome, associated with thick, tenacious meconium, occurs in approximately two percent of deliveries, with an associated 25% perinatal mortality (140). Despite vigorous suctioning of the newborn nose and pharynx during delivery, the incidence of the syndrome has not changed, presumably because deep inhalation of meconium occurs prior to birth (141). In cases of thick meconium with no documented fetal distress, intrauterine infusion of up to 1000 ml of 0.9% saline can prevent fetal acidosis (142) and decrease meconium below the cords and the incidence of neonatal meconium aspiration syndrome (142–143). This procedure appears to have potential value and, therefore, requires further evaluation.

Procedure

Following identification of pregnancies with oligohydramnios associated with repetitive decelerations or thick meconium staining of the amniotic fluid in early labor, an intrauterine pressure catheter is introduced into the amniotic cavity. Approximately 200 ml (up to 1000 ml with meconium) is infused at 20–25 ml/min through the catheter. If a slower infusion rate is used (10–15 ml/hr), it is unnecessary to warm the saline (135). Some operators suggest that a second intrauterine pressure monitor be inserted to allow continuous pressure readings to be made simultaneously during the procedure to identify uterine hypertonus (144). A single or continuous infusion may be performed to increase amniotic fluid levels into the normal range (measured by ultrasound) (145), or six hourly repeat infusions have been described for the management of thick meconium (143).

Complications

Although cord prolapse has been listed as a potential complication of amnioinfusion, no increased incidence has been reported in the small series published so far. Hypertonus should not occur if uterine pressures do not increase excessively (144). Chorioamnionitis has not been described as a problem. A case of maternal respiratory failure has been reported in association with amnioinfusion in labor, but a cause and effect relationship has not been established (146). Overall, the procedure appears to be safe as long as the precautions of accurate fluid balance, fetal heart rate, and uterine pressure monitoring are made.

THERAPEUTIC REDUCTION AMNIOCENTESIS

Hydramnios is a complication of pregnancy associated with a poor perinatal outcome (147). Some of the loss can be attributed to the underlying pathology, such as congenital malformations, neural tube defects, tracheoesophageal fistulae, diaphragmatic hernia, duodenal atresia, but a significant component is secondary to preterm labor with death resulting from immaturity. A list of disorders associated with hydramnios is shown in Table 12-9.

With improved diabetic management and the introduction of Rh prophylaxis using, hydramnios associated with these conditions is now rare. Therefore, the poor perinatal outcome associated with twin pregnancies and hydramnios has become more prominent, and methods for improved management are sought. More detailed discussion in specific reference to multiple gestation is found in chapter 11.

Table 12-9 Conditions Associated with Hydramnios

Idiopathic

Diabetes Mellitus

RBC Isoimmunization

Multiple Pregnancy
Twin to twin transfusion

Congenital Abnormalities
CNS   Renal
Obstructive gastrointestinal
Respiratory   Skeletal
Congenital infections

Nonimmune Hydrops

Placental Chorioangiomas

Definition

Hydramnios is defined on ultrasound as a vertical fluid pocket measurement of >8 cm. Strict guidelines have not yet been adopted, but maximum pockets of 8–12 cm may be classified as mild, 12–18 cm as moderate, and >18 cm as severe (gross) hydramnios. Further ultrasound criteria for hydramnios (as opposed to one "generous" pocket) are: fetus floating freely (not touching anterior uterine wall), uterine contour round (as opposed to flattened oval), and placenta attenuated, with a tense maternal abdomen (Figure 12-15).

In the stuck twin syndrome, one twin is visualized immediately adjacent to the uterine wall within a sac devoid of amniotic fluid. The dividing membrane between the two sacs is adherent to this fetus (the smaller donor), while the other fetus (the larger recipient) has associated hydramnios secondary to increased urine output from the high output cardiovascular state (148), and may be hydropic secondary to cardiac

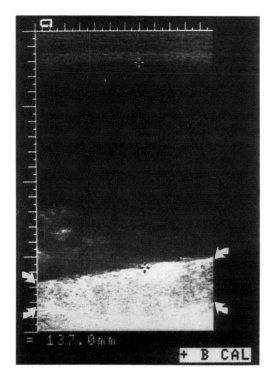

Figure 12-15   Hydramnios of moderately severe extent, with maximum vertical dimension of 13.7 cm shown here. The fetus lies completely out of the frame and the posterior placenta is seriously attenuated (arrows).

failure (Figure 12-16). Increased intrauterine pressure makes the placenta of the stuck twin thin and compressed. Hydramnios in these situations is often in the severe range, with associated uterine distension, irritability, advanced cervical effacement, and maternal symptoms.

Including "stuck twin," the incidence of the hydramnios is 0.2–1.6% of all pregnancies (149). Traditionally, the condition has been divided by the speed of onset (acute or chronic), with the former occurring in two percent of all cases (150). Acute hydramnios usually develops during the second trimester and most commonly is associated with twin to twin transfusion syndrome.

Physiological Studies

Amniotic pressure normally increases with increasing gestational age but is not dependent on parity or multiple pregnancy (151). Women with hydramnios, particularly with a vertical pool measurement of ≥ 15 cm, exhibit dramatically increased amniotic pressures over normal levels (152). Preterm labor almost invariably occurs in these cases of uterine overdistension concurrent with maternal distress from respiratory and cardiovascular embarrassment. Removal of a small amount of fluid transabdominally rapidly reduces the amniotic pressure. It has been suggested that only small amounts of fluid need to be removed to normalize amniotic pressure and, thus, decrease the tendency towards preterm labor (152).

Management

When a diagnosis of hydramnios is confirmed by ultrasound, detailed fetal examination must be done to exclude the many anomalies that may be associated. These include general conditions, such as CNS, ventral wall, and multiple anomalies, and specific defects affecting swallowing, facial clefts, oropharyngeal masses, tracheoesophageal fistulas, and intestinal atresias at all levels, and the urinary tract. Provided diagnosis is normal, specific therapy is directed towards identified underlying causes, such as diabetes mellitus or Rhesus isoimmunization. Alternatively, in cases where no antenatal correction of the underlying pathophysiology is available and yet further fetal maturity is essential for survival, e.g., congenital malformations requiring postnatal corrective surgery, methods to reduce amniotic fluid volume and pressure have been used. These include reduction amniocentesis (153), indomethacin therapy

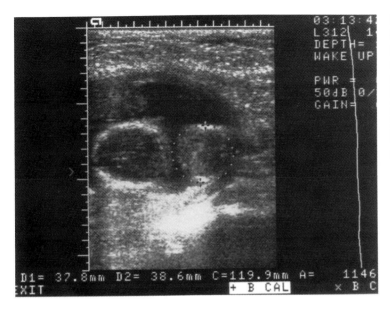

Figure 12-16 "Stuck" twin. Size difference between the larger (L) twin and his small (R) brother is readily apparent. No membrane is seen on this scan because all the fluid visible belongs to (L), the membrane being tightly bound against twin (R).

(154,155), applied to both single and multiple gestations, and under preliminary evaluation, laser coagulation of the placental circulation (156), which is exclusive to twin gestation at this point.

Clinical Reports

Reduction amniocentesis was first described in 1933 (157), and subsequently, isolated reports have shown some success for the technique to prevent preterm labor and improve perinatal survival (153,158–161). Nevertheless, there are many who consider the procedure to be limited because of the rapid reaccumulation of fluid, which ultimately makes any gain in gestational age small (162). Initially, a Drew-Smythe catheter was recommended to remove the amniotic fluid (163), but this soon was discouraged as preterm labor ensued (153). Subsequently, the procedure has been performed transabdominally. Controversy exists as to whether a large volume of fluid should be removed (decompression amniocentesis) or a smaller volume at greater fre-

quency. Two case reports describe the outcome of two or more successive pregnancies requiring reduction amniocentesis in a single woman. These showed an improved outcome in the pregnancies in which small volumes of fluid were removed compared to those in which decompression amniocentesis was performed (153,164). Recent series have shown that with aggressive reduction amniocentesis, perinatal survival can be greater than 70% (165,166). Nevertheless, a concurrent series, in which a similar technique was used, showed only a 37% perinatal survival rate (167). Different selection of cases may account for these differences.

Several case reports have described "normalization" of amniotic fluid levels in both sacs subsequent to reduction amniocentesis in twins, and occasionally, the situation has stabilized to enable no further intervention until mid-late third trimester delivery (161). In some situations, this is clearly the result of associated improvement of the stuck twin, with resumption of significant urine production. In other cases, it is likely that perforation of both sacs occurs because the membranes of the stuck twin are wrapped against the uterine wall. The fluid of the donor twin may then move freely from one sac to the other.

Technical Aspects

Following cleaning of the skin, an 18–20 gauge spinal needle is inserted into the amniotic sac of the twin with hydramnios at a site localized by ultrasound. For decompression amniocentesis, fluid is withdrawn until the amniotic fluid pool is < 8 cm on ultrasound scan. The speed at which the fluid should be withdrawn has not been determined. One recent study stated that 6.5 liters were removed in two hours (167), whereas another described "rapid removal" of volumes up to five liters (165). Others still consider that only small volumes need to be removed to achieve the desired decrease in amniotic pressure (152). In view of the high risks of rupture of membranes and/or membrane dissection, it may be wise to use insertion sites as far apart as possible for subsequent punctures. Reducing needle manipulation by attachment of tubing, stopcocks, or even surgical suction devices may also prevent membrane tearing. Most of the recent studies did not use prophylactic tocolytic cover but introduced it with any sign of preterm labor. Frequent ultrasound assessment, at least twice weekly, is then required to assess the fetal state(s). Fluid reaccumulation, enough to precipitate preterm labor or compromise the donor twin, would indicate the need for a repeat amniocentesis.

Problems and Complications

Expectant management of acute twin to twin transfusion syndrome has shown almost a 100% perinatal mortality (168),

and in addition, causes some risk to maternal status, including cardiac decompensation and obstructive renal failure (168–169). Reduction amniocentesis does entail some risks, including precipitation of preterm labor or PROM, but as preterm delivery is almost inevitable with no intervention, little is to be lost. Furthermore, maternal discomfort and respiratory embarrassment is relieved. Repeated procedures through the same areas often lead to progressive degrees of membrane stripping from the anterior wall of the uterus. In twin gestations, this can lead to the membranes of both sacs as well as one or both cords becoming completely entangled as shown in Figure 12-17. Placental abruption has been stated as a risk following rapid decompression of the uterus but this has mainly been reported with membrane rupture in labor or following the delivery of a first twin.

The main concern of using reduction amniocentesis for early therapy (18–24 weeks) in the stuck twin syndrome is that delivery may be delayed three to four weeks to allow fetal survival but at the cost of high perinatal morbidity. Data on singleton pregnancies treated by reduction amniocentesis is generally hampered by lack of ultrasound data or by convincing evidence that net therapeutic benefit is clear. In general, severe hydramnios with a normal single fetus occurs at a reasonably mature gestation, so one or two procedures, at most, are occasionally required.

Conclusions

Depending on the pathophysiology of the placental bed vascular communications, reduction amniocentesis may allow stabilization of the twin-twin transfusion process enough to enable both twins to gain maturity in a less compromised intrauterine

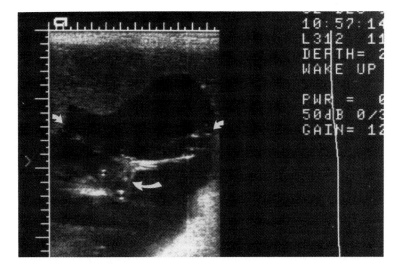

Figure 12-17 Serial amniocentesis for severe twin-twin transfusion syndrome led to this complication. The membranes (diamnionic, monochorionic) are separated from each other and both cords are entangled in the two sets of amnion, at large arrow. The two cord insertions (small arrows) are drawn toward the central knot, buckling the placentas.

environment. Any advantage is an improvement over the 100% perinatal mortality of expectant management alone. A large multicenter randomized trial would be required to address the technical questions of how much and how quickly the fluid should be removed. Further study of these techniques in other less critical situations is necessary to establish their value.

A complete discussion of indomethacin and hydramnios is not appropriate here, but this is a clear example of maternal medication given for its uterine and fetal effects. As opposed to its role as a tocolytic in premature labor, the role of indomethacin in severe hydramnios is based on its ability to reduce fetal and blood flow and, therefore, amniotic fluid production. Limitations in both data and timing are similar to reduction amniocentesis, in singleton pregnancies.

With regard to indomethacin and twins, the original work was primarily done in unusual cases where both sacs had excessive amniotic fluid (Figure 12-18) (154), a situation not at all analogous to the imbalance of twin-twin transfusion. It may well be that the apparent safety demonstrated with

that use of indomethacin is not implicit in a situation where rapid shifts in flow, preexisting hypertension, anemia, hyperviscosity, and hypersensitive vascular systems may be profoundly affected by prostaglandin inhibition.

LASER COAGULATION OF THE PLACENTAL CIRCULATION

In cases of circulatory imbalance between twins, or potentially between a single fetus and a placental tumor, division of vessels within and on the surface of the placenta to interrupt communication and correct the imbalance, would theoretically address the underlying pathophysiology of this condition. The technique, using fetoscopically directed laser, was first described in experimental situations using sheep (170) and rhesus monkey models (170–171). The latter has a hemochorial placenta, with some similarities to the human. The placenta in these animals is discoidal, even in singleton pregnancies, with communicating vessels between the discs. In eight of 12 procedures, division of the com-

Figure 12-18 Twins with premature labor (cervix 4 cm dilated, 90% effaced) with bilateral hydramnios. Indomethacin 200 ml daily, tapered to 100 mg daily, given over four weeks, extended this pregnancy from 27 to nearly 32 weeks. During therapy, the cervix lengthened and closed (60% effaced and closed after 10 days). [Reprinted with permission of Lange, Harman, and Ash 1989 (154)]

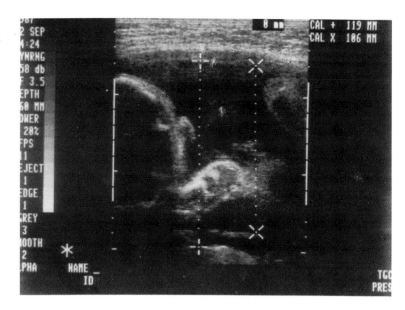

municating vessels resulted in the second disc being small and underdeveloped at the time of delivery, with no evidence of extensive maternal tissue damage around the area of laser coagulation.

In 1990, this group reported three cases of twin to twin transfusion in women who underwent the procedure at 18–23 weeks gestation (155). The pregnancies continued for six–11.5 weeks, and four of six fetuses were born alive and survived. One procedure was complicated by a placental vessel perforation and was discontinued following loss of visualization. No maternal injuries occurred and no infants were shown to have laser-induced eye damage. Placental examination showed small nodules at the laser impact site. Recently, this group has reported their results in a further 22 pregnancies (172). In 19 cases, laser coagulation was performed in addition to concurrent amniotic fluid reduction. Furthermore, in all cases, the women were administered indomethacin for three days (pre- and postlaser). Of those delivered (18/19), 56% of the twins have survived, and 78% of the women have at least one survivor.

Technique (155)

The technique involves fetoscopically-directed neodymium-yttrium-aluminium-garnet (Nd-YAG) laser coagulation to the placental vessels considered to underlie the pathology. The Nd-YAG laser is used because it functions through a fluid medium, and it is an efficient coagulator (173). The gestational age should be between 18–28 weeks, the placenta posterior, and hydramnios present in one sac.

With ultrasound guidance, an abdominal incision is made into the abdomen overlying the placental insertion of the cord of the recipient fetus. A stab wound is made into the uterus and the fetoscope is inserted. A longer rigid fetoscope is required because of the distance through a hydramniotic sac to a posterior placenta. The laser fiber is then passed through a sideport of the fetoscope.

Once the cord insertion of the recipient is identified, vessels that course over the placental surface towards the other sac are followed. The designated vessels are coagulated over one cm for two to three seconds, with the fiber held at a 0.5–1 cm distance from the site. When all the vessels have been coagulated, the fetoscope is removed and the incisions are sutured. The procedure is covered by indomethacin for three days (200mg daily).

Complications

The main problem limiting the procedure has been blood contamination of the amniotic fluid secondary to the hysterotomy incision. No maternal or fetal injuries, specifically laser damage to the fetal eye, have been reported. In one of the animal experiments, placental abruption occurred immediately following insertion of the fetoscope, a risk with any overdistended uterus.

Conclusions

This intervention seems an innovative, if very invasive, method for correcting the underlying pathophysiology of twin to twin transfusion syndrome. Nevertheless, reduction amniocentesis and indomethacin were used concurrently in most cases, and therefore, both of these interventions themselves may have contributed significantly to the outcome. Furthermore, it is probably simplistic to expect the vascular communications to be solely on the surface of the placenta, and, therefore, amenable to therapy. This procedure awaits evaluation from other groups in controlled trials, but it appears to have promise in certain situations. If its efficacy is accepted, the procedure will be confined to specialist centers that may make transfer of acute cases difficult.

DIRECT FETAL ALIMENTATION

Therapy for IUGR has always been a primary focus of obstetrics/perinatology. In the past decade, not only has a wealth of information become available by direct fetal testing (174), but access to the fetal compartment has raised the possibility of bypassing the placenta altogether and providing essential nutrients directly to the fetus (175–177).

Initial therapeutic attempts utilized access to the amniotic cavity. When amino acid solutions, sugars, or proteins are infused into the amniotic fluid, normal fetal swallowing results in digestion and incorporation of the infused nutrients. Amino acid clearance likely includes nonenteric clearance as well, with transit across membranes into the umbilical cord and into the placenta. A number of attempts have been made to supplement growth-retarded fetuses, especially using essential amino acids, but those experimental procedures have a large number of drawbacks (178). An excellent review of past experience with intra-amniotic fetal feeding is found in Harding and Charlton, 1989 (179), while recent research has centered on the animal model (180–181).

Clinical attempts to feed growth-retarded fetuses in this fashion have been reported. Amino acid solutions were infused intra-amniotically every one to three days (50 ml) in cases with clinical and ultrasound evidence of deficient growth. In 10 cases reported (182), growth was demonstrated in six of 11 fetuses once the infusions were begun. While such regimes have been applied by other groups, no data on fetal impact (as opposed to estriol excretion or birthweight) were reported. A single case of direct fetal feeding (183) has apparently not been duplicated. In that case, an indwelling intraperitoneal fetal catheter was connected to an extrauterine reservoir in the maternal abdominal wall. Continuous "TPN" (amino acids and vitamins) were administered until the membranes ruptured after nine days, at 34½ weeks gestation. Fetal growth over the interval was not shown. Birthweight was >2.0 kg.

There are many problems with these early studies. All relied on clinical evidence and biparietal diameter measurements, both quite inadequate as uncorroborated indices of growth. The duration of study was too short to measure growth reliably, even in a normally-growing group, let alone fetuses growing at low rates, in most of the cases. There are not enough cases; there are no controls; most of the cases would be resolved uneventfully by observation and/or delivery, with modern neonatal care; and the proposed mechanism of action is limited by knowledge that fetal swallowing is an activity that diminishes as compromise becomes more apparent and accounts for only 10–15% of fetal nutrition in normal circumstances (184).

Finally, since the evidence is fragile that fetal growth is likely to respond to increased substrate at any rate, the apparent danger of such regimes is worrisome. In fetuses who may actually have chosen not to grow because of placental, uterine, or extrauterine forces, obligating them to process energy-consuming and waste-producing substrate may be harmful (178). Among the fetal functional tests noted earlier (Table 12-7) was the glucose challenge evaluated by Nicolini (185). In growth-retarded fetuses, supplementary glucose was an obligation, not a gift: pH dropped as anaerobic metabolism produced lacticacidemia.

The ongoing research in oxygen therapy (186,187), bed-rest regimes, maternal nutritional supplement, and even placentotrophic hormones (188) may produce signifi-

cant benefit in specific subgroups—such studies are in development. A few infants may have improved outcome from direct nutritional therapy, but this approach is strictly experimental at the moment. Much more data with observations on normal fetuses as well as the nutritionally-deprived are essential.

FETAL STEM CELL TRANSPLANTS

A broad array of hereditable conditions has been successfully treated by bone marrow transplantation. These include *erythrocyte disorders*, such as β-thalassemia, or sickle cell disease, *lymphocyte disorders*, such as the multiple forms of severe combined immunododeficiency syndrome, *granulocyte defects*, such as Chediak-Higashi syndrome, *reticuloendothelial metabolic disorders*—the *mucopolysaccharidoses*, e.g., Maroteaux-Lamy, arylsulfatase-β deficiency and the *mucolipidoses*, e.g., metachromatic leukodystrophy, arylsulfatase-A deficiency and *abnormal osteoclast function*, seen in infantile malignant osteopetrosis (189). Successful treatment of these disorders in the postnatal period has led many groups to application of the theory and practicalities of hematopoietic stem cell transplants to the fetal patient (189–192).

Various animal models have been used to show that mutant forms or specifically-injured offspring can be redeemed by in utero stem cell therapy. Using hematopoietic stem cell (HSC) transplants at varying (but always early) gestations, researchers have shown engraftment by donor HSC in mice (193), sheep (194), monkeys (193,195,196), and in the laboratory, using human fetal liver cells to generate immunocompetent lymphocytes (197,198).

At the same time, much recent research has defined the origins and fetal development of the immune system (199–204). This research has clearly detailed a progression of maturation and expressivity (as monoclonal antibody-recognized surface markers) throughout fetal life (199,200). There are clear reasons why fetal liver HSC may be advantageous as donor tissue in virtually all such situations. (Fetal liver HSC are T-cell free, the liver containing T-lymphocyte precursors that are immunologically "naive," whereas adult marrow HSC must be processed to remove the "educated" lymphocyte component to avert rejection of the graft or the disastrous consequences of graft-versus-host disease.) Further, detailed fetal studies have shown that development of lymphocytes capable of graft-versus-host responses (post-thymic T-lymphocytes) occurs at 18–20 weeks, as detectable in fetal liver. Progressive steps in lymphocyte responsiveness to mitogens, or antigenic stimuli, begin much earlier, so the eight to 10 week fetus seems to be the best source of the least immunocompetent HSC. As can be seen from Table 12-10 (193,205–210), the only survivors of fetal engraftment to date have been fetal liver HSC recipients. With release of the NIH proscription on fetal tissue research in 1993, this area is certain to develop even more rapidly.

Two further areas are of specific concern to the fetal patient, i.e., HSC recipient. Firstly, the diagnosis must be made. This is primarily based on a history of a previously affected sibling, although carrier states are clear indicators for several of these disorders. Specific markers (or their abnormal absence) must be reliably available for evaluation. For example, while many markers, e.g., CD7, HLA ABC and DR antigens, are expressed on HSC in fetal livers by eight to 10 weeks, others, e.g., IgE receptors on B-lymphocytes, or *many* of the T-cell receptors, are not recognized in circulating fetal lymphocytes until 20–22 weeks (198,200). Prenatal diagnosis of these disorders is fa-

cilitated by careful analysis of affected individuals in the family and is now possible for virtually all of this group of disorders. Against a background of enhanced knowledge about normal fetuses at varying gestations (211,212), precise diagnosis is usually available from fetal blood at 18–20 weeks gestation.

Once the diagnosis is made with certainty, technical factors are the second area of concern. Reference to Table 12-10 suggests there are too few human cases upon which to base therapeutic decisions. However, several factors suggest the 20–22-week mark as optimal. Both intravenous and intraperitoneal routes are available then. The fetus is still reasonably immunologically passive, and graft rejection is probably less likely than at term. The smaller fetus clearly requires a much smaller volume of fetal liver HSC, mandated by the optimal seven to eight week fetal donor. Interval testing may allow detection of engraftment as early as 24 weeks, thus preventing pregnancy termination. Further, there is likely much more room in the depleted marrow at 20 weeks than the seeded marrow of the more advanced fetus to receive the HSC. It is notable, however, that in the two varieties of immunodeficiency successfully engrafted to date, later HSC transplant was possible, perhaps facilitated by the host's deficiency.

Technical Considerations

This is an area where very few centers have the necessary expertise to refine the fetal liver HSC for donation, make the diagnosis of more than the most classic forms, or monitor the subtle beginnings of fetal engraftment. After that, however, standard techniques of ultrasound-directed intraperitoneal and/or intravascular transfusion have been utilized. It is not clear how the recipient is first engrafted, although the case

Table 12-10 Fetal Stem Cell Transplants

A. Engraftment Demonstrated

Disorder	Stem Cell	Route	Gestation	Result	Ref (Yr)
Bare lymphocyte syndrome	Fetal liver / thymus cells	IV	28 weeks	Engraftment, survival, normal cell-mediated immunity	206 (1989)
(SCID) Severe combined immunodeficiency	Fetal liver	IV	26 weeks	Engraftment, incomplete effect but "normal life at home"	207 (1992)
β-Thalassemia	Fetal liver	IP	12 weeks	Engraftment, not curative Small % HbA production	208 (1992)
α-Thalassemia	Maternal bone marrow	IP	18 weeks	No circulating HbA at 23 wks– TOP; Autopsy = microscopic engraftment	193 (1990)

B. No Engraftment Demonstrated

Disorder	Stem Cell	Route	Gestation	Result	Ref (Yr)
Rh disease	Maternal bone marrow	IP	17 weeks	No engraftment. Survived due to fetal transfusions.	205 (1986)
SCID	Maternal marrow	IP/IV	20 weeks	No engraftment—TOP	209 (1992)
Chediak-Higashi	Maternal marrow	IP	19 weeks	Liveborn—no engraftment	209 (1992)
β-Thalassemia	Fetal liver	IV	17 weeks	Procedural fetal death	207 (1992)
β-Thalassemia	Paternal marrow	IP/IV*	25 weeks	Liveborn—no engraftment	210 (1992)
Metachromatic leukodystrophy	Paternal marrow /	IP/IV	34 weeks	Both liveborn, no engraftment	210 (1992)
	Sibling marrow	IP	23 weeks		

IV = intravenous - umbilical vein except (*) intrahepatic.
IP = intraperitoneal.
HbA = Normal adult hemoglobin.
TOP = Termination of pregnancy.

at UCSF demonstrated widespread extramedullary hematopoiesis, suggesting engraftment of many organs (193). Over 200 postnatal fetal liver HSC transplants in 58 patients resulted in effective bone marrow and extramedullary engraftment after intravenous infusion (213). Given the importance of the microenvironments of both the thymus and bone marrow in processing lymphocyte precursors, it is likely that at least part of successful engraftment takes place in the organs normally involved.

Future Applications

None of these disorders is very common. Most are self-limited by voluntary infertility of the affected family. Engraftment may treat or ameliorate the disease but does not alter the inheritance patterns. The techniques are, as Touraine has stated, "unprecedented" (213) and, therefore, completely unknown. The techniques cross many ethical boundaries in procuring the donor HSC, deciding which diseases to treat, and diverting valuable resources. All of these tissues must be addressed fully before fetal stem cell therapy can advance safely.

Once this demanding agenda is met, however, the potential is immense. Not only can the HSC result in beneficial engraftment to produce a direct hematologic effect, it also may well be possible to use these progenitors to carry intact/normal genetic information to reverse the broad range of all genetic disorders (214). Thus, fetal liver HSC engraftment may enjoy even broader application as a vector for human gene therapy.

FETAL SURGICAL PROCEDURES

A number of intrauterine fetal surgical procedures has been recorded in the litera-

ture (Table 12-11) (215–221). These procedures have some common elements: (a) severe congenital anomalies with serious mortality if untreated, (b) reliable antenatal ultrasound diagnosis (structural anomalies) by midtrimester, (c) singleton fetus with proven normal karyotype, (d) neonatal surgical remedy seriously impaired by the original condition, and (e) reasonable expectancy of normal life if the repair is successful.

It is clear that there will be many differences on the basis of the specific entities, but it is interesting to note that one investigating team provides the large majority of reports. At UCSF, the team led by Michael Harrison has provided meticulous surgical research using innovative animal models, looked with care at the contemporary "natural history" of neonatal management of the particular defect concerned, prospectively outlined the specific rationale for their highly-invasive procedures, and provided unstinting detail in reports of clinical application (94,222–225). While not all groups have followed this example, there are, in fact, very few examples of the poorly-considered human experiments feared by many public, i.e., talk-show, commentators. Dr. Manning provides a balanced assessment of fetal surgical procedures; that analysis will not be repeated here. Some common concerns do need to be addressed, however:

Rationale for intervention This is usually that neonatal management is so unsuccessful because of the extremes of the disease or that intrauterine progression of the disease without treatment yields an unsalvageable infant. Both scenarios are inherently fleeting—rapid neonatal advances and/or much less invasive intrauterine approaches will alter or negate the rationale so

Table 12-11 Fetal Surgical Procedures

Operative Procedure	Fetal Condition	Ref.	Rationale	N*	Outcome
Ventriculoamniotic shunt	Cerebral ventriculomegaly	215	Prevent progressive brain injury	<50	Improved survival + no change in brain injury = increased number of severe handicap
Vesicoamniotic shunt	Posterior urethral obstruction	216	Prevent/reverse pulmonary hypoplasia; ameliorate urinary tract damage	>200	>50% long-term survival, many with chronic renal impairment
	Other urinary tract obstruction	217	As above.	<50	No effect on disease prognosis
Pleuroamniotic shunt	? Thoracic duct occlusion Bilateral pleural effusion	218	Reverse anasarca/hydrops; ? Allow resumption of normal lung development	<100	>75% long-term survival if no undetected heart anomaly
	Pulmonary tumors	**	? As above	<10	No effect on disease prognosis
Tumor resection	Sacrococcygeal teratoma	219	Fetal high-output heart failure precludes maturity/neonatal treatment	1	Fetal recovery, premature labor, neonatal death
Hernia reduction, diaphragm patch	Diaphragmatic hernia	220	Reversal of lethal pulmonary hypoplasia	<20	A few intact survivors have resulted in the latest cohort
Open fetal vesicostomy or ureterostomy	Urethral obstruction	221	Vesicoamniotic shunts sometimes fail	<10	Survival no better than closed shunting, with serious maternal sequelae

*In the literature, in the Fetal Surgery Registry, and reported to the Fetal Medicine and Surgery Society.
**See preceding discussion, "Cavity Drainage and Lung Biopsy."

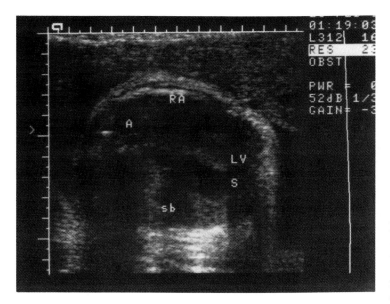

Figure 12-19 Congenital diaphragmatic hernia, originally diagnosed at 18 weeks gestation. Normal karyotype confirmed, spontaneous onset of labor ensued at 39 weeks. Neonatal management included immediate paralysis, sedation, conventional ventilation using "preductal" cutaneous O_2 saturation monitoring, and delayed repair (day five of life) with diaphragmatic patch required. The infant has survived intact. A = aorta; RA = right atrium; LV = left ventricle, illustrating pronounced right-sided diversion of heart by hernia contents; S = stomach; sb = small bowel.

compelling just a few years earlier (Figure 12-19). A column headed "Proven superiority vs. neonatal management" in Table 12-11 would have NO beside every major procedure.

Analysis of results Promising results by one group with a sophisticated background of pediatric surgery and animal research are not automatically duplicated anywhere else. The lack of multicenter experience and the small number of cases in any specific category prevent decisive critique in many cases.

Long-term maternal morbidity These disorders are not associated with medically-measured maternal infertility. Mid-trimester hysterotomy, however, confers a lasting maternal liability that may include repeated very premature delivery, abnormal placental invasion, hemorrhage, uterine rupture, and hysterectomy (226–227).

Open operations vs. closed puncture-techniques In view of the previous paragraph, maternal concerns clearly favor puncture techniques. There are caveats here. (A) Of course, detailed complicated operations are not *yet* possible via intrauterine endoscopic, i.e., puncture, techniques (228). (See also Table 12-4 and the associated discussion.) The lesson of open fetal exchange transfusion for severe Rh diseases (229), which procedure withered and vanished in the face of improving sophistication with needle techniques for intraperitoneal and then, intravascular transfusion, is appropriate here. (B) If a large number of serial punctures are needed to replace a single hysterotomy, the advantage may disappear. (C) Improvements in techniques and technology of fetal and maternal monitoring during open techniques may well improve the safety and success of open fetal surgery (113).

The family Ethical concerns are ubiquitous in this entire text. The need for pre- and postprocedure dialogue, information, and support is clear and critical. At the same time, all of those involved may be coerced (subtly or not, depending on our level of conviction about the lethality and potential reversibility of the procedure) by the chance that "everything can be made right." On clear, sober, second thought, more than 40% of hemophilia carriers (recurrence risk 25%) would not "consider going through prenatal diagnosis in the future" (230). With a recurrence risk of virtually zero, one wonders what families of fetal surgery patients would say in retrospect.

Surgery of the Perinate

A number of situations may present where neonatal respiration is either precarious or completely impossible unless the airway is secured by surgical means. Such cases include cervical or oropharyngeal teratomas, cystic hygromas, and other anterior cervical tumors. In these situations, the fetal head and neck have been exposed by cesarean section incision, but the baby has been left undelivered while the airway was secured with endotracheal intubation (231,232). With vaginal delivery, immediate attention to the airway, by chest needling for bilateral pleural effusions and by tracheostomy for laryngeal atresia, have both resulted in healthy survivors in our institution (Figure 12-20). If the pediatric surgeon is in the delivery room and the procedure is done immediately, the unclamped cord provides the essential life-line, facilitated by the mother breathing high-concentration oxygen. In four cases (three chest tubes, one tracheostomy), rapid surgery has taken place in the narrow window after delivery and before cord spasm and placental separation. Further, we now drain at least one side of bilateral pleural effusions in the labor suite

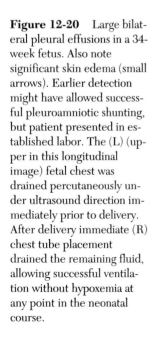
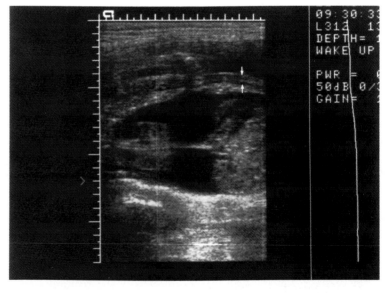

Figure 12-20 Large bilateral pleural effusions in a 34-week fetus. Also note significant skin edema (small arrows). Earlier detection might have allowed successful pleuroamniotic shunting, but patient presented in established labor. The (L) (upper in this longitudinal image) fetal chest was drained percutaneously under ultrasound direction immediately prior to delivery. After delivery immediate (R) chest tube placement drained the remaining fluid, allowing successful ventilation without hypoxemia at any point in the neonatal course.

immediately prior to induction of labor, or elective cesarean section. A final example of a truly perinatal procedure is the infusion of pancuronium 0.2 mg/kg predicted fetal weight intravenously immediately prior to cesarean section in the fetus with congenital diaphragmatic hernia. This results in a paralyzed fetus/paralyzed newborn. While immediate intubation is obviously required, the stomach will thus remain empty, chest wall and voluntary resistance are removed, and the sedation/paralysis technique of neonatal management can be initiated at time zero (233).

Fetal Surgery: The Future

Clarification of current applications is important before large-scale expansion is undertaken, a principle evident in the recent contributions of the UCSF Group. Research of utmost value in the characteristics and mechanisms of fetal wound healing and innovations in maintenance of animal models have recently become available (113,234). This research suggests that fetal wounds heal without scarring, raising attractive possibilities about intrauterine repair of cleft lip, facial anomalies, cavernous hemangiomas, and so on that may well be addressed in the future. Of more critical interest are the life-and-death issues of CNS abnormalities, especially open neural tube defects (Figure 12-21). The meticulous animal experiment detailed by Maria Michejda (235) certainly suggests that detailed surgical debridement with facilitated repair, perhaps with bone paste, perhaps with electrical stimulation of muscle and nerve tissue via permanent implants, may be able to convert spina bifida to a normal situation. It may well be that a clean excision will pave the way for the amazing reparative powers of the fetus, with restoration of normal tissue. Preliminary work in early fetal sheep in our lab has shown some individuals who have recovered from lumbar spinal cord transection to walk as newborn lambs 40–50 days later (236) (Figure 12-22).

Heart defects may also be a consideration for early fetal surgery. Although the first at-

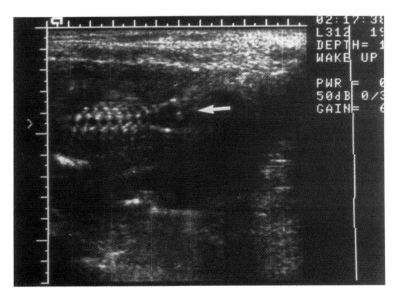

Figure 12-21 Severe spina bifida with broad flaring of dysraphic bones and visible strands of neural tissue (arrow). Is this lesion reparable? See text.

Figure 12-22 Post-mortem examination of lamb who underwent complete dorsal laminectomy and lumbar spinal cord transection at 100 days gestation but walked at delivery (151 days). Note significant boney callus (arrow) and spinal cord repair (probe) across the area of resection.

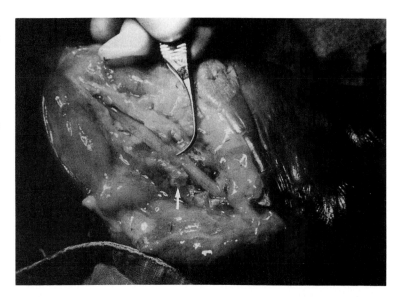

tempts (noted in the section on cardiac procedures) have not been successful, this is an area of active research.

To balance these speculations, there undoubtedly will be major progress in nonsurgical approaches to these difficult problems. At the time of publication of this book, the United States moratorium on fetal tissue research has been repealed, a large expansion of current knowledge is anticipated in both the medical side and in the broad social/ethical considerations that surround it.

SELECTIVE FETICIDE

Various terms have been associated with these interventions, including selective reduction, multifetal reduction, selective embryocide, selective termination, and selective feticide. Reduction of the number of embryos or fetuses in multiple pregnancy can be divided into two groups. Those which occur in the first trimester to reduce high order multiple pregnancies will be referred to here as multifetal reduction. The

term selective is erroneous in this situation because no embryo is selected for termination. No information is available regarding sex, karyotype, or any other individual feature—only the position of the sac is important. Procedures in the second trimester, performed on a specific abnormal fetus in discordant twins or triplets, are properly termed selective terminated. The approach to these two procedures differs in philosophy, ethics, technique, and management.

Multifetal Reduction

Professor Nicolini has dealt with the principles of the procedures and compelling reasons for multifetal reduction. To highlight the place of this established procedure, consider the ethical issues:

1. This couple has a history of infertility and may be unable to conceive again.
2. They have undergone emotionally exhausting and expensive therapy to arrive at this stage.
3. The perinatal outlook for a pregnancy with four or more embryos is poor.

4. The mother is placed in a situation of considerable risk by the pregnancy as well.
5. The ongoing pregnancy will utilize expensive obstetric, neonatal, and, possibly, pediatric resources, which may limit the amount of care available to other singleton pregnancies.

Therefore, the available options are to:

1. Continue the pregnancy
2. Terminate the pregnancy
3. Reduce embryo number

(The reader should refer to a comprehensive article that covers these issues (237). A recent review of perinatologists' and neonatologists' views on multifetal reduction showed that most considered the procedure acceptable in certain situations (238). The initial pregnancy number had to be four or more, reduced to two.)

These eight factors present many possibilities as perinatology enters the twenty-first century. Advancement in infertility treatment, with higher yield per embryo replaced for example, would make replacing four or more unnecessary and reduce dramatically the frequency of unacceptably high fetal numbers. Among options for management, an example of the potential for rapid change is that therapeutic interventions based on better understanding of the mechanisms of premature cervical changes of premature labor, may make intact survival more likely. It is certain, therefore, that these procedures will remain under development.

In addition to the transabdominal approaches that are technically refined, the advent of high-resolution vaginal sonography makes transvaginal needling procedures the subject of current investigation. The transvaginal approach is preferred by some because it can be performed earlier (around 8–11 weeks gestation), the clarity of the individual sacs is greater due to the smaller distance between the vaginal probe and uterus, and the needle only needs one insertion into the uterus (239–241). The vaginal probe is inserted into the posterior fornix, and using a guided needle, avoiding the cervix, the uterus and embryonic sacs are entered.

Whether the procedure is done abdominally or transvaginally, a number of methods have been used once the needle is clearly visualized within a given sac. *Aspiration* of the embryonic sac contents, may result in a change of uterine volume, which may stimulate spontaneous abortion (242). *Direct fetal injury* and *fetal exsanguination* (by cardiac puncture or rupture of a major vessel) (243), are no longer used because certainty of death was sometimes difficult owing to limited vision secondary to the procedure (244) and because simpler and more successful techniques are now available. *Air embolism* produces marked echogenicity of the embryo, interfering with the procedure without allowing certainty that the embryo is dead (245). *Injection of lethal substances* into the region of the embryonic heart is usually effective (246,247). Saline, potassium chloride, or lignocaine have all been used, with KCl being the most successful.

If the number of fetuses terminated is to be three or more, some prefer a two-stage reduction, allowing for enlargement of the remaining sacs in the interval, but experienced operators can usually complete the procedure on a single occasion (246,248).

SELECTIVE TERMINATION

As noted, the principles underlying this procedure are quite different from the earlier reduction of embryos and are thoroughly discussed in the chapter on twins. In the context of this chapter, the continued accumulation of experience and expertise will likely confirm several issues: (a) KCl injection is most effective (Figure 12-23) (249); (b) there is an upper gestational age limit (20 weeks) for safety; (c) only twin or triplet pregnancies where the circulation of the abnormal twin is *proven* to be absolutely separate from the other(s) are considered; and (d) detailed multidisciplinary counselling and support must precede and follow the procedure. Finally, in situations where only an abnormal karyotype is present, some other method to identify the affected twin should be used immediately prior to the procedure. For procedural details, the reader is referred to Professor Nicolini's chapter.

FETECTOMY

"Selective delivery" by hysterotomy has been performed in twins with discordance for cytogenetic abnormality (250) and the acardiac fetal malformation (251,252), with subsequent delivery of the normal twin during the third trimester. Other methods of selective termination (described earlier) are not appropriate for termination of the acardiac twin fetus because of the vascular connections between the two fetuses.

Procedure

Hysterotomy has been performed between 19 and 26 weeks gestation. The uterine incision is made under ultrasound guidance over the abnormal fetus, avoiding the placenta. The fetus is delivered, and the umbilical cord is doubly ligated with nonabsorbable suture, close to the placental insertion site. The uterine incision is then closed in two layers, with the addition of sterile saline to replace amniotic fluid. Intensive tocolytic therapy, using several agents simultaneously, is required for several weeks. Delivery of the normal fetus is by lower segment cesarean section, the timing controlled by preterm labor onset.

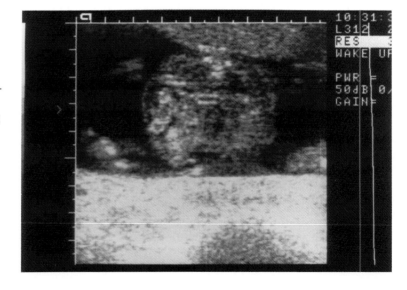

Figure 12-23 Intracardiac and pericardial KCl infusion produces this distorted echogenic appearance within the fetal chest. Selective feticide was the option selected after extensive multidisciplinary counselling due to discordance for severe spina bifida, hydrocephalus, and other anomalies in twins.

Conclusion

Fetectomy may be successful to produce one normal twin, but the associated maternal morbidity and subsequent risks are high. Reported complications include placental abruption, PROM, and maternal pulmonary edema (252). These risks, in addition to the complications of prolonged hospitalization and tocolytic therapy, must be considered before attempting such a procedure.

SUMMARY

A broad array of approaches, instruments, and techniques is surveyed in this chapter. Its goal will have been achieved if the reader has the impression that all things are possible in the arena of fetal surgical procedures. Some of these procedures will have very short half-lives as newer fetal procedures or, more likely, maternal procedures, enable better, safer fetal evaluation. Many of them will never reach broad application but will remain important, even life-saving, in critical instances. Only through critical appraisal initiated by open discussion will we sort out the significant advances from the unnecessarily meddlesome, among these novel invasive techniques.

References

1. Moore KL. The developing human. Toronto: WB Saunders, 1982;111–129.
2. Westin B. Technique and estimation of oxygenation of the human fetus in utero by means of hysterophotography. Acta Paediatrica 1957;46:117–124.
3. MacKenzie IZ. Transcervical fetoscopy. The Lancet 1974;ii:346–347.
4. Gallinat A, Lueken RP, Lindemann HJ. A preliminary report about transcervical embryoscopy. Endoscopy 1978;10:47–50.
5. Dumez Y. Embryoscopy and congenital malformations. Presented at the International Conference on Chorionic Villus Sampling and Early Prenatal Diagnosis, May 28–29, 1988, Athens, Greece.
6. Ghirardini G. Embryoscopy: old technique new for the 1990s? Am J Obstet Gynecol 1991;164:1361–1362.
7. Cullen MT, Reece EA, Whetham J, Hobbins JC. Embryoscopy: description and utility of a new technique. Am J Obstet Gynecol 1990; 162:82–86.
8. Cullen MT, Whetham J, Viscarello RR, Reece EA, Sanchez-Ramos L, Hobbins JC. Transcervical endoscopic verification of congenital anomalies in the second trimester of pregnancy. Am J Obstet Gynecol 1991;165:95–97.
9. Reece EA, Rotmensch S, Whetham J, Cullen M, Hobbins JC. Embryoscopy: a closer look at first-trimester diagnosis and treatment. Am J Obstet Gynecol 1992;166:775–780.
10. Rotmensch S, Reece EA, Hobbins JC. Embryoscopy and fetoscopy. In: Iffy L, Apuzzio JJ, Vintzileos AM, eds. Operative Obstetrics. 2nd ed. New York: McGraw-Hill, 1992;11:114–123.
11. Quintero RA, Romero R, Mahoney MJ, Abuhamad A, Vecchio M, Holden J, Hobbins JC. Embryoscopic demonstration of hemorrhagic lesions on the human embryo after placental trauma. Am J Obstet Gynecol 1993;168:756–759.
12. Lindsay DJ, Lovett IS, Lyons EA, Levi CS, Zheng X-H, Holt SC, Dashefsky SM. Yolk sac diameter and shape at endovaginal US: predictors of pregnancy outcome in the first trimester. Radiology 1992; 183:115–118.
13. Westin B. Hysteroscopy in early pregnancy. The Lancet (Letter) 1954;ii:872.
14. Mandelbaum, Pontarelli DA, Brushenko A. Amnioscopy for prenatal transfusion. Am J Obstet Gynecol 1967;98(8):1140–1143.
15. Valenti C. Endoamnioscopy and fetal biopsy: a new technique. Am J Obstet Gynecol 1972;114:561–564.
16. Scrimgeour JB. Other techniques for antenatal diagnosis. In: Emery AEH, ed.

Antenatal diagnosis of genetic disease. Edinburgh: Churchill Livingstone, 1973; 4:40–57.

17. Hobbins JC, Mahoney MJ, Goldstein LA. New method of intrauterine evaluation by the combined use of fetoscopy and ultrasound. Am J Obstet Gynecol 1974;118: 1069–1072.

18. Laurence KM, Pearson JF, Prosser R, Richards C, Rocker I. Fetoscopy followed by live birth. The Lancet 1974;i: 1120–1121.

19. Benzie RJ, Doran TA. The "fetoscope"— A new clinical tool for prenatal genetic diagnosis. Am J Obstet Gynecol 1975;121: 460–464.

20. Benzie RJ, Malone RM, Miskin M, Rudd NL, Schofield PA. Prenatal diagnosis by fetoscopy with subsequent normal delivery: report of a case. Am J Obstet Gynecol 1976;126:287–288.

21. Hobbins JC, Mahoney MJ. Fetoscopy in continuing pregnancies. Am J Obstet Gynecol 1977;129:440–442.

22. Rodeck CH, Campbell S. Early prenatal diagnosis of neural-tube defects by ultrasound-guided fetoscopy. The Lancet 1978; i:1128–1129.

23. Patrick JE, Perry TB, Kinch RAH. Fetoscopy and fetal blood sampling: a percutaneous approach. Am J Obstet Gynecol 1974;119: 539–542.

24. Hobbins JC, Mahoney MJ. In utero diagnosis of hemoglobinopathies. N Engl J Med 1974;290:1065–1067.

25. Rodeck CH, Campbell S. Sampling pure fetal blood by fetoscopy in second trimester of pregnancy. Br Med J 1978;2:728–730.

26. Rodeck CH. Fetoscopy guided by real-time ultrasound for pure fetal blood samples, fetal skin samples, and examination of the fetus in utero. Br J Obstet Gynaecol 1980; 87:449–456.

27. Rodeck CH, Mibashan RS, Abramowicz J, Campbell S. Selective feticide of the affected twin by fetoscopic air embolism. Prenat Diagn 1982;2:189–194.

28. Schwartz DB, Zweibel WJ, Donovan D, Arbogast RL. Fetoscopic visualization in second-trimester pregnancies. Am J Obstet Gynecol 1983;145:51–55.

29. Filkins K, Benzie RJ. Fetoscopy. Clin Obstet Gynecol 1983;26:339–346.

30. Rodeck CH, Nicolaides KH. Ultrasound-guided invasive procedures in obstetrics and gynecology. Clinic Obstet Gynecol 1983;10:515–539.

31. Rauskolb R. Fetoscopy. J Perinat Med 1983; 11:223–231.

32. Rodeck CH, Nicolaides KH, Warsof SL, Fysh WJ, Gamsu HR, Kemp JR. The management of severe Rhesus isoimmunization by fetoscopic intravascular transfusions. Am J Obstet Gynecol 1984;150: 769–774.

33. Rodeck CH, Nicolaides KH. Fetoscopy and fetal tissue sampling. Br Med Bull 1983; 39:332–337.

34. Golbus MS, McGonigle KF, Goldberg JD, Filly RA, Callen PW, Anderson RL. Fetal tissue sampling. The San Francisco experience with 190 pregnancies. West J Med 1989; 150:423–430.

35. Shulman LP, Elias S. Percutaneous umbilical blood sampling, fetal skin sampling, and fetal liver biopsy. Semin Perinatol 1990;14: 456–464.

36. Levin MD, McNeil DE, Kaback MM, Frazer RE, Okada DM, Hobel CJ. Second-trimester fetoscopy and fetal blood sampling: current limitations and problems. Am J Obstet Gynecol 1974;120:937–943.

37. Rodeck CH, Campbell S. Umbilical cord insertion as source of pure fetal blood for prenatal diagnosis. The Lancet (Letter) 1979;i:1244–1255.

38. Rodeck CH, Nicolaides KH. The use of fetoscopy for prenatal diagnosis and treatment. Sem Perinat 1983;7:118–124.

39. Fairweather DVI, Ward RHT, Modell B. Obstetric aspects of mid-trimester fetal blood sampling by needling or fetoscopy. Br J Obstet Gynaecol 1980;87:87–99.

40. Hertogs K, Nicolini U, Tzannatos C, Rodeck CH. The safety of fetoscopy: (I). Effect of umbilical vessel puncture on the fetal heart rate and cord histology. Prenat Diagn 1983;3:91–96.

41. Nicolaides KH, Koullapis EN, Rodeck CH. The safety of fetoscopy: (II). Effect on maternal plasma levels of 13,14-dihydro-15-oxo-prostaglandinF2α. Prenat Diagn 1983; 3:97–100.
42. Rodeck CH, Nicolaides KH. Fetoscopy. Br Med Bull 1986;42:296–300.
43. Rodeck CH, Patrick AD, Pembrey ME, Tzannatos C, Whitfield AE. Fetal liver biopsy for prenatal diagnosis of ornithine carbamyl transferase deficiency. The Lancet 1982;ii:297–299.
44. Holzgreve W, Golbus MS. Prenatal diagnosis of ornithine transcarbamylase deficiency utilizing fetal liver biopsy. Am J Hum Genet 1984;36:320–328.
45. Sereni LP, Bachmann C, Pfister U, Buscaglia M, Nicolini U. Prenatal diagnosis of carbamyl-phosphate synthetase deficiency by fetal liver biopsy. Prenat Diagn 1988;8:307–309.
46. Murotsuki J, Uehara S, Okamura K, Yaiima A, Kikuchi M, Oura T, Miyabayashi S. Prenatal diagnosis of carbamyl phosphate synthetase deficiency by fetal liver biopsy. Acata Obstet Gynaecol Jpn 1991;43:1613–1616.
47. Golbus MS, Simpson TJ, Koresawa M, Appelman ZVI, Alpers CE. The prenatal determination of glucose-6-phosphatase activity by fetal liver biopsy. Prenatal Diagn 1988;8:401–404.
48. Danpure CJ. Peroxisomal alanine: glyoxylate aminotransferase and prenatal diagnosis of primary hyperoxaluria type 1. The Lancet 1986;ii(8516):1168.
49. Arulkumaran S, Rodeck CH. Invasive prenatal diagnostic techniques. Fetal Med Rev 1990;2:171–185.
50. Hyland K, Surtees AH, Rodeck C, Clayton PT. Aromatic L-amino acid decarboxylase deficiency: clinical features, diagnosis, and treatment of a new inborn error of neurotransmitter amine synthesis. Neurology 1992;42:1980–1988.
51. Mibashan RS, Rodeck CH, Thumpston JK, Edwards RJ, Singer JD, White JM, Campbell S. Plasma assay of fetal factors VIIIC and IX for prenatal diagnosis of haemophilia. The Lancet 1979; 1309–1311.
52. Simpson GF, Sun NH, Golbus MS. Changes in maternal serum alpha-fetoprotein levels associated with intrauterine genetic diagnostic procedures. Prenatal Diagn 1984; 4:207–211.
53. Nussbaum RL, Boggs BA, Beaudet AL, Doyle S, Potter JL, O'Brien WE. New mutation and prenatal diagnosis in ornithine transcarbamylase deficiency. Am J Hum Genet 1986;38:149–158.
54. Fox J, Hack AM, Fenton WA, Golbus MS, Winter S, Kalousek F, Rozen R, Brusilow SW, Rosenberg LE. Prenatal diagnosis of ornithine transcarbamylase deficiency with use of DNA polymorphisms. New Engl J Med 1986;315:1205–1208.
55. Rodeck CH, Eady RAJ, Gosden CM. Prenatal diagnosis of epidermolysis bullosa letalsis. The Lancet 1980;i:949–952.
56. Anton-Lamprecht I. Prenatal diagnosis of genetic disorders of the skin by means of electron microscopy. Hum Genet 1981;59:392–405.
57. Fine J-D, Eady RAJ, Levy ML, et al. Prenatal diagnosis of dominant and recessive dystrophic epidermolysis bullosa: application and limitations in the use of KF-1 and LH 7:2 monoclonal antibodies and immunofluorescence mapping technique. J Invest Dermatol 1988;91:465–471.
58. Holbrook KA, Wapner R, Jackson L, Zaeri N. Diagnosis and prenatal diagnosis of epidermolysis bullosa herpetiformis (Dowling-Meara) in a mother, two affected children, and an affected fetus. Prenat Diagn 1992; 12:725–739.
59. Perry TB, Holbrook KA, Hoff MS, et al. Prenatal diagnosis of congenital non-bullous ichthyosiform erythroderma (lamellar ichthyosis). Prenat Diagn 1987;7:145–155.
60. Golbus MS, Sagebiel RW, Filly RA, Grindhart TD, Hall JG. Prenatal diagnosis of congenital bullous ichthyosiform erythroderma (epidermolytic hyperkeratosis) by fetal skin biopsy. N Engl J Med 1980; 302:93–95.

61. Elias S, Mazur M, Sabbagha R, Esterly NB, Simpson JL. Prenatal diagnosis of harlequin ichthyosis. Clin Genet 1980;17:275–280.

62. Kousseff BG, Matsuoka LY, Stenn KS, et al. Prenatal diagnosis of Sjögren-Larsson syndrome. J Pediatr 1982;101:998–1001.

63. Arnold M-L, Rauskolb R, Anton-Lamprecht I, Schinzel A, Schmid W. Prenatal diagnosis of anhidrotic ectodermal dysplasia. Prenat Diagn 1984;4:85–98.

64. Eady RAJ, Gunner DB, Garner A, Rodeck, CH. Prenatal diagnosis of oculocutaneous albinism by electron microscopy of fetal skin. J Invest Derm 1983;80:210–212.

65. Arnold M-L, Anton-Lamprecht I. Problems in prenatal diagnosis of the ichthyosis congenita group. Hum Genet 1985;71:301–311.

66. Kohlschutter A, Rauskolb R, Goebel HH, Anton-Lamprecht I, Albrecht R, Klein H. Probable exclusion of juvenile neuronal ceroid lipofuscinosis in a fetus at risk: an interim report. Prenat Diagn 1989;9:289–292.

67. Elias S, Esterly NB. Prenatal diagnosis of hereditary skin disorders. Clin Obstet Gynecol 1981;24:1069–1087.

68. Lofberg L, Gustavii B. Technical difficulties in fetal skin sampling. Acta Obstet Gynecol Scand 1982;61:505–507.

69. Bakharev VA, Aivazyan A, Karetnikova NA, Mordovtsev VN, Yantovsky YUR. Fetal skin biopsy in prenatal diagnosis of some genodermatoses. Prenat Diagn 1990;10:1–12.

70. Kurjak A, Alfirevic Z, Jurkovic D. Ultrasonically-guided fetal tissue biopsy. Acta Obstet Gynecol Scand 1987;66:523–527.

71. Buckshee K, Parveen S, Mittal S, Verma K, Singh M. Percutaneous ultrasound-guided fetal skin biopsy: a new approach. Int J Gynecol Obstet 1991;34:267–270.

72. Zonana J, Schinzel A, Upadhyaya M, Thomas NST, Anton-Lamprecht I, Harper PS. Prenatal diagnosis of X-linked hypohydrotic ectodermal dysplasia by linkage analysis. Am J Med Genet 1990;35:132–135.

73. Happle R, Stekhoven JH, Hamel BC, Kollee LA, Nijhuis JG, Anton-Lamprecht I, Steijlen PM. Restrictive dermopathy in two brothers. Arch Dermatol 1992;128:232–235.

74. Hamel BC, Happle R, Steylen PM, et al. False-negative prenatal diagnosis of restrictive dermopathy. Am J Med Genet 1992;44:824–826.

75. Nazzaro V. Normal development of human fetal skin. G Ital Dermatol Venereol 1989;124:421–427.

76. Boot PM, Rowden G, Walsh N. The distribution of Merkel cells in human fetal and adult skin. Am J Dermatopath 1992;14:391–396.

77. Eady RAJ, Gunner DB, Tidman MJ, et al. Rapid processing of fetal skin for prenatal diagnosis by light and electron microscopy. J Clin Pathol 1984;37:636–638.

78. Eady RAJ. Fetoscopy and fetal skin biopsy for prenatal diagnosis of genetic skin disorders. Semin Dermatol 1988;7:2–8.

79. Heagerty AHM, Kennedy AR, Gunner DB, Eady RAJ. Rapid prenatal diagnosis and exclusion of epidermolysis bullosa using novel antibody probes. J Invest Dermatol 1986;86:603–605.

80. Hausser I, Anton-Lamprecht I. Prenatal diagnosis of genodermatoses by ultrastructural diagnostic markers in extraembryonic tissues: defective hemidesmosomes in amnion epithelium of fetuses affected with epidermolysis bullosa Herlitz type (an alternative prenatal diagnosis in certain cases). Hum Genet 1990;85:367–375.

81. Eady RAJ, Gunner DB, Lake BD, et al. Prenatal diagnosis of genetic skin disease using fetal skin biopsy: 10 years' experience. Br J Dermatol 1990;123:37.

82. Shulman LP, Elias S, Emerson DS, Phillips OP, Simpson JL. Minimal fetomaternal transfusion in ultrasound-guided fetal skin sampling. Prenat Diagn 1991;11:924–927.

83. Gustavii B, Lofberg L, Henriksson KG. Fetal muscle biopsy. Acta Obstet Gynecol Scand 1983;62:369–371.

84. Evans M, Greb A, Kunkel LM, et al. In utero fetal muscle biopsy for the diagnosis of Duchenne muscular dystrophy. Am J 1991;165:728–732.

85. Kuller JA, Hoffman EP, Fries MH, Golbus MS. Prenatal diagnosis of Duchenne mus-

cular dystrophy by fetal muscle biopsy. Hum Genet 1992;35–40.

86. Morcos SF, Lobb MO. The antenatal diagnoses by ultrasonography of type III congenital cystic adenomatoid malformation of the lung. Case report, Br J Obstet Gynaecol 1986;1002–1005.

87. Rodeck CH, Nicolaides KH. Fetal tissue biopsy: techniques and indications. Fetal Ther 1986;46–58.

88. Chao A, Monoson RF. Neonatal death despite fetal therapy for cystic adenomatoid malformation. Case report. J Reproduct Med 1990;35:655–657.

89. Clark SL, Vitale DJ, Minton SD, et al. Successful fetal therapy for cystic adenomatoid malformation associated with second trimester hydrops. Am J Obstet Gynecol 1987;157:294–295.

90. Nimrod C, Nicholson S, Davies D, Harder J, Dodd G, Sauve R. Pulmonary hypoplasia testing in clinical obstetrics. Am J Obstet Gynecol 1988;158(2):277–280.

91. Wigglesworth JS, Hislop AA, Desai R. Biochemical and morphometric analyses in hypoplastic lungs. Pediatr Pathol 1991;11: 537–549.

92. Bronshtein M, Bar-Hava I, Blumenfeld I, Bejar J, Toder V, Blumenfeld Z. The difference between septated and nonseptated nuchal cystic hygroma in the early second trimester. Obstet Gynecol 1993;81: 683–687.

93. Campbell WA, Yamase HT, Salafia CA, Vintzileos AM, Rodis JF. Fetal renal biopsy: technique development. Fetal diagnosis and therapy 1993;8:135–143.

94. Adzick NS, Harrison MR, Glick PL, Flake AW. Fetal urinary tract obstruction: experimental pathophysiology. Semin Perinat 1985;9:79–90.

95. Gore RM, Callen PW, Filly RA, Harrison MR, Golbus MS. Prenatal percutaneous antegrade pyelography in posterior urethral valves: sonographic guidance. AJR 1982;139:994–996.

96. Kirkinen P, Jouppila P, Tuononen S, Paavilainen T. Repeated transabdominal renocenteses in a case of fetal hydronephrotic kidney. Am J Obstet Gynecol 1982;142: 1049–1052.

97. Redwine FO, Pertes RE, Cruinkshank DP. Reversal of polyhydramnios by drainage of a fetal renal cyst. Case report. J Reprod Med Obstet Gynecol 1983;28: 421–423.

98. Kyle P, Lange IR, Menticoglou SM, Harman CR, Manning FA. Intrauterine thoracentesis of fetal cystic lung malformations. Fet Diagn Ther 1994;9:84–87.

99. Adzick NS, Harrison MR, Glick PL, et al. Fetal cystic adenomatoid malformation: prenatal diagnosis and natural history. J Pediatr Surg 1985;20:483–488.

100. Avni EF, Vanderelst A, Van Gansbeke D, et al. Antenatal diagnosis of pulmonary tumours: report of two cases. Pediatr Radiol 1986;16:190–192.

101. Slotnick RN, McGahan J, Milio L, Schwartz M, Ablin D. Antenatal diagnosis and treatment of fetal bronchopulmonary sequestration. Fetal Diagn Ther 1990;5:33–39.

102. Shozu M, Akasofu K, Iida K, Harada T. Treatment of an antenatally diagnosed fetal ovarian cyst by needle aspiration during the neonatal period. Arch Gynecol Obstet 1991;249(2):103–106.

103. Suita S, Handa N, Nakano H. Antenatally detected ovarian cysts—a therapeutic dilemma. Early human development 1992; 29:363–367.

104. Weiner C. Cordocentesis. Obstet Gynecol Clin NA 1988;15:283–301.

105. Hallak M, Moise KJ Jr, Hesketh DE, Cano LE, Carpenter RJ Jr. Intravascular transfusion of fetuses with Rhesus incompatibility: prediction of fetal outcome by changes in umbilical venous pressure. Obstet Gynecol 1992;80:286–290.

106. Weiner CP, Heilskov J, Pelzer G, Grant S, Wenstrom K, Williamson RA. Am J Obstet Gynecol 1989;161:714–717.

107. Johnson P, Sharland G, Allan LD, Tynan MJ, Maxwell DJ. Umbilical venous pressure in nonimmune hydrops fetalis: Correlation with cardiac size. Am J Obstet Gynecol 1992;167:1309–1313.

108. Harman CR. Antenatal fetal monitoring: abnormalities of fetal behaviour. In: James D, Steer P, Weiner C, Gonik B, eds. High-Risk Pregnancy: Management Options. London: WB Saunders, 1993, (in press).

109. Harman CR, Menticoglou S, Pillai M. Intravenous fetal fluid challenge in the evaluation of absolute obigohydramnios. Fet Diag Ther 1994, (in press).

110. Harman CR, Menticoglou S, Pollock J, Manning F, Bowman JM. Human fetal pO_2 responses to maternal oxygenation. Am J Obstet Gynecol 1994, (in press).

111. Harman CR, Menticoglou S, Manning F, Pillai M. Fetal oxygen uptake—a test of placental reserve. Am J Obstet Gynecol 1994, (in press).

112. Personal Communication: Quay SC, Sonus Pharmaceuticals, Costa Mesa, Ca. (Reported in Diagnostic Imaging SCAN, 1993;Vol 7, #8, May 5, and Advance for Radiologic Science Professionals 1993;Vol 6, #17, April 26.)

113. Jennings RW, Adzick NS, Longaker MT, Lorenz HP, Estes JM, Harrison MR. New techniques in fetal surgery. J Pediatr Surg 1992;27(10);1329–1333.

114. Westgren M, Selbing A, Stangenberg M. Fetal intracardiac transfusions in patients with severe Rhesus isoimmunisation. Br Med J 1988;296:885–886.

115. Westgren M, Selbing A, Stangenberg M, Phillips R. Acid-base status in fetal heart blood in erythroblastotic fetuses: a study with special reference to the effect of transfusions with adult blood. Am J Obstet Gynecol 1989;160:1134–1138.

116. Antsaklis AI, Papantoniou NE, Mesogitis SA, Koutra PT, Vintzileos AM, Aravantinos DI. Cardiocentesis: an alternative method of fetal blood sampling for the prenatal diagnosis of hemoglobinopathies. Am J Obstet Gynecol 1992; 79:630–633.

117. Lindenberg S, Andersen AM, Thomsen SG, Van der Hagen, CB. Prenatal diagnosis of the fragile X syndrome (Martin-Bell's syndrome). Ugeskr-Laeg 1986; 148:134–135.

118. Murotsuki J, Okamura K, Iwamoto M, et al. Hematological values in fetal blood by cordocentesis. Acta Obstet Gynaecol Jpn 1992;44:638–642.

119. Thorpe-Beeston JG, Nicolaides KH, Feelton CV, Butler J, McGregor AM. Maturation of the secretion of thyroid hormone and thyroid-stimulating hormone in the fetus. New Engl J Med 1991;324:532–536.

120. Harman CR, Manning FA, Menticoglou S, Bowman J. Fetal exsanguination at intravascular transfusion. Proc Soc Obstet Gynecol Canada 1990:(Abstract).

121. Ash KM, Mibashan RS, Nicolaides KH. Diagnosis and treatment of feto-maternal hemorrhage in a fetus with homozygous von Willebrand's disease. Fetal Ther 1988; 3:189–191.

122. Benatar A, Vaughan J, Nicolini U, Trotter S, Corrin B, Lincoln C. Prenatal pericardiocentesis: its role in the management of intrapericardial teratoma. Am J Obstet Gynecol 1992;79:856–858.

123. Strasburger JF, Carpenter R, Smith RT, Deter R, Garson A. Fetal transthoracic pacing for advanced hydrops fetalis secondary to complete atrioventricular block. J Am Coll Cardio (in press).

124. Allan LD. Arrhythmias. In: Allan LD, ed. Manual of fetal echocardiography. Lancaster: MTP Press Ltd 1993;11:156–168.

125. Maxwell D, Allan L, Tynan MJ. Balloon dilatation of the aortic valve in the fetus: a report of two cases. Br Heart J 1991;65: 256–258.

126. Gembruch U, Hansmann M. Artificial instillation of amniotic fluid as a new technique for the diagnostic evaluation of cases of oligohydramnios. Prenat Diag 1988;8:33–45.

127. Fisk NM, Ronderos-Dumit D, Soliani A, Nicolini U, Vaughan J, Rodeck CH. Diagnostic and therapeutic transabdominal amnioinfusion in olighydramnios. Obstet Gynecol 1991;78:270–278.

128. Nicolini U, Monni G. Intestinal obstruction in babies exposed in utero to methylene blue. The Lancet 1990;336: 1258–1259.

129. van der Pol JG, Wolf H, Boer K, et al. Jejunal atresia related to the use of methylene blue in genetic amniocentesis in twins. Br J Obstet Gynaecol 1992;99: 141–143.

130. Nicolini U, Fisk NM, Rodeck CH, Talbert DG, Wigglesworth JS. Low amniotic fluid pressure—Is this the cause of pulmonary hypoplasia? Am J Obstet Gynecol 1989; 161:1098–1101.

131. Hansmann M, Chatterjee MS, Schuh S, Gembruch U, Bald R. Multiple antepartum amnioinfusions in selected cases of oligohydramnios. J Reprod Med 1991;36: 847–851.

132. University of British Columbia. Grace Maternity Hospital Perinatal Group, Vancouver. Canadian Press (CP) Reports; Canadian Broadcasting Corporation (CBC) Reports, April, 1993.

133. Imanaka M, Ogita S, Sugawa T. Saline solution amnioinfusion for oligoyhdramnios after premature rupture of the membranes. Am J Obstet Gynecol 1989;161: 102–106.

134. Ogita S, Imanaka M, Matsumoto M, Oka T, Sugawa T. Transcervical amnioinfusion of antibiotics: a basic study for managing premature rupture of membranes. Am J Obstet Gynecol 1988;158:23–27.

135. Miyazaki FS, Taylor NA. Saline amnioinfusion for relief of variable or prolonged decelerations. Am J Obstet Gynecol 1983; 146:670–678.

136. Miyazaki FS, Nevarez F. Saline amnioinfusion for relief of repetitive variable decelerations: a prospective randomized study. Am J Obstet Gynecol 1985;153: 301–306.

137. Nageotte MP, Freeman RK, Garite TJ, Dorchester W. Prophylactic intrapartum amnioinfusion in patients with preterm premature rupture of membranes. Am J Obstet Gynecol 1985;153:557–562.

138. Nageotte MP, Bertucci L, Towers CV, Lagrew DL, Modanlou H. Prophylactic amnioinfusion in pregnancies complicated by oligohydramnios: a prospective study. Obstet Gynecol 1991;77:677–680.

139. Goodlin RC. Was there really a difference with amnioinfusion? Am J Obstet Gynecol 1991;164:235.

140. Ting P, Brady JP. Tracheal suction in meconium aspiration. Am J Obstet Gynecol 1975;122:767–771.

141. Davis RO, Philips JB, Harris BA, Wilson ER, Huddleston JF. Fetal meconuium aspiration syndrome occurring despite airway management considered appropriate. Am J Obstet Gynecol 1985;151: 731–736.

142. Sadfovsky Y, Amon E, Bade ME, Petrie RH. Prophylactic amnioinfusion during labor complicated by meconium: a preliminary report. Am J Obstet Gynecol 1989; 161:613–617.

143. Wenstrom KD, Parsons MT. The prevention of meconium aspiration in labor using amnioinfusion. Obstet Gynecol 1989;73: 647–651.

144. Posner MD, Ballagh SA, Paul RH. The effect of amnioinfusion on uterine pressure and activity: a preliminary report. Am J Obstet Gynecol 1990;163:813–818.

145. Strong TH, Hetzler G, Paul RH. Amniotic fluid volume increase after amnioinfusion of a fixed volume. Am J Obstet Gynecol 1990;162:746–748.

146. Dragich DA, Ross AF, Chestnut DH, Wenstrom K. Respiratory failure associated with amnioinfusion during labor. Anesth Analg 1991;72:549–551.

147. Chamberlain PF, Manning FA, Morrison I, Harman CR, Lange IR. Ultrasound evaluation of amniotic fluid. II. The relationship of increased amniotic fluid volume to perinatal outcome. Am J Obstet Gynecol 1984;150:250–254.

148. Kirshon B. Fetal urine output in hydramnios. Obstet Gynecol 1989;73:240–242.

149. Phelan JP, Martin GI. Polyhydramnios: fetal and neonatal implications. Clin Perinatol 1989;16:987–994.

150. Queenan JT, Gadow EC. Polyhydramnios: chronic versus acute. Am J Obstet Gynecol 1970;108:349–354.

151. Fisk NM, Ronderos-Dumit D, Tannirandorn Y, Nicolini U, Talbert D. Normal am-

niotic pressure throughout gestation. Br J Obstet Gynaecol 1992;99:18–22.

152. Fisk NM, Tannirandorn Y, Nicolini U, Talbert DG, Rodeck CH. Amniotic pressure in disorders of amniotic fluid volume. Obstet Gynecol 1990;76:210–214.

153. Erskine JP. A case of acute hydramnios successfully treated by abdominal paracentesis. J Obstet Gynaecol Br Emp 1944;5:549–551.

154. Lange IR, Harman CR, Ash KM, Manning FA, Menticoglou S. Twin with hydramnios: treating premature labor at source. Am J Obstet Gynecol 1989;160:552–557.

155. Kirshon B, Mari G, Moise KJ, Wasserstrum N. J Reprod Med Obstet Gynecol 1990; 35:529–532.

156. DeLia JE, Cruikshank DP, Keye WR. Fetoscopic neodymium:yag laser occlusion of placental vessels in severe twin-twin transfusion syndrome. Obstet Gynecol 1990;75:1046–1052.

157. Rivett LC. Hydramnios. J Obstet Gynaecol Br. Empire 1933;40:522–538.

158. Brandt GR. Acute hydramnios treated by abdominal paracentesis. J Obstet Gynaecol Br Empire 1958;65:61–63.

159. Brandt AJ, Bates JS. Transabdominal amniocentesis in hydramnios. Obstet Gynecol 1961;17:392–394.

160. Pitkin RM. Acute polyhydramnios recurrent in successive pregnancies. Obstet Gynecol 1976;48:42s–43s.

161. Wax JR, Blakemore KJ, Blohm P, Callan NA. Stuck twin with cotwin nonimmune hydrops: successful treatment by amniocentesis. Fetal Diagn Ther 1991;6: 126–131.

162. Bebbington MW, Wittman BK. Fetal transfusion syndrome: antenatal factors predicting outcome. Am J Obstet Gynecol 1989;160:913–915.

163. Eden TW, Holland E. Manual of Obstetrics. London: Churchill, 1937;166.

164. Queenan JT. Recurrent acute polyhydramnios. Am J Obstet Gynecol 1970;106: 625–626.

165. Elliot JP, Urig MA, Clewell WH. Aggressive therapeutic amniocentesis for treatment of twin-twin transfusion syndrome. Obstet Gynecol 1991;77:537–540.

166. Reisner DP, Mahony BS, Petty CN, Nyberg DA, Zingheim MA. Stuck twin syndrome: outcome in 38 consecutive cases. Am J Obstet Gynecol 1993;168:382.

167. Saunders NJ, Snijders RJM, Nicolaides KH. Therapeutic amniocentesis in twin-twin transfusion syndrome appearing in the second trimester of pregnancy. Am J Obstet Gynecol 1992;166:820–824.

168. Weir PE, Ratten GJ, Beischer NA. Acute polyhydramnios—a complication of monozygous twin pregnancy. Br J Obstet Gynaecol 1979;86:849–853.

169. Vintzileos AM, Turner GW, Campbell WA, Weinbaum PJ, Ward SM, Nochimson DJ. Polyhydramnios and obstructive renal failure: a case report and review of the literature. Am J Obstet Gynecol 1985;152: 883–885.

170. DeLia JE, Rogers JG, Dixon JA. Treatment of placental vasculature with a neodymium-YAG laser via fetoscopy. Am J Obstet Gynecol 1985;151:1126–1127.

171. DeLia JE, Cukierski MA, Lundergan DK, Kochenour NK. Neodymium-yttrium-aluminium-garnet laser occlusion of Rhesus placental vasculature via fetoscopy. Am J Obstet Gynecol 1989;160:485–489.

172. DeLia JE, Kuhlmann R, Harstad T, Cruikshank D. Twin-twin transfusion syndrome treated by fetoscopic neodymium-yag laser occlusion of chorioangiopagus. Am J Obstet Gynecol 1993;168:308.

173. O'Brien SJ, Miller DV. The contact neodymium-yttrium-aluminium garnet laser. Clin Orthoped 1990;252:95–100.

174. Soothill PW, Ajayi RA, Nicolaides KN. Fetal biochemistry in growth retardation. Early Hum Dev 1992;29:91–97.

175. Johnson MP, Evans MI. Intrauterine growth retardation: pathophysiology and possibilities for intrauterine treatment. Fetal Therapy 1987;2:109–122.

176. Harding J, Liu L, Evans P, Oliver M, Gluckman P. Intrauterine feeding of growth-retarded fetus: can we help? Early Hum Dev 1992;29:193–197.

177. Economides DL, Nicolaides KH, Gahl WA, Bernardini I, Bottoms S, Evans M. Cordocentesis in the diagnosis of intrauterine starvation. Am J Obstet Gynecol 1989;161:1004–1008.

178. Harding JE, Owens JA, Robinson JS. Should we try to supplement the growth-retarded fetus? A cautionary tale. Br J Obstet Gynaecol 1992;99:707–710.

179. Harding JE, Charlton V. Treatment of the growth-retarded fetus by augmentation of substrate supply. Sem Perinat 1989;13:211–223.

180. Flake AW, Villa RL, Adzick NS, Harrison MR. Transamniotic fetal feeding. II. A model of intrauterine growth retardation using the relationship of "natural runting" to uterine position. J Pediatr Surg 1987;22:816–819.

181. Flake AW, Villa-Troyer RL, Adzick NS, Harrison MR. Transamniotic fetal feeding. III. The effect of nutrient infusion on fetal growth retardation. J Pediatr Surg 1986;21:481–484.

182. The following reports were cited by Harding and Charlton (179) but are no longer available:
   (A) Renaud R, Kirschtetter L, Koehl C, et al. Amino acid intra-amniotic injections. In: Persianinov LS, Chervakova TV, Presl J, eds. Recent progress in obstetrics and gynaecology. Amsterdam: Excerpta Medica 1974;234–256.
   (B) Renaud R, Vincendon G, Boog G, et al. Injections intra-amniotiques d'acides amines dans les cas de malnutrition foetale. Premiers resultats. J Gynecol Obstet Biol Reprod 1972;1:231–244.
   (C) Massobrio M, Margaria E, Campograne M, et al. Treatment of severe fetoplacental insufficiency by means of intra-amniotic injection of amino acids. In: Salvadori B, ed. Therapy of feto-placental insufficiency. Berlin: Springer-Verlag, 1975:296–301.

183. Saling E. Versuch einer neuen Kompensatorischen versorgung des hypotrophen

feten. Geburtsch u Frauenheilk 1987;47:90–92.

184. Pitkin RM, Reynolds WA. Fetal ingestion and metabolism of amniotic fluid protein. Am J Obstet Gynecol 1975;123:356–363.

185. Nicolini U, Hubinont C, Santolaya J, Fisk NM, Rodeck CH Effects of fetal intravenous glucose challenge in normal and growth-retarded fetuses. Horm Meta Res 1990;22:426–430.

186. Battaglia C, Artini PG, D'Ambrogio G, Galli PA, Segre A, Genazzani AR. Maternal hyperoxygenation in the treatment of intrauterine growth retardation. Am J Obstet Gynecol 1992;167:430–435.

187. Nicolaides KH, Campbell S, Bradley RJ, Bilardo CM, Soothill PW, Gibb D. Maternal oxygen therapy for intrauterine growth retardation. The Lancet 1987;1:942–945.

188. Kurjak A, Zmijanac J. Antepartum and intrapartum management of the growth-retarded fetus. Clin Obstet Gynecol 1992;35:185–193.

189. Farah SB, Simpson TJ, Golbus MS. Hematopoietic stem cells for the treatment of genetic disease. Clin Obstet Gynecol 1986;29(3):543–550.

190. Crombleholme TM, Langer JC, Harrison MR, Zanjani ED. Transplantation of fetal cells. Am J Obstet Gynecol 1991;164:218–230.

191. Gale RP. Fetal liver transplants. Bone Marrow Transplant 1992;9(S1):118–120.

192. Touraine J-L. In utero transplantation of fetal liver stem cells in humans. Blood Cells 1991;17:379–387.

193. Golbus MS, Cowan MJ. In utero stem cell transplantation. J Perinat Med 1990:Suppl I:38.

194. Crombleholme TM, Harrison MR, Zanjani ED. In utero transplantation of hematopoietic stem cells in sheep: the role of T cells in engraftment and graft-versus-host disease. J Pediatr Surgery 1990;25(8):885–892.

195. Harrison MR, Crombleholme TM, Tarantal AF, Slotnick RN, Golbus MS, Zanjani ED. In utero transplantation of fetal liver haemopoietic stem cells in monkeys. The Lancet 1989;2:1425–1427.

196. Roodman GD, Kuehl TJ, Vandeberg JL, Muirhead DY. In utero bone marrow transplantation of fetal baboons with mismatched adult baboon marrow. Blood Cells 1991;17:367–375.

197. Ikuta K, Uchida N, Friedman J, Weissman IL. Lymphocyte development from stem cells. Annual Rev Immunol 1992;10: 759–783.

198. Ikuta K, Kina T, MacNeil I, Uchida N, Peault B, Chien Y-H, Weissman IL. Development of γδ T-cell subsets from fetal hematopoietic stem cells. Ann New York Acad Sci 1992;651:21–32.

199. Tavassoli M. Embryonic and fetal hemopoiesis: an overview. Blood Cells 1991; 1:269–281.

200. Prindull G. Early embryonal/fetal lymphopoietic ontogeny and leukemogenesis. Ann Hematol 1991;63:291–296.

201. Liu C-P, Auerbach R. Ontogeny of murine T cells: thymus-regulated development of T cell receptor-bearing cells derived from embryonic yolk sac. Eur J Immunol 1991;21:1849–1855.

202. Than S, Inaba M, Inaba K, Fukuba Y, Adachi Y, Ikehara S. Origin of thymic and peritoneal Ly-1 B cells. Eur J Immunol 1992;22:1299–1303.

203. Ikuta K, Weissman IL. The junctional modifications of a T cell receptor Y chain are determined at the level of thymic precursors. J Exp Med 1991;174:1279–1282.

204. Nagy A, Gocza E, Diaz EM, Prideaux VR, Ivanyi E, Markkula M, Rossant J. Embryonic stem cells alone are able to support fetal development in the mouse. Development 1990;110:815–821.

205. Linch DC, Rodeck CH, Nicolaides K, et al. Attempted bone marrow transplantation in a 17-week fetus. The Lancet 1986;2:1453.

206. Touraine JL, Raudrant D, Royo C, et al. In utero transplantation of stem cells in a patient with the bare lymphocyte syndrome. The Lancet 1989;1:1382.

207. Touraine JL. Rationale and results of in vitro transplants of stem cells in humans. Bone Marrow Transplant 1992;10(S1): 121–126.

208. Touraine J-L. In utero tansplantation of fetal liver stem cells into human fetuses. Hum Reprod 1992;7(1):44–48.

209. Diukman R, Golbus MS. In utero stem cell therapy. J Reprod Med 1992;37(7): 515–520.

210. Slavin S, Naparstek E, Ziegler M, Lewin A. Clinical application of intrauterine bone marrow transplantation for treatment of genetic diseases—feasibility studies. Bone Marrow Transplant 1992;9(S1):189–190.

211. Andreux JP, Renard M, Daffos F, Forestier F. Erythropoietic progenitor cells in human fetal blood. Nouv Rev Fr Haematol 1991;33:223–226.

212. Liang D-C, Ma S-W, Lin-Chu M, Lan C-C. Granulocyte/macrophage colony-forming units from cord blood of premature and full-term neonates: its role in ontogeny of human hemopoiesis. Ped Res 1988;24: 701–702.

213. Touraine J-L, Raudrant D, Vullo C, et al. New developments in stem cell transplantation with special reference to the first in utero transplants in humans. Bone Marrow Transplant 1991;3:92–97.

214. Karson EM, Polvino W, Anderson WF. Prospects for human gene therapy. J Reprod Med 1992;37:508–514.

215. Manning FA, Harrison RR, Rodeck CR. Catheter shunts for fetal hydronephrosis and hydrocephalus: report of the International Fetal Surgery Registry. N Engl J Med 1986;315:336–340.

216. Manning FA. The fetus with obstructive uropathy: the Fetal Surgery Registry. In: Harrison MR, Golbus MS, Filly RA, eds. The unborn patient: prenatal diagnosis and treatment. Philadelphia: WB Saunders, 1990:394–398.

217. Manning FA, Harman CR, Lange IR, Brown R, Decter A, MacDonald N. Antepartum chronic fetal vesicoamniotic shunts for obstructive uropathy: a report of two cases. Am J Obstet Gynecol 1983; 145:819–822.

218. Nicolaides KH, Azar GB. Thoracoamniotic shunting. Fetal Diagn Ther 1990; 5:153–164.

219. Langer JC, Harrison MR, Schmidt KG, et al. Fetal hydrops and death from sacrococcygeal teratoma: rationale for test surgery. Am J Obstet Gynecol 1989;160:1145–1150.
220. Harrison MR, Langer JC, Adzick NS, et al. The correction of congenital diaphragmatic hernia in utero. V. Initial clinical experience. J Pediatr Surg 1990;25:45–57.
221. Crombleholme TM, Harrison MR, Langer JC, et al. Early experience with open fetal surgery for congenital hydronephrosis. J Pediatr Surg 1988;23:1114–1121.
222. Harrison MR, Nakayama DK, Noall R, de-Lorimier AA. Correction of congenital hydronephrosis in utero. II. Decompression reverses the effects of obstruction on the fetal lung and urinary tract. J Pediatr Surg 1982;17:965–974.
223. Glick PL, Harrison MR, Noall RA, Villa RL. Correction of congenital hydronephrosis in utero. III. Early mid-trimester ureteral obstruction produces renal dysplasia. J Pediatr Surg 1984;18:681–682.
224. Glick PL, Harrison MR, Adzick NS. Correction of congenital hydronephrosis in utero. IV. In utero decompression prevents renal dysplasia. J Pediatr Surg 1984;19:649–657.
225. Glick PL, Harrison MR, Golbus MS, et al. Management of the fetus with obstructive hydronephrosis. II. Prognostic criteria and selection for treatment. J Pediatr Surg 1985;20:376–387.
226. Longaker MT, Golbus MS, Filly RA, Rosen MA, Chang SW, Harrison MR. Maternal outcome after open fetal surgery: a review of the first 17 human cases. JAMA 1991;265;737–741.
227. Dewhurst C. The ruptured cesarean section scar. J Obstet Gynaecol Br Commonw 1957;74:113–118.
228. Estes JM, MacGillivray TE, Hedrick MH, Adzick NS, Harrison MR. Fetoscopic surgery for the treatment of congenital anomalies. J Pediatr Surg 1992;27:950–954.
229. Adamsons K Jr, Freda VJ, James LS, Towell ME. Prenatal treatment of erythroblastosis fetalis following hysterotomy. Pediatrics 1965;35:848–855.
230. Tedgard U, Ljung R, McNeil T, Tedgard E, Schwartz. How do carriers of hemophilia experience prenatal diagnosis (PND)? Acta Paediatr Scand 1989;78:692–700.
231. Kelly MF, Berenholz L, Rizzo KA, Greco R, Wolfson P, Zwillenberg DA. Approach for oxygenation of the newborn with airway obstruction due to a cervical mass. Ann Otol Rhinol Laryngol 1990;99:179–182.
232. Langer JC, Tabb T, Thompson P, Paes BA, Caco CC. Management of prenatally diagnosed tracheal obstruction: access to the airway in utero prior to delivery. Fetal Diagn Ther 1992;7:12–16.
233. Harman CR, Kosseim M, Casiro O, Menticoglou S, Manning FA. Successful management of congenital diaphragmatic hernia does not require antenatal fetal surgery. Proc Soc Obstet Gynecol Canada 1991:Abstract #53.
234. Longaker MT, Adzick NS. The biology of fetal wound healing: a review. Plast Reconstr Surg 1991;87:788–798.
235. Michejda M. Antenatal treatment of central nervous system defects: current and future developments in experimental therapies. Fetal Ther 1989;4(S1):108–131.
236. Manning FA, Harman CR, Lange IR. Experimental surgical ovine fetal neural tube defect: preliminary observation. Proc Soc Obstet Gynecol Canada 1984:Abstract.
237. Evans MI, Fletcher JC, Zador IE, Newton BW, Quigg MH, Stuyk CD. Selective and first-trimester termination in octuplet and quadruplet pregnancies: clinical and ethical issues. Obstet Gynecol 1988;71:289–296.
238. Evans MI, Drugan A, Bottoms SF, Platt LD, Rodeck CA, Hansmann M. Attitudes on the ethics of abortion, sex selection, and selective pregnancy termination among health care professionals, ethicists, and clergy likely to encounter such situations. Am J Obstet Gynecol 1991;164:1092–1099.
239. Itskovitz J, Boldes R, Thaler I, Levron J, Rottem S, Brandes JM. First trimester selective reduction in multiple pregnancy guided by transvaginal sonography. J Clin Ultrasound 1990;18:323–327.

240. Gonen Y, Blankier J, Casper RF. Transvaginal ultrasound in selective embryo reduction for multiple pregnancy. Obstet Gynecol 1990;75:720–722.

241. Timor-Tritsch I, Peisner DB, Monteagudo A. Vaginal sonographic puncture procedures. In: Timor-Tritsch IE, Rottem S, eds. Transvaginal sonography. 2nd ed. New York: Elsevier Science Publishing, 1991; 16:427–492.

242. Evans MI, May M, Fletcher JC. Multifetal pregnancy reduction and selective termination. In: Iffy L, Apuzzio JJ, Vintzileos AM, eds. Operative Obstetrics, 2nd ed. New York: McGraw-Hill, 1992:165–171.

243. Petres RE. Letter. N Engl J Med 1981; 305:1218–1219.

244. Kanhai HHH, Van Rijssel EJC, Meerman RJ, Gravenhorst J. Selective termination in quintuplet pregnancy during first trimester. The Lancet 1986;1:1447.

245. Dommergues M, Nisand I, Mandelbrot L, Isfer E, Radunovic N. Embryo reduction in multifetal pregnancies after infertility therapy: obstetrical risks and perinatal benefits are related to operative strategy. Fertil Steril 1991;55:805–811.

246. Lynch L, Berkowitz RL, Chitkara U, Alvarez M. First-trimester transabdominal multifetal pregnancy reduction: a report of 85 cases. Obstet Gynecol 1990;75:735–738.

247. Tabsh KMA. Transabdominal multifetal pregnancy reduction: report of 40 cases. Obstet Gynecol 1990;75:739–741.

248. Farquharson DF, Wittman BK, Hansmann M, Yuen BH, Baldwin VJ, Lindahl S. Management of quintuplet pregnancy by selective embryocide. Am J Obstet Gynecol 1988;158:413–416.

249. Evans MI, Goldberg JD, Dumez Y, Wapner RJ, Lynch L, Dock BS. Efficacy of second trimester selective termination (ST) for fetal abnormalities: international collaborative experience among the world's largest centers. Am J Obstet Gynecol 1993;168:307.

250. Beck L, Terinde R, Dolff M. Zwillingsschwangerschaft mit frier Trisomie 21 eines Kindes; Sectio parva mit entfernung des Kranken und spatere Geburt des gesunden Kindes. Geburtshilfe Frauenheilkd 1980;40:397–400.

251. Robie GF, Payne GG, Morgan MA. Selective delivery of an acardiac, acephalic twin. N Engl J Med 1989;320:512–513.

252. Fries MH, Goldberg JD, Golbus MS. Treatment of acardiac-acephalus twin gestations by hysterotomy and selective delivery. Obstet Gynecol 1992;79:601–604.

ETHICAL FRONTIERS IN INVASIVE FETAL THERAPY

FRANK A. CHERVENAK
LAURENCE B. MCCULLOUGH

13

RELEVANCE OF MEDICAL ETHICS

We live in an era characterized by rapid, often startling advances in medical technologies and their applications in the development of diagnostic and therapeutic innovations. Nowhere is this more true than in the subspecialty of maternal-fetal medicine. Preimplantation embryos can be sustained ex utero, and the capacity to manipulate their genetic and gross structures and functions will only increase in the coming years. We are now able to obtain fixed and real-time images of the fetus from very early in gestation, to obtain fetal tissue for analysis or transplantation shortly thereafter, and to treat fetal anomalies in the latter months of pregnancy. Finally, a battery of diagnostic and therapeutic interventions is available for intrapartum management of pregnancy for fetal and maternal indications. In summary, maternal-fetal medicine is increasingly in the position to do routinely for the fetus what other specialties and subspecialties do: undertake a wide array of diagnostic and therapeutic interventions and conduct research on new interventions. In other words, the fetus seems just as much a patient as any other patient, save for its locale in utero (1–5). Indeed, references to the fetus as a patient have become commonplace in the literature and practice of maternal-fetal medicine (6–13).

Interestingly, the concept and language of the fetus as patient have developed more as a byproduct of technological advances than as a result of careful reflection on the concept of the fetus as patient and its clinical implications. As a consequence, the concept of the fetus as patient has not been carefully examined, especially in its ethical dimensions. As a further consequence, the clinical implications of the concept are unclear. The purpose of this chapter is to provide a careful examination of the concept of the fetus as patient and on that basis to identify its ethical implications for invasive fetal testing and treatment.

LANGUAGE OF CONCEPTS OF MEDICAL ETHICS: A PRIMER

To think of the fetus—or any human being, for that matter—as a patient is to employ the language and concepts of medical ethics. Indeed, concern for protecting and promoting the interests of the patient has constituted the foundation for medical ethics and, thus, for medicine since the days of the Hippocratic oath and its accompanying texts.

In the ancient version of the oath, the physician swears by Apollo and the Greek gods and goddesses to do what will benefit the sick, while preventing harm to them (14). In the technical language of ethics, the oath should be understood as asserting beneficence-based ethical obligations to patients: The physician is to act in such a way as to produce a greater balance of goods over harms, as those goods and harms are understood from a clinical perspective (15,16). Over the centuries, the definition of these goods and harms has been undertaken on the basis of what medicine as a profession can claim as its competencies. In our time, the authors believe that, on this basis, the goods that medicine is competent to achieve are the prevention of premature death and the prevention, cure, or, at least, management of disease, injury, handicap, and unnecessary pain and suffering (16). Pain and suffering are sometimes a necessary price to be paid in the attempt to achieve the other goods of medicine. When pain and suffering occur in the absence of achieving those goods, pain and suffering become unnecessary. Acting on these goods provides concrete meaning to the fundamental ethical obligation of protecting and promoting the interests of patients.

Beneficence-based clinical judgment and ethical obligations were the whole of medical ethics until the dawn of our own century. Under the influences of the common law and philosophical ethics, medical ethics has increasingly come to acknowledge and emphasize the importance of the patient's perspective on his or her interests and what should count as protecting and promoting his or her interests (17). Patients form their judgments about their interests on the basis of their own values and express those judgments in value-based preferences. The ethical principle of respect for autonomy translates this fact into autonomy-based ethical obligations: to acknowledge the integrity of the patient's values in his or her life; to elicit the patient's value-based preferences; and to assist the patient to put his or her preference(s) into effect.

Following a well-established and respected ethical theory (18), the authors take the view that autonomy-based obligations are theoretically equally weighted with beneficence-based obligations. As a consequence, the former cannot be thought automatically to override the latter, nor vice versa. This view of beneficence-based and autonomy-based obligations has been defended in the literature of medical ethics (15,16) and obstetric ethics (19,20), a subspecialty of medical ethics.

The concepts of autonomy-based clinical judgment and ethical obligations and of beneficence-based clinical judgment and ethical obligations provide a framework in terms of which the concept of the fetus as patient can be articulated and its clinical implications identified in terms of concrete ethical obligations to the fetus and to the pregnant woman (19). The distinctive feature of maternal-fetal medicine is that there are sometimes two patients and ethical obligations and both must be identified and negotiated (19). The main implications with which we shall be concerned are two intertwined issues: the informed consent process and when invasive management of fetal anomalies and problems should be regarded as standard of care.

THE FETUS AS PATIENT: AN ETHICAL CONCEPT

A Failed Approach

One prominent approach to the analysis of the concept of the fetus as patient has involved attempts to show whether or not the fetus has independent moral status (21–30). Independent moral status for the fetus would mean that one or more characteristics that the fetus possesses in and of itself and, therefore, independently of the pregnant woman or any other factor, generate and, therefore, ground obligations to the fetus on the part of the pregnant woman and her physician.

A wide range of intrinsic characteristics has been nominated for this role, e.g., moment of conception, implantation, central nervous system development, quickening, and the moment of birth (31–33). Given the variability of proposed characteristics, it should come as no surprise that there is a wide range of views about when the fetus acquires independent moral status. Some take the view that the fetus has independent moral status from the moment of conception or implantation (34–36). Others believe that independent moral status is acquired in degrees, thus resulting in graded moral status (28,30). Still others hold, at least by implication, that the fetus never has independent moral status so long as it is in utero (29).

Despite a voluminous theological and philosophical literature on this subject that, literally, spans the centuries, there has been no consensus agreement on a single authoritative account of the independent moral status of the fetus (37,38). This outcome should surprise no one, given the absence of a single methodology that would be authoritative for all of the markedly diverse theological and philosophical schools of thought involved in this endless debate. In the absence of such a methodology, consensus is impossible. For consensus ever to be possible, intramural and transmural debates about such a final authority within and between theological and philosophical traditions would have to be resolved in a way satisfactory to all. This is an inconceivable event. It is best, therefore, to abandon futile attempts to understand the fetus as patient in terms of independent moral status of the fetus and turn to an alternative approach. This approach makes it possible to identify ethically distinct senses of the fetus as patient and their clinical implications. We need to ask not, "Does the fetus have independent moral status?" but, as Warnock puts it, "How ought we to treat the fetus?" (39,40)

An Alternative Approach

This alternative approach begins with the recognition that being a patient does not require that one possesses independent moral status (27). Rather, being a patient means that one can benefit from the applications of the clinical skills of the physician. Put more precisely, a human being without independent moral status is properly regarded as a patient when two conditions are met: that a human being (a) is presented to the physician (b) for the purpose of applying clinical interventions that are reliably expected to be efficacious, in that they are reliably expected to result in a greater balance of goods over harms for the human being in question.

In other words, someone is a patient when a physician has beneficence-based ethical obligations to that individual. There have been some beneficence-based discussions of the fetus as patient (41,42). However, there is a need to clarify the senses in which beneficence-based approaches illuminate the concept of the fetus as patient.

We begin as follows. Because the independent moral status of the fetus cannot be established, there can be no autonomy-based obligations to the fetus. To clarify the concept of the fetus as patient, it is, therefore, appropriate to turn to an account of when there are beneficence-based obligations to the fetus.

The authors have argued elsewhere that beneficence-based obligations to the fetus exist when the fetus *can become* a child (19). That is, the fetus is a patient when medical interventions, whether diagnostic or therapeutic, reasonably can be expected to result in a greater balance of goods over harms for the child the fetus can become. The ethical significance of the concept of the fetus as patient, therefore, depends on links that can be established between the fetus and the child it can become.

The Viable Fetus as a Patient

One such link is *viability*, establishing a basis for the first ethical sense of the fetus as patient. Viability, however, cannot be understood as an intrinsic property of the fetus because viability must be understood in terms of both biological and technological factors (38,43,44). Both factors are required for a viable fetus to exist ex utero and, thus, become a child, the offspring of its parent(s). Interestingly, these two factors do not exist as a function of the autonomy of the pregnant woman. When a fetus is viable, i.e., when it is of sufficient maturity so that it can survive into the neonatal period and become a child given the availability of the requisite technological support, the fetus is a patient (45). Any beneficence-based obligations to the viable fetus must, of course, be balanced against beneficence-based and autonomy-based obligations to the pregnant woman (19).

Viability thus exists partly as a function of biomedical and technological capacities, which are different in different parts of the world. As a consequence, there can, at the present time, be no world-wide uniform gestational age to define viability. In the United States, the authors believe, viability presently occurs at approximately 24 weeks gestational age (46).

The Previable Fetus as a Patient

The only possible link between the previable fetus and the child it can become is the pregnant woman's autonomy, which provides the sole basis for the second ethical sense of the fetus as patient. This is because technological factors cannot result in the previable fetus becoming a child. This is simply what previable means. A link, therefore, between a fetus and the child it can become, when the fetus is previable, can be established only by the pregnant woman's decision to confer the status of being a patient on her previable fetus. The previable fetus, therefore, because it cannot reliably be thought to possess independent moral status, has no claim to the status of being a patient independently of the pregnant woman's autonomy. It follows, therefore, that the pregnant woman is free to withhold, confer, or, having once conferred, withdraw the status of being a patient on or from her previable fetus according to her own values. In other words,

the previable fetus is a patient solely *as a function of the pregnant woman's autonomy* (45).

A subset of the second sense of the fetus as patient includes in vitro embryos. It might, at first, seem that the in vitro embryo is a patient because such an embryo is surely presented to the physician. However, for there to be beneficence-based obligations to a human being without independent moral status, it also must be the case that the medical interventions are reliably expected to be efficacious.

Simply being presented to a physician does not make the in vitro embryo a patient. This is because, in terms of beneficence, whether the fetus is a patient depends as well on links that can be established between the fetus and the child it can become. Therefore, the reasonableness of medical interventions on the in vitro embryo depends on whether that embryo later becomes viable. Otherwise, no benefit of such intervention can meaningfully be said to result. An in vitro embryo, therefore, becomes viable only when it survives in vitro cell division, transfer, implantation, and subsequent gestation to such a time as it becomes viable.

This process of achieving viability occurs only in vivo and is, therefore, entirely dependent on the woman's decision regarding the status of the fetus(es) as a patient, should assisted conception successfully result in the gestation of the previable fetus(es). Whether an in vitro embryo will become a viable fetus and whether medical intervention on such an embryo will benefit the fetus are both functions of the pregnant woman's decision to withhold, confer, or, having once conferred, withdraw the moral status of being a patient on or from the previable fetus(es) that might result from assisted conception. Therefore, it is appropriate to regard the in vitro embryo as a previable fetus rather than as a viable fetus. As a consequence, any in vitro embryo(s) should be regarded as a patient only when the woman into whose reproductive tract the embryo(s) will be transferred confers that status (45).

In summary, the viable fetus is a patient. The previable fetus, including the in vitro embryo, is a patient solely as a function of the exercise of the woman's autonomy.

INFORMED CONSENT AND WHEN INVASIVE FETAL MANAGEMENT SHOULD BE REGARDED AS STANDARD CARE

We turn now to a discussion of the clinical implications of the concept of the fetus as patient. The usual account of informed consent in the medical ethics literature describes three elements in the process. They are (1) the disclosure of an adequate amount of information by the physician to the patient, (2) the understanding of that information by the patient, and (3) a voluntary choice by the patient for or against treatment (17).

This account suffers from at least two serious inadequacies. First, it assumes that there is no role for beneficence-based clinical judgment on the part of the physician. Instead, the physician is understood simply, and incorrectly, as a technically knowledgeable purveyor of information, not as a professional committed to the interests of the patient. Second, it assumes that all of us, when we become patients, are fully capable of participating at all times in this process, possessing an autonomy that requires no assistance or empowerment by the physician.

The authors propose an alternative account of informed consent, one that avoids these deficiencies and is expressed in terms

that can be translated directly into clinical practice in the following six steps: (1) the physician starts the process by finding out how much the pregnant woman knows about her fetus's condition, its diagnosis, available alternatives, and the prognosis of each alternative; (2) the physician corrects factual errors and incompleteness in the patient's fund of knowledge; (3) the physician provides and explains his or her clinical judgment about the fetus's condition and all available management strategies, including doing nothing; (4) the physician works with the patient to develop as complete a picture as possible of her fetus's condition and available alternatives; (5) the physician helps the patient, as needed or requested, identify her relevant values and beliefs; and (6) the physician helps the patient evaluate alternatives in terms of those values and beliefs (47).

The crucial issue at this stage of the informed consent process concerns what sort of recommendations, if any, the physician may make regarding invasive management of the fetus's condition. This issue can only be addressed in terms of two more fundamental considerations: when should invasive management of the fetus be regarded as standard of care and when should such management be considered experimental. When such management is reliably judged to be standard of care, directive counseling in the form of a recommendation of invasive management is ethically justified. When such management is reliably judged to be experimental, only non-directive counseling is ethically justified.

Whether invasive fetal management can be judged to be standard of care depends on the fulfillment of three considerations. These considerations are ethically justified on the basis of the concept of the fetus as patient.

First, such management must reliably be thought, on the basis of documented clinical experience, to benefit the child that the fetus can become. Recall that the ethical content of this concept is to be understood not simply in terms of simple physical accessibility but also in terms of whether clinical interventions on the fetus are reliably thought to be efficacious, in that they are reliably expected to result in a greater balance of goods over harms for the child the fetus can become. Satisfying both conditions establishes standard of care in its initial beneficence-based sense.

This standard, however, cannot be completely understood until its autonomy-based dimensions are considered. This leads to the second and third considerations.

Second, the pregnant woman is under no ethical obligation to confer the status of being a patient on her previable fetus simply because there is an invasive fetal management that meets a beneficence-based standard of care. Whether such management is in fact to be judged standard of care for her fetus is entirely a function of the pregnant woman's autonomy. That is, satisfying both beneficence-based and autonomy-based conditions are necessary for invasive fetal management to be reliably judged to be standard of care for previable fetuses.

The same is true for the third consideration, which concerns invasive fetal management of the viable fetus. Such a fetus is properly judged to be a patient. However, as noted above, beneficence-based obligations to the fetus must be balanced against beneficence-based and autonomy-based obligations to the pregnant woman. This is because of a factual consideration—invasive fetal management necessarily involves physical and, perhaps, mental health risks to the pregnant woman—and an ethical consideration—she is ethically obligated only to accept reasonable risks to

herself in order to attempt to benefit her fetus (19,48).

Therapy for the Viable Fetus

There is no simple algorithm by which a pregnant woman or her physician can reach the judgment that she is obligated to accept risk to herself on behalf of her fetus. In the authors' view, such an ethical obligation, which should be automatically equated with a legal obligation, exists when three criteria are satisfied. The first criterion concerns the outcome of the procedure for the fetus and the child it can become. The other two criteria concern risks of harm for the fetus and the child it can become as well as the pregnant woman. The three criteria are the following: (A) invasive management of the viable fetus has a very high probability of being life-saving or of preventing serious and irreversible disease, injury, or handicap for the fetus and for the child the fetus can become; (B) such management involves low mortality risk and low or manageable risk of serious disease, injury, or handicap to the fetus and the child it can become; and (C) the mortality risk to the pregnant woman is very low, and the risk of disease, injury, or handicap to the pregnant woman is low or manageable. The justifications for these criteria are both beneficence-based and autonomy-based. When A and B are satisfied, there is a clear and substantial net benefit to the fetus and the child it can become. When C is satisfied, there is not a clear and substantial net harm to the pregnant woman. Given the expected net benefit to the fetus and the low risk of harm to the pregnant woman, the latter are risks she should reasonably be expected to accept (19). This moral fact shapes her autonomy. Under beneficence-based and autonomy-based clinical judgment, therefore, treatment of the fetus is warranted. The burden of ethical proof seems to rest with those who would propose further ethical obligations when one or more of these three criteria cannot be satisfied, which is a matter of further careful reflection and debate.

When the pregnant woman is ethically obligated to accept invasive fetal management of her viable fetus, such management is ethically, not necessarily legally judged to be standard of care. Any forms of invasive fetal management for which an ethical obligation as defined above on the part of the pregnant woman to accept them cannot be established must be regarded as experimental.

We are now in a position to complete our description of the remainder of the informed consent process. That remainder in the case of the viable fetus differs from the case of the previable fetus.

In the case of the viable fetus, the physician is ethically justified in recommending standard of care invasive fetal management. There is a vital role in the process for the exercise of the woman's autonomy in assessing the risks and benefits to herself and to her fetus. These matters should be explained carefully to the pregnant woman. The benefits and risks of both invasive and noninvasive fetal management should be explained without bias, to the extent humanly possible, to the pregnant woman. She should be given time to reflect on her own and to reach her own decision.

How should the physician respond if the pregnant woman rejects standard of care invasive fetal management of a viable fetus? Certainly, informed consent as an ongoing dialogue with the pregnant woman should be the first approach. In undertaking the next step, negotiation, the physician should acknowledge and take into account the pregnant woman's assessment of the risks and benefits of invasive fetal management to herself and her fetus. It is justified to go beyond negotiation to respectful persuasion

and perhaps even to an ethics committee as part of a preventive ethics clinical strategy (49). Whether resort should be made to legal intervention is a matter of considerable dispute in the literature on the intrapartum management of pregnancy (50–53). Given the newness of invasive fetal management and the fact that few forms of such management satisfy the above defined ethical standard of care, it is unclear how courts might respond. It is also unclear whether resort to legal intervention bodes well for the future development of still experimental forms of fetal management.

Experimental management, that is, situations in which one or more of the above-mentioned criteria are not satisfied, of the viable fetus can be offered to the pregnant woman. Unlike the case of standard of care management, there is no ethical justification to recommend either because there is not a clear net benefit to the fetus or there is a clear net harm to the pregnant woman. Moreover, experimental management can be offered with ethical confidence only if there is a formal, scientifically sound protocol for the research and that protocol has been approved by the appropriate institutional review board. Obviously, discussion of experimental invasive fetal management with the pregnant woman should be rigorously nondirective.

Therapy for the Previable Fetus

There are two subgroups of previable fetuses. The first comprises those upon whom the pregnant woman has conferred the status of being a patient. When she has done so and the above-mentioned ethical criteria are also satisfied, standard of care invasive fetal management should be recommended on the basis of the beneficence-based and autonomy-based justification described above. This situation is directly analogous to the viable fetus, and the strategies discussed above apply.

When the pregnant woman withholds or withdraws the status of being a patient from her previable fetus, the situation is directly analogous to experimental fetal therapy. This is so because there is no ethical obligation on the part of the pregnant woman or the physician to regard the previable fetus as a patient. It follows that any discussion of invasive fetal management must be strictly nondirective.

The authors are aware that some researchers may take the view that our ethical analysis of the informed consent process is unrealistic because of the strong, perhaps even coercive, psychological pressure pregnant women may experience when confronted with an imperiled pregnancy and the availability of invasive fetal management. To the contrary, the authors are well aware of such a phenomenon and have sought to address its main ethical implication, namely, the possible impairment of the exercise of the pregnant woman's autonomy. Indeed, our emphasis on the place and importance of nondirective counseling is meant precisely as the most powerful antidote to such impairment. In other words, there is no reason whatever to believe, and substantial ethical stakes in not acting on the belief, that such self-imposed, psychological pressure is in all cases irreversible and, therefore, irresistible. Physicians should beware of the paternalism, indeed possible sexism, implicit in such a belief.

SUMMARY

In this chapter we have attempted to provide ethical guidance to the application in clinical practice of invasive fetal management. We have done so first by examining the concept of the fetus as patient, in the course of which the distinction between the viable and the previable fetus was found to be ethically significant. We then showed how this distinction should shape the informed consent process and clinical judgment as to when invasive fetal management should reliably be judged to be standard of care and when such management should reliably be judged to be experimental.

References

1. Harrison MR, Golbus MS, Filly RA. The Unborn Patient. New York: Grune & Stratton, 1984.
2. Liley AW. The fetus as a personality. Aust N Zeal J Psych 1972;6:99–105.
3. American Academy of Pediatrics Committee on Bioethics. Fetal therapy: ethical considerations. Pediatrics 1988;81:898–899.
4. American College of Obstetricians and Gynecologists. Committee on Ethics. Patient choice: maternal-fetal conflict. Washington, D.C. American College of Obstetricians and Gynecologists, 1987.
5. American College of Obstetricians and Gynecologists. Technical Bulletin. Ethical decision-making in obstetrics and gynecology. Washington, D.C. American College of Obstetricians and Gynecologists, 1989.
6. Mahoney MJ. Fetal-maternal relationship. In: Reich WT, ed. Encyclopedia of Bioethics, New York: Macmillan, 1978.
7. Fletcher JC. The fetus as patient; ethical issues. JAMA 1981;246:772–773.
8. Pritchard JA, MacDonald PC, Gant NF. Williams Obstetrics. 17th ed. Norwalk: Appleton-Century-Crofts, 1985, xi.
9. Shinn RL. The fetus as patient: a philosophical and ethical perspective. In Milunski A, Annas GJ, eds. Genetics and the Law III New York: Plenum Press, 1985.
10. Murray TH. Moral obligations to the not-yet born: the fetus as patient. Clin Perinatol 1987;14:313–328.
11. Mahoney MJ. The fetus as patient. West J Med 1989;150:517–540.

12. Newton ER. The fetus as patient. Med Clin NA 1989;73:517–540.
13. Walters L. Ethical issues in intrauterine diagnosis and therapy. Fet Ther 1986;1: 32–37.
14. Edelstein L. The Hippocratic oath: text, translation, and interpretation. In: Temkin O, Temkin CL, eds. Ancient medicine: selected papers of Ludwig Edelstein. Baltimore: The John Hopkins Press, 1967, 3–63.
15. Beauchamp TL, Childress JF. Principles of Biomedical Ethics. 3rd ed. New York: Oxford University Press, 1989.
16. Beauchamp TL, McCullough LB. Medical ethics: the moral responsibilities of physicians. Englewood Cliffs: Prentice-Hall, 1984.
17. Faden R, Beauchamp TL. History and theory of informed consent. New York: Oxford University Press, 1986.
18. Ross WD. The Right and the Good. Oxford: Clarendon Press, 1930.
19. Chervenak FA, McCullough LB. Perinatal ethics: a practical method of analysis of obligations to mother and fetus. Obstet Gynecol 1985;66:442–446.
20. Field DR, Gates EA, Creasy RK, et al. Maternal brain death during pregnancy: medical and ethical issues. JAMA 1988; 260:816–822.
21. Engelhardt HT, Jr. The Foundations of Bioethics. New York: Oxford University Press, 1986.
22. Strong C. Ethical conflicts between mother and fetus in obstetrics. Clin Perinatol 1987;14:313–328.
23. Anderson G, Strong C. The premature breech: cesarean section or trial of labor? J Med Ethics 1988;14:18–24.
24. Ford NM. When did I begin? Conception of the human individual in history, philosophy, and science. Cambridge, England: Cambridge University Press, 1988.
25. Strong C, Anderson G. The moral status of the near-term fetus. J Med Ethics 1989; 15:25–27.
26. Fleming L. The moral status of the fetus: a reappraisal. Bioethics 1987;1:15–34.
27. Ruddick W, Wilcox W. Operating on the fetus. Hastings Cent Report 1982;12:10–14.
28. Dunstan GR. The moral status of the human embryo. A tradition recalled. J Med Ethics 1984;10:38–44.
29. Elias S, Annas GJ. Reproductive genetics and the law. Chicago: Year Book Medical Publishers, 1987.
30. Evans MI, Fletcher JC, Zador IE, et al. Selective first-trimester termination in octuplet and quadruplet pregnancies: clinical and ethical issues. Obstet Gynecol 1988; 71:289–296.
31. Curran CE. Abortion: contemporary debate in philosophical and religious ethics. In: Reich WT, ed. Encyclopedia of Bioethics. New York: Macmillan, 1978, 17–26.
32. Noonan JT, ed. The morality of abortion. Cambridge: Harvard University Press, 1970.
33. Hellegers AE. Fetal development. Theological Studies 1970;31:3–9.
34. Noonan JT. A private choice. Abortion in America in the seventies. New York: The Free Press, 1979.
35. Bopp J, ed. Restoring the right to life: the human life amendment. Provo: Brigham Young University, 1984.
36. Bopp J, ed. Human life and health care ethics. Frederick, Maryland: University Publications of America, 1985.
37. Callahan S, Callahan D, eds: Abortion: Understanding Differences. New York: Plenum Press, 1984.
38. Roe v. Wade, 410 US 113 (1973).
39. Warnock M. Do human cells have rights? Bioethics 1987;1:1–14.
40. Hare RM. An ambiguity in Warnock. Bioethics 1987;1:175–178.
41. Fletcher JC. Ethics and trends in applied human genetics. Birth defects: original article series 1983;19:143–158.
42. Fletcher JC. Ethical considerations. In: Harrison MR, Golbus MS, Filly RA, eds. The unborn patient. New York: Grune & Stratton, 159–170.
43. Fost N, Chudwin D, Wikker D. The limited moral significance of fetal viability. Hastings Cent Rep 1980;10:10–13.

44. Mahowald M. Beyond abortion: refusal of cesarean section. Bioethics 1989;3:106–121.

45. Chervenak FA, McCullough LB. Does obstetric ethics have any role in the obstetrician's response to the abortion controversy? Am J Obstet Gynecol 1990;163:1425–1429.

46. Hack M, Fanaroff AA. Outcomes of extremely low birth weight infants between 1982 and 1988. N Engl J Med 1989; 321:1642–1647.

47. McCullough LB. An ethical model for improving the patient-physician relationship. Inquiry 1988;25:454–468.

48. Chervenak FA, McCullough LB. An ethically justified, clinically comprehensive management strategy for third-trimester pregnancies complicated by fetal anomalies. Obstet Gynecol 1990;75:311–316.

49. Chervenak FA, McCullough LB. Clinical guides to preventing ethical conflicts between pregnant women and their physicians. Am J Obstet Gynecol 1990; 162:303–307.

50. Annas GJ. Protecting the liberty of pregnant patients. N Engl J Med 1988;316: 1213–1214.

51. Nelson LJ, Milliken N. Compelled treatment of the pregnant woman: life, liberty, and law in conflict. JAMA 1988;259: 1060–1066.

52. Chervenak FA, McCullough LB. Justified limits on refusing intervention. Hastings Cent Rep 1992;21:12–18.

53. McCullough LB, Chervenack FA. Ethics in Obstetrics and Gynecology. New York: Oxford University Press, 1994.

FETAL BLOOD SAMPLING: NECESSARY INVESTIGATION OR NEEDLESS INVASION?

14

SAVAS M. MENTICOGLOU

Few would deny that the advent of fetal blood sampling under ultrasound guidance has been a "turning point" (1) or a "major force" (2) in the development of fetal medicine and has now made the fetus almost as accessible as the neonate or adult. Fetal blood sampling has become almost "a complementary routine examination" (3) because it is simple and minimally invasive for the mother, it is usually not technically difficult, there is a high success rate in obtaining the sample, the procedure can be performed from the thirteenth week of pregnancy until labor, it is repeatable, it has a low incidence of complications and fetal loss rate, and no other fetal tissue provides such a wealth of cytogenetic, hematological, biochemical, and other information.

Nevertheless, fetal blood sampling is not an innocuous procedure. It would be misleading to claim that it is an inordinately dangerous procedure. Nevertheless, it is equally misleading to suggest that the procedure is little riskier than amniocentesis (4,5). It is not proper to compare the risks of fetal blood sampling, performed in single centers by highly skilled experts under continuous ultrasound guidance usually beyond 20 weeks gestation, with amniocentesis series over a decade old, performed by a pool of individuals without ultrasound guidance and usually done before 20 weeks gestation. Like should be compared with like. In a 10-year period comprising nearly 1000 amniocenteses performed by a team of five individuals for the determination of ΔOD450 for alloimmune disease, there were no fetal losses attributable to the procedure (personal communication, Dr. J. Bowman, Rh Institute, Winnipeg). There are complications associated with fetal blood sampling that by the nature of the procedure must perforce occur with greater frequency than amniocentesis: (1) amnionitis and fetal sepsis (5–12), because

prolonged procedure times and multiple needle insertions are needed more often than with amniocentesis (3,8); (2) fetal death due to cord hematoma even in the absence of transfusions (13–15); (3) fetal exsanguination (16-18); and (4) fetal bradycardia leading to death (3) or to emergency cesarean section (19-21). Indeed, the increased risk of the procedure is acknowledged (by a member of the group that introduced the procedure to North America), by the admonition that the procedure should be performed after fetal viability is reached close to an operating room if an emergency cesarean section becomes necessary for fetal distress (22).

The originator of the technique acknowledges in his hands a procedure-related risk of fetal loss of 0.4% (3). The fetal blood sampling registry reports a procedure-related loss rate of 1% in over 5000 procedures (Fifth International Conference: Percutaneous Fetal Umbilical Blood Sampling, Philadelphia, October 22–23, 1990). Smaller loss rates than this have compelled some authorities to say it is unacceptable to continue performing midforceps, vaginal breech, or macrosomic fetus deliveries. However, it sometimes appears that because fetal blood sampling is a new and exciting procedure, a 1% loss rate per procedure is accepted with equanimity.

In the enthusiasm that greets many new medical procedures, there is a danger that doing the procedure receives more attention than if and when to do the procedure. The value of a procedure is a balance between the information it provides (or the benefit it confers) versus the costs in getting the information or benefit. Many of the benefits of modern medicine would be unavailable if reasonable steps in diagnosis and therapy were withheld because of possible risks. However, from reading the literature and listening to other fetal medicine specialists at conferences and at informal discussions, this writer has received the impression that fetal blood sampling is done too often for unconvincing indications.

Fetal blood sampling under ultrasound guidance is an invaluable technique—if it is used in the right circumstances. The dilemma, of course, is that everyone has different ideas of what the right circumstances are, and this writer acknowledges that much of what follows is a personal opinion. The purpose of this chapter is to inject a cautionary note against the overenthusiastic application of this procedure to what seems like every obstetrical situation.

FETAL BLOOD SAMPLING FOR ALLOIMMUNE HEMOLYTIC DISEASE

The superiority of the intravascular route to transfuse fetuses with alloimmune hemolytic anemia is clear (23). The role of which procedure, fetal blood sampling or amniocentesis, should be used to follow the fetus at risk of significant anemia is not.

In pregnancies at risk for alloimmune hemolytic anemia, some authorities recommend the routine use of fetal blood sampling instead of amniocentesis as early as 18 to 20 weeks gestation (2,4,5,24). The arguments used to favor fetal blood sampling instead of amniocentesis are as follows: (1) if the fetus is negative for the antigen in question, this can be determined with one invasive procedure (the fetal blood sample) and the patient can be discharged to normal care, whereas with amniocentesis, the fetus would be exposed to perhaps four to six unnecessary procedures; and (2) if the fetus is positive for the antigen in question, fetal blood sampling gives an immediate and accurate reflection of the fetal hemoglobin, whereas amniotic fluid ΔOD450 reflects the degree of hemolysis and not necessarily the fetal hemoglobin.

The objection against ΔOD450 determinations is that in a certain proportion of cases, especially in the second trimester, they may give misleading information (24,25). One possibility is that a high zone 2 or zone 3 ΔOD450 may provoke unnecessary treatment of a nonanemic fetus or even of a fetus that is antigen negative. This was a problem more in the era of intraperitoneal transfusions; now such a ΔOD450 reading would quite properly lead to a fetal blood sample to determine fetal blood type and hemoglobin. The more worrisome accusation against ΔOD450 determination is that a low reading may give false reassurance that the fetus is well, whereas there may be severe anemia, even hydrops. Since the presence of ascites and other hydropic changes is detectable with ultrasound, the problem comes down to the possibility of a falsely low ΔOD450 reading when the fetus is severely anemic but not hydropic.

Without question, a single ΔOD450 reading taken in isolation can be misleading, especially in the second trimester. However, in a pregnancy in which one is worried enough to start amniocentesis in the second trimester, one would naturally follow the fetus closely with ultrasound observations and repeated ΔOD450 readings. If there was a recent dramatic rise in maternal antibody titer or if there was a clearly rising upward trend in the ΔOD450 readings in a mother with historically demonstrated virulent antibody, even if the value per se was not in a dangerous zone, then these patients would be selected for fetal blood sampling (see Figure 14-1). For example, one report (24) described seven cases where the ΔOD450 was in Liley zone 2 and gave false reassurance about the fetal condition when, in fact, the fetal hematocrit was low and transfusion or delivery was indicated. However, in five of these seven cases, the anemia was modest (hematocrit $\geq$ 23), and in two cases where

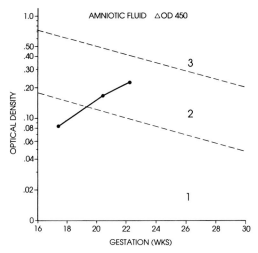

Figure 14-1 Serial ΔOD450 readings. During first pregnancy, mother found to have anti-c, presumably the result of transfusion for tonsillectomy as a child; labor induced at 34 weeks for zone 3 fluid, cord hemoglobin 50 g/L. In the next pregnancy, the previous history and the steep rise in ΔOD450 from 17 to 22 weeks prompted a fetal blood sampling at 23 weeks, even though the ΔOD450 was only 55% zone 2. The fetal hemoglobin was 47 g/L.

the anemia was severe, the trend of ΔOD450 would have prompted a fetal blood sample. In the first case, the hematocrit was found to be 12 at 22 weeks, but the ΔOD450 had risen from zone 1 at 18 weeks to 75% zone 2 at 22 weeks. In the second case, the hematocrit was 16 at 23 weeks; but the ΔOD450 had gone from 60% zone 2 to 80% zone 2 in just one week.

Reliance on serial ΔOD450 and on ultrasound observations of the fetus with selected instead of routine fetal blood sampling may risk identifying the fetus for transfusion when he is more anemic or even has mild ascites. However, this is not a serious problem in terms of ultimate outcome because, unlike the situation with intraperitoneal transfusion where the sicker the fetus, the less effective the treatment, with intravascular transfusion, the outcome is

good as long as the fetus is not moribund to start with (23).

Although the use of routine fetal blood sampling may eliminate some of the empiricism of ultrasound observation and serial ΔOD450 readings, there are certain disadvantages. A routine blood sample at 18 to 22 weeks means exposing the fetus to what is probably a greater risk than would an amniocentesis at the same gestation. If the fetus is antigen-negative, it is not known whether having one procedure which is more invasive is safer than perhaps several amniocenteses. If the fetus is antigen-positive but not anemic, one has not gained much since multiple blood samples or amnioceteses will still be needed. In one center of excellence (5), there were three procedure-related deaths in 19 cases where routine fetal blood sampling was performed for the determination of fetal antigen and anemia in the second trimester. Although this high loss rate is the exception rather than the rule, it certainly indicates that fetal blood sampling in the early secondtrimester is potentially risky. Even if there is no direct procedure-related complication, there remains the definite risk of accidentally aggravating a mild or moderate hemolytic anemia, which seems more common with fetal blood sampling than with amniocentesis (26–28). A fetomaternal hemorrhage could induce further maternal sensitization to fetal antigens and aggravate mild disease to serious disease or oblige earlier transfusions than would otherwise be necessary in cases of more serious disease. Examples of such calamities, with their ominous implications for subsequent pregnancies, are illustrated in Figures 14-2 and 14-3.

The case for routine fetal blood sampling in alloimmune hemolytic anemia is not established. At this time, it is not clear that the increased information provided by fetal blood sampling and the possible reduction

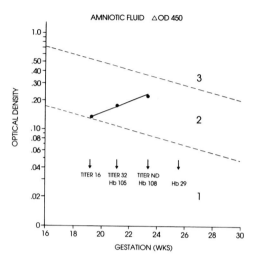

Figure 14-2 Hazard of fetal blood sampling. Mother sensitized, presumably as a result of multiple blood products received for severe burns when a small child. At 19 weeks gestation anti-D titer 16, ΔOD450 at zone 1- zone 2 boundary. At 21 weeks, titer 32, ΔOD450 30% zone 2, and fetal blood sampling showed a hemoglobin of 105 g/L, bilirubin 25 μmol/L. At 23 4/7 weeks, titer not done, ΔOD450 60% zone 2, fetal hemoglobin 108 g/L, bilirubin 35 μmol/L. The post procedure Kleihauer was positive. At next evaluation at 25 4/7 weeks, the fetus was moribund with ascites. Fetal hemoglobin was 29 g/L and fetus died during attempted transfusion. Titer 2048. The dramatic increase in titer may well have been precipitated by the fetal blood samples at 21 and 23 1/2 weeks.

in the number of procedures needed in some cases compensate for the increased risk per procedure and the chances of making the disease worse.

FETAL BLOOD SAMPLING FOR ULTRASOUND-DETECTED MALFORMATIONS

In many series, the most frequent use of fetal blood sampling has been to obtain a rapid karyotype. The advantage of fetal

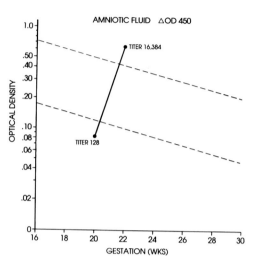

Figure 14-3 Hazard of fetal blood sampling. Mother found to be sensitized at end of first pregnancy. In next pregnancy, anti-D-titer 128 at 20 weeks, unsuccessful attempts to obtain fetal blood sample, ΔOD450 0.084. One week later (21 weeks), titer 16,384. At 22 weeks, fetus had ascites, ΔOD450 0.626. Fetus dead by time of arrival in our unit 12 hours later. The massive rise in titer between 20 and 21 weeks and the dramatic rise in ΔOD450 were probably the consequences of the attempted fetal blood sampling.

blood sampling over amniocentesis is that the karyotype from fetal lymphocytes is available in two to three days instead of the possibly two- to three-week wait from cultured amniocytes.

There are certain structural malformations detectable with ultrasound that are associated with a high likelihood of fetal chromosomal abnormality; examples are cystic hygroma, omphalocele, duodenal atresia, heart anomaly, obstructive uropathy, and nonimmune hydrops (29–31). If the anomaly is thought to be consistent with postnatal surgical repair and/or survival, then a karyotype is important to management (32). An abnormal karyotype may obviate the need for cesarean section for fetal indications or the need to deliver in a referral center away from home.

The desirability of a karyotype in these instances, however, does not mean that the riskier procedure of fetal blood sampling should be automatically chosen over amniocentesis. The discovery of a ventricular septal defect or an omphalocele at 28 weeks in a patient not in threatened premature labor is unlikely to impact on obstetrical management for many weeks. There would seem to be little urgency in obtaining the karyotype within 72 hours and little to be lost by waiting for the results from amniocentesis. This conservative approach is especially important when the indication for obtaining the karyotype is associated with only a marginal risk of chromosomal anomaly, for example, isolated hydramnios, isolated unilateral hydronephrosis, single umbilical artery without other anomaly, or isolated choroid plexus cysts. As an example, one study (33) suggests that the finding of an enlarged fetal renal pelvis (pyelectasis) is associated with a 3.3% incidence of Down's syndrome, so it may be argued that a karyotype is desirable for obstetric management. Leave aside for a moment the fact that the fetus in no way benefits from having its karyotype known. Suppose this ultrasound finding is detected in a normally-grown fetus without other anomalies at 33 weeks gestation and the fetus is in cephalic presentation. Assume the likelihood of premature labor before 36 weeks is 3% and the chance of needing a cesarean section for fetal indications is 10%. Assume, furthermore, the morally questionable position that a cesarean section would not be done for fetal indications if the fetus were known to have Down's syndrome. The chance that this fetus would have Down's syndrome and that premature labor would ensue before the results of the karyotype from amniocentesis

were available and that an otherwise necessary cesarean section would be avoided for the mother would be

$$\frac{1}{30} \times \frac{1}{33} \times \frac{1}{10} = \frac{1}{9900}.$$

Estimates of this nature can be derived for various combinations of the type of anomaly, the stage of gestation and likelihood of premature delivery, and the likelihood that obstetrical circumstances or the type of anomaly may lead to a cesarean section. This estimate should always be set against the risk of the fetal blood sampling procedure. One should always ask oneself how often the 10 or 14 days difference between rapid karyotype from fetal blood sampling and from amniocentesis will actually benefit the mother; it will almost never benefit the fetus.

Discussions elsewhere have considered the benefits of cordocentesis over amniocentesis to be marginal in many situations (34,35). Indeed, there are only three clinical scenarios where a rapid karyotype from fetal blood sampling for structural malformations may be warranted. The first is where the nature of the anomaly, e.g., obstructive uropathy, obstructive hydrocephalus, diaphragmatic hernia, sacrococcygeal teratoma, may prompt consideration of in utero surgical interventions, which carry much higher risks to fetus and mother than the blood sampling procedure itself. The second is the detection of a serious anomaly, such as hydrocephalus or omphalocele, quite late in the pregnancy, when the knowledge of the karyotype may significantly impact on the likelihood of a cesarean section being done. The third is the discovery of a fetal anomaly (or the presentation of a woman at increased risk for chromosomal anomaly because of age or low serum alpha-fetoprotein) very close to the legal limit of termination, where the results of amniocentesis may be available too late. The fact that fetal blood sampling is now feasible as early as 12 weeks gestation (1,36) should not lead to the temptation to use it as a substitute for amniocentesis at early gestations. The contention that a fetal blood sampling for karyotype at 17 weeks gestation for, say, advanced maternal age is better than amniocentesis because if termination were chosen, it would be easier at 17 weeks than at 20 weeks is only theoretic (37), since maternal risks of termination are largely the same at these gestations, and procedure-related fetal loss rates are higher than after amniocentesis (1,38).

Indeed, if it is urgent to obtain a rapid karyotype, it may be preferable to obtain a placental biopsy for direct chromosomal preparation; whether this is safer than fetal blood sampling is not clear. Furthermore, new culturing techniques for amniotic fluid can reduce markedly the time required to get a karyotype. By means of sampling single mitotic cells from growing amniotic fluid cultures ("pipette method") a reliable karyotype can be obtained in five to seven days (39,40).

FETAL BLOOD SAMPLING FOR EVALUATION OF HYPOXEMIA AND ACIDEMIA

Just as fetal scalp sampling is used to assess fetal well-being during labor, so fetal blood sampling under ultrasound guidance has been proposed to assess fetal health before labor, especially in cases of small-for-gestational-age (SGA) fetuses. It is now generally known that some fetuses may be chronically hypoxemic and/or acidotic before labor (41–43). The identification of such

a fetus before antepartum death or damage occurs or before the additional stress of labor is added is important. The whole essence of antepartum fetal monitoring is to identify which fetus is sick now or is going to get sick soon. Fetal blood sampling would, at first sight, appear to be the most direct way to make this determination. However, if one accepts that there are fetal risks associated with fetal blood sampling, then this invasive procedure is justified only if it provides not only more accurate but also more useful information than less invasive or noninvasive methods of assessing the fetus. Fetal blood sampling must be measured against the more commonly used methods—the nonstress test [NST], the biophysical score [BPS], and Doppler analysis of the fetal circulation.

There is no compelling reason to perform fetal blood sampling to assess the fetal oxygenation and acid-base status when the NST is reactive or the BPS is normal. Fetal death after a reactive NST is a most unusual occurrence (44,45), usually related to a factor other than that for which testing was undertaken and, even more so, when the amniotic fluid volume is assessed and is also normal (46,47). Similarly, when the BPS is normal, fetal death is very rare (48,49). In a study (50) of 67 SGA third trimester fetuses where the antepartum fetal heart rate (FHR) pattern was correlated with blood gas values obtained at fetal blood sampling, none of the 52 fetuses with a reactive pattern by 60 minutes of recording were acidotic, although four were mildly hypoxemic. In another study (51) of 14 severely growth-retarded fetuses, a reactive FHR tracing was always associated with a pH > 2.5th centile. One study (42) related the results of the fetal biophysical profile with the umbilical cord arterial pH at the time of elective cesarean section and found that if the acute markers of fetal condition (NST, fetal breathing movements, fetal gross body movements, and fetal tone) were all normal, then the fetus was never acidotic.

When the NST is truly nonreactive [false-positives having been eliminated by extended testing time (52–54) and allowance made for interpretation at early gestational ages (55–57)] and the nonreactivity cannot be accounted for by maternal drug intoxication, fetal anemia, or fetal anomaly, then the fetus is very likely to be seriously compromised (41,52–54). If ultrasound observation at this point shows, in addition, the absence of fetal breathing movements and gross body movements during a 60-minute observation (BPS, 0 to 4, depending on the volume of amniotic fluid and the presence or absence of fetal tone), then the fetus is almost certain to be severely acidotic (42,58). Between 24 and 28 weeks, healthy fetuses never go more than 24 minutes without gross body movements; indeed, absence of body movements for more than 15 minutes is extremely rare before 30 weeks (59,60). Beyond 30 weeks, the longest period a healthy fetus will go without moving is 75 minutes, and there is a 99% chance of seeing gross body movements within a 45-minute time period (61). Prolonged fetal inactivity as assessed by a nonreactive NST and corroborated by ultrasound observation indicates that the fetus is sick. Fetal blood sampling for blood gas analysis is not needed to tell us this.

It can be argued, however, that if a test of fetal well-being has no gradation between normoxemia and severe acidosis, between good health and serious compromise, the result is only black or white, if at the first sign of abnormality, the fetus is about to die, then, in this case, the test is not a reliable method of predicting forthcoming impairment, and this is where fetal blood gas analysis can play a role. However, just as fetuses usually do not die quickly, without

warning, but deteriorate over days, so this deterioration is reflected in the NST and BPS. The healthy fetus has organized flurries of activity reflected in normal variability with frequent accelerations that fuse; as deterioration occurs, the accelerations become widely spaced with decreased variability; then, occasional late or variable decelerations appear; and finally, accelerations disappear completely (41,62,63). One study (50) showed that whereas a normal reactive FHR pattern can sometimes be present with a fetal pO_2 value in the lower normal range, moderate to severe fetal hypoxemia is associated with changes in the FHR pattern before severe acidosis occurs. Similarly, work relating the fetal BPS to umbilical cord artery pH at the time of elective cesarean section (42) and to blood gas values at fetal blood sampling in severely growth-retarded fetuses (51) shows that the BPS can predict the degree of fetal acidosis, with mild acidosis reflected in a loss of FHR reactivity and loss of fetal breathing movements first, and only in advanced acidosis are fetal gross body movements and tone compromised.

Further information about fetal oxygenation is available noninvasively. Amniotic fluid volume reflects the chronic state of fetal well-being (64); a reduced or absent amount indicates that the fetus is producing less urine and less lung fluid, presumably from redistribution of cardiac output away from the kidneys and lungs consequent to hypoxemia (65–67). Possibly, a more precise reflection of the current state of fetal oxygenation is to estimate, by ultrasound observation of changing bladder volumes, the actual urine output per hour. It has been shown that the worse the hypoxemia, the lower the hourly fetal urine output (68). Similarly, examining the fetal blood flow velocity waveforms of the umbilical artery, descending aorta, and cerebral vessels can indicate whether redistribution of blood flow is occurring, again presumably due to chronic hypoxia (69–71). Using a combination of the BPS, observation of bladder filling, and Doppler studies, one can obtain within 30 to 60 minutes a very good indication of fetal oxygenation.

It may be argued that this approach is too empiric; that the exact "scientific" knowledge of the fetal pO_2, PCO_2, and pH obtainable through fetal blood sampling is preferable and can provide a better guide to management. However, it is very arguable whether a single biochemical measurement can provide a better description of the fetal condition than careful observation of fetal behavior. The problem with fetal blood sampling is that it gives us information at only one point in time; therefore, one cannot predict how fast the fetus is going to become too sick to stay in utero. Serial fetal blood samplings do not seem to be as practical an approach as careful serial observations of the fetus; and the fetus that one is worried about enough to perform a fetal blood sampling (because of, say, severe intrauterine growth retardation or absent end-diastolic velocity) is the fetus that one should be worried about enough to examine once or even twice a day.

The few cases detailed in the literature where fetal blood sampling was performed to determine fetal acid-base status illustrate that, generally, the procedure was either unnecessary or misleading. One report (72) described three cases of fetal blood gas analysis for abnormal FHR patterns. In one case, the blood sample was performed because of ambiguities in the FHR tracing at 24 weeks gestation; the result was reassuring, but even though interpretation of FHR tracings at this gestation is indeed often problematic, the ambiguity could probably have been resolved by ultrasound observation of fetal gross body movements (56,59). In the

second case, a blood sample was done because of numerous late decelerations during tocolytic treatment of premature labor at 27 weeks; although the results were normal, an urgent cesarean had to be done anyway 24 hours later because of a sustained fetal bradycardia, emphasizing, as the authors note, that fetal blood gas analysis reflects fetal status at the time of sampling only and does not obviate the need for continued careful fetal surveillance when conditions are changing. In the third case, a BPS of 0 at 29 weeks prompted a fetal blood sampling for blood gas analysis and showed the fetus to be severely hypoxemic and acidotic, an entirely predictable result (58). What would the authors of the report have done if the blood gas results were normal, but repeated observation still showed a BPS of 0? A recent case in our unit emphasized for us the greater value of observing the fetus rather than paying attention to numbers. A woman with ruptured membranes at 27 weeks was being treated expectantly in hospital. She complained of decreased fetal movement, and a one hour BPS was 0. An emergency cesarean section was performed without prior fetal blood sampling, and we were chagrined when the umbilical cord blood gases were normal, thinking that we had delivered a 27-week fetus needlessly. The explanation for the BPS of 0 became evident when the neonate showed the clinical features of sepsis and the blood culture at birth was positive for E. coli. Had one done a fetal blood sample and obtained a normal blood gas result, there may have been lethal procrastination.

Another investigator (73) performed fetal blood sampling in 10 fetuses less than 32 weeks gestation with severe growth retardation and "pathological" FHR tracings. In two fetuses, the pH was normal and urgent delivery by cesarean was avoided. In these two cases, the FHR tracing improved over the subsequent hours, and the authors acknowledge that a biophysical profile would probably have clarified the situation and avoided the need for fetal blood sampling or cesarean section for a false-positive FHR trace. In another report (74), fetal blood sampling was performed in six fetuses with absent or reversed flow in the umbilical artery, and five fetuses were found to be acidotic by nonlaboring norms; however, all five fetuses had either a BPS ≤ 4 or a positive oxytocin challenge test, and the sixth nonacidotic fetus developed overt fetal acidosis and distress on the FHR tracing within a week. One writer (75) described a fetal blood sampling done at 27 weeks because of severe preeclampsia and absent end-diastolic velocity in the umbilical artery and aorta. The pH was 7.36 in the umbilical vein, but three days later, an urgent cesarean section had to be done because of repetitive late decelerations on the NST and the umbilical vein pH was 7.04. Again, this illustrates that, in some cases, an extended margin of safety cannot be guaranteed with any test (NST, BPS, fetal blood gas analysis) when there is worsening maternal disease or other changing conditions, and if one is worried enough to do a fetal blood sample, one will have to watch the fetus very carefully even if the blood gas result is normal.

It is this writer's judgment that the obstetrician with extensive experience in assessing the welfare of the fetus by FHR testing, ultrasound observation of fetal activity and amniotic fluid volume, and Doppler waveform analysis of the fetal circulation will almost never need to resort to fetal blood sampling to determine if and when to intervene. Fetuses who are going to get sick in utero generally get sick gradually, and the obstetrician gets a better sense of when to intervene by watching the fetus closely than by doing a fetal blood sample at one point in this progression. Indeed, a recent study (76)

concluded that acid-base determination could not predict outcome in growth-retarded fetuses.

In the end, the real question comes down to this: even if mild fetal hypoxia or acidosis is present when conventional tests of fetal well-being are normal, does it matter (4)? The NST and BPS reflect fetal brain function and are probably more important than blood gas results from the umbilical cord. However, if it does turn out that fetal hypoxemia is causing some intrauterine neurological damage even when the NST and biophysical profile are normal, then perhaps, fetal blood gas analysis will be useful. Or, if watching the fetus closely means waiting sometimes until fetal motility is reduced (77) or there are FHR changes (50), if this also leads to some neurological damage, then again, fetal blood sampling may become important. However, one would have to weigh this possible (and, for now, still theoretic) advantage for some fetuses against the appreciable number of invasive procedures that would have to be done needlessly in healthy fetuses and the probable appreciable rise in prematurity related morbidity and mortality to which such an approach would give rise (50).

FETAL BLOOD SAMPLING FOR EVALUATION OF PLATELET COUNT

The thrombocytopenic fetus is at risk of intracranial hemorrhage. For perinatal alloimmune thrombocytopenia, the reasons to use fetal blood sampling to diagnose thrombocytopenia are logical and compelling; for autoimmune thrombocytopenia, the role of fetal blood sampling is unsettled.

Perinatal alloimmune thrombocytopenia (PAIT) is caused by a platelet-incompatible situation between the mother and the fetus that has resulted in immunization of the mother against fetal platelets and consequent fetal thrombocytopenia. The thrombocytopenia is usually already present by mid-gestation (78). Intracranial hemorrhage occurs in some 25% of cases and usually leads to death or serious neurologic sequelae. Many of these instances of intracranial hemorrhage occur remote from term and cannot be prevented by elective cesarean section before labor. In one study (79) of 130 cases of PAIT, 10% were associated with antepartum intracranial bleeding, evident by third trimester ultrasonography or at birth, when ultrasound or computed tomographic examination of the neonatal head revealed hydrocephalus or porencephalic cyst. Another report (80) identified at least five instances of in utero intracranial hemorrhage among 88 cases of PAIT. If a woman has had one child affected with PAIT, the recurrence rate is 88% (81). Such a high recurrence rate and serious frequent sequelae would, however, only justify prenatal diagnosis by blood sampling immediately before delivery (to plan for mode of delivery)—if no efficient treatment could be offered earlier in pregnancy. However, since antenatal therapy is available—either frequent platelet transfusions to the fetus (82,83) or administration of IVIgG and/or dexamethasone to the mother (84)—that may raise the fetal platelet count and prevent these bad fetal outcomes, fetal blood sampling becomes not only justified but necessary to properly manage these cases.

Less certain is the role of fetal blood sampling in women who are at risk of delivering a child with PAIT but who have not had an affected child. It is estimated that in a Caucasian population the incidence of at-risk PL^{A1}-negative pregnancies (a PL^{A1}-negative mother with PL^{A1}-positive fetus) is about one in 50, and in about half of affected families, it is the first PL^{A1}-positive child who is affected (79,80). If a screening program to identify women having the at risk phenotype were instituted (85), the question would arise whether fetal blood sampling to identify the small percent of thrombocytopenic fetuses would be justified, not only because of the direct procedure-related risks of sampling but also because sampling may risk immunizing a woman not yet immunized.

In cases of autoimmune thrombocytopenia (ITP), the case for fetal blood sampling is not plain to see. Antepartum intracranial hemorrhage is exceedingly rare in the fetuses of mothers with ITP. Therefore, if there is a role for fetal blood sampling to determine fetal platelet count, it would be near the time of delivery, so that the mode of delivery, cesarean section or vaginal, can be planned. An important point is to avoid fetal blood sampling in cases of "pseudo" or "gestational" ITP, where mild maternal thrombocytopenia has been detected by routine lab tests (86–90). Several studies have shown that in asymptomatic pregnant women who are thrombocytopenic but have no history of ITP, the chance of delivering a neonate with a platelet count <50,000 is practically zero (86,88,89). In one report (19) of 21 fetal blood samplings performed to evaluate fetal platelet counts in pregnant patients with presumed ITP, only four women had a bona fide history of ITP. In another report (91) of 19 fetal blood samplings for this indication, 12 of 19 women were identified through prenatal screening, although the subsequent course in two of these 12 women suggests that they had the real disease. Although unexpected asymptomatic thrombocytopenia in the mother can be consistent with a diagnosis of ITP, the likelihood that this is indeed the case and that the fetus will be thrombocytopenic

Table 14-1   Frequency of Thrombocytopenia at
Birth when Mother has ITP

Study	Number patients with history ITP before pregnancy	Number of newborns with platelet count <50,000
Samuels (89)	88	18
Christiaens (93)	28	2
Burrows (94)	61	3
Ballem (95)	24	7

and that the fetus will be injured during delivery is almost certainly less than the risks of fetal blood sampling.

In bona fide cases of ITP, the dilemma is that we do not have clear answers to the most basic questions (92): (1) how often do pregnant women with ITP deliver thrombocytopenic infants? and (2) how often do these thrombocytopenic infants have intracranial hemorrhage develop as a result of the birth process? The results of four recent reports (89,93–95) with respect to the first question are summarized in Table 14-1. The answer to the second question is even more difficult. It is difficult to find reports of intracranial hemorrhage in infants of mothers with ITP. It is not clear if this is because of a reluctance to report bad outcomes, because intracranial hemorrhage is rare even if the thrombocytopenic fetus is delivered vaginally, or because, perhaps, most women with ITP are delivered by cesarean section. However, a recent report (89) of 88 women with a history of ITP before pregnancy showed that the only two cases of neonatal intracranial hemorrhage occurred among the 17 women delivered vaginally, and in both cases the neonatal platelet count on the day of delivery was <100,000. Therefore, it seems the risk of intracranial hemorrhage is real and, notwithstanding a recent report

(94) that does not even recommend fetal scalp platelet sampling in labor let alone antepartum fetal blood sampling, some estimate of fetal platelet count is desirable before allowing vaginal delivery.

The choice is between fetal blood sampling before labor starts and fetal scalp platelet count in labor once the cervix has dilated sufficiently and the head is low enough in the pelvis to perform the procedure. A purported advantage (19,91) of antepartum fetal blood sampling over intrapartum fetal scalp sampling is that several hours of latent phase labor may be needed before fetal scalp sampling is feasible and this labor may cause an intracranial hemorrhage that would have been avoidable with fetal blood sampling. This writer suspects this argument is describing theory more than reality. A more telling argument in favor of fetal blood sampling is that it is likely to lead to fewer cesarean sections for mothers with ITP; because fetal scalp platelet sampling is difficult to perform and because it often leads to falsely low fetal platelet counts (94,96,97), many inappropriate cesarean sections are done. However, fetal blood sampling should ideally be judged not by its maternal benefits but by its fetal risks and benefits. Fetal blood sampling is not risk-free to the fetus (or to the mother). When blood sampling has been done for this indication, emergency cesarean section has been necessary in some cases because of severe fetal bradycardia (19,20,98). A reasonable compromise is as follows. If the blood sample looks like it will be straightforward to get, e.g., because of a clearly visible target through an anterior placenta, and the procedure is going easily and emergency cesarean section is available in the event of a problem, then fetal blood sampling is reasonable to attempt. However, if one anticipates or encounters any difficulty, it is better to desist and to opt for scalp sampling in labor. Common sense is more important in this case than to do the test that appears most scientific and fashionable.

FETAL BLOOD SAMPLING FOR NONIMMUNE HYDROPS FETALIS

Nonimmune hydrops fetalis (NIHF) has been described as "an obvious indication for fetal blood sampling" (99). This is probably because hydrops fetalis is a nonspecific finding of many fetal abnormalities and diseases, and fetal blood sampling makes possible the diagnosis of some of its diverse chromosomal, hematologic, infectious, and metabolic etiologies. Furthermore, NIHF is often an indication that the life of the fetus is in danger and quick diagnosis is felt to be imperative.

Nevertheless, a few cautions are in order. Some authorities (100) continue to include as cases of NIHF some fetuses with pleural effusions only or ascites only, without edema. A unilateral pleural effusion is not an emergency, and one can usually wait for the karyotype result from amniocentesis. Ascites alone can have the same etiology as hydrops fetalis and may sometimes be its earliest manifestation, but often intraperitoneal fluid is the result of local intra-abdominal causes, e.g., ruptured bladder or kidney, perforated intestinal or-gans, ruptured ovarian cyst, spontaneous chyloperitoneum (101), or, sometimes, an isolated finding of transient nature (102). Even when ascites is an early manifestation of a more systemic problem, such as an in utero infection, congenital heart anomaly (103), or lupus serositis (104), ascites is not as immediately life-threatening as is NIHF, and one usually has time to discover the etiology by the less invasive means of examining ma-ternal blood, careful ultrasound examination and amniocentesis.

When one has a bona fide case of NIHF but ultrasound reveals an obvious structural malformation or syndrome, the outlook for fetal/neonatal survival is very bleak (100,105,106), whether the karyotype is normal or not. One may argue that, in these cases, fetal blood sampling is not going to make things any worse, but if the fetus is going to die anyway, there is no point having the death blamed on the procedure. Indeed, if one gets severe bradycardia or excessive bleeding as a result of the procedure, the sudden emergency may prompt an urgent cesarean section that more sober reflection would avoid. The only ultrasound visible structural abnormalities associated with NIHF that seem to offer some hope of survival are not malformations, but tumors, cases of space-occupying thoracic lesions (107) or sacrococcygeal teratomas (108,109), and these are not associated with chromosomal anomalies often enough to warrant karyotype by fetal blood sampling—unless in utero surgery is planned.

One of the two causes of NIHF with reasonable prospects for survival is fetal tachycardia in the absence of associated cardiac structural malformations. Fetal blood sampling is unnecessary in these cases. It may be helpful to determine fetal thyroid status with blood sampling in the rare case of maternal Graves' disease treated with thyroidectomy or radioactive ablation in the past, although an empiric trial of maternal antithyroid medication is probably warranted in these cases. In the more usual cases of supraventricular tachycardia, in cases where rhythm control is difficult to achieve, there may be a strong temptation to treat directly via the fetal intravascular route. However, unless the fetus is hydropic and moribund, this temptation should be resisted as direct administration of antiarrhythmic drugs to the fetus can result in irreversible fetal asystole (110,111). Indeed, in these situations, intraperitoneal administration of drugs is effective and safe (112).

There is one circumstance where fetal blood sampling must be done. This is in cases of NIHF where maternal serum studies, ultrasound, echocardiography, and FHR monitoring have not revealed an etiology, that is, one has a case of idiopathic hydrops. The concern is that one not miss the second very treatable cause of NIHF, namely, fetal anemia, due either to fetomaternal hemorrhage (113,114) or human parvovirus B19 infection (115–118). Although one would anticipate most cases of fetomaternal hemorrhage to be detectable by Kleihauer-Betke staining, it is possible that in situations of maternal-fetal ABO incompatibility, there may be no fetal cells left in the circulation. Similarly, although one would think that fetal anemia due to B19 infection would be associated with maternal serology positive for IgM, by the time fetal hydrops appears, the IgM may have disappeared (118,119).

FETAL BLOOD SAMPLING FOR ACQUIRED FETAL INFECTION

The value of fetal blood sampling in cases of possible fetal infection depends on the particular infection under consideration.

With respect to rubella, at first consideration, there does not appear to be any benefit to the fetus by fetal blood sampling. If the individual fetus turns out not to be infected, then he has been exposed to the risk of the procedure without benefit to himself. If the fetus is infected, there is no available treatment and he is likely to be aborted. However, the ability provided by fetal blood sampling to discriminate with reasonable reliability between infected and noninfected fetus (by measurement of rubella-specific

IgM between 20 and 24 weeks) will probably save many more noninfected fetuses, which might otherwise have been aborted (120–122), than will be lost by the procedure itself.

The same applies with respect to toxoplasmosis infection. In infected mothers treated with spiramycin, more than 90% of fetuses will not be infected (123). But, the consequences of fetal infection can be so disastrous for the fetus that, if there was not a reasonable assurance that the fetus was not infected, many noninfected fetuses would be aborted (124). Although most cases of congenital toxoplasmosis can be identified by inoculation of amniotic fluid into mice or by tissue culture using amniotic fluid samples (125,126), in some cases *T. gondii* is detected only in fetal blood (127), so fetal blood sampling is necessary for the time being if the maximum number of cases are to be identified. In addition to preventing the termination of noninfected fetuses, the documentation that a fetus has been infected justifies the use of additional antiparasite medication, namely, the combination of pyrimethamine and sulfonamide, since the proven consequences of fetal infection are more serious than the theoretical risks of teratogenicity for the fetus (124,128).

Fetal blood sampling has very little role in the diagnosis of fetal cytomegalovirus (CMV) infection. Amniocentesis and culture of the amniotic fluid for the virus is easy and safe and gives a result within days. In infants with congenital infection, whether symptomatic or not, viruria is universal at birth (129,130) so that one would expect that amniotic fluid, which is largely composed of fetal urine, would be positive for CMV if the fetus were infected. This supposition has been borne out in a recent review (131). If an initial amniotic fluid culture were negative but further assurance were needed, this would probably be better achieved by further negative amniotic fluid cultures than by a single negative fetal blood serology test.

There is no compelling reason to perform fetal blood sampling in pregnant women with syphilis; this is an example of doing a test for curiosity's sake (132). The mother has to be treated regardless of the fetal result, and the treatment for the mother is also the appropriate treatment for the fetus.

There is also very little role for fetal blood sampling in pregnancies complicated by maternal B19 parvovirus infection. In a prospective study (133) of 39 pregnant women with recent B19 paravovirus infection, the only adverse outcome possibly related to the infection was one spontaneous abortion. Human B19 parvovirus infection does not appear to cause congenital defects, so it is not essential to determine if the fetus is infected. What is important is to perform very frequent ultrasound examinations in order to detect fetal ascites, the precursor of hydrops. This finding mandates fetal blood sampling because it may indicate the fetus is anemic as a result of the infection and may benefit from transfusions.

The role of fetal blood sampling in HIV-seropositive mothers is very problematic. As with rubella and toxoplasmosis, if fetal blood tests suggest the fetus is not infected, then elective abortion of noninfected fetuses would be limited (134). However, there are some problems. One is that since studies of cord blood at birth have failed to identify all babies who developed immunodeficiency in the first years of life, fetal blood studies may similarly miss instances of infected fetuses (134,135). As well, the fetus may become infected after the sampling is done. More telling an argument against fetal blood sampling, however, may be the risk that a previously noninfected fetus could be infected by exposure to maternal blood at the time of the sampling (135,136).

FETAL BLOOD SAMPLING FOR INTRAUTERINE GROWTH RETARDATION (IUGR) AND ABNORMAL AMNIOTIC FLUID VOLUMES

In the case of severe oligohydramnios without visible fetal kidneys or bladder at a gestation where extrauterine survival is possible, the two possible diagnoses have completely different implications for the fetus and the mother. If renal agenesis is responsible for the findings, the fetal outlook is hopeless and interventions on fetal behalf that may jeopardize the mother are unwarranted. If, however, the explanation for the ultrasound findings is a seriously compromised fetus that is redistributing blood flow away from structurally normal kidneys (65,66,137), then urgent delivery, probably by cesarean section, is necessary for fetal indications. This writer has made a false-positive diagnosis of renal agenesis, and this has been reported by others (138,139). Since the consequence of such a false-positive diagnosis of renal agenesis is that a salvageable fetus may be "written off," it is imperative that efforts be made to disprove the diagnosis of renal agenesis. This may require artificial instillation of amniotic fluid (140) or intraperitoneal infusion of fluid (141). If these do not demonstrate fetal kidneys, then one should consider the infusion of saline and furosemide directly into the fetal circulation (32). In these cases, if the alternative is to make a diagnosis of renal agenesis, there is nothing to lose and possibly something to gain by invading the fetal circulation. At a *previable* gestation, a precise diagnosis is unnecessary and invasive tests are best deferred. If the reason for the oligohydramnios and nonvisualized kidneys and bladder is fetal compromise, the fetus is likely to die within a few days and there is no point in having the death blamed on the invasive procedure.

The same reasoning applies to fetal blood sampling for karyotype or blood gas studies in fetuses with early severe IUGR, with or without oligohydramnios. If the fetus is thought to be too immature or too small to deliver even if the chromosomes are normal or the blood gas studies abnormal, then doing this risky procedure for curiosity's sake is unconscionable. Either one should wait until a gestation or size is reached when one would intervene for fetal reasons, or one should do a placental biopsy, which is probably less risky than a blood sample for compromised fetuses (142). This writer thinks there are two circumstances where one could reasonably argue for fetal blood sampling in cases of early severe IUGR without evident structural anomalies. If there is a strong suspicion of triploidy, either on the basis of placental architecture or maternal signs of preeclampsia, then an early karyotype is warranted lest the mother be subjected needlessly to the risks of preeclampsia by continuing to carry a pregnancy with a hopeless outlook. As well, if maternal oxygen administration turns out to be beneficial in fetuses with early severe IUGR, then fetal blood sampling to evaluate whether an improvement in fetal oxygenation is achieved would be imperative before subjecting the mother to this prolonged therapy.

Fetal blood sampling for IUGR detected in the third trimester is problematic. When there is an obvious maternal cause, such as preeclampsia, cyanotic heart disease, or lupus anticoagulant, the procedure is unnecessary. Even without a maternal cause, a third trimester IUGR fetus free of structural malformations is very unlikely to have a chromosomal anomaly (31,111). If a karyotype is nevertheless thought necessary, an amniotic fluid specimen will generally be satisfactory. If there is no amniotic fluid available or if the fetal condition is thought to be so precarious as to preclude waiting for amniotic fluid results and one feels that a karyotype is necessary before recommending delivery, then one should proceed to a placental biopsy since a direct preparation of placental villi can provide a result within hours, and this approach minimizes the risk of a chromosomally normal fetus dying during the wait for the karyotype results from cultured lymphocytes, as has been reported (76).

The combination of severe IUGR and hydramnios is unusual and sometimes indicates a serious chromosomal abnormality (29), although if this were the case, some sort of structural anomaly would probably be evident (143). One should base one's decision on whether to proceed with amniocentesis or blood sampling for karyotype by judging how likely a decision for delivery is to arise before amniotic fluid results are available.

Hydramnios as the sole abnormal ultrasound finding does not warrant fetal blood sampling. Although one writer (99) found that two of four fetuses evaluated for hydramnios using fetal blood sampling had a karyotype abnormality, this seems to be an unusual situation. One series (144) identified only one abnormal karyotype in 59 sonographically-identified cases of idiopathic hydramnios and another series (31), only one out of 61. If a karyotype is thought necessary, the safer procedure, amniocentesis, is preferable in view of the low yield of abnormal karyotypes.

FETAL BLOOD SAMPLING FOR THE EVALUATION OF MEDICAL THERAPY

There are certain situations where fetal blood sampling is indicated to monitor the effect of various therapeutic interventions.

This is because it is unreasonable to subject the mother to the inconvenience, e.g., of prolonged maternal hyperoxygenation for severe fetal IUGR (145), or the risks, e.g., of corticosteroid use in an attempt to improve fetal platelet count in ITP (146,147), if the efficacy of the treatment is uncertain. In other cases, the efficacy of maternal drug treatment, e.g., the use of maternal digoxin administration for fetal tachycardia, can be observed directly with ultrasound or be ascertained by less invasive means, e.g., by measurement of amniotic fluid 17-OH progesterone in cases of dexamethasone treatment of congenital adrenal hyperplasia, making fetal blood sampling superfluous.

The role of fetal blood sampling for this sort of indication can be profitably examined in cases of possible fetal thyrotoxicosis. If a pregnant woman has been treated in the past for Graves' disease by either surgical or radioactive iodine ablation of the thyroid gland and if she is not currently receiving antithyroid drugs, then the fetus may be at risk for hyperthyroidism if maternal thyroid-stimulating immunoglobulins are still present that can traverse the placenta and stimulate the fetal thyroid (148). The consequences of fetal thyrotoxicosis can be serious (148,149). If there is sustained fetal tachycardia or cardiomegaly, then an empiric decision to treat the fetus via the mother, without fetal blood sampling, is reasonable. However, if there are no or only relatively nonspecific findings of fetal thyrotoxicosis, such as IUGR, then fetal blood sampling to make or refute the diagnosis is advisable, since antithyroid drugs are not innocuous (150,151).

If the mother is receiving antithyroid drugs to control her Graves' disease, then fetal blood sampling to assess fetal thyroid status and modulate propylthiouracil dose

is, although superficially attractive, actually needlessly meddlesome. If the mother on antithyroid medications is not clinically hyperthyroid, neither will the fetus be. If the mother is clinically hyperthyroid, she will need more medication regardless of the fetal thyroid status (152). It is true that the fetus exposed to antithyroid medications may have some suppression of its thyroid gland, but this is not a serious problem since there is no evidence that mild intrauterine hypothyroidism has any serious neonatal consequences or long-term effects (152,153). In cases of fetal goiter (154), where the potential treatments (antithyroid drugs or thyroxine) are mutually exclusive (155), fetal blood sampling is valuable, but these cases are rare.

CONCLUSION

The pioneer of fetal blood sampling under ultrasound guidance was being modest when he opined that "this new procedure could . . . initiate an important field of new investigation" (156). Indeed, the opportunities for fetal diagnosis and therapy that this procedure has made possible now make it realistic to speak of the field of fetal medicine and to speak of the fetus as our "unborn patient."

However, this exciting advance is not without its problems; there are real risks with this procedure. If we are to regard the fetus as our patient, then we should endeavor to accord the fetus the same protection as all patients in medicine. We should try as much as possible to adhere to the rule that "a potentially injurious diagnostic procedure should be carried out only when its possible benefit to that patient justifies the risk" (157). Since, in the case of fetal blood sampling, it is the fetus that bears almost all the risk, the prime consideration before undertaking the procedure should be whether the fetus is likely to benefit from the information obtained. Of course, obstetrics is unlike all other fields of medicine since there are two patients to consider, and sometimes fetal blood sampling benefits the mother and not the fetus. But, the necessity for compromise in some cases should nevertheless not let us abandon the principle that, ideally, for the fetus, the benefits of the blood sampling should outweigh the risks. Fetal blood sampling should not be done for curiosity's sake. Fetal blood sampling should not be done if the information is not essential or if it can be obtained at lesser cost by ultrasound or amniocentesis. Fetal blood sampling should not be done just for the sake of thoroughness, that is, just because one expects one's peers to suggest it. Fetal blood sampling should not be done just to enhance one's reputation as a specialist.

Obtaining a fetal blood sample is a matter of technique. Deciding if and when to obtain a fetal blood sample is a matter of judgment. The interests of our fetal patients are best served when good technique is married to good judgment.

References

1. Orlandi F, Damiani G, Jakil C, Lauricella S, Bertolino O, Maggio A. The risks of early cordocentesis (12-21 weeks): analysis of 500 procedures. Prenat Diagn 1990;10(7):425–428.
2. Weiner CP. The role of cordocentesis in fetal diagnosis. Clin Obstet Gynecol 1988;31(2):285–292.
3. Daffos F. Fetal blood sampling. Ann Rev Med 1989;40:319–329.
4. Soothill PW. Cordocentesis: role in assessment of fetal condition. Clin Perinatol 1989;16(3):755–770.
5. Reece EA, Copel JA, Scioscia AL, Grannum PAT, DeGennaro N, Hobbins JC. Diagnostic fetal umbilical blood sampling in the management of isoimmunization. Am J Obstet Gynecol 1988;159(5):1057–1062.
6. Shalev E, Dan U, Weiner E, Romano S, Giselevitz J, Mashiach S. Prenatal diagnosis using sonographic-guided cordocentesis. J Perinat Med 1989;17(6):393-398.
7. Barss VA, Benacerraf BR, Frigoletto FD, et al. Management of isoimmunized pregnancy by use of intravascular techniques. Am J Obstet Gynecol 1988;159(4):932–937.
8. Wilkins I, Mezrow G, Lynch L, Bottone EJ, Berkowitz RL. Amnionitis and life-threatening respiratory distress after percutaneous umbilical blood sampling. Am J Obstet Gynecol 1989;160(2):427–428.
9. Ludomirski A, Weiner S. Percutaneous fetal umbilical blood sampling. Clin Obstet Gynecol 1988;31(1):19–26.
10. Donnenfeld AE, Wiseman B, Lavi E, Weiner S. Prenatal diagnosis of thrombocytopenia-absent radius syndrome by ultrasound and cordocentesis. Prenat Diagn 1990;10(1):29–35.
11. Boulot P, Deschamps F, Lefort G, et al. Pure fetal blood samples obtained by cordocentesis: technical aspects of 322 cases. Prenat Diagn 1990;10(2):93–100.
12. McColgin SW, Hess LW, Martin RW, Martin JN, Morrison JC. Group B streptococcal sepsis and death in utero following funipuncture. Obstet Gynecol 1989;74(3, part 2):464–465.
13. Hogge WA, Thiagarajah S, Brenbridge AN, Harbert GM. Fetal evaluation by percutaneous blood sampling. Am J Obstet Gynecol 1988;158(1):132–136.
14. Jauniaux E, Donner C, Simon P, Vanesse M, Hustin J, Rodesch F. Pathologic aspects of the umbilical cord after precutaneous umbilical blood sampling. Obstet Gynecol 1989;73(2):215–218.
15. Chenard E, Bastide A, Fraser WD. Umbilical cord hematoma following diagnostic funipuncture. Obstet Gynecol 1990;76(5, part 2):994–996.

16. Harman CR, Bowman JM, Menticoglou SM, Pollock JM, Manning FA. Profound fetal thrombocytopenia in Rhesus disease: serious hazard at intravascular transfusion [letter]. The Lancet 1988;2(8613): 741–742.
17. Maeda H, Shimokawa H, Satoh S, et al. Safety of cordocentesis under ultrasound guidance for fetal blood sampling. Acta Obst Gynaec Jpn 1990;42(2):199–202.
18. Rightmire DA, Ertmoed EE. Fetal exsanguination following umbilical cord blood sampling [abstract 336]. Am J Obstet Gynecol 1991;164 (1,part 2):339.
19. Moise KJ, Carpenter RJ, Cotton DB, Wasserstrum N, Kirshon B, Cano L. Percutaneous umbilical cord blood sampling in the evaluation of fetal platelet counts in pregnant patients with autoimmune thrombocytopenia purpura. Obstet Gynecol 1988;72 (3, part 1):346–350.
20. Moise KJ, Cano LE, Sala DJ. Resolution of severe thrombocytopenia in a pregnant patient with Rhesus-negative blood with autoimmune thrombocytopenia purpura after intravenous Rhesus immune globulin. Am J Obstet Gynecol 1990;162(5):1237–1238.
21. Donner C, Simon Ph, Avni F, Jauniaux E, Rodesch F. Diagnostic cordocentesis: two years of experience. Eur J Obstet Gynecol Reprod Biol 1989;31:119–125.
22. Romero R, Athanassiadis AP, Inati M. Fetal blood sampling. In: Fleischer AC, Romero R, Manning FA, Jeanty P, James AE, eds. The principles and practice of ultrasonography in obstetrics and gynecology. 4th ed. Norwalk, Connecticut: Appleton & Lange, 1991, 455–473.
23. Harman CR, Bowman JM, Manning FA, Menticoglou SM. Intrauterine transfusion—intraperitoneal versus intravascular approach: a case-control comparison. Am J Obstet Gynecol 1990;162(4):1053–1059.
24. MacKenzie IZ, Bowell PJ, Castle BM, Selinger M, Ferguson JF. Serial fetal blood sampling for the management of pregnancies complicated by severe Rhesus (D) isoimmunization. Br J Obstet Gynaecol 1988;95(8):753–758.
25. Nicolaides KH, Rodeck CH, Mibashan RS, Kemp JR. Have Liley charts outlived their usefulness? Am J Obstet Gynecol 1986; 155(1):90–94.
26. Bowell PJ, Selinger M, Ferguson J, Giles J, MacKenzie IZ. Antenatal fetal blood sampling for the management of alloimmunized pregnancies: effect upon maternal anti-D potency levels. Br J Obstet Gynaecol 1988;95(8):759–764.
27. Weiner C, Grant S, Hudson J, Williamson R, Wenstrom K. Effect of diagnostic and therapeutic cordocentesis on maternal serum alpha-fetoprotein concentration. Am J Obstet Gynecol 1989;161(3):706–708.
28. Nicolini U, Kochenour NK, Greco P, et al. Consequences of fetomaternal hemorrhage after intrauterine transfusion. Br Med J 1988;297(6660):1379–1381.
29. Eydoux P, Choiset A, Le Porrier N, et al. Chromosomal prenatal diagnosis: study of 936 cases of intrauterine abnormalities after ultrasound assessment. Prenat Diagn 1989; 9(4):255–268.
30. Rizzo N, Pittalis MC, Pilu G, Orsini LF, Perolo A, Bovicelli L. Prenatal karyotyping in malformed fetuses. Prenat Diagn 1990; 10(1):17–23.
31. Vamos E, Elmer C, Levi S, et al. Interet du diagnostic chromosomique prenatal en cas d'anomalies foetales: resultats obtenus dans 468 grossesses pathologiques. Rev Med Brux 1990;11:231–235.
32. Nicolaides KH, Rodeck CH, Gosden CM. Rapid karyotyping in nonlethal fetal malformations. The Lancet 1986;1(8476): 283–287.
33. Benacerraf BR, Mandell J, Estroff JA, Harlow BL, Frigoletto FD. Fetal pyelectasis: a possible association with Down's syndrome. Obstet Gynecol 1990;76(1):58–60.
34. Rightmire DA. Discussion. Of: Shah DM, Roussis P, Ulm J, Jeanty P, Boehm FH. Cordocentesis for rapid karyotyping. Am J Obstet Gynecol 1990;162(6):1548–1553.
35. Moise KJ. Discussion. Of: Shah DM, Roussis P, Ulm J, Jeanty P, Boehm FH. Cordocentesis for rapid karyotyping. Am J Obstet Gynecol 1990;162(6):1548–1553.

36. Orlandi F, Damiami G, Jakil C, et al. Clinical results and fetal biochemical data in 140 early second trimester diagnostic cordocenteses. Acta Eur Fertil 1987;18(5):329–333.

37. Thoulon JM. L'amniocentese face a la choriocentese (prelevement de villosites choriales) et a la cordocentese (prelevement de sang foetal). Rev Fr Gynecol Obstet 1990;85(2):101–104.

38. Levi Setti PE, Buscaglia M, Ferrazzi E, Zuliani G, Ghisoni L, Pardi G. Valutazione del rischio fetale dopo prelievo di sangue ecoguidato dal cordone ombelicale nel II trimestre di gravidanza. Ann Ost Gin Med Perin 1989;110(2):98–104.

39. Claussen U, Klein R, Schmidt M. A pipette method for rapid karyotyping in prenatal diagnosis. Prenat Diagn 1986;6(6):401–408.

40. Hentemann M, Rauskolb R, Ulbrich R, Bartles I. Abnormal pregnancy sonogram and chromosomal anomalies; four years' experience with rapid karyotyping. Prenat Diagn 1989;9(9):605–612.

41. Visser GHA, Redman CWG, Huisjes HJ, Turnbull AC. Nonstressed antepartum heart rate monitoring: implications of decelerations after spontaneous contractions. Am J Obstet Gynecol 1980;138(4):429–435.

42. Vintzileos AM, Gaffney SE, Salinger LM, Campbell WA, Nochimson DJ. The relationship between fetal biophysical profile and cord pH in patients undergoing cesarean section before the onset of labor. Obstet Gynecol 1987;70(2):196–201.

43. Soothill PW, Nicolaides KH, Campbell S. Prenatal asphyxia, hyperlacticaemia, hypoglycemia, and erythroblastosis in growth-retarded fetuses. Br Med J 1987;294(6579): 1051–1053.

44. Schifrin BS, Foye G, Amato J, Kates R, MacKenna J. Routine fetal heart rate monitoring in the antepartum period. Obstet Gynecol 1979;54(1):21–25.

45. Phelan JP. The nonstress test: a review of 3000 tests. Am J Obstet Gynecol 1981; 139(1):7–10.

46. Rutherford SE, Phelan JP, Smith CV, Jacobs N. The four-quadrant assessment of amniotic fluid volume: an adjunct to antepartum fetal heart rate testing. Obstet Gynecol 1987;70(3,part 1):353–356.

47. Eden RD, Seifert LS, Kodack LD, Trofatter KF, Killam AP, Gall SA. A modified biophysical profile for antenatal fetal surveillance. Obstet Gynecol 1988;71(3):365–369.

48. Manning FA, Morrison I, Harman CR, Lange IR, Menticoglou S. Fetal assessment based on fetal biophysical prolice scoring: experience in 19,221 referred high-risk pregnancies: II. An analysis of false-negative fetal deaths. Am J Obstet Gynecol 1987:157(4,part 1):880–884.

49. Baskett TF, Allen AC, Gray JH, Young DC, Young LM. Fetal biophysical profile and perinatal death. Obstet Gynecol 1987; 70(3,part 1):357–360.

50. Visser GHA, Sadovsky G, Nicolaides KH. Antepartum heart rate patterns in small-for-gestational-age third-trimester fetuses: correlations with blood gas values obtained at cordocentesis. Am J Obstet Gynecol 1990;162(3):698–703.

51. Ribbert LSM, Snijders RJM, Nicolaides KH, Visser GHA. Relationship of fetal biophysical profile and blood gas values at cordocentesis in severely growth-retarded fetuses. Am J Obstet Gynecol 1990;163(2):569–571.

52. Brown R, Patrick J. The nonstress test: how long is enough? Am J Obstet Gynecol 1981;141(6):646–651.

53. Leveno KJ, Williams ML, DePalma RT, Whalley PJ. Perinatal outcome in the absence of antepartum fetal heart rate acceleration. Obstet Gynecol 1983;61(3):347–355.

54. Devoe LD, McKenzie J, Searle NS, Sherline DM. Clinical sequelae of the extended nonstress test. Am J Obstet Gynecol 1985; 151(8):1074–1078.

55. Gagnon R, Campbell K, Hunse C, Patrick J. Patterns of human fetal heart rate accelerations from 26 weeks to term. Am J Obstet Gynecol 1987;157(3):743–748.

56. Baskett TF. Gestational age and fetal biophysical assessment. Am J Obstet Gynecol 1988;158(2):332–334.

57. Castillo RA, Devoe LD, Arthur M, Searle N, Metheny WP, Reudrich DA. The preterm nonstress test: effects of gestational age and

length of study. Am J Obstet Gynecol 1989;160(1):172–175.

58. Manning FA, Harman CR, Morrison I, Menticoglou S. Fetal assessment based on fetal biophysical profile scoring: III. Positive predictive accuracy of the very abnormal test (biophysical profile score = 0). Am J Obstet Gynecol 1990;162(2):398–402.

59. Nasello-Paterson C, Natale R, Connors G. Ultrasonic evaluation of fetal body movements over 24 hours in the human fetus at 24 to 28 weeks gestation. Am J Obstet Gynecol 1988;158(2):312–316.

60. Drogtrop AP, Ubels R, Nijhuis JG. The association between fetal body movements, eye movements, and heart rate patterns in pregnancies between 25 and 30 weeks of gestation. Early Hum Dev 1990; 23(1): 67–73.

61. Patrick J, Campbell K, Carmichael L, Natale R, Richardson B. Patterns of gross fetal body movements over 24-hour observation intervals during the last 10 weeks of pregnancy. Am J Obstet Gynecol 1982;142(4): 363–371.

62. Schifrin BS, Clement D. Routine antepartum fetal heart rate monitoring. In: Spencer JAD, ed. Fetal monitoring: physiology and techniques of antenatal and intrapartum assessment. Philadelphia: FA Davis, 1989: 98–103.

63. Brioschi PA, Extermann P, Terracina D, Neil C, Mao WT, Beguin F. Antepartum nonstress fetal heart rate monitoring: systematic analysis of baseline patterns and decelerations as an adjunct to reactivity. Am J Obstet Gynecol 1985;153(6):633–637.

64. Manning FA. Dynamic ultrasound-based fetal assessment. The fetal biophysical profile score. In: Fleischer AC, Romero R, Manning FA, Jeanty P, James AE, eds. The principles and practice of ultrasonography in obstetrics and gynecology. 4th ed. Norwalk, Connecticut: Appleton & Lange, 1991:417–428.

65. Peeters LLH, Sheldon RE, Jones MD, Makowski EL, Meschia G. Blood flow to fetal organs as a function of arterial oxygen content. Am J Obstet Gynecol 1979; 135(5):637–646.

66. Sheldon RE, Peeters LLH, Jones MD, Makowski EL, Meschia G. Redistribution of cardiac output and oxygen delivery in the hypoxemic fetal lamb. Am J Obstet Gynecol 1979;135(8):1071–1078.

67. Block BSB, Llanos AJ, Creasy RK. Responses of the growth-retarded fetus to acute hypoxemia. Am J Obstet Gynecol 1984;148(7):878–885.

68. Nicolaides KH, Peters MT, Vyas S, Rabinowitz R, Rosen DJD, Campbell S. Relation to rate of urine production to oxygen tensions in small-for-gestational-age fetuses. Am J Obstet Gynecol 1990;162(2):387–391.

69. Wladimiroff JW, Wijngaard JAGW vd, Degani S, Noordam MJ, van Eyck J, Tonge HM. Cerebral and umbilical arterial blood flow velocity waveforms in normal and growth-retarded pregnancies. Obstet Gynecol 1987;69(5):705–709.

70. Stewart P, Wladimiroff JW, Stijnen T. Blood flow velocity waveforms from the fetal external iliac artery as a measure of lower extremity vascular resistance. Br J Obstet Gynaecol 1990;97(5):425–430.

71. Vyas S, Nicolaides KH, Bower S, Campbell S. Middle cerebral artery flow velocity waveforms in fetal hypoxaemia. Br J Obstet Gynaecol 1990;97(9):797–803.

72. Shah DM, Boehm FH. Fetal blood gas analysis from cordocentesis for abnormal fetal heart rate patterns. Am J Obstet Gynecol 1989;161(2):374–376.

73. Pearce JM, Chamberlain GVP. Ultrasonically-guided percutaneous umbilical blood sampling in the management of intrauterine growth retardation. Br J Obstet Gynaecol 1987;94(4):318–321.

74. Weiner CP. The relationship between the umbilical artery systolic/diastolic ratio and umbilical blood gas measurements in specimens obtained by cordocentesis. Am J Obstet Gynecol 1990;162(5):1198–1202.

75. Warren W, Ronkin S, Chayen B, Needleman L, Wapner RJ. Absence of end-diastolic umbilical artery blood flow predicts poor

fetal outcome despite normal blood gases. Am J Obstet Gynecol 1989;160(1):197.

76. Nicolini U, Nicolaidis P, Fisk WM, et al. Limited role of fetal blood sampling in prediction of outcome in intrauterine growth retardation. The Lancet 1990;336: 768–772.

77. Bekedam DJ, Visser GHA, Mulder EJH, Polemann-Weesjes G. Heart rate variation and movement incidence in growth-retarded fetuses: the significance of antenatal late heart rate decelerations. Am J Obstet Gynecol 1987;157(1):126–133.

78. Daffos F, Forestier F, Kaplan C, Cox W. Prenatal diagnosis and management of bleeding disorders with fetal blood sampling. Am J Obstet Gynecol 1988;158(4): 939–946.

79. Reznikoff-Etievant MF. Management of alloimmune neonatal and antenatal thrombocytopenia. Vox Sang 1988;55(4):193–201.

80. Mueller-Eckhardt C, Kiefel V, Grubert A, et al. Three-hundred-forty-eight cases of suspected neonatal alloimmune thrombocytopenia. The Lancet 1989;1(8634):363–366.

81. Muller JY, Kaplan C, Reznikoff-Etievant MF, et al. In utero fetal sampling in neonatal alloimmune thrombocytopenia: justification and usefulness. Curr Stud Hematol Blood Transf 1988;54:127–135.

82. Nicolini U, Tannirandorn Y, Gonzalez P, et al. Continuing controversy in alloimmune thrombocytopenia: fetal hyperimmunoglobulinemia fails to prevent thrombocytopenia. Am J Obstet Gynecol 1990; 163(4, part 1):1144–1146.

83. Murphy MF, Pullon HWH, Metcalfe P, et al. Management of fetal alloimmune thrombocytopenia by weekly in utero platelet transfusions. Vox Sang 1990;58(1):45–49.

84. Bussel JP, Berkowitz RL, McFarland JG, et al. Antenatal treatment of neonatal alloimmune thrombocytopenia. N Engl J Med 1988;319(21):1374–1378.

85. Gafni A, Blanchette VS. Screening for neonatal alloimmune thrombocytopenia: an economic perspective. Curr Stud Hematol Blood Transf 1988;54:140–147.

86. Nagey DA, Alger LS, Edelman BB, Heyman MR, Pupkin MJ, Crenshaw C. Reacting appropriately to thrombocytopenia in pregnancy. S Med J 1986;79(11):1385–1388.

87. Hart D, Dunetz C, Nardi M, Porges RF, Weiss A, Karpatkin M. An epidemic of maternal thrombocytopenia associated with elevated antiplatelet antibody: platelet count and antiplatelet antibody in 116 consecutive pregnancies: relationship to neonatal platelet count. Am J Obstet Gynecol 1986;154(4):878–883.

88. Burrows RF, Kelton JG. Thrombocytopenia at delivery: a prospective survey of 6715 deliveries. Am J Obstet Gynecol 1990; 162(3):731–734.

89. Samuels P, Bussel JB, Braitman LE, et al. Estimation of the risk of thrombocytopenia in the offspring of pregnant women with presumed immune thrombocytopenic purpura. N Engl J Med 1990;323(4):229–235.

90. Aster RH. "Gestational" thrombocytopenia: a plea for conservative management. N Engl J Med 1990;323(4):264–266.

91. Scioscia AL, Grannum PAT, Copel JA, Hobbins JC. The use of percutaneous umbilical blood sampling in immune thrombocytopenic purpura. Am J Obstet Gynecol 1988;159(5):1066–1068.

92. Bussel JB. Management of infants of mothers with immune thrombocytopenic purpura. J Pediatr 1988;113(3):497–499.

93. Christiaens GCML, Nieuwenhuis HK, von dem Borne AEGKr, et al. Idiopathic thrombocytopenic purpura in pregnancy: a randomized trial on the effect of antenatal low dose corticosteroids on neonatal platelet count. Br J Obstet Gynaecol 1990; 97(10):893–898.

94. Burrows RF, Kelton JG. Low fetal risks in pregnancies associated with idiopathic thrombocytopenic purpura. Am J Obstet Gynecol 1990;163(4, part 1):1147–1150.

95. Ballem PJ, Buskard N, Wittmann BK, Wilson RD, Effer S, Farquharson D. ITP in pregnancy: use of the bleeding time as an indicator for treatment. Blut 1989;59(1): 132–135.

96. Christiaens GCML, Helmerhorst FM. Validity of intrapartum diagnosis of fetal thrombocytopenia. Am J Obstet Gynecol 1987;157(4, part 1):864–865.

97. Dan U, Barkai G, David B, Goldenberg M, Kukkia E, Mashiach S. Management of labor in patients with idiopathic thrombocytopenic purpura. Gynecol Obstet Invest 1989;27(4):193–196.

98. Pielet BW, Socol ML, MacGregor SN, Ney JA, Dooley SL. Cordocentesis: an appraisal of risks. Am J Obstet Gynecol 1988;159(6):1497–1500.

99. Weiner CP. Cordocentesis. Obstet Gynecol Clin NA 1988;15(2):283–301.

100. Holzgreve W. The fetus with nonimmune hydrops. In: Harrison MR, Golbus MS, Filly RA, eds. The unborn patient; prenatal diagnosis and treatment. 2nd ed. Philadelphia: Saunders, 1990:228–245.

101. Machin GA. Diseases causing fetal and neonatal ascites. Pediatr Pathol 1985;4(3–4):195–211.

102. Winn HN, Stiller R, Grannum PAT, Crane JC, Coster B, Romero R. Isolated fetal ascites: prenatal diagnosis and management. Am J Perinatol 1990;7(4):370–373.

103. Allan L, Little D, Campbell S, Whitehead MI. Fetal ascites associated with congenital heart disease. Br J Obstet Gynaecol 1981;88(4):453–455.

104. Bierman FZ, Baxi L, Jaffe I, Driscoll J. Fetal hydrops and congenital complete heart block: response to maternal steroid therapy. J Pediatr 1988;112(4):646–648.

105. Hansmann M, Gembruch U, Bald R. Management of the fetus with nonimmune hydrops. In: Harrison MR, Golbus MS, Filly RA, eds. The unborn patient: prenatal diagnosis and treatment. 2nd ed. Philadelphia: Saunders, 1990:246–248.

106. Machin GA. Hydrops revisited: literature review of 1414 cases published in the 1980s. Am J Med Genet 1989;34(3):366–390.

107. Clark SL, Vitale DJ, Minton SD, Stoddard RA, Sabey PL. Successful fetal therapy for cystic adenomatoid malformation associated with second trimester hydrops. Am J Obstet Gynecol 1987;157(2):294–295.

108. Langer JC, Harrison MR, Schmidt KG, et al. Fetal hydrops and death from sacrococcygeal teratoma: rationale for fetal surgery. Am J Obstet Gynecol 1989;160(5, part 1):1145–1150.

109. Nakayama DK. Survival in a fetus with sacrococcygeal teratoma and hydrops. Am J Obstet Gynecol 1990;163(2):682.

110. Maxwell DJ, Crawford DC, Curry PV, Tynan MJ, Allan LD. Obstetric importance, diagnosis, and management of fetal tachycardias. Br Med J 1988;297(6641):107–110.

111. Donner C, Simon Ph, Gosselin F, et al. La cordocentese: experience des 391 premiers prelevements. Rev Med Brux 1990;11:217–222.

112. Gembruch U, Hansmann M, Redel DA, Bald R. Intrauterine therapy of fetal tachyarrhythmias: intraperitoneal administration of antiarrhythmic drugs to the fetus in fetal tachyarrhythmias with severe hydrops fetalis. J Perinat Med 1989;16(1):39–44.

113. Saltzman DH, Frigoletto FD, Harlow BL, Barss VA, Benacerraf BR. Sonographic evaluation of hydrops fetalis. Obstet Gynecol 1989;74(1):106–111.

114. Cardwell MS. Successful treatment of hydrops fetalis caused by fetomaternal hemorrhage: a case report. Am J Obstet Gynecol 1988;158(1):131–132.

115. Schwarz TF, Roggendorf M, Hottentrager B, et al. Human parvovirus B19 infection in pregnancy [letter]. The Lancet 1988;2(8610):566–567.

116. Rodis JF, Hovick TJ Jr, Quinn DL, Rosengren SS, Tattersall P. Human parvovirus infection in pregnancy. Obstet Gynecol 1988;72(5):733–738.

117. Maeda H, Shimokawa H, Satoh S, Nakano H, Nunoue T. Nonimmunologic hydrops fetalis resulting from intrauterine human parvovirus B-19 infection: report of two cases. Obstet Gynecol 1988;72(3,part 2):482–485.

118. Peters MT, Nicolaides KH. Cordocentesis for the diagnosis and treatment of human fetal parvovirus infection. Obstet Gynecol 1990;75(3,part 2):501–504.

119. Bernstein IM, Capeless EL. Elevated maternal serum alpha-fetoprotein and hydrops fetalis in association with fetal parvovirus B-19 infection. Obstet Gynecol 1989;74(3,part 2):456–457.

120. Miller E, Cradock-Watson JE, Pollock TM. Consequences of confirmed maternal rubella at successive stages of pregnancy. The Lancet 1982;2(8302):781–784.

121. Nicolaides KH. Cordocentesis. Clin Obstet Gynecol 1988;31(1):123–135.

122. Hsieh FJ, Ko TM, Chang FM, Chen HY, Kao ML, Furng MH. Percutaneous ultrasound-guided fetal blood sampling: experience in the first 100 cases. Taiwan I Hsueh Hui Tsa Chih 1989;88(2):137–142.

123. Hohlfeld P, Daffos F, Thulliez P, et al. Fetal toxoplasmosis: outcome of pregnancy and infant follow-up after in utero treatment. J Pediatr 1989;115(5,part 1): 765–769.

124. Couvreur J, Desmonts G. Toxoplasmosis. In: MacLeod CL, ed. Parasitic infections in pregnancy and the newborn. Oxford: Oxford University Press, 1988.

125. Derouin F, Thulliez P, Candolfi E, Daffos F, Forestier F. Early prenatal diagnosis of congenital toxoplasmosis using amniotic fluid samples and tissue culture. Eur J Clin Microbiol Infect Dis 1988;7(3):423–425.

126. Foulon W, Naessens A, Mahler T, de Waele M, de Catte L, de Meuter F. Prenatal diagnosis of congenital toxoplasmosis. Obstet Gynecol 1990;76(5,part 1):769–772.

127. Daffos F, Forestier F, Capella-Pavlovsky M, et al. Prenatal management of 746 pregnancies at risk for congenital toxoplasmosis. N Engl J Med 1988;318(5):271–275.

128. Cook GC. *Toxoplasma gondii* infection: a potential danger to the unborn fetus and AIDS sufferer. Q J Med 1990;74:3–19.

129. Stagno S, Pass RF, Dworsky ME, Alford CA Jr. Congenital and perinatal cytomegalovirus infections. In: Amstey MS, ed. Virus infection in pregnancy. Orlando: Harcourt Brace Jovanovich, 1984:103–105.

130. Overall JC. Viral infections of the fetus and neonate. In: Feigin RD, Cherry JD, eds. Textbook of pediatric infectious diseases, 2nd ed. vol. 1. Philadelphia: WB Saunders, 1987, 977–981.

131. Grose C, Weiner CP. Prenatal diagnosis of congenital cytomegalovirus infection: two decades later. Am J Obstet Gynecol 1990;163(2):447–450.

132. Peters M, Harstad T, Sanchez P, Norgard M, Goldberg M, Wendel G. Prenatal diagnosis of congenital syphilis [abstract 322]. Am J Obstet Gynecol 1991;164(1, part 2):335.

133. Rodis JF, Quinn DL, Gary GW, et al. Management and outcomes of pregnancies complicated by human B19 parvovirus infection: a prospective study. Am J Obstet Gynecol 1990;163(4,part 1):1168–1171.

134. Plebani A, Biolchini A, Bucceri A, Buscaglia M, Pardi G, Semprini AE. Prenatal immune status of fetuses of HIV-seropositive mothers. Gynecol Obstet Invest 1990;29(2):108–111.

135. Daffos F, Forestier F, Mandelbrot L, Pialoux G, Rey MA, Brun-Vezinet F. Prenatal diagnosis of HIV infection: two attempts using fetal blood sampling. J Acquir Immune Defic Syndr 1989; 2(2):205–207.

136. Grose C, Itani O, Weiner CP. Prenatal diagnosis of fetal infection: advances from amniocentesis to cordocentesis—congenital toxoplasmosis, rubella, cytomegalovirus, varicella virus, parvovirus, and human immunodeficiency virus. Pediatr Infect Dis J 1989;8(7):459–468.

137. Steele BT, Paes B, Towell ME, Hunter DJS. Fetal renal failure associated with intrauterine growth retardation. Am J Obstet Gynecol 1988;159(5):1200–1202.

138. Romero R, Cullen M, Grannum P, et al. Antenatal diagnosis of renal anomalies with ultrasound. III. Bilateral renal agenesis. Am J Obstet Gynecol 1985;151(1): 38–43.

139. Hackeloer BJ, Waldenfels HV, Martin K, Hamburg D. Treatment and results of oligohydramnios by instillation of artificial amniotic fluid (150 cases). Presented at the 5th annual meeting of the international fetal medicine and surgery society, Bonn, West Germany, 1988.

140. Gembruch U, Hansmann M. Artificial instillation of amniotic fluid as a new technique for the diagnostic evaluation of
cases of oligohydramnios. Prenat Diagn
1988;8(1):33–45.

141. Nicolini U, Santolaya J, Hubinont C, Fisk
N, Maxwell D, Rodeck C. Visualization of
fetal intra-abdominal organs in second-
trimester severe oligohydramnios by intraperitoneal infusion. Prenat Diagn
1989;9(3):191–194.

142. Weiner CP. Pathogenesis, evaluation, and
potential treatments for severe, early-
onset growth retardation. Semin Perinatol
1989;13(4):320–327.

143. Wladimiroff JW, Stewart PA, Reuss A,
Sachs ES. Cardiac and extracardiac anomalies as indicators for trisomies 13 and 18:
a prenatal ultrasound study. Prenat Diagn
1989;9(7):515–520.

144. Landy HJ, Isada NB, Larsen JW. Genetic
implications of idiopathic hydramnios.
Am J Obstet Gynecol 1987;157(1):114–117.

145. Nicolaides KH, Campbell S, Bradley RJ,
Bilardo CM, Soothill PW, Gibb D. Maternal oxygen therapy for intrauterine
growth retardation. The Lancet 1987;
1(8539):942–945.

146. Blanchette VS, Sacher RA, Ballem PJ,
Bussel JB, Imbach P. Commentary on the
management of autoimmune thrombocytopenia during pregnancy and in the neonatal period. Blut 1989;59(1):121–123.

147. Daffos F. The fetus at risk for thrombocytopenia. In: Harrison MR, Golbus MS,
Filly RA, eds. The unborn patient: prenatal
diagnosis and treatment. 2nd ed. Philadelphia: WB Saunders, 1990:210–214.

148. Bruinse HW, Vermeulen-Meiners C, Wit
JM. Fetal treatment for thyrotoxicosis in
nonthyrotoxic pregnant women. Fetal
Ther 1988;3(3):152–157.

149. Page DV, Brady K, Mitchell J, Pehrson J,
Wade G. The pathology of intrauterine
thyrotoxicosis: two case reports. Obstet
Gynecol 1988; 72(3,part 2):479–481.

150. Porreco RP, Bloch CA. Fetal blood sampling in the management of intrauterine
thyrotoxicosis. Obstet Gynecol 1990;
76(3,part 2):509–512.

151. Wenstrom KD, Weiner CP, Williamson
RA, Grant SS. Prenatal diagnosis of fetal
hyperthyroidism using funipuncture. Obstet Gynecol 1990;76(3,part 2):513–517.

152. Davis LE, Lucas MJ, Hankins GDV, Roark
ML, Cunningham FG. Thyrotoxicosis
complicating pregnancy. Am J Obstet Gynecol 1989;160(1):63–70.

153. Momotani N, Noh J, Oyanagi H, Ishikawa
N, Ito K. Antithyroid drug therapy for
Graves' disease during pregnancy: opti-
mal regimen for fetal thyroid status. N
Engl J Med 1986;315(1):24–28.

154. Davidson KM, Richards DS, Schatz DA,
Fisher DA. Successful in utero treatment
of fetal goiter and hypothyroidism. N
Engl J Med 1991;324(8):543–546.

155. Utiger RD. Recognition of thyroid disease
in the fetus. N Engl J Med 1991;324(8):
559–561.

156. Daffos F, Capella-Pavlovsky M, Forestier
F. Fetal blood sampling during pregnancy with use of a needle guided by
ultrasound: a study of 606 consecutive
cases. Am J Obstet Gynecol 1985;153(6):
655–660.

157. Beeson PB. On becoming a clinician. In:
Beeson PB, McDermott W, Wyngaarden
JB, eds. Cecil textbook of medicine. 15th
ed. Philadelphia: WB Saunders, 1979, 1–3.

THE FUTURE OF INTRAUTERINE SURGERY: A CRITICAL APPRAISAL

FRANK A. MANNING

We are at present in the midst of a fundamental change in human medicine, occurring as a consequence of recognition of a new patient, the fetus. Beginning in the late 1970s, this new era of fetal medicine began to emerge, ushered in by the advent of high resolution dynamic ultrasound imaging methods. The cadence of events in the field has been dramatic. In a few short years, a relatively passive observational and diagnostic stance has evolved to a highly active state that includes an extensive invasive diagnostic/therapeutic armamentarium. It is this state, being able to invade the heretofore sacrosanct fetal environment with the intent of correcting a congenital condition or acquired problem (with the expectation of a lifelong cure), that has stirred great interest and controversy.

The range of these invasive therapeutic maneuvers, collectively described by the provocative although not entirely appropriate term, *fetal surgery,* has expanded quickly from the original descriptions of ultrasound-guided percutaneous needle placement and shunt delivery for obstructive fetal lesions, to exceedingly complex open fetal surgical procedures and even intrauterine endoscopy-guided laser therapies. The concept of fetal surgery is unique to medicine, for nowhere else is there a circumstance where operating on one patient carries with it potential risk for another. Nowhere else in medicine is there a circumstance where the risk of "wrongful life" is greater. On the other hand, there is no circumstance in surgery where a patient has more perfect corporeal support systems, healing mechanisms, and potential for lifelong benefits. The issue to be discussed is the balancing of these risks and benefits. This requires the critical appraisal of techniques, present and future, that may alter the natural history of fetal disease.

Selection Criteria

The initial apparent successes with daring imaginative intrauterine rescue maneuvers for the fetus with certain anomalies, such as obstructive uropathies (1,2), ventriculomegaly (3,4), and diaphragmatic hernia (5), sparked widespread optimism in both general society and, in particular, the medical society. Over time, it has now become evident that the benefits of such therapies are not universal but rather sporadic (6,7,8), that the therapies themselves can create morbidity and mortality (6,7,9), that there may be significant disparity between immediate and long-term results (6), and that there may be potential risk to maternal health with subsequent pregnancies (9). There is now clear and visible risk that the failure of the results to meet expectations will result in disenchantment with the concepts of fetal therapies, ultimately relegating these advances to the category of failed clinical experiments. The counter force is equally obvious in the development and implementation of rational case selection criteria such that in the individual case, a therapeutic benefit of measurable clinical significance will likely occur.

Development and refinement of such selective criteria have been critical steps in extrauterine medicine and surgery and, appropriately, need now be considered for the intrauterine patient. At a minimum, these four criteria must include:

(1) Identification of a Discrete Fetal Disease or Disease Process

All clinical evidence points to the premise that the more certain is the diagnosis, the more certain is the selection of the appropriate therapy. Thus, for example, in fetuses presenting with lower urinary tract obstructive uropathies, whereas chronic in utero vesicoamniotic shunting may yield an overall 40% survival (10), the survival for a specific diagnosis may range from 20% for urethral atresia to 85% for posterior urethral valve syndrome (8). For either diagnosis, diversion therapy is likely to correct signs of disease (vesicomegaly, hydronephrosis, oligohydramnios), but the effect of such therapy on the underlying sinister characteristics of the disease process (renal dysgenesis, pulmonary hypoplasia) will vary widely. Similarly, with the fetal anemias, whereas intravascular fetal blood transfusion will restore normal circulating hemoglobin levels in all transfused anemic fetuses and will ultimately correct the signs of chronic anemia (edema, ascites), the beneficial effects in the alloimmune fetus, e.g., Rh disease, are readily apparent (95% survival), whereas in the fetus with certain congenital hemoglobinopathies, e.g., alpha-thalassemia, the effect will be negligible (0% survival). It is, therefore, evident that the therapy must be directed towards a disease and not to the signs of the disease.

(2) Determination of Disease Severity
and Prognosis

The severity of the fetal disease process at first diagnosis and, therefore, the assignment of an immediate prognosis is a key first determinant in selection of cases most likely to benefit from in utero therapeutic maneuvers. Ultrasound organ imaging alone or in combination with an invasive fetal diagnostic procedure, e.g., fetal vesicocentesis for urine analysis, is the primary method for prognosis assignment; as expected, a range of predicted outcome occurs. At one extreme of distribution, a hopeless prognosis may be assigned, ending all consideration of therapy. Such a hopeless prognosis may be the result of observed end-stage vital organ disruption as,

for example, with obstructive uropathy and bilateral multicystic dysplastic renal disease (Figure 15-1A,B), as a result of measured irreversible vital organ dysfunction as, for example, with isotonic hyponatremic fetal urine in cases of obstructive uropathy (11), or as a result of association with other lethal anomalies as either observed, e.g., diaphragmatic hernia associated with major cardiac anomaly (12) or as determined by an invasive procedure, e.g., obstructive uropathy associated with Trisomy 18 (10).

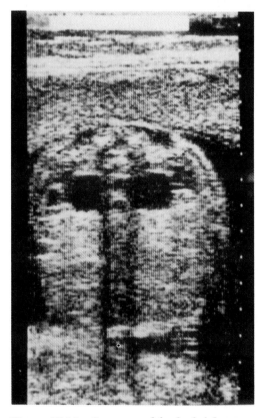

Figure 15-1A   Sonogram of the fetal abdomen at the level of the kidneys demonstrating the presence of multiple renal cysts of varying size bilaterally. Note the presence of some amniotic fluid. Disease was progressive in the fetus culminating in early neonatal death.

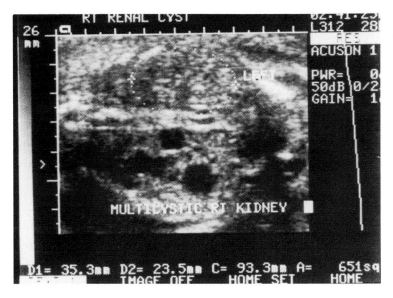

Figure 15-1B Sonogram in a coronal plane demonstrating unilateral multicystic dysplasia of the kidney. Note the multiple irregular cysts causing generalized renomegaly.

Similarly, at the other end of the spectrum, the prognosis for a particular anomaly may be deemed so positive regardless of intervention that therapy, while possible, is withheld. An example of this rare occurrence may be isolated unilateral fetal pleural effusion due to impaired lymphatic damage or chylothorax. Management of such cases by observation only, with avoidance of invasive drainage or shunting maneuver in fetal life, and planned immediate postnatal decompressing thoracocentesis has been associated with intact survival (13). In contrast, effusions that are bilateral, large, and associated with hydrops fetalis yield a much more sinister prognosis, and in such cases, decompression may be indicated and beneficial. Among such cases, it is of interest to note that pulmonary hypoplasia, a complication postulated to be frequent or even expected with prolonged lung compression, is not common (14).

(3) Evaluation of Progressive Pathophysiology

After recognition of a specific fetal disease process that is amenable to in utero therapy and determination that such therapy is likely to be of benefit, it then becomes critical to determine when such therapy should be instituted. Monitoring of progressive pathophysiology becomes a next key step in case selection.

Pathophysiological processes in the fetus are subject to unique modifications that are not found in extrauterine life. Firstly, the effect of a disease process on the fetal organ systems will be muted or even masked entirely by parallel compensatory placental function. Thus, for example, pulmonary hypoplasia, a frequent complication of obstructive uropathies and diaphragmatic hernia and the most common cause of postnatal death in such conditions (9,10) has no apparent effect on the fetus in utero. This standard viewpoint has recently been challenged, suggesting pulmonary hypoplasia in utero may alter fetal renal development (15). Similarly, progressive renal failure in utero secondary to chronic obstruction does not produce azotemia in the fetus provided placental function remains intact. Secondly, the rate of progression of fetal disease must be considered in the context of fetal organ system maturation (aging), and these factors are considered in light of the direct risks attendant to invasive fetal therapies. At present, it is generally held to be true that the procedure-related risk for a given treatment, e.g., surgical urinary bladder diversion, will always be greater for intrauterine procedures than for extrauterine procedures. Hence, when disease severity and progression permit, in utero therapy is deferred in favor of advancing maturity, delivery, and neonatal surgery. This principle may not hold for future therapies. Thus, for example, if the promise of stem cell therapy is confirmed, it is likely that the risk of therapy for the very immature and immunologically naive fetus will be less than for the postnatal infant who will require obliteration of the immune system prior to treatment.

Thirdly, the pathophysiological processes of the fetus may be a direct consequence of *fetal* status. The alloimmune disease model is the best example of this relationship. Delivery severs the maternal-fetal interface, abruptly halting the progressive pathophysiology; provided the neonate can compensate for the residual hemolysis and bilirubin load, the disease process will resolve completely. Similarly, the pathophysiology of isolated pleural effusion secondary to lymphatic obstruction is altered by transition from fetal to neonatal life: lung inflation by air and changed intrathoracic pressure dynamics facilitate lymphatic channel function and, thereby, over time, eliminate the effusions (16).

The contemporary methods available to monitor progressive pathophysiology vary by disease condition. In some conditions, for example, the alloimmune anemias, a battery of biochemical, hematological, and biophysical tests are available that yield an extremely accurate measure of disease progression; in such conditions, unnecessary fetal intervention with iatrogenic procedural risk or the converse, failure to intervene soon enough to avert serious or even lethal disease, should now be very rare. Unfortunately, for most of the developmental anomalous conditions considered amenable to in utero therapy, methods of monitoring pathophysiology are either nonexistent or are based upon relatively imprecise morphometric and morphological assessment of target organ systems. Thus, for example, progressive accurate measurement of degrees of pulmonary hypoplasia is not possible despite the obvious clinical importance of such information. Similarly, measurement of degrees of urinary tract dilatation and renal morphology in cases of obstructive uropathy offer, at best, only an estimate of residual function and reversibility (17). At present, these methods are prone to serious inaccuracies. Development of better methods to monitor end organ effects of various fetal anomalous conditions will be a key step in case selection and advancement of fetal surgery.

(4) Evaluation and Comparison of Procedural Risks

For all fetal invasive therapeutic procedures, there are inherent serious and potentially lethal complications for all involved patients, the fetus, the mother, and, occasionally, an otherwise normal intrauterine sibling. Given the unique nature of these complications and their potential severity, both immediate and life long, when a prenatal invasive therapy is contemplated, it is mandatory to weigh the risks to all patients involved, comparing those risks to those attendant to postnatal therapy of the affected neonate alone. Such a balance, comparing risks for two (or more) to the usually better understood risks for one, is unique to fetal invasive therapies and remains difficult and inexact. This risk comparison is then contrasted with potential benefit, proven or surmised, yielding a rational management plan.

Complications of prenatal invasive therapy may be either common (universal) to all or most procedures or may be unique (specific) to a given method. Universal risks for ultrasound-guided intrauterine fetal needling procedures include maternal and fetal infection, traumatic rupture of membranes, premature labor and delivery, abruption, and transplacental hemorrhage. Fetal infections have included lethal gonococcal ventriculitis after ventriculoamniotic shunt placement and *E. coli* septicemia following attempted vesicoamniotic shunting (10). Further, given the difficulty in culturing of anaerobes from amniotic fluid/fetal and placental tissue, it is likely that a proportion of unexplained fetal deaths after invasive procedures had an infectious etiology. Serious maternal infection is less common, although total hysterectomy and loss of reproductive future and near-fatal adult respiratory distress syndrome have occurred as the consequence of Group B streptococcal infection after needling of the umbilical vein (Berkowitz R, personal communication, 1987). The complications of spontaneous rupture of membranes, premature labor, premature delivery, and neonatal death secondary to immaturity have been reported in most series of therapeutic needling procedures (18). Traumatic abruption with fetal death and the potential for maternal death has occurred, as has massive silent fetomaternal hemorrhage, exsanguination, and fetal death.

In addition to universal risks, there are many specific procedural risks that need to be considered in the implementation of a treatment strategy. Procedure-specific complications with guided-needle therapies include brain stem trauma and immediate fetal death ("pithing") during attempts at

ventriculoamniotic shunt placement (6), umbilical cord hematoma and cord occlusion at the time of intravascular transfusion (19), embolic fetal cerebral hemiparesis and fetal cortical necrosis with porencephalic cyst formation following intravascular transfusion (20), fetal exsanguination secondary to laceration of fetal pelvic side wall vessels and laceration of hepatic vessels during intraperitoneal transfusion (Bowman JM, Manning FA, Harman CR, unpublished observation), and sacral nerve root damage and foot drop sequelae following attempts at fetal intramuscular injection of neuromuscular blocker (21). These serious complications are directly procedure-related and not the consequence of our former inability to image targets accurately.

The most invasive of the therapies, hysterotomy with primary fetal repair (open fetal surgery), has both an increased incidence of some universal risks, e.g., premature labor is reported as 100% (9), as well as obvious procedure-specific risks. The latter include the rare but nonetheless real risks to the mother, such as anesthetic death, emboli, and uncontrollable hemorrhage. Further, it must be remembered that open fetal surgery in the fecund woman with normal future reproductive expectations commits this patient to repetitive operative deliveries because of the relatively radical incision utilized. Hence, the cumulative risk of these complications can only be summarized at the end of a reproductive career.

Maternal risks associated with open fetal surgery have been studied in the primate model (22), but as yet, there is not sufficient human experience by which risks may be assigned. Experience with other forms of uterine surgery may offer some insight to these risks. A full thickness incision of the upper (muscular) uterine segment, as occurs with the hysterotomy technique described for open fetal surgery, causes permanent weakening in wall integrity, and risk of rupture in subsequent pregnancies is high. The most extensive experience with pregnancy following full thickness incision occurs in patients undergoing classical cesarean section; in these patients, the incidence of uterine rupture was 2.2, fetal mortality exceeded 50%, and maternal mortality was 5% (23).

It is important to note that upper segment and lower segment incision complications are dissimilar. Upper segment incisions tend to rupture and tear *across* tissue planes and vessels, often with hemorrhagic sequelae, whereas lower uterine scars are prone to dehiscence, a slowly progressive separation *along* tissue planes parallel to the vessels, not associated with bleeding of significance unless there is extension into the broad ligament. Given that a), there may be up to a 10-fold increase in maternal mortality comparing upper and lower segment incisions (5% versus 0.5% respectively), and b), an unaffected sibling in a subsequent pregnancy has a risk of fetal death of 50/1000 (calculated as 50% fetal mortality among the 10% of cases of uterine rupture), a rate up to 10-fold the expected, it is somewhat surprising to discern minimal significance attached to potential maternal risks by proponents of these open methods (9). Open fetal surgery also causes specific immediate fetal risks; fetal death secondary to exsanguination, infection, and venous occlusion are reported (9).

The neonatal risks of surgical procedures remain, of course, confined to the affected neonate and do not extend to its mother or unaffected siblings. It is generally held to be true that neonatal surgical risks are always less than fetal risks and usually to a considerable degree. It follows, therefore, that provided a therapeutic benefit of approximately equal value may be expected with either fetal or neonatal surgery, then the less complicated neonatal route is the appropri-

ate choice. While this point may seem obvious in the light of current knowledge, such was not always the case—there are several reports of invasive fetal procedures in fetuses in mid- to late third trimester at a time when adequate extrauterine adaptation would be the norm (10). It remains important to evaluate carefully the risk of prematurity and to include these risks within the decision process. As intact extrauterine survival continues to occur at even earlier fetal ages, it remains important to incorporate improving survival curves with the decision process.

The relationship of these risks to potential benefits is central to the decision process as to if and when to initiate a form of invasive therapy. One means of assessing potential benefits has been to use animal models, primarily ovine or primate, to attempt to recreate the pathophysiology and then determine the benefits, if any, of timed therapeutic intervention. Several investigations using the ovine fetus have shown that urinary tract obstruction can cause renal lesions ranging from a multicystic dysplastic-type lesion to simple hydronephrosis and varying degrees of oligohydramnios and lung hypoplasia, and these gestational age-related effects can be ameliorated or even reversed by removing the obstructive process (24–27). Experimental diaphragmatic hernia in the ovine fetus can cause degrees of pulmonary hypoplasia that may be overcome by subsequent repair (28–30). Experimental obstructive hydrocephalus created by an intense periductal inflammatory fibrosis in the ovine fetus can cause progressive compression and thinning of cerebral tissue, an effect reversed by placement of a ventriculoamniotic shunt (31). These pure surgical lesions in otherwise normal fetuses produce a mimicking of pathophysiology and a reversibility of effect that supports the notion that similar benefits would occur in the affected human fetus. While such a line of reasoning is attractive, the complexities of the human disease, often mutlifactoral and rarely due to a lesion discrete in nature, make comparisons more difficult than is immediately apparent. The cumulative experience for treated human cases confirms that the animal experiments do not always approximate the clinical diseases (10).

Application of Selection Criteria:
Clinical Models

Management of fetal alloimmune disease is the best clinical model to underscore the significance and interplay of selection criteria. Notwithstanding that the relatively higher frequency, repetitive history, and availability of a maternal marker makes screening for alloimmune disease routinely possible (a prospect not likely in the near future for sporadic, potentially treatable anomalous conditions), the key to the remarkable success with therapy for the anemic fetus has been the ability to select, almost perfectly, the fetus *in need* of therapy. Since the invasive method of fetal transfusion is not without measurable risk—the procedure-related mortality for intraperitoneal transfusion is 3–5% (32) and for intravascular transfusion is 1–2% (33)—the importance of reserving therapy for fetuses who truly require it is obvious.

There are at least four discrete well-established markers of disease severity and progression: amniotic fluid bilirubin concentration ($\Delta OD450$) reflecting rate of hemolysis (34); fetal hemoglobin concentration reflecting the final balance between red cell production and destruction; ultrasound derived fetal pathomorphological signs, such as effusions in serous cavities or edema reflecting organ response (35); and ultrasound derived biophysical monitoring reflecting CNS adaptation to chronic compromise (36). Other fetal indices, especially biochemical and hematologic patterns now regularly obtained by cordocentesis, are under investigation and show promise. Working these markers in concert permits extremely accurate differentiation between grades of severity and rates of progression, thereby maximizing the timing and effect of definitive therapy, fetal transfusion.

No such prognostic and monitoring systems exist for any of the fetal structural anomalous conditions considered in contemporary medicine to be amenable to invasive therapy. To date, the anomalous model closest to the alloimmune model is obstructive uropathy in which renal tubular damage may be assessed by fetal urine electrolyte analysis (11), chiefly sodium, chloride and osmolality, the glomerular damage may be assessed by urine protein, chiefly beta-2-microglobulins (37), and pathomorphological signs (renal calcification, multiple cyst formation) are determined by serial ultrasound observations (17). It is important to note that renal failure is rarely the cause of perinatal death with these conditions (Table 15-1), variation of clinical significance in urinalysis is likely (8), and determination of a defined accurate threshold of fetal urinary excretion, below which survival is unlikely, remains elusive.

The principal cause of death in fetuses with obstructive uropathies is pulmonary insufficiency, thought to be due chiefly to alveolar hypoplasia but also due to deficient development of the pulmonary vascular systems. Detection and determination of the extent of pulmonary hypoplasia, an obvious critical step in case selection, has been notoriously difficult. Lung morphometrics, even with very high resolution ultrasound or MRI techniques, has proven generally inconclusive, except in the extremes of distribution. Both critical clinical assignment

Table 15-1   Fetal Obstructive Uropathy: Primary Diagnosis* and Outcome in 98 Cases (to June, 1991)

Primary Diagnosis	No. of Cases	% of Total	No. of Survivors	% Survival by Diagnosis
Posterior urethral valve syndrome	31	31.6	22	70.96
Karyotype abnormality	7	7.14	0	0
Renal dysplasia by ultrasound	6	6.12	0	0
Urethral atresia	8	8.2	1	12.5
"Prune-belly" syndrome	5	5.10	4	80
?	1	1.00	1	100
Cloacal anomalies	1	1.00	0	0
Ureteropelvic function obstruction	2	2.04	2	100
Unknown etiology	37	37.8	10	27
Total	98	100.0	40	40.8

errors, that is, assigning a lethal prognosis with subsequent intact survival, and the converse expectation of adequate postnatal pulmonary function ending with neonatal death due to pulmonary insufficiency, have occurred. Recently, we have studied high resolution broad band color spectral analysis of Doppler flow velocities of lung perfusion as a means to differentiate the lung of the normal fetus from that with pulmonary hypoplasia. Initial results were encouraging, suggesting that the presence or absence of measured Doppler shift velocities within pulmonary parenchyma were predictive. As our experience has increased, the validity of these relationships is now seriously questioned.

CONGENITAL DIAPHRAGMATIC HERNIA—IS FETAL SURGERY JUSTIFIED?

Congenital diaphragmatic hernia is a relatively uncommon fetal lesion (estimated incidence 0.03 to 0.05% of births) (38) characterized by abnormal migration of abdominal contents to within the thoracic cavity. Clinical, pathological, and pathophysiological aspects of the condition are well understood. This condition is one for which open fetal surgery has been touted: consideration of selection criteria as discussed in the previous section seems warranted.

Firstly, congenital diaphragmatic hernia is not necessarily or even usually a discrete disease entity; in slightly more than half the reported cases, the condition is associated with other anomalies, most commonly cardiac but also including other tissue plane closure defects (neural tube, oropharyngeal, abdominal wall) and chromosomal abnormalities, including trisomies 13, 18, and 21 (12,39). A detailed fetal anatomical survey by high resolution dynamic ultrasound methods and fetal karyotype determination is, therefore, required as a minimum for case selection. Even then, serious and potentially lethal anomalies, especially cardiac, may be missed. Secondly, and of extreme importance, disease severity at diagnosis, disease progression, and prognosis assignment cannot be determined reliably at present. The actual prenatal diagnosis of an existing isolated congenital diaphragmatic hernia is not difficult in the hands of an experienced ultrasonographer since the intrathoracic echolucent and/or echodense masses associated with mediastinal shift and abdominal concavity are overt and pathognomonic (Figure 15-2). However, the relationship between the physical definition of the defect and hernia, and the extent of lung damage as manifest by alveolar hypoplasia, pulmonary vascular hypoplasia and hyperactivity, or both, is neither simple nor direct and does not lend itself to

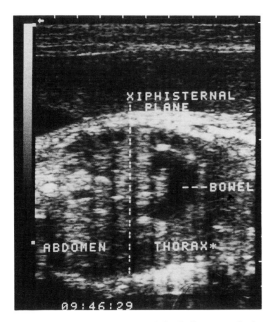

Figure 15-2 Sonogram of fetal thorax and abdomen in the midline longitudinal plane. Note the echolucency within the fetal thorax, the result of fluid accumulation within the herniated bowel. Congenital diaphragmatic hernia of this degree is easily recognized by the experienced ultrasonographer. This affected fetus died at birth from pulmonary insufficiency despite surgical repair of the defect.

meaningful examination by conventional techniques.

Proposed disease-specific selection criteria, such as hydramnios (presumed a consequence of partial obstruction or impaired function of the herniated fetal gut), stomach or bowel loop dilatation, or early gestational age (38), have identified most fetuses destined to die from the condition in retrospective studies. These criteria have not held up in prospective studies, however (12). Further, newer concepts of postnatal care, including delayed repair, diminish the predictive accuracy of these fetal prognostic criteria. The converse, that is, recognition of the fetus with diaphragmatic hernia but with no or minimal lung damage and, therefore, neither in need of or likely to benefit from fetal surgery, is even more difficult. Accordingly, except in extreme cases, prognosis assignment for this condition is largely guesswork.

The pathophysiology of isolated congenital diaphragmatic hernia is not easily monitored nor understood. In animal models, the creation of a diaphragmatic defect with bowel herniation causes pulmonary hypoplasia and interval repair ameliorates the lesion severity (29,30). Similarly, an implant of an iatrogenic intrathoracic mass, such as an inflated balloon, causes reversible changes to lung growth and morphology (28,29). Extrapolation of these ovine data to the human circumstance may not be simple. There are overt altricial differences between the lamb and human fetus and between the embryonic state of natural occurrence and the fetal age of surgical creation. There are also clear differences in timing, magnitude, and duration of the pulmonary compressive effects hypothesized. In the human fetus, we have observed diaphragmatic hernia with apparent sliding characteristics by which the extent of mediastinal deviation and intrathoracic herniation may vary in a waxing and waning fashion over days (14). Similarly, we have observed fetuses in whom multiple detailed observations yielded no evidence of herniation, followed by abrupt appearance at 27 weeks gestation (unpublished observation).

Open fetal surgery for congenital diaphragmatic hernia, that is, maternal laparotomy and hysterotomy followed by fetal thoracotomy, laparotomy, or both, with reduction of the hernia, then suturing or patching the diaphragm, has been reported (5). To date, there are eight cases reported in the literature (9), yielding one survivor (gross survival rate 12.5%) but also two perinates whose deaths seemed unrelated or indirectly related to the primary diagnosis. Intraoperative death occurred in three fetuses and postoperative death in one fetus, yielding a procedural-specific death rate of 50%. One fetus survived the procedure but died at birth from pulmonary hypoplasia and is, therefore, classified as a treatment failure. In fetuses who survived the operative period, the interval between repair and delivery ranged from one–10 weeks; the fetus with the longest interval died from pulmonary hypoplasia while the single survivor had an interval of seven weeks between repair and delivery. All postoperative fetal "survivors" had uterine irritability requiring tocolytics, and all delivered prematurely (range of age at delivery 28–34 weeks). One mother delivered vaginally eight days after the fetal repair, and the remainder were delivered by cesarean section. There were no maternal deaths. Three of these eight women have completed a subsequent pregnancy of which one has experienced uterine rupture with survival of both mother and child.

The importance and clinical relevance of these data depend critically upon the risk to benefit appraisal. Using the animal data

bank, these experiences approximate the experimental results, suggesting that an amelioration or reversal of lethal pathophysiology occurred in at least three cases (the survivor plus the two nonpulmonary deaths) and, in best light, in those fetuses for whom repair is possible, that is, those without liver herniation, survival could be as high as 75% (three possible of four postoperative survivors). This survival rate contrasts favorably with the same group's reported experience of 75% mortality among 20 untreated cases and, therefore, might justify the experienced serious maternal morbidity, such as subsequent uterine rupture.

Subsequent to this report, as of July 1, 1991, there have been an additional five cases (four from San Francisco, one from Paris) reported at the International Fetal Medicine and Surgery Society meeting in Phoenix—four of these fetuses survived. The cumulative survival rate with inclusion of these cases is now 38% (five of 13 cases). What is deficient in this best case argument is a description of outcome among cases referred for therapy but not treated for reasons other than selection criteria. It is likely that such patients exist since Longaker et al., in their description of their first 17 cases of fetal surgery for various conditions, including diaphragmatic hernia, report more than 300 patients with prenatally diagnosed anatomical lesions were referred to their center for fetal treatment, although categorization by diagnosis is not given (9).

While this group has not reported yet on their most recent experience in untreated fetal disease, others have. Harman et al., from the University of Manitoba, reported on perinatal outcome among 15 fetuses with an accurate prenatal diagnosis of congenital diaphragmatic hernia. Referral to the Fetal Treatment Program a the University of California in San Francisco was a consideration for these cases, and counselling was offered, but none elected for this option. These 15 cases met all the ultrasound criteria proffered to indicate extreme risk of lethality, that is, gross hydramnios, diagnosis at less than 28 weeks gestation, dilated stomach within the fetal chest and, in retrospect, a defect of sufficient size to preclude simple suturing and requiring a synthetic patch. Antenatal diagnosis did not specifically influence obstetric management. The expectation was towards spontaneous onset of parturition, vaginal delivery unless contraindicated by obstetric factors or fetal factors other than the diaphragmatic defect, prolonged neonatal stabilization and support, early neonatal paralysis and mechanical ventilation based on preductal oxygen saturation, significant sedation, and minimized handling, with delayed repair (on average on day five). Ten of these 15 fetuses (67%) survived. Four of the five deaths were due to pulmonary hypoplasia, and one death

was due to nonpulmonary causes. The incidence of premature delivery (<36 weeks) was 20% (three cases), and there was no specific diagnosis-related maternal morbidity.

Thorpe-Beeston et al. described outcome in 36 fetuses with congenital diaphragmatic hernia diagnosed from as early as 18 weeks gestation (12). Seventeen of these 36 (47%) had isolated hernia not associated with chromosomal or other anomalies. Fifteen of the 17 elected to continue pregnancy yielding nine survivors (survival rate 60%).

Against this background, the benefits of open fetal surgery for congenital diaphragmatic hernia are subject to rigorous challenge (Table 15-2). It seems reasonable to conclude, based on this comparison, that open fetal surgery for this condition does not enhance perinatal survival, but does convey discrete immediate and long-term potential maternal complications, and, therefore, cannot be justified. The definitive answer to this controversy must come from a prospective randomized trial.

Table 15-2   Outcome in Congenital Diaphragmatic Hernia: Untreated Cases vs. Cases Treated by Open Fetal Surgery

Variable	Treated Cases* (UCSF) (9)	Nontreated** (U of Man) (42)	Non-treated (King's College)
No. of fetuses	12	15	15
Stillbirths	4 (33.3%)	0	—
Premature delivery (<36 weeks)	12 (100%)	3 (20%)	—
Tocolysis	12 (100%)	0	—
Liveborn	8	15	15
Immediate neonatal death (pulmonary hypoplasia/insufficiency)	1	4	6
Nonpulmonary neonatal death	2	1	—
Long-term survival	5 (41%)	10 (67%)	9 (60%)
Subsequent maternal morbidity	1 of 3 (33.3%)	N/A	N/A

* Includes eight published cases and four verbally reported at the Annual International Fetal Medicine and Surgery Society Meeting, Phoenix, June 1991
** Diagnosis-therapy specific

FETAL OBSTRUCTIVE HYDROCEPHALUS—IS INVASIVE THERAPY JUSTIFIED?

Before the introduction of ultrasound, fetal hydrocephalus was a diagnosis that for the most part was made either at the time of delivery or because of dystocia requiring decompression. With the introduction of ultrasound, it became possible to establish the diagnosis early in the evolution of the ventriculomegaly and before cephalomegaly was evident. There are few fetal diagnoses in which the progression of a disease process is more apparent, and consequently, almost coincident with the dissemination of dynamic ultrasound methods, came reports of attempts at in utero correction of hydrocephalus. These were initially by serial decompressive ventriculocentesis (3) and then by valved ventriculoamniotic shunt placement in utero (4).

Forty-one fetuses with progressive hydrocephalus were treated and reported to the fetal surgery registry under the auspices of the International Fetal Medicine and Surgery Society (10). Review of these case results offers important insights into problems unique to the concepts of invasive fetal procedures (6). Firstly, ventriculomegaly is a distinct example of a single clinical sign with multiple etiologies, multiple associations, and variable clinical significance. Among the 41 treated cases, aqueductal stenosis, a diagnosis of exclusion, was most commonly assigned (77% of cases), but a range of other CNS lesions were observed (Table 14-1). The immediate prognosis could not then, nor can it today, be fixed with certainty based on the clinical sign of ventriculomegaly alone. Nor could the progressive pathophysiology be plotted with certainty, since spontaneous arrest was known to occur (41) and a relationship between either the degree of ventriculomegaly or the extent of cerebral mantle compression and long-term cognitive function is neither simple nor direct.

Cerebral ventriculomegaly is often not a discreet abnormality; major anomalies of organ systems other than the CNS are common (13%) and contributed heavily to morbidity (10). Further, related CNS anomalies, such as myelomeningocoele with Arnold-Chiari-type ventriculomegaly, compound outcome. Assignment of prognosis based on survival statistics only and not the quality of survival give a very misleading slant to the experience. Gross survival was sharply increased with in utero shunting; 34 of 41 treated fetuses survived (84%), whereas in 87 comparable untreated fetuses gleaned from the literature, only 27 survived (31%). The in utero therapy was not without immediate risk. The procedure-related mortality was 9.75% and included fetal death due to direct trauma, infection, and premature labor.

However, it is the survivor morbidity results that cast this method in its most unfavorable light. Among the 34 fetuses who survived after in utero shunting, only 12 were thought to be neurologically normal at initial follow-up (35%), and in the ensuing years, at least five of these children now exhibit major cognitive delay and other functional disorders. Therefore, the ongoing intact survival rate is now, at best, 20–25%. The handicap among survivors has often been severe and has included functional disorders, such as cortical blindness (23%), seizure disorder (15%), and spastic diplegia (9%). Most of these survivors (23 of 34, 68%) exhibit serious cognitive delay. Identification of matching natural history cases is difficult and, at best, approximate. Survival among the 87 reported cases in 22%, and normal development is 19.5% (42,43,44). In comparison, neonates born with overt hydrocephalus and treated immediately thereafter have an 87% survival rate, and 66% of these survivors were normal at follow-up (45). In the latter group, the exclusion of those who died before or during labor introduces a powerful selection bias. Based upon these unfavorable comparisons, an informal moratorium on this form of fetal therapy has occurred, and as of July 1991, there has been a four-year period during which no new cases have been reported. It would seem that on the basis of current knowledge and techniques, there is no clinical justification for this procedure .

SUMMARY

The advent of methods to image the fetus, initially crude and static, now sophisticated and dynamic and soon likely to be colored and three-dimensional, have made it possible to recognize fetal structural disease, sample fetal fluids and tissues, evaluate disease etiology and severity and, in some instances, guide placement of products, e.g., blood, and devices, e.g., shunts, meant to eliminate or ameliorate the underlying disease processes. In some instances, for example, with alloimmune anemias, the results have been dramatic and spectacular. In other instances, for example, obstructive ventriculomegaly, the benefits of therapy have been at best obscure and at worst nonexistent.

For the majority of proposed therapies, the risk to benefit ratio does not fall at the extremes of distribution, nearly all good or nearly all bad, but rather remains undetermined. The basis for this ambiguity does not stem from the inability to recognize risk. Virtually all fetal invasive procedures will yield lethal complications given sufficient experience. The ambiguity in the efficacy of fetal surgery arises from the inability to define benefit. It is an unfortunate fact that dis-

ease recognition and therapy innovations occurred almost simultaneously, spurred by a priori clinical reasoning and by technical feasibility. To some degree, the fact that it was possible to alter a sign of fetal disease became a justification for the therapeutic attempt regardless of attendant risk. For the ultrasound-guided percutaneous procedures, the procedural risk is largely confined to the fetus. Such will not be the case for open fetal surgery. For these procedures, a measurable maternal risk will apply.

The ability to treat is not an indication to treat, nor is it a guarantee of efficacy. Alternately, as eloquently penned by the late Sir William Liley, "Since there is no precedent for anything until it is done for the first time, progress and improvement (in fetal therapy) will be inevitable" (46). The key step in the continued advancement of fetal surgery must now be the mature decision to subject all present and future therapies to prospective randomized trials. Given the relatively infrequent occurrence of most of the conditions for which therapy has been attempted or postulated, it seems likely that cooperative multicenter trials will be the only method to achieve these goals. Regrettably, until such proper trials are organized and completed, fetal surgery remains experimental, potentially dangerous, and of unproven value.

References

1. Harrison MR, Golbus MS, Filly RA, et al. In utero treatment of urinary tract obstruction. Am J Obstet Gynecol 1982;142:383–388.
2. Manning FA, Harman CR, Lange IR, et al. Antepartum chronic vesicoamniotic shunts for obstructive uropathy. Am J Obstet Gynecol 1983;145:819–822.
3. Birnholz JC, Frigoletto F. Antenatal treatment of hydrocephalus. N Engl J Med 1984; 304:1021–1023.

4. Clewell WH, Johnson ML, Meier PR, et al. A surgical approach to the treatment of fetal hydrocephalus. N Engl J Med 1982;306: 1320–1325.

5. Harrison MR, Langer JC, Adzick NS, et al. The correction of congenital diaphragmatic hernia in utero. V. Initial clinical experience. J Pediatr Surg 1990;25:47–57.

6. Manning FA. The fetus with ventriculomegaly: The Fetal Surgery Registry. In: Harrison MR, Golbus MS, Filly RA, eds. The unborn patient: prenatal diagnosis and treatment. 2nd. edition. Philadelphia: WB Saunders, 1990, 448–452.

7. Manning FA. The fetus with obstructive uropathy: The Fetal Surgery Registry. In: Harrison MR, Golbus MS, Filly RA, eds. The unborn patient: prenatal diagnosis and treatment. 2nd. ed. Philadelphia: WB Saunders, 1990, 394–398.

8. Albar H, Manning FA. Fetal obstructive uropathy (see chapter 10 this book).

9. Longaker MT, Golbus MS, Filly RA, et al. Maternal outcome after open fetal surgery: a review of the first 17 human cases. JAMA 1991;265:737–741.

10. Manning FA, Harrison MR, Rodeck CR, et al. Catheter shunts for fetal hydronephrosis and hydrocephalus: report of the International Fetal Surgery Registry. N Engl J Med 1986;315:336–340.

11. Glick PL, Harrison MR, Golbus MS, et al. Management of the fetus with obstructive hydronephrosis. II. Prognostic criteria and selection for treatment. J Pediatr Surg 1985; 20:376–387.

12. Thorpe-Beeston SG, Gosden CM, Nicolaides KA. Prenatal diagnosis of congenital diaphragmatic hernia: associated malformation and chromosomal defects. Fetal Therapy 1989;4:21–28.

13. Lange IR, Manning FA. Antenatal diagnosis of congenital pleural effusions. Am J Obstet Gynecol 1981;140:839–840.

14. Longaker MT, Laberge JM, Darsereau J, et al. Primary fetal hydrothorax: natural history and management. J Ped Surg 1989; 24:578–576.

15. Siehert JR, Benjamin DR, Juul S, et al. Urinary tract anomalies associated with congenital diaphragmatic defects. Am J Med Genet 1990;37:1–5.

16. Chernick V, Reed MH. Pneumothorax and chylothorax in the neonatal period. J Pediatr 1970;76:624–632.

17. Mahoney BS, Filly RA, Callen PW, et al. Sonographic evaluation of fetal renal dysplasia. Radiology 1984;152:143–146.

18. Daffos, F. Fetal Blood Sampling. In: Harrison MR, Golbus MS, Filly RA, eds. The unborn patient: prenatal diagnosis and treatment. 2nd. edition. Philadelphia: WB Saunders, 1990:75–81.

19. Moise KJ Jr, Carpenter RJ Jr, Huhta JC, et al. Umbilical cord hematoma secondary to intravascular transfusion for Rh alloimunization. Fetal Therapy 1987;2:65–70.

20. Dildy GA III, Smith LG, Moise KJ, et al. Porencephalic cyst: a complication of fetal intravascular transfusion. Am J Obstet Gynecol 1991;165:76–78.

21. Moise KJ. The use of fetal neuromuscular blockade during intrauterine procedures. Am J Obstet Gynecol 1987;157:874–879.

22. Adzick NS, Harrison MR, Glick PL, et al. Fetal surgery in the primate III: Maternal outcome after fetal surgery. J Pediatr Surg 1986; 21:477–480.

23. Dewhurst C. The ruptured cesarean section scar. J Obstet Gynaecol Br Commonw 1957; 74:113–118.

24. Harrison MR, Ross NA, Noall R, et al. Correction of congenital hydronephrosis I: The model: fetal urethral obstruction produces hydronephrosis and pulmonary hypoplasia in fetal lambs. J Pediatr Surg 1983;18: 247–256.

25. Harrison MR, Nakayama DK, Noall R, et al. Correction of congenital hydronephrosis in utero. II. Decompression reverses the effects of obstruction on the fetal lung and urinary tract. J Pediatr Surg 1982;17: 965–974.

26. Glick PL, Harrison MR, Adzick NS, et al. Correction of congenital hydronephrosis in utero III. Early midtrimester ureteral ob-

struction produces renal dysplasia. J Pediatr Surg 1984;18:681–682.

27. Glick PL, Harrison MR, Adzick NS, et al. Correction of congenital hydronephrosis in utero IV. In utero decompression prevents renal dysplasia. J Pediatr Surg 1984;19: 649–657.

28. Harrison MR, Jester JA, Ross NA. Correction of congenital diaphragmatic hernia I: The model: intrathoracic balloon produces fetal pulmonary hypoplasia. Surgery 1980; 88:174–182.

29. Harrison MR, Bressack MA, Chung AM, et al. Correction of congenital diaphragmatic hernia II: Simulated correction permits fetal lung growth with survival at birth. Surgery 1980;88:260–268.

30. Harrison MR, Ross NA, deLorimer AA. Correction of congenital diaphragmatic hernia in utero III. Development of a successful technique using abdominoplasty to avoid compromise of umbilical blood flow. J Pediatr Surg 1981;16:934–942.

31. Nakayama DK, Harrison MR, Berger MJ, et al. Correction of congenital hydrocephalus in utero I: The model: intracisternal kaolin produces hydrocephalus in fetal lambs and rhesus monkeys. J Pediatr Surg 1983; 18:331–338.

32. Bowman JM, Manning FA. Intrauterine fetal transfusion: Winnipeg 1982. Obstet Gynecol 1982;61:203–209.

33. Harman CR, Bowman JM, Manning FA, et al. Intrauterine transfusion—intraperitoneal versus intravascular approach: a case control comparison. Am J Obstet Gynecol 1990;162:1053–1059.

34. Bowman JM. The management of RH-isoimmunization. Obstet Gynecol 1978;52: 1–16.

35. Harman CR. Ultrasound in the management of the alloimmunized pregnancy. In: Fleischer AC, Romero R, Manning FA, Jeanty P, James AE Jr, eds. The principles and practice of ultrasound in obstetrics and gynecology. 4th edition. Norwalk: Appleton, Lange, 1991:393–416.

36. Harman CR, Manning FA, Bowman JM, et al. Use of intravascular transfusion to treat hydrops foetalis in a moribund fetus. Can Med Assoc J 1988;138:827–830.

37. Dumez Y, Revillon Y, Dommergues M, et al. Long-term predictive value of fetal renal function. Proc. International Fetal Medicine and Surgery Society, Annual Meeting, Bonn 1988.

38. Butler N, Claireaux C. Congenital diaphragmatic hernia as a cause of perinatal mortality. The Lancet 1962;1:659–663.

39. Adzick NS, Harrison MR, Glick PL, et al. Diaphragmatic hernia in the fetus: prenatal diagnosis and outcome in 94 cases. J Pediatr Surg 1985;20:315–319.

40. Harman CR, Kosseim M, Casiro O, et al. Successful management of congenital diaphragmatic hernia does not require antenatal fetal surgery. Proc Soc Obstet Gynecol Can, Annual Meeting, Toronto, 1991.

41. Murphy S, Das P, Grant DN, et al. Importance of neurosurgical consultation after ultrasound diagnosis of fetal hydrocephalus. Br Med J 1984;289:1212–1213.

42. Glick PL, Harrison MR, Nakayama DK, et al. Management of ventriculomegaly in the fetus. J Pediatr 1984;105:97–105.

43. Chervenak FA, Duncan C, Ment LR, et al. Outcome of fetal ventriculomegaly. The Lancet. 1984;2:199179–181.

44. Clewell WH, Meier PR, Manchester DK, et al. Ventriculomegaly: evaluation and management. Sem Perinatol 1985;9:98–102.

45. McCullough DC, Balzer-Martin LA. Current prognosis in overt neonatal hydrocephalus. J Neurosurg 1982;57:378.

46. Liley, W. Prologue. In: Harrison MR, Golbus MS, Filly RA, eds. The unborn patient: prenatal diagnosis and treatment. Norwalk: Appleton & Lange, 1990:xi.

INDEX